RESEARCHING
HEALTH

Sara Miller McCune founded SAGE Publishing in 1965 to support the dissemination of usable knowledge and educate a global community. SAGE publishes more than 1000 journals and over 800 new books each year, spanning a wide range of subject areas. Our growing selection of library products includes archives, data, case studies and video. SAGE remains majority owned by our founder and after her lifetime will become owned by a charitable trust that secures the company's continued independence.

Los Angeles | London | New Delhi | Singapore | Washington DC | Melbourne

3RD EDITION

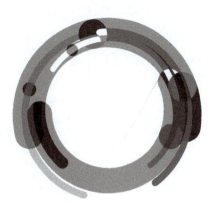

RESEARCHING HEALTH

QUALITATIVE, QUANTITATIVE AND MIXED METHODS

EDITED BY

MIKE SAKS & JUDITH ALLSOP

SAGE

Los Angeles | London | New Delhi
Singapore | Washington DC | Melbourne

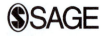

Los Angeles | London | New Delhi
Singapore | Washington DC | Melbourne

SAGE Publications Ltd
1 Oliver's Yard
55 City Road
London EC1Y 1SP

SAGE Publications Inc.
2455 Teller Road
Thousand Oaks, California 91320

SAGE Publications India Pvt Ltd
B 1/I 1 Mohan Cooperative Industrial Area
Mathura Road
New Delhi 110 044

SAGE Publications Asia-Pacific Pte Ltd
3 Church Street
#10-04 Samsung Hub
Singapore 049483

Editor: Alex Clabburn
Editorial assistant: Jade Grogan
Production editor: Rachel Burrows
Marketing manager: George Kimble
Cover design: Wendy Scott
Typeset by: C&M Digitals (P) Ltd, Chennai, India
Printed in the UK

Editorial arrangement © Mike Saks and Judith Allsop 2019

Chapter 1 © Mike Saks and Judith Allsop 2019
Chapter 2 © Judith Allsop and Mike Saks 2019
Chapter 3 © Judith Allsop 2019
Chapter 4 © Kathryn Jones 2019
Chapter 5 © Lara Maestripieri, Arianna Radin and Elena Spina 2019
Chapter 6 © Andy Alaszeswki 2019
Chapter 7 © Jacqueline Low 2019
Chapter 8 © David Hughes 2019
Chapter 9 © Judith Green 2019
Chapter 10 © Heather Waterman 2019
Chapter 11 © Miwako Hosada 2019
Chapter 12 © Nichola Shackleton, Martin von Randow and Lara Greaves 2019
Chapter 13 © Michael Calnan 2019
Chapter 14 © George Lewith and Paul Little 2019
Chapter 15 © A. Niroshan Siriwardena 2019
Chapter 16 © Steve Parrott and Alan Maynard 2019
Chapter 17 © George Argyrous 2019
Chapter 18 © Ian Kirkpatrick and Gianluca Veronesi 2019
Chapter 19 © Priscilla Alderson 2019
Chapter 20 © Teresa Carvalho and Tiago Correia 2019
Chapter 21 © Anneliese Synnot and Sophie Hill 2019
Chapter 22 © Viola Burau 2019
Chapter 23 © A. Paul Williams and Janet M. Lum 2019
Chapter 24 © Jonathan Tritter 2019
Chapter 25 © Denis Anthony 2019
Chapter 26 © Judith Allsop and Mike Saks 2019
Chapter 27 © Mike Saks and Judith Allsop 2019

First edition published 2008. Reprinted 2010 and twice in 2011. Second edition published 2013. Reprinted 2014, 2015, 2016 and 2017. This third edition first published 2019

Library of Congress Control Number: 2018958415

British Library Cataloguing in Publication data

A catalogue record for this book is available from the British Library

ISBN 978-1-5264-2428-0
ISBN 978-1-5264-2429-7 (pbk)

At SAGE we take sustainability seriously. Most of our products are printed in the UK using responsibly sourced papers and boards. When we print overseas we ensure sustainable papers are used as measured by the PREPS grading system. We undertake an annual audit to monitor our sustainability.

Contents

Figures

Tables

About the Editors

Mike Saks is Emeritus Professor at the University of Suffolk and Visiting Professor at the University of Lincoln and the Royal Veterinary College, University of London, UK, as well as the University of Toronto, Canada. He has published many books, chapters and articles on health, professions, regulation and research methods – and advises governments on these subjects internationally.

Judith Allsop is Visiting Professor at the University of Lincoln and Professor Emerita at London South Bank University, UK. She has researched and published works on health policy, patient and user groups, complaints and medical regulation. She has advised central government on these topics.

About the Contributors

Andy Alaszewski is Emeritus Professor at the University of Kent, UK. He is an applied social scientist who has researched individual experiences of illness and disability and the nature of risk in health and social care. He has published widely on qualitative research methods.

Priscilla Alderson is Professor Emerita of Childhood Studies, University College London, UK, where she convenes courses on critical realism. Her recent sole-authored and co-edited books are about the politics of childhood and the ethics of research with children and young people.

Denis Anthony is Emeritus Professor at the University of Leeds, Professor of Health and Social Care at the University of Derby and Fellow of the Royal Statistical Society, UK. He is an adult and mental health nurse, who works in health research, largely as a statistician.

George Argyrous has taught economics, research methods and statistics at the University of New South Wales, Australia, and the Australia and New Zealand School of Government. He has published articles on topics including the use and abuse of statistics and consulted with many government agencies/private companies on quantitative analysis, especially involving the use of SPSS.

Viola Burau is Associate Professor in the Department of Public Health/Political Science, Aarhus University, Denmark. She has extensive experience in health services research, especially relating to health policy reform, health services organization and change, health care professions and cross-country comparison. She has published widely on these topics, including numerous articles in international, peer-reviewed journals.

Michael Calnan is Professor of Medical Sociology in the School of Social Policy, Sociology and Social Research at the University of Kent, UK. He has researched and published in books and journals on a wide range of health-related topics, in the UK and internationally.

Teresa Carvalho is Associate Professor at the University of Aveiro, Portugal, where she is a senior researcher at the Centre for Research in Higher Education Policies. She is a member of the European Sociological Association Executive Committee. She has participated in several multidisciplinary research projects and published widely in international journals and books on professionalism and managerialism in health and higher education.

Tiago Correia is Assistant Professor and Research Fellow at ISCTE-Lisbon University Institute, Portugal, where he coordinates undergraduate and graduate courses on the sociology of health and illness, health policies and medical epistemology. On these subjects, he has published extensively, conducted research projects and acted as a policy adviser.

Lara Greaves is a Lecturer in New Zealand Politics at the University of Auckland, New Zealand. Her research is in the broad area of political psychology. Her particular focuses are indigenous (Māori) identity, sexual orientation, survey research, and political attitudes and behaviour.

Judith Green is Professor of Sociology of Health in the School of Population Health and Environmental Sciences, at King's College London, UK, where she is part of the Social Sciences and Urban Public Health Institute. She has researched and published extensively on public health, health services research and methodology.

Sophie Hill is an Associate Professor and Head of the Centre for Health Communication and Participation at La Trobe University, Australia. She is also the Joint Coordinating Editor of Cochrane Consumers and Communication.

Miwako Hosoda is Professor and Vice-President of Seisa University, Japan. She is also President of the Asia Pacific Sociological Association and the International Sociological Association Research Committee on the Sociology of Health, as well as a member of the Board of Trustees of the Japan Foundation of Cancer Research. She has undertaken research observing human relations in health care in Japan and the United States.

David Hughes is Professor of Health Policy at Swansea University, UK. He has utilized qualitative methods to research in such areas as rationing and resource allocation, NHS contracting, patient choice, and patient and public involvement. He has also completed field studies of the roll-out of universal health care coverage reforms in Thailand.

Kathryn Jones is Senior Research Fellow in the Department of Politics and Public Policy, De Montfort University, UK. Her main research interests are patient and public involvement, health system reform and the links between patients' organizations and the pharmaceutical industry. She has published in journals such as *Sociology of Health and Illness* and *Social Science and Medicine*.

Ian Kirkpatrick is the Monash Warwick Professor of Healthcare Improvement and Implementation Science (Organizational Studies) at Warwick Business School, UK. His research interests are in the management, organization and performance of health services, both in the UK and internationally. He is also involved in research focusing on other professional services, including management consulting, law and professional and trade associations in the United States.

George Lewith is the late Professor of Health Research in the Academic Unit of Primary Care and Population Sciences in the School of Medicine at the University of Southampton, UK. He was a well-published and prominent researcher and practitioner of complementary and alternative medicine.

Paul Little is Professor of Primary Care Research at the University of Southampton, UK, and has been a general practitioner for twenty years. He is a Fellow of the Academy of Medical Sciences, a National Institute of Health Research (NIHR) Senior Investigator (Emeritus) and Director of the NIHR Programme Grants for Applied Research Funding Board. His expertise is in pragmatic trial design and the development of complex interventions.

Jacqueline Low is Professor of Sociology at the University of New Brunswick, Canada. She has expertise in qualitative methodology, symbolic interactionism and the sociology of health. She has published widely in books and journals on subjects ranging from deviance, health and symbolic interactionism to the concept of theoretical saturation.

Janet M. Lum is Professor in Politics and Public Administration, Ryerson University, Canada. She leads the Canadian Research Network for Care in the Community, a knowledge mobilization network that leverages international best practices and translates research ideas into policy action. Her research focuses on home and community care for vulnerable populations.

Lara Maestripieri is a Marie Skłodowska-Curie Fellow at the Institute of Government and Public Policies at the Universitat Autònoma Barcelona, Spain. Her main interests in research and publication are labour transformation in post-industrial society – in particular, marginalized groups like women and the young in labour markets, social innovation and emerging professions.

Alan Maynard is the late Emeritus Professor of Health Economics in the Department of Health Sciences at the University of York, UK. His research interests were in economic aspects of health workforce planning, health care reform, incentive systems, addiction policies and the regulation of industry in areas such as pharmaceuticals.

Steve Parrott works as a health economist in the Department of Health Sciences and previously the Centre for Health Economics at the University of York, UK. He heads the economics of mental health and addiction research and has undertaken many economic evaluations of smoking cessation and alcohol interventions and published extensively in the addiction field.

Arianna Radin is Research Fellow at the University of Bergamo, Italy, in the field of sociology of health and sociology of professions. Her interests in research are ageing, information and communication technology in health and social care and science, technology and society. She is a board member of the European Sociological Association Research Network of Sociology of Health and Illness.

Martin von Randow is a data analyst at the University of Auckland, New Zealand. He has instructed on quantitative methods via software, with postgraduate classes in sociology, politics and social work, and has been involved in discussions internationally on best practice in this area.

Nichola Shackleton is a Senior Research Fellow at the University of Auckland, New Zealand. She is a social scientist specializing in quantitative research methods and social statistics. Her research interests include measuring and reducing inequalities in child and adolescent health, longitudinal data analysis and latent variable modelling.

A. Niroshan Siriwardena is Professor of Primary and Prehospital Health Care at the University of Lincoln, UK, where his expertise is in quality improvement and implementation science. He trained in medicine at St Bartholomew's Hospital, London, general practice in Lincolnshire, and research at Nottingham University and De Montfort University.

Elena Spina is a Research Fellow at Università Politecnica delle Marche, Italy. Her main field of interest is the sociology of professions. She focuses on social and health professions with a particular emphasis on both the generational and gender dimensions. She has published widely in leading journals in the social sciences and health professional fields.

Anneliese Synnot is currently exploring stakeholder involvement in systematic reviews through doctoral studies at the Centre for Health Communication and Participation, La Trobe University, Australia. She also works as a Research Fellow at Cochrane Australia, Monash University.

Jonathan Tritter is Professor of Sociology and Policy and Pro Vice Chancellor and Executive Dean of the School of Languages and Social Sciences at Aston University, UK. His research focuses on service user and citizen involvement in research, and service development and policy. He has a particular interest in focus group methodology and cross-national comparative research.

Gianluca Veronesi is Professor of Healthcare Management at the School of Economics, Finance and Management, University of Bristol, UK. His research focuses on the relationship between governance and management structures and the characteristics and performance of health care organizations, in terms of both effectiveness and efficiency – mainly employing quantitative research methods.

Heather Waterman is Professor of Nursing and Ophthalmology at Cardiff University, UK. She is a longstanding health services researcher with interests in promoting the self-care of patients with long-term conditions, especially concerning loss of sight. Her methodological expertise is in action research and she has led, or collaborated on, several externally funded research projects.

A. Paul Williams is Emeritus Professor of Health Policy, Institute of Health Policy, Management and Evaluation, University of Toronto, Canada. His research focuses on access to, and the cost-effectiveness of, community-based care for vulnerable groups and individuals, including older persons at risk of institutionalization, persons with disabilities and children with complex medical needs.

Publisher's Acknowledgements

The publishers are grateful to the following academics for their contribution to the third edition of the book at the proposal stage:

Jan Davison-Fischer, Oxford Brookes University, UK

Ye Htut, Flinders University, Australia

Leena Panicker, Charles Darwin University, Australia

Souraya Sidani, Ryerson University, Canada

Grace Spencer, Anglia Ruskin University, UK

Penelope Stanford, University of Manchester, UK

The publishers are grateful to all third-parties for permission to reproduce the following material:

Figure 4.1 Screen shot from Mendeley Reference Managing Software for AHRC Scoping Review. Hamalainen, L. and Jones, K. (2011) 'Conceptualising community as a social fix, argument and persuasion in health, housing and local governance'. Available at: https://connected-communities.org/index.php/project_resources/conceptualising-community-as-a-social-fix-argument-and-persuasion-in-health-housing-and-local-governance/

Figure 13.1 Clarifying concepts: Descending the ladder of abstraction. De Vaus, D. (2002) *Surveys in Social Research*, 5th edition. London: Routledge.

Figure 13.3 Public levels of trust in health services staff: Putting the interests of patients above the convenience of organizations. Calnan, M. and Rowe, R. (2008) *Trust Matters in Health Care*. Buckingham: Open University Press.

Figure 13.4 Study design for upper-limb pain sufferers. Calnan, M., Wainwright, D., O'Neill, C., Winterbottom, A. and Watkins, A. (2005) 'Lay evaluation of health care: The case of upper limb pain', *Health Expectations* 8(2): 149–60.

Figure 13.5 Response rates for upper-limb pain sufferers. Calnan, M., Wainwright, D., O'Neill, C., Winterbottom, A. and Watkins, A. (2005) 'Lay evaluation of health care: The case of upper limb pain', *Health Expectations* 8(2): 149–60.

Figure 14.1 Patient recruitment in a study of homeopathic proving. Brien, S., Lewith, G. T. and Bryant, T. (2003) 'Ultramolecular homoeopathy has no observable clinical effects: a randomized, double-blind, placebo-controlled proving trial of Belladonna C30', *British Journal of Clinical Pharmacology 56*: 562–8.

About the Online Resources

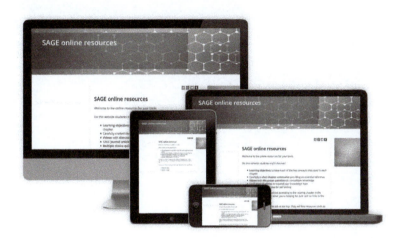

Visit the companion website at **https://study.sagepub.com/saks_allsop3e** to find a range of teaching and learning material for instructors and students, including the following:

For instructors

- **Teaching notes:** Password-protected teaching notes with chapter overviews, key themes, summaries and seminar topics for discussion.
- **PowerPoint slides:** Slides for each chapter neatly summarize the main points in the teaching notes and make a great visual aid for teaching.

For students

- **Chapter summaries and contributor biographies:** These are designed to give a comprehensive overview of the book by chapter with associated contributor details.
- **SAGE online readings:** Free access to two journal articles for each chapter and further online readings reinforcing chapter themes – along with weblinks as appropriate.
- **Key concepts:** A list of key terms in health research that appear in the book.
- **Study skills:** Suggestions for further reading from SAGE books and other material to enhance generic study skills for researching health.

The editors wish to thank Dr Kathryn Jones for her assistance in compiling this website.

PART I
Conducting Health Research

1

Introduction to Researching Health

MIKE SAKS AND JUDITH ALLSOP

Chapter objectives

- To highlight the value of sound research and research processes in health care
- To create awareness of the range of approaches used in conducting research
- To explain the relevance of health research to students, researchers, health professionals and policy makers
- To show the international dimensions of research – following the trend for a convergence of health research principles across modern societies
- To give a broad overview of the book in terms of both its individual parts and its chapters – as well as the case studies, exercises and further reading it provides.

Introduction

We live in an age of fake news, when 'facts' are disputed, so well-conducted research has never been more important. Research that is poorly constructed wastes time and resources – and research that does not use rigorous and well-founded practice can have a damaging effect on individuals and society. In this book, we aim to provide the ground rules for research and studies undertaken in the field of health. We cover research in both the clinical and the social sciences. Our view is that students, researchers, health professionals and policy makers should have an understanding of the methodologies and methods employed across the whole spectrum of research. Even if those undertaking or assessing research have chosen or favour a particular method to carry out a specific project, they should still be acquainted with other methods and the kind of knowledge that these different methods produce. They should also be able to evaluate whether a project has been carried out sufficiently well to support the findings put forward.

The findings of research should be based on evidence, and evidence in turn must be based on sound research processes – even when there are challenges (Brown, Crawford and Hicks 2003). In this light:

- Undergraduate and postgraduate students and others should acquire the tools to assess how research findings have been reached and know how to 'read' a journal paper and other research output with a critical eye.
- If researchers plan to carry out a project themselves, they should be in a position to choose the tools that are most applicable to answering their research question. This means knowing how to select from the range available and to acquire the particular skills they will need.
- Most projects will in practice use a number of methods to collect and analyse data and require some ability to handle numbers as well as text. There is no clear quantitative and qualitative divide – the two are not mutually exclusive.
- In the workplace, health professionals and policy makers must also be able to evaluate the quality of research findings. Such findings provide the basis for making decisions and/or providing advice to parties including policy makers, clients and patients.

To assist with these issues, the contributors to this book draw on their long experience of undertaking research. They provide many examples to show best practice and discuss how to deal with the difficult issues that can occur in conducting high-quality research.

This third edition of the book aims to provide an extended and updated guide to the range of ways in which readers may approach researching health. The volume contains a number of key improvements from the second edition following extensive international peer review. There are new chapters on the principles of health research, methods of sampling in qualitative health research, qualitative data analysis, using secondary data in health research, identity in health research, online research in health and evaluating health research to reflect the developing interests of those directly engaged in, studying and/or assessing research in health. In addition, all the existing chapters have been updated with new material. There is more emphasis on interdisciplinary health research as well as mixed methods – which now appear as separate chapters rather than as a single chapter. The expanded number of chapters overall, as compared to both the first and second edition of *Researching Health*, draw on a wider array of top-quality contributors – hailing from a diverse international range of eight different countries – including Australia, Canada, Denmark, Italy, Japan, New Zealand, Portugal and the United Kingdom (UK).

The development of the book

The book unfolds in a coherent and well-defined manner. After the opening chapters in Part I on how to conduct health research, Part II examines how qualitative methods have been used to research health, illness and the delivery of services in health care settings. In Part III, the quantitative methods used in health research to investigate health, illness and treatment for disease, and to assess the costs and benefits of interventions in health care, are discussed. In both of these sections, the aim is to describe the use of various methods in practice; the type of questions each method is intended to address; and the strengths and weaknesses of each approach. This is followed by a consideration of the challenges likely to be encountered in carrying out research.

The book then turns in Part IV to consider selected issues in health research that have emerged as under-researched areas, such as that of identity, and where current research practice has faced a critical challenge, leading to ongoing debate. Questions about how to ensure ethical research practice and how to involve those who use health care in the research process remain areas of importance, but conflicts of interest may arise. For example, the interests of researchers may run counter to those of people who are the subjects of research. Moreover, even if there is agreement that ethics is a central issue in health research, and that a partnership between researchers and health care users offers a way forward, there are still practical problems about how this can best be achieved. This is especially sensitive in a comparative international context and in the era of the internet, and research issues that emerge in both of these areas are directly addressed in this section.

The concluding chapters, in Part V, crystallize the core themes of the book by focusing on applying health research, addressing specifically the issues of writing a research proposal, writing up research projects and disseminating findings. The final chapter also discusses how to evaluate health research papers and how to evaluate policy change. Throughout the book, we have aimed to engage with the practical problems of conducting research. In so doing, each of the ensuing chapters provides case study examples of health research in practice, drawn from the authors' own research where appropriate. Our aim is to help readers to carry out their own research projects and, in so doing, draw on the research of others in their work.

Research into health – and, by extension, illness and disease – can be focused at many different levels in the historic and contemporary context: to name but a few, from the individual to the community, from the activities of patients as health producers to the contribution of informal carers, and from health care assistants with brief training to fully-fledged health professionals in the labour force. Health research can provide a critique to challenge existing policies and practice as well as being supportive of positive client-centred change on the ground in practice. As such, those concerned with research into health care may operate in a local, national and/or international context. This is reflected in the range of research undertaken in the health field, as well as in its applicability to different layers of government policy.

Research in policy and practice

From this viewpoint, we would emphasize that health research using a range of methods may be undertaken not only to gain an understanding of health, illness and disease in contemporary society, but also to contribute to policy development. In this regard, there has been a major change in the culture of health services in the developed world. Not only have clinical interventions become more evidence-based, but policy makers are more inclined to pivot their policies on interventions that are most effective (Kuhlmann and Saks 2008). Clinical science centred on a biomedical model of disease has made a considerable contribution to developing evidence for treatment based on clinical trials and experimental methods. This is witnessed by the Cochrane Collaboration, for example, which, since its establishment, has driven the growth of international centres for preparing, maintaining and disseminating systematic reviews in health care, typically based on randomized controlled trials (RCTs) (Cassels 2015).

In the UK specifically, governments over the past two decades from the Blairite New Labour onwards have put an emphasis on the maxim: 'what counts is what works' (Rawnsley 2001), following the position in many other countries. In the clinical care arena, this is illustrated by such developments as the now re-titled National Institute for Health and Care Excellence (NICE), which produces clinical guidelines based on research evidence. NICE has a remit to reconsider the funding of interventions that are not effective. For balance, it also has a Citizens Council with representatives of consumers and there is a network to support health consumer groups to submit evidence. This publishes reports for time to time – such as on societal values in reaching decisions about funding treatment interventions and the trade-off between equity and efficiency (Citizens Council 2014). Both clinical and policy research have benefited from unprecedented levels of research funding to evaluate interventions and to carry out pilot projects in the UK, following international trends. The National Institute of Health Research (NIHR) Research and Development Programme, directed by the Department of Health, has made substantial research funds available for work on policy priorities such as the cause, care, cure and prevention of dementia and surgical interventions and their outcomes in the search for good practice (Ham 2017).

Another aspect of the expansion and diversification of health research lies in the changing division of labour in health care and the expansion in the occupational groups providing specialist services. Nurses and doctors are the largest of the professional groups providing care in the UK, alongside a multiplicity of other health practitioners. As well as the nine statutory councils in medicine and elsewhere, the Health and Care Professions Council regulates 16 different health professions (Allsop and Jones 2018). There are also voluntary registers for support workers providing curative and caring services (Saks and Allsop 2007). It is expected that, as part of their training, practitioners will learn to evaluate the research evidence underlying their practice, keep up to date with advancements in knowledge and contribute to new knowledge.

However, there is continuing debate and controversy about the validity and utility of the evidence base for clinical and policy guidelines on the efficacy of treatments and the appropriateness of the services provided. Although evolution has been fast, some areas remain under-researched and not all developments have been based on sound research evidence – often to the cost of individuals and/or the wider community, as exemplified in the operation of aspects of the pharmaceutical industry (see Goldacre 2013). The negative consequences of poorly conducted research in health can be illustrated in the more specific case of research into the MMR vaccine set out in Box 1.1.

Box 1.1   The cost of poor research: The case of MMR vaccine

In 1998 *The Lancet* published a study by Dr Andrew Wakefield that suggested a link between MMR, a vaccine against measles, mumps and rubella, and autism. The study was based on 12 cases with no control group but received wide publicity. Subsequent studies demonstrated that there was no link between the vaccine and autism – or indeed other conditions, such as bowel disease. The original research was flawed. Wakefield was struck off the medical register for fraud. However, for some decades afterwards in the UK, immunization rates fell. This left non-immunized children and adults at risk of illnesses that could have severe side-effects. It also led to a reduction in population immunity.

Source: www.nhs.uk/conditions/mmr-vaccines

There have also been differences of opinion about the appropriate balance between clinical and more social science-oriented research and the role of lay people in providing a perspective and form of knowledge distinct from those of health professionals – as well as about the ethical issues raised in health research. What is apparent is that, both nationally and internationally, work on policy issues such as professional governance can be as important for health care users as clinical research itself, although the two are clearly interrelated. However, we note that the contribution of research has developed unevenly in practice. The prime beneficiary of funds for evidence-based research in the health service in the UK at least has been conventional, hospital-based acute care, following the establishment and expansion of scientific medicine (Le Fanu 2011). In contrast, many areas, from nursing (Witz and Annandale 2006) and primary care (Goodyear-Smith and Mash 2016) to complementary and alternative medicine (Saks 2015a) and mental health (Slade and Priebe 2006), have not had the same level of investment in research.

The readership, objectives and focus of the book

In this context, the main readership of this book is intended to be health researchers, academics working in the health field, health care managers, and health practitioners from doctors, nurses and midwives to pharmacists and physiotherapists, together with students on health and health-related programmes. In this latter regard, it is designed to appeal to those working on courses at a higher undergraduate and postgraduate level who are taking research methods programmes or are qualified health professionals. Although based largely on research undertaken in the UK, the intention has been to give the book a broader, more cosmopolitan, dimension with contributors from a greater range of other modern societies with more advanced research capabilities, including North America, the Antipodes and Asia as well as from a wider European context. This provides the reader with access to examples of health research undertaken in other countries, underlining the trend towards a shared health research agenda drawing on similar principles and methods that have developed across national boundaries. We have acknowledged this further as editors by including Chapter 22, which is dedicated to exploring how to conduct comparative health research by looking at single issues across countries. Although the comparative method presents many challenges, there is much to be learnt from policy and practice in other countries. The challenge of funding health care and developing effective policies in the community and elsewhere are shared issues in an international context.

The book has been planned to be clear, accessible and oriented to practice. It provides a distinctive overview in a critical, but constructive, manner of research in the health field. This differentiates it from a number of more general research texts (as exemplified by Argyrous 2011; Bryman 2016; Silverman 2014). Unlike many books in the health research field, this volume focuses on the wide range of methods used to research health and health services. It also does not focus on a closely defined set of qualitative or quantitative research methods (see, for instance, more specialized texts such as Bruce and Pope 2018; Green and Thorogood 2018; Scott and Mazhindu 2014), aim to be a research text directed at very specific groups of health practitioners (see, for example, Ernst 2012; Gerrish and Lathlean 2015; Harvey and Land 2017) or strive to provide research tools for particular practice contexts, such as clinical hospital-based medicine or primary care (as illustrated by Cosby, DiClemente and Salazar 2006; Piantadosi 2017; Saks, Williams and Hancock 2000). Instead, this text aims to discuss how the range of health research methods can be applied more generally and the issues that they raise – albeit in a way that applies to the various contexts in which those researching health or drawing on research about health operate.

Despite its length, of course no single book can cover in detail all areas of health research. The references in each chapter, therefore, act as a guide to additional study. This complements the recommended further reading and online sources given for each chapter. Contributors not only cover the technical issues related to their areas but, where appropriate, illustrate their accounts with reference to their own personal experience of conducting health research, highlighting its pleasures and pitfalls. The chapters also contain case studies where relevant and conclude with a problem-solving exercise to encourage readers to demonstrate how theory, methods and data interrelate. In addition, where helpful, chapters are cross-referenced to each other to assist readers in navigating the text. It is therefore distinct from, but complementary to, such widely used texts by Bowling (2014) and Bowling and Ebrahim (2005), which take a multidisciplinary approach to health research.

In putting this volume together, the editors bring much experience of both writing and editing books on many aspects of health, applying research methods to health and receiving funding from bodies such as the Departments of Health, Medical Research Council, the Wellcome Trust, the Economic and Social Research Council and the European Union. Research projects in which they have engaged mutually or separately include using research methods in relation to primary care, professional regulation, orthodox and alternative medicine, consumers in health care, quality assurance in health care and comparative health care (see, for example, Allsop and Saks 2002; Allsop and Jones 2018; Baggott, Allsop and Jones 2005; Kuhlmann, Allsop and Saks 2009; Saks 2005, 2015b). They also bring wide experience of examining doctoral research nationally and internationally. They have acted as book series editors for research monographs and edited collections, commissioning research and reviewing research protocols and evaluating research reports through their membership of a range of government policy and research committees. Their experience is complemented by that of the broad span of nationally and internationally recognized specialists in different forms of health research, who have written the specific chapters that make up this text. As an edited collection with a consistent format, the book has the added advantage of drawing on a range of contributions from leading experts in the field.

The organization of the book

As noted earlier, the book has been organized into five parts. The first part starts with contributions on 'Conducting Health Research'. Aside from Chapter 1, the introduction to the volume, the editors, Mike Saks and Judith Allsop, have also contributed Chapter 2 on the principles of research relevant to conducting all forms of health research. Chapter 3, written by Judith Allsop, is on the strategies involved in designing and planning health research. This chapter examines the different methodological paradigms used in the production of research knowledge and focuses on outlining and evaluating aspects of the more quantitative positivist and more qualitative interpretivist approaches. Chapter 4, by Kathryn Jones, on undertaking literature reviews in health, is also of generic relevance. She considers two main types of literature review – the narrative and the systematic review – before describing techniques for undertaking a comprehensive search and offering guidance on how best to present an analysis of the literature.

Contributors in the next two parts of the book on 'Qualitative Methods and Health' and 'Quantitative Methods and Health' variously give attention to why particular research methods should be employed; what kind of research questions could be addressed by specific methods; and how the data are gathered using different methods, including data coding, analysis and presentation. The main areas that authors address in each chapter on research methods include, with varying degrees of emphasis, the following:

- Definition/elaboration of the research method to be considered
- The rationale for employing the type of research method concerned
- Examples of employing the research method in practice
- The strengths and weaknesses of the research method in question
- The resources required to apply the method in practice
- Issues involved in the coding/analysis of data using the research method
- The identification, writing up and presentation of the findings
- Questions that are appropriate to critically appraise the method
- How to evaluate the findings of research studies that use the method
- Ethics issues related to the method concerned.

Within this framework, the second part of the book on 'Qualitative Methods and Health' covers a broad span of chapters on research methods written by seasoned qualitative researchers in the field. In Chapter 5, Lara Maestripieri, Arianna Radin and Elena Spina consider methods of sampling in qualitative health research. Andy Alaszewski then examines, in Chapter 6, the ways in which documents have been and can be used for health research. He describes the nature of documentary research, identifying the resource base needed, assessing the research issues for which it is most appropriate and considering how documentary data can best be analysed. In Chapter 7, Jacqueline Low looks at parallel issues related to the increasing use of unstructured interviews, including their advantages and disadvantages, the recruitment of participants and the techniques of both carrying them out and assessing and presenting the data that they produce. While a range of observational methods, including unobtrusive measures, are used in researching health, David Hughes, in Chapter 8, provides a specific outline of, and justification for, the use of participant observation in health research and the insights it can bring. Judith Green, in Chapter 9, considers the use of focus groups in research into health, examining aspects of the employment of such groups, from their strengths and weaknesses to the resources they require and the ethical issues that they raise. Action research in health is addressed in Chapter 10 by Heather Waterman, who discusses some of the challenges of action research and how these difficulties can be overcome with positive effects on health and health care. Finally, in Chapter 11, Miwako Hosoda examines the important task of qualitative data analysis in health research.

The third part of the book on 'Quantitative Methods and Health' draws on the experience of a range of well-established authors, this time in the quantitative area. It begins with Chapter 12 from Nichola Shackleton, Martin von Randow and Lara Greaves, which sets out the fundamental aspects of health sampling methods, with primary reference to probability sampling, and draws on a number of examples from the health field. Michael Calnan, in Chapter 13, explains the nature of quantitative survey methods in health research, and describes how to go about using these methods. This chapter is linked to the previous one in so far as sampling is usually employed in conducting large-scale questionnaire surveys. The basic concepts and principles related to RCTs are then outlined by George Lewith and Paul Little in Chapter 14. Niroshan Siriwardena complements this contribution in Chapter 15 by providing insights into experimental and quasi-experimental methods, which offer alternatives to the RCT in health research. In Chapter 16 Steve Parrott and Alan Maynard write on the ever more important use of economics in health research. In this chapter, among other things, a research framework is set out for appraising evidence on cost and effectiveness to inform difficult rationing choices in health care. In Chapter 17 George Argyrous describes and evaluates a range of basic statistical methods to analyse the quantitative data derived from these and other sources in health research. Ian Kirkpatrick and Gianluca Veronesi then complete this section in Chapter 18 by examining the use of secondary data in researching health care managers, with a particular focus on the increasing employment of 'Big Data', which in this chapter draws on the large data sets available from UK Departments of Health sources.

The next part of the book deals with a selection of topical issues in health research. Contributors consider a number of contemporary challenges for researchers working in the health field. In the context of the wide range of research methods discussed, they variously:

- Define the issues involved
- Consider the advantages and disadvantages of different approaches
- Outline how the issues can best be addressed
- Illustrate these points with examples of their own work in the area concerned
- Discuss the politics of the process of applying research methods in health in their field.

Accordingly, the fourth part of the book on 'Issues in Health Research' starts with a discussion in Chapter 19 of the important question of ethics in health research. Here Priscilla Alderson considers the merits of various approaches to ethics review and governance, including how ethical issues can best be addressed in health research. In Chapter 20 Teresa Carvalho and Tiago Correia examine the issues involved in researching identity in the health field, including areas such as gender and ethnicity. Given the importance of users in lobbying for particular causes, it is appropriate that Anneliese Synnot and Sophie Hill next examine the nature and characteristics of user engagement in health research in Chapter 21. Chapter 22, as previously indicated, is on comparative health research. Here Viola Burau points out the range of international challenges to health research and how these can be tackled. In Chapter 23 Paul Williams and Janet Lum draw on their experience of interdisciplinary health research in highlighting the benefits and drawbacks of this form of research. Jonathan Tritter then focuses more specifically on the pros and cons of employing mixed methods in health research in Chapter 24. This part of the text ends with Chapter 25, by Denis Anthony, on the highly topical method of online research in health. Health researchers increasingly depend on online research methods in conducting studies, and he discusses making data available through technological developments as well as the benefits and limitations of using these sources.

Finally, the book finishes with a short fifth part on 'Applying Health Research', which includes two chapters by the editors. Chapter 26 centres on the skills involved in writing up a range of forms of health research, including how to write a research proposal and how to write up research findings for assessment. Chapter 27 concentrates on the all-important tasks of disseminating and evaluating different forms of health research, bringing together the key strands of the book into a focused conclusion.

Key themes in researching health

In this volume, several strong, substantive and interlinked contemporary themes emerge across the various chapters, in addition to the consideration of a range of quantitative and qualitative research methods. Two particular interrelated themes are highlighted here to illustrate the multidimensional nature of this volume. They include, first, the role of health care users, both patients and carers, in contributing to the research process and, second, the ethics of research in health. Health care users can contribute at all stages of the research process, from helping to determine topics for research to contributing to the publication and dissemination of research findings. They should be considered as participants and partners in health research and are drawn into research in different ways in different projects. There are now both institutions and regulations to ensure that patients give their informed consent to taking part in research and that they understand what will be involved when they participate, as well as rules to protect confidentiality and anonymity. Nevertheless, there are still underlying issues about power relationships in the research process and debates about whether research is done 'on' or 'for' health care users. There are therefore powerful arguments in favour of trying to ensure that users are active participants in health research, although their involvement poses a range of ethical, scientific and administrative problems that are discussed at different points in this book.

One major methodological theme that also runs through this text is that many current research projects use a mixture of methods. They are also often multidisciplinary or, now more commonly, interdisciplinary. This raises issues of how data collected using different methods can be analysed and integrated into the whole. In many respects, these kinds of approaches sit uneasily with the traditional model of lone researchers pursuing their own interest and making a career and reputation based on individual publications. The final part of the text will assist singleton researchers and those working in research teams in developing and presenting their work. However, there is no doubt that undertaking collaborative research in teams is now a more typical setting for the career health researcher. While this can often pose management problems, there are many benefits that flow from working together in a team, as the more general experience of interprofessional working in health and other fields amply demonstrates (see, for instance, Day 2007). A number of chapters comment on the implications of this more collective way of working.

Conclusion

Research, in principle, and with some caveats, benefits those involved with health, whether as provider, producer or user. This is a very good reason, in its own right, for conducting research into health. So too is the sheer exhilaration of engaging in health research that can further disciplinary and interdisciplinary knowledge, even where there is no obvious application. However, as we note above, the contribution of research in the health field has developed unevenly in practice. We trust that this book will contribute to areas of health research hitherto under-resourced, as well as more generally. While opportunities for health research are increasing – notwithstanding the challenging national and global economic climate in which resources are often restricted, even in the more developed countries – the onus on researchers to produce robust results based on sound methods has never been greater (Kuhlmann and Saks 2008). Producing well-considered and rigorous results will also be vital if researchers are to make a positive input to policy formation in the fast-changing health field locally, nationally and internationally. We hope that this book on researching health, together with its supportive website, will assist in this critical process – in shaping the health strategies and activities that lie ahead at all levels and across a wide range of settings.

We should finally like to record our thanks to the contributors, as well as all members of the team at Sage – not least Rachel Burrows, Alex Clabburn and Jade Grogan – without whom this third edition of the book would not have been possible. Special reference too needs to be made to Kathryn Jones, who not only has written a chapter in the volume, but also has played a key role in developing the supporting material on the accompanying website. Whatever position you occupy in relation to health and health care – whether as a user, student, academic, practitioner, manager or policy maker – it is our wish that the book will be helpful to you in researching health, both now and in the future.

Recommended further reading

This text provides a useful set of readings on mixed methods in research for health professionals: Andrew, S. and Halcomb, E. J. (eds) (2009) *Mixed Methods Research for Nursing and the Health Sciences*. Chichester: Wiley-Blackwell.

This book gives a clear description of a range of selected health research methods and has been produced in a fourth edition to reflect new methodological and other developments:

Bowling, A. (2014) *Research Methods in Health: Investigating Health and Health Services*, 4th edition. Maidenhead: Open University Press.

This book contains a useful set of further readings that will help researchers from different disciplines work together in health research:
Bowling, A. and Ebrahim, S. (eds) (2005) *Handbook of Health Research Methods: Investigation, Measurement and Analysis*. Maidenhead: Open University Press.

References

Allsop, J. and Jones, K. (2018) 'Regulating the regulators: The rise of the United Kingdom Professional Standards Regulatory Authority', in M. J. Chamberlain, M. Dent and M. Saks (eds), *Professional Health Regulation in the Public Interest: International Perspectives*. Bristol: Policy Press.

Allsop, J. and Saks, M. (eds) (2002) *Regulating the Health Professions*. London: Sage.

Argyrous, G. (2011) *Statistics for Research*, 2nd edition. London: Sage.

Baggott, R., Allsop, J. and Jones, K. (2005) *Speaking for Patients and Carers: Health Consumer Groups and the Policy Process*. Basingstoke: Palgrave.

Bowling, A. (2014) *Research Methods in Health: Investigating Health and Health Services*, 4th edition. Maidenhead: Open University Press.

Bowling, A. and Ebrahim, S. (eds) (2005) *Handbook of Health Research Methods: Investigation, Measurement and Analysis*. Maidenhead: Open University Press.

Brown, B., Crawford, P. and Hicks, C. (2003) *Evidence-based Research: Dilemmas and Debates in Health Care*. Maidenhead: Open University Press.

Bruce, N. and Pope, D. (2018) *Quantitative Methods for Health Research: A Practical Interactive Guide to Epidemiology and Statistics*, 2nd edition. Chichester: Wiley-Blackwell.

Bryman, A. (2016) *Social Research Methods*, 5th edition. Oxford: Oxford University Press.

Cassels, A. (2015) *The Cochrane Collaboration: Medicine's Best-Kept Secret*. Victoria: Agio Publishing House.

Citizens Council (2014) *Report on Societal Values in Trade-offs between Equity and Efficiency*. London: NICE.

Cosby, R. A., DiClemente, R. J. and Salazar, L. F. (eds) (2006) *Research Methods in Health Promotion*. San Francisco, CA: Wiley.

Day, J. (2007) *Interprofessional Working: An Essential Guide for Health and Social Care Practitioners*. Andover: Cengage Learning.

Ernst, E. (2012) *Understanding Research in Complementary and Alternative Medicine: A Guide to Reading and Analysing Research in Health Care*. London: EMS Publishing.

Gerrish, K. and Lathlean, J. (2015) *The Research Process in Nursing*, 7th edition. Chichester: Wiley-Blackwell.

Goldacre, B. (2013) *Bad Pharma: How Drug Companies Mislead Doctors and Harm Patients*. New York: Farrar, Straus and Giroux.

Goodyear-Smith, F. and Mash, B. (2016) *International Perspectives on Primary Care Research*. Boca Raton, FL: CRC Press.

Green, J. and Thorogood, N. (2018) *Qualitative Methods for Health Research*. London: Sage.

Ham, C. (2017) *Health Policy in Britain: The Politics and Organization of the National Health Service*. Abingdon: Routledge.

Harvey, M. and Land, L. (2017) *Research Methods for Nurses and Midwives: Theory and Practice*. London: Sage.

Kuhlmann, E., Allsop, J. and Saks, M. (2009) 'Professional governance and public control: A comparison of healthcare in the United Kingdom and Germany', *Current Sociology*, 57: 511–28.

Kuhlmann, E. and Saks, M. (eds) (2008) *Rethinking Professional Governance: International Directions in Healthcare*. Bristol: Policy Press.

Le Fanu, J. (2011) *The Rise and Fall of Modern Medicine*, 2nd edition. London: Abacus.

Piantadosi, S. (2017) *Clinical Trials: A Methodologic Perspective*, 3rd edition. Chichester: John Wiley-Blackwell.

Rawnsley, A. (2001) *Servants of the People: The Inside of New Labour*, 2nd edition. London: Hamish Hamilton.

Saks, M. (2005) 'Improving the research base of complementary and alternative medicine', Editorial, *Complementary Therapies in Clinical Practice*, 11: 1–3.

Saks, M. (2015a) 'Health policy and complementary and alternative medicine', in E. Kuhlmann, R. Blank, I. Bourgeault and C. Wendt (eds), *The Palgrave International Handbook of Healthcare Policy and Governance*. Basingstoke: Palgrave Macmillan.

Saks, M. (2015b) *The Professions, State and the Market: Medicine in Britain, the United States and Russia*. Abingdon: Routledge.

Saks, M. and Allsop, J. (2007) 'Social policy, professional regulation and health support work in the United Kingdom', *Social Policy and Society*, 6(2): 165–77.

Saks, M., Williams, M. and Hancock, B. (eds) (2000) *Developing Research in Primary Care*. Abingdon: Radcliffe Medical Press.

Scott, I. and Mazhindu, D. (2014) *Statistics for Health Care Professionals*, 2nd edition. London: Sage.

Silverman, D. (2014) *Interpreting Qualitative Data*, 4th edition. London: Sage.

Slade, M. and Priebe, S. (2006) *Choosing Methods in Mental Health Research: Mental Health Research from Theory to Practice*. London: Routledge.

Witz, A. and Annandale, E. (2006) 'The challenge of nursing', in J. Gabe, D. Kelleher and G. Williams (eds), *Challenging Medicine*, 2nd edition. London: Routledge.

2

Principles of Health Research

JUDITH ALLSOP AND MIKE SAKS

Chapter objectives

- To demonstrate the aim and principles of health research
- To outline the scope of health research, showing recent trends
- To introduce the concept of induction and deduction
- To consider the types of research design
- To consider the research process, the principles to follow and how to choose research questions.

Introduction

As editors, we believe that two principles underlie all research. First, research is about producing new insights and new knowledge by setting answerable research questions, collecting data in a systematic way, analysing research questions intelligently and rigorously, and identifying patterns and establishing associations. In this way, researchers may contribute to a greater understanding of both individual health and collective health behaviour, the role and impact of health providers, and the options for delivering health services to communities. In putting together the book, we believe:

> Research is about illumination. If we don't succeed in that we have failed. If a person reads something and doesn't feel any wiser, then why was it done? Research should fire curiosity and

the imagination. … If people feel research illuminates their understanding and gets into their thinking, then it's of use. (Richardson, Jackson and Sykes 1990: 75)

The second principle is that the findings produced by research are always contingent on the context in which the research is carried out, the methods used, and how the data have been analysed and interpreted. We therefore think that it is incumbent upon the researcher to be explicit and transparent about these elements in the research process. New knowledge or insights occur in small steps. Often studies need to be replicated and/or reanalysed and revisited before findings can be said to be soundly based. All research results are subject to reinterpretation and review. In this sense, the production of new knowledge is a collective enterprise and each researcher, even if working alone, is part of a wider research community. Although there is no single organization that covers all researchers in health and/or other fields, there are both formal and informal rules that govern research. These are outlined and assessed in the various chapters in this volume.

What is health research?

Health research takes many forms from basic scientific and social research to applied clinical research. What, though, is 'research' in the health context? At its most general level the conventions of health research can be viewed as work conducted to develop knowledge based on available evidence, following certain rules and procedures. However, as Henn, Weinstein and Foard (2006) point out, what is to count as knowledge and how we acquire that knowledge is a contested area. Most significantly, there are different beliefs and assumptions that shape what is studied, how research is conducted, what methodology and methods are used to test knowledge claims, as well as how the findings from research should be interpreted. It is important to distinguish between methodology and methods. The former refers to a research strategy, while methods are tools for data collection and can be either quantitative or qualitative. It is fundamental to understand assumptions made between different approaches to research, termed positivism and interpretivism, as these frame what are considered as acceptable ways of carrying out research. They are more fully discussed in Chapter 3.

The scope of health research is broad. It covers scholarly research carried out within the natural and clinical sciences as well as the social sciences – each of which draws on a wide range of theoretical frameworks and related concepts. On the one hand, there are the natural sciences, with disciplines such as anatomy, biology, chemistry, physiology and physics, on which research in clinical areas of health tend to be based. Then, there are the social science disciplines, such as history, politics, psychology, sociology and policy analysis, which contribute to understanding the social context of health and health care. Economics as well as statistics also makes a vital contribution to health research across clinical science and social science projects as they provide techniques to measure and assess the strength of research findings and to compare outcomes. Economic models may be used to assess the cost-effectiveness of interventions, for example in surgical interventions for the treatment of coronary heart disease (Bowling 2014). Each has a distinct approach and so too do the related disciplines of epidemiology and translational research. The former has a focus on the distribution of diseases and the health of populations. Research findings can also contribute to the development of new products such as medicines. They can assess the suitability of existing devices such as wheelchairs, and explore the use of digital technologies to enable people to receive health care in their own home (see, for example, Davies and Newman 2012).

These various disciplines use a range of methods in health research. These can be grouped into qualitative or quantitative methods (see, for instance, Bourgeault, Dingwall and de Vries 2010; Bruce and Pope 2018, respectively). Each type is based on a different set of assumptions (or paradigms) that provide a philosophical and methodological basis for using the method in the health field. In the past, there was a divide between the two – as a number of the chapters in this book highlight. Some research projects, particularly larger and well-funded projects, now use a mixture of methods (Andrew and Halcomb 2009). In these circumstances, it is vital for the researcher to understand what kind of knowledge each type of method produces, what kind of evidence supports the interpretation of findings from research data and how different kinds of evidence may or may not be linked together in practice. How to mix methods is discussed by Cresswell and Plano Clark (2017), and in the health context in particular is considered in various chapters of this book.

Conceptualizing health: The social and natural sciences

The conceptualization of health in research is now considered further by comparing and contrasting the ways in which this is seen through the lens of the social and natural sciences, which provide rather different perspectives.

The contribution of the social sciences

Almost all societies are concerned with maintaining health, treating illness and caring for people who are dependent. Issues of reproduction and birth, dying and death are central concerns. However, in the social sciences health and illness have been conceptualized in different ways. For social scientists undertaking research, the meaning of these concepts is a matter for investigation and this has been carried out using the range of both qualitative and quantitative methods. In an early study of how lifestyle can affect health, Blaxter (2010) explored the interrelationship in a survey-based empirical study to investigate whether the social conditions in which people lived were more important than lifestyle factors such as smoking and exercise.

What people understand by health and illness is subjective and what social groups see as the causes of ill health and their approach to health work are socially constructed and are likely to be embedded in a framework of meaning shaped by a specific social context. There have been many empirical studies of how such views differ. Herzlich (1973) and Stacey (1988) provide early illustrative examples of qualitative studies across different societies. Currently, there are many national and international studies based on quantitative surveys on health and health behaviour providing longitudinal data for researchers. Recent examples are the European Quality of Life Survey, so far conducted periodically between 2003 and 2016 (Ahrendt et al. 2018), and the Survey of Healthy Behaviour and Wellbeing (Rainville 2016).

Turner (2003) charts the manner in which the concepts of health and illness have changed historically, from early societies where ideas are linked to spiritual notions of purity and danger, to the now dominant biomedical, scientific and professional definitions that focus on disease and pathology and on the body and body parts. Moreover, in contemporary society, health can be viewed as a moral norm defining a socially constructed, prescriptive standard that tends towards an ideal of wellbeing or social functioning. Within this perspective, illness is usually conceptualized as the obverse of health, although we know that the way people in different social groups define health depends on variables such as social class, gender, ethnic group and age (Scambler 2008).

In their studies of heath and illness, sociologists tend to focus on the study of social groups in society and have adopted different theoretical perspectives. A foundational theoretical study is the account by Parsons (1951) of the 'sick role' as a system for the social control of illness in society. In a development of this perspective, other social scientists have seen illness as a socially sanctioned, but legitimated, role that is socially patterned through the interpretations of the individuals themselves and significant others. Family, friends and health providers influence and legitimate, or not, the patient pathway through to diagnosis and treatment. This is an arena where health care users, clinicians and health providers interact. Whereas many early sociological studies focused on professional dominance in health care work, health can also be conceptualized as a form of co-production between health care users, carers and professionals (Realpe and Wallace 2010).

Taking an interactionist perspective, Goffman (1968) showed how people with certain conditions are stigmatized in society and the effect on their sense of identity. This line of inquiry has led to a body of work about people with specific illnesses, both physical and mental. Qualitative studies include an influential account by Bury (1982), who investigated the disruption caused by chronic illness and the subsequent process of adjustment. More recently, Monaghan and Gabe (2016) published their insightful research on young people with asthma, and Hudson and colleagues (2016) reported on the impact of endometriosis on women and their partners.

Another line of research using both qualitative and quantitative methods has been the study of pathways through the health care system. An illustration of a qualitative study is provided by an analysis by Hudson and Culley (2015) of people who cross country borders in the search for fertility treatment. Both gender and ethnicity have been shown to affect access to health care and pathways through treatment. Edited texts by Kuhlmann and Annandale (2012) on gender and health care and by Ingleby and colleagues (2012) on the health and experiences of migrants and ethnic minorities contain contributions exemplifying quantitative and qualitative studies in this field.

Among psychologists, who tend to focus on individual and small-group behaviour, theoretical viewpoints about health cover a wide range. Some psychologists, such as Maslow (1954) and his followers, have considered human motivation in terms of the hierarchy of needs. These range from basic concerns about physiological functioning and safety to a search for esteem and self-actualization. Others have engaged in the assessment of the impact of psychosocial factors on a variety of illnesses (Cassileth et al. 1984). More recently, the interest of psychologists has focused on the relationship between stress and health (Lovallo 2005), health practitioner–client interaction (Purtilo, Haddad and Doherty 2014), and the role of psychology in providing an explanation of the onset of specific health conditions (Straub 2011).

A major area of investigation for social scientists across countries has been on the inequalities in the incidence of disease and illness, especially in relation to class, gender, ethnicity and region in both societal and global contexts (see, for instance, Evans, Barer and Marmor 1994; Lenard and Straehle 2012). In this area, researchers have mainly used quantitative methods to map inequalities and, in epidemiological studies, the incidence and causes of disease and illness. These have been complemented by qualitative studies, not least in relation to psychosocial aspects of health and illness (Bartlett 2017).

Other classic studies take the wider distribution of social and economic power as a starting point for their analysis of health care provision and health care systems. Navarro (1986) is an example of a Marxist analysis of factors influencing access and the availability of health care to different social groups in the United States in particular. Social science writers in this field sometimes use their analyses as a platform for discussions about human justice and to argue for policies that combat poverty and meet the health needs of all social groups (as illustrated by Smith and Bambra 2016).

Health care politics and the interplay of the interests of the state, the medical profession and health care users as patients and carers has also been a major theme for health researchers and policy analysts. Saks (2015a) has analysed from a neo-Weberian viewpoint the influence of the medical profession as an interest group on health inequalities in Britain and the United States. Gabe, Kelleher and Williams (2006) and Kuhlmann and Saks (2008) consider shifts in national and international health care governance. Other studies have focused on the more recent influence and role of social movements in health care (Allsop, Baggott and Jones 2004).

The challenges for policy makers in health care in most countries are well known: rising health care costs, fuelled by population increase and technical innovation; the demographic imbalance, with an increasing proportion of elderly people compared to the working population; and the persistent inequalities in access and outcomes. Yet, a feature of health systems is resistance to change. This is partly due to conflicting interests in the politics of health, but also to the size and complexity of health care delivery systems. Can health research contribute to a greater understanding of the barriers to change and what policies facilitate both efficiency and effectiveness? State policies have supported organizational change and increased the power of managers, but evidence on the benefits of this shift is limited, with many instances of perverse incentives. Greener and colleagues (2014) suggest a way forward for health research through a careful comparative analysis of specific organizational change programmes that have had positive benefits and, where they have not, to investigate the factors that contribute to cost/benefit outcomes. This requires a focus on a detailed analysis of both programme and context. For example, why did policy incentives to increase quality and productivity improve outcomes in general practice in the United Kingdom, but were less evident in hospital care?

Other scholars have used Normalization Process Theory to develop a qualitative method to assess the factors that facilitate or impede the implementation of new policy interventions (May and Finch 2009). Initially developed to assess the implementation of new technologies, it provides a middle-range theory that sets out a framework of factors that have been shown to support the implementation of new policy interventions (May 2009). To be embedded in practice, participants must understand the purpose of the innovation; they must support the change as worthwhile; and it must be seen as compatible with their working lives. These propositions provide a framework that has been used more widely to identify the factors that have facilitated the implementation of policy changes across a number of settings (McEvoy et al. 2013).

Biomedicine and the medical model

From the viewpoint of the natural and clinical sciences, there has been a greater emphasis on the identification and classification of disease categories, with the biomedical, scientific and professional emphasis on pathology and on the body and body parts. These provide the basis for diagnosis, prognosis and treatment. The causes of mortality and morbidity are defined in terms of diseases and objective clinical pathology, with a distinction between the normal and abnormal (as exemplified by Damjanov 2012). These are the basis of the medical model of ill health, which is clearly set out by Neighbors and Tannehill-Jones (2009). The approach focuses less on personal and social contexts of health and more on the biomedical frame of reference, in subjects ranging from infectious diseases (Török, Moran and Cooke 2009) to the implications of genetic structures for the disease process (Panno 2010).

The biomedical model and the medical gaze, which emerged with the birth of the clinic over two centuries ago (Foucault 2003), is rooted in the belief that wellbeing is an objective and measurable state. Yet one of the anomalies in contemporary practice is that patients' subjective perception of personal wellbeing may be discordant with their 'objective' health status. For example, a person can feel ill without medical science being able to detect disease and many people live with pathologies of which they are unaware (Bowling 2014). These two points of view, the objective and the subjective, are said to differ ontologically – that is, they take opposed positions about what is 'real'. Does reality exist in the mind of the beholder or is there an objective reality in the material world that is there to be discovered? Researchers should be able to identify which approach they are taking as this can influence the methodology they choose to investigate a research question.

To be sure, the biomedical model of orthodox medicine currently dominates and is heavily state-supported in modern societies. While it has brought many benefits through the use of drugs and surgery – and, more recently through such innovations as STEM cell science (Le Fanu 2011) – its ascendance as contemporary orthodoxy is historically contingent. During the seventeenth and eighteenth centuries effective remedies were few in a more plural health system, but the doctor listened to the patient in a form of 'bedside medicine' that was available at least to the better off. This was overtaken in the later nineteenth century in Europe, by, first, 'hospital medicine', based on classifying diseases generically in the emergent hospital system, and then in the twentieth century by 'laboratory medicine'. In the latter, the body was seen primarily as a complex of cells and a symptom-bearing organism, resulting in the patient voice becoming peripheral, and diagnoses were based on the analysis of blood and other samples at a distance by laboratory technicians (Saks 2002).

Although scientific biomedicine based on a natural science model is dominant, it operates alongside other medical systems and practices. From the perspective of people who use services, some are accessed as alternative systems and others are seen as complementary to orthodox medicine. This explains the term 'complementary and alternative medicine' (CAM), which consists of a diverse range of therapies outside the mainstream, from aromatherapy and crystal therapy to acupuncture and homoeopathy. These do not share a common philosophy but tend to be ideologically positioned more towards the 'holistic' end of the spectrum, in which the subjective views of clients and mind–body links are usually regarded by their proponents as more central to treatment than in orthodox medicine. Despite their growing popularity among members of the public – especially where orthodox medicine has little to offer, as in chronic conditions – they are marginalized in the politics of health care (Saks 2015b). Alternative medical systems and practices co-exist with orthodox medicine in most societies and complementary medical systems, as the name implies, may be recognized through state registration. The extent of recognition varies between countries. In France, for example, hydrotherapies in rehabilitation are funded through the state insurance system, while in the United States there is also funding through insurance schemes of chiropractic and osteopathy, which have become professionalized and underwritten by state licensing (Saks 2015c).

The perspective of proponents of the more holistic CAM therapies has implications for the research methods employed. In assessing the relative efficacy of therapies, orthodox clinical research has placed a heavy emphasis on quantitative methods in general and randomized controlled trials (RCTs) in particular. The latter follow a standard protocol with a control group to be compared with a group that receives the intervention, which is more fully discussed in Chapter 14. Some CAM therapists also place emphasis on this perspective and follow standard RCT procedures, but others challenge these assumptions and argue that more qualitative forms of assessment based on subjective client feedback should be more fully taken into account (Saks 2006). CAM treatments are typically targeted more on individual clients in the context of their lives and values rather than on their presenting physical symptoms.

Nonetheless, reference to the widespread use of RCTs in biomedicine over the past few decades accentuates that there has been a major change in the culture of health services in the developed world. Clinical interventions have therefore become more evidence-based. This has led to an emphasis on the assessment of the efficacy and cost-effectiveness of particular interventions and technologies in treating patients. Evidence-based medicine initially drew on indicators from the biomedical sciences. Increasingly, though, they have started to become focused on additional indicators, such as social functioning, patient-perceived health status and quality of life measures (Kane and Radosevich 2011), thus reducing some of the original polarity between CAM and orthodox therapies.

What are the principles of the health research process?

In terms of the principles of health research, the following aspects need to be considered: the different types of reasoning, the main forms of research design, starting the research process, theories and concepts in health research, and the key factors guiding such research.

Types of reasoning in health research

In terms of the underpinning of health research, there are two mainstream starting points for research. These are based on contrasting forms of reasoning, as outlined in Bryman (2016). On the one hand, there is research that tests theory and, on the other hand, there is research that builds theory. The first uses *deductive* reasoning, the second *inductive* reasoning. The logic of biomedical research and social research using quantitative methods begins with a hypothesis or a proposition drawn from a tested body of theory that underpins a research question. Data are collected, and the findings may support, refine or refute the research question and the underlying theory. This follows a *deductive* form of reasoning – from theory to testing. The alternative is to build theory from data by drawing out patterns and generalizations from the data themselves. Then, on the basis of these, the aim is to arrive at a theory or explanation through an *inductive* form of reasoning. This is a logic followed in data collection using qualitative methods where little is known. Why is it that some mothers refuse to have their children immunized for measles, even when they may know that this disease can have serious consequences? On the basis of qualitative interviews, the researcher may be able to identify assumptions about biomedicine and relate these to education or social class. The logic of these two forms of reasoning is shown in Figure 2.1.

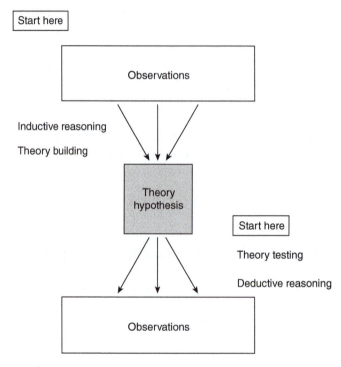

FIGURE 2.1   Forms of reasoning in health research: Inductive and deductive

Source: De Vaus (2002: 6)

Science-based research and quantitative methods tend to be deductive. Existing studies indicate a hypothesis to be tested. Exploratory research and qualitative methods collect data on a research question about which they are curious and where an initial literature search suggests there is a gap in knowledge. The link to theory is developed in the process of analysis from patterns observed in the data. Dyson and Brown (2006) provide a useful contribution to understanding the contribution of theory to applied health research.

This brings us to the more practical aspects of doing research by introducing the concept of research design, followed by a discussion of the early stages of the research process. Prior to starting on a research project, three questions must be addressed:

- What is my research question?
- What research design am I using to address the question?
- What methods am I going to use and are they quantitative or qualitative, or both?

First, we consider research design and methods.

Research design: The main forms

Research design is a way of organizing a project to provide evidence for answering a question. It refers to the structure, or architecture, of a project: the analogy of a building has been used to express the concept of a research design. Buildings have a particular structure to suit their purpose. There will be guidelines and principles to be followed in their construction (methodology). Various methods (quantitative or qualitative, or a mixture of both) will be used to construct the building and certain materials (instruments) will be required. The purpose of the analogy is to make a distinction between a research design and research methods (De Vaus 2002). A commonly used typology is a distinction between designs that are experimental or quasi-experimental, cross-sectional, case studies, longitudinal (they take place over time) or comparative. The overall design of a project should be mapped out before deciding on particular methods for data collection. For each category of design, a range of quantitative or qualitative methods may be used. As can be seen in Box 2.1, a particular design does not predetermine what methods are used.

Box 2.1   Different types of design in health research

Experiments are set up to test a hypothesis and they are more common in the clinical sciences and psychological studies. In essence, experiments seek to introduce an independent variable and control for a range of other variables in one of two or more groups in a before-and-after study. If there is a control group, this allows for a causal explanation of the effect of introducing the independent variable. An RCT that is double-blinded is the most highly developed form of experiment. It is known that not blinding a trial introduces bias (Schulz et al. 1995). Experiments are rare in sociology and social policy due to the difficulties in setting up a control group and manipulating the independent variable, although they may be used in psychological studies. For instance, if we wished to test the effect of social class on health status, it would not be possible to do this through an experiment because social class is an attribution that cannot be changed. It is also ethically contentious to have a control group where a known-to-be effective treatment is denied to participants. However, there have been examples of experiments in some areas of public policy that have offered incentives, exerted peer pressure or provided targeted information to nudge people into

(Continued)

(Continued)

changing their behaviour (John et al. 2011). There may also be opportunities for a nimble researcher to study naturally occurring situations. For example, when, during a school vaccination session, one of two batches of ampoules contained one and a half times the standard measure due to a labelling error, an opportunity arose to compare the two groups at intervals to check for a specified range of side-effects.

Cross-sectional designs refer to studies that require the collection of data from a number of subjects/objects over a specified and short time period. This would include surveys of different kinds. The aim is to establish an association between variables, such as gender and the use of acupuncture, and to draw inferences. Methods can be quantitative, where questionnaires or structured interviewing are used to collect data from more than one, and often a very large number of, respondents. The aim is to capture variation. If the methods are sound, and the number sufficient, findings can be extrapolated to larger populations. Data can also be collected using qualitative methods, such as documentary evidence or observation. The aim is to select particular criteria to establish similarity and difference across the units being analysed to make generalizations.

Case study designs focus on a single organization, place or person as the subject of research. The case is the unit of analysis, and the research methods focus on the circumstances, dynamics and complexity of a single or small number of cases. Yin (2018) defines five types of case: the critical, the unique, the typical, the revelatory and the longitudinal. An example of a unique case study is the research by Korman and Glennerster (1990) on the process of closing a large mental handicap hospital. A number of methods were used to collect both quantitative and qualitative data. Bryman (2016) warns that the term 'case study' is often used loosely. Some so-called case studies are in fact cross-sectional studies.

Longitudinal designs study phenomena over time. They require a significant investment of resources and large teams, so they are unlikely to be used by student researchers. The National Child Development Study (www.esds.ac.uk/longitudinal/access/ncds) is an example of a longitudinal study that has generated a raft of publications. Data were collected on a sample of children born in one week in 1958 and then followed up at intervals subsequently. The design allows for a number of very interesting and profound questions about the influence of childhood events or smoking, for instance on health in adult life (Wadsworth 1991).

Comparative designs are based on the value of studying similarity and difference between two or more contrasting cases. Typically, the same phenomenon is compared within two or more contrasting socio-cultural settings, such as institutions, customs, traditions and values. Studies may be cross-national, cross-regional or cross-institutional. Studies use the same methods for data collection in each setting. For example, there can be a secondary analysis of national data followed by data collection through a questionnaire or observation. If the study is cross-national, particular problems can arise in identifying key concepts and asking whether these can be compared across settings. For example, the procedures that are carried out in a hospital or in the community may differ between countries. It is important to be sure that the unit of comparison refers to the same phenomenon. This is discussed in Chapter 22.

As Table 2.1 shows, a range of methods may be used within any of the design types described in Box 2.1.

TABLE 2.1 The range of methods in types of research design

Design type	Experiment	Cross-sectional	Case study	Longitudinal	Comparative
Method of data	Questionnaire	Questionnaire	Questionnaire	Questionnaire	Questionnaire
Method of data	Interview	Interview	Interview	Interview	Interview
Method of data	Observation	Observation	Observation	Observation	Observation
Method of data	Document analysis	Document analysis	Document analysis	Document analysis	Document analysis

Source: De Vaus (2002: 10)

Starting the research process

This chapter concludes with some general guidelines on starting a small-scale research study. These are further elaborated in Chapter 26, which discusses the shape of a research proposal and writing up health research. The research question is critical because it will determine the aims and objectives of a project, the scope of the literature review, and will influence the design and methods for data collection and analysis. It will suggest explicitly or implicitly a body of theory relevant to researching a topic.

Students often find pinning down a research question difficult. A particular topic may be a starting point, but this must be refined down. There are likely to be both what and why questions. A question is likely to be answerable if it is explicit, focused and feasible. Your own life, experience and interests may provoke questions or ideas may come from your immediate circle of friends and family. Almost everyone has experience of episodes of health and illness, has looked after others who have been ill or has used health services. You may have read something that identifies a puzzle or a gap in knowledge. Curiosity about why things are as they are, and persistence in working through ideas, then finding out what has already been written, can help in refining research questions. These should be clear, focused and concise, and be answerable through data collection. Denscombe (2017) describes types of research question, which are shown with examples in Box 2.2.

Box 2.2 Types of research question

The types of research questions are as follows:

Descriptive – A phenomenon is described: What is X and what form does it take? What visual images do hospices use in their advertisements? Why are these used?

Explanatory – The causes and consequences are explained. What is causing or what has caused an outcome? What are the explanations for an increase in obesity in the United Kingdom or other country?

Evaluative – Did an intervention bring benefits? What are the short- and long-term effects of taking HRT to alleviate discomfort during the menopause? What have been the outcomes of a project in health area X to encourage pregnant women to stop smoking?

Comparative – How do A and B differ in relation to X? How does the system for dealing with complaints from patients in hospital A compare to hospital B? What are the outcomes?

Predictive – An outcome is predicted. Have predicted benefits occurred? Have there been unwanted/undesirable side-effects?

Here research questions should be:

- Significant in terms of addressing real-world events
- A problem answerable through research
- A question that has not been answered.

There are examples of how to develop research questions by sharing your ideas with others at the end of the chapter. Chapter 26 gives further examples.

The practical advice is to pick an area of interest first and then look at the relevant literature. The process is iterative – zig-zag between reading, note taking and thinking about theory and methods. Who has carried out research on a topic before? What theories and concepts have been used? What research methods have been used? What have been the main findings? Are there any gaps in knowledge? If you find a study that has been done well, could this model be used to address a different population group, a different illness, or a different organization or policy area? It is worth taking time to frame the question in a way that makes the research feasible and interesting but also has the potential to make a contribution to knowledge. Your literature review should include studies that have used a variety of methods.

The chapters in this book provide examples of qualitative methods such as the use of documents, unstructured and semi-structured interviews, participant observation, focus groups and action research. They also provide examples of quantitative methods such as surveys, experimental methods including RCTs, as well as methods used in economics and to analyse secondary data.

Theory and concepts in health research

In general terms, theories tend to be discipline-based and describe findings that have been observed in earlier research. In clinical research, questions are typically narrow and the research instruments and measures used will be quantitative and well founded as valid measures of the phenomenon under investigation. In qualitative research, theories aid data analysis. Although some theories are too general or abstract to be of use to student researchers or even more experienced researchers, they can be indicative of where to look. Middle-range theories may be more relevant. These can be identified from the literature.

During a literature review, researchers should notice the concepts used and how these are defined as this can lead to identifying relevant theories. A concept is an abstract idea or generalization based on things observed in the real world. We have already discussed the concepts related to health, illness and health work, and have shown that, in consequence, definitions differ. This does not inhibit communication in day-to-day life as people have a general understanding of terms. When doing research, differences in definitions can contribute to a literature review and provide a basis for developing an argument – particularly if there is disagreement between authors. You will find that concepts abound in health research literature. For example, hospital culture, bureaucracy, health technology, carers and the caring professions are all concepts that require discussion. Researchers can note differences and select their preferred definition.

Key factors guiding health research

In health research, the onus is on researchers to produce robust results based on sound methods. This chapter concludes with definitions of some central factors that should guide the conduct of research whatever method is used. In order to add to knowledge, research should be carried out in a way that is as rigorous as possible to produce findings that are *reliable, replicable* and *valid*. These relate to the quality of and the robustness of findings and are outlined in Box 2.3.

Finally, ethical practice in health research is of central importance. This relates to how research has been done – that is, to the robustness of the findings, the truth-telling in the research process, the claims made in presenting findings and, not least, how the researcher has sought to safeguard the interests of research participants in collecting data. Research involves responsibilities to the bodies funding and enabling research, and to the constituencies and the public who draw on research findings. Research projects that are well structured, feasible and cost-effective benefit the public. Research findings should be presented critically, and alternative explanations should be considered.

Box 2.3 Reliability, replicability and validity

These important factors in health research can be outlined as follows:

Reliability in research refers to the tools or measures used to make assess-ments of the research data. Some measures are unreliable because they are poorly defined or inconsistent in what they measure. A tape measure is reliable as it provides a consistent measurement of distance each time it is used. The Short Form 36 (SF-36) is tool designed to measure health status. It asks a series of questions on physical, social and emotional functioning and has been tested for consistency and is considered reliable. However, most measures require a degree of interpretation.

Replicability is a question that is asked in research. It means is it possible to repeat the study? If a study is described well enough to allow it to be repeated, it can be used to confirm or refute previous findings. If there is the same result, this strengthens a knowledge claim. The term is particularly applicable in biomedical research using quantitative methods. As will be discussed in the next chapter, studies are more difficult to replicate exactly in the social sciences.

Validity refers to the soundness of the research findings. Will the research design and the chosen methods answer the research question? Are the findings of a study drawn from the evidence presented and are the conclusions that are made justified?

Clearly, the interests of participants in health research should be protected. A few projects have involved serious violations of ethical principles, leading to harm to participants. It is now incumbent on all researchers in social as well as biomedical research to ensure, if permission to proceed is given, that there is no harm to participants, that their consent is obtained to take part in research and that the anonymity of participants is protected. There is also an expectation, particularly in social and policy research, that participants can and should contribute to the research process from the inception of a project and its design, through to developing research instruments, taking part in the project and being informed of the findings, including the opportunity to comment and provide feedback. There are underlying issues about power relationships in the research process. Researchers must respect participants as persons, be aware of vulnerabilities where sensitive issues are being discussed and avoid any form of coercion. In the more informal research methods, coercion can take subtle forms such as asking leading questions and straying into areas that are not part of the project. Researchers should also not put themselves at risk in doing research.

Conclusion

In discussing the principles of health research, this chapter has indicated the range and scope of research on health and health care. A number of disciplines may be drawn on to provide theories and concepts to formulate research questions. Some illustrations have been given of studies undertaken within both the natural and social sciences. These studies may develop from observing or collecting data and then formulating a theory to explain patterns of behaviour, or theories may be tested through data collection. We have argued that researchers must be thoughtful about the design they choose to pursue their research project. There are a limited number of options to follow, but then a variety of methodologies and methods may be adopted to carry out an investigation. The latter should be selected to suit both the question chosen and personal preference. A number of principles have been referred to that should govern the conduct of all health research. These relate to both the substance and ethics of the research process. On the one hand, findings must be soundly-based in order to add to knowledge. On the other, collecting data involves personal relations with people whose interests and dignity should be respected.

Exercise 2.1   Engaging in health research

- Choose a research topic for health research and present it to colleagues (as a group or in pairs), describing it in one sentence. Construct three possible research questions from this topic and discuss.
- Search for three texts related to one of these questions and write a short paper examining the methods used in these papers and how the question has been answered. Are there any gaps in the argument? If so, what are they?

Recommended further reading

This book provides a strong general grounding in social research methods, albeit it is not specifically oriented to health:
Bryman, A. (2016) *Social Research Methods*, 5th edition. Oxford: Oxford University Press.

This useful guide will help researchers engage in designing and conducting mixed methods research:

Cresswell, J. W. and Plano Clark, V. L. (2017) *Designing and Conducting Mixed Methods Research*, 3rd edition. London: Sage.

This book provides a straightforward introductory overview covering the whole research process, with a particular focus on health:

Jacobsen, K. H. (2017) *Introduction to Health Research Methods: A Practical Guide*, 2nd edition. Burlington, MA: Jones & Bartlett Learning.

References

Ahrendt, D., Anderson, A., Dubois, H., Jungblut, J.-M., Leončikas, T., Sándor, E. and Pöntinen, E. (2018) *The European Quality of Life Survey 2016: Overview Report*. Luxemburg: Eurofound.

Allsop, J., Baggott, R. and Jones, K. (2004) 'Health consumer groups: A new social movement?', *Sociology of Health and Illness*, *26*(6): 737–56.

Andrew, S. and Halcomb, E. J. (eds) (2009) *Mixed Methods Research for Nursing and the Health Sciences*. Chichester: Wiley-Blackwell.

Bartlett, M. (2017) *Health Inequality: An Introduction to Concepts, Theories and Methods*, 2nd edition. Cambridge: Polity Press.

Blaxter M. (2010) *Health*, 2nd edition. Cambridge: Polity Press.

Bourgeault, I., Dingwall, R. and de Vries, R. (eds) (2010) *The SAGE Handbook of Qualitative Methods in Health Research*. London: Sage.

Bowling, A. (2014) *Research Methods in Health: Investigating Health and Health Services*, 4th edition. Maidenhead: Open University Press.

Bruce, N. and Pope, D. (2018) *Quantitative Methods for Health Research: A Practical Interactive Guide to Epidemiology and Statistics*, 2nd edition. Chichester: Wiley-Blackwell.

Bryman, A. (2016) *Social Research Methods*, 5th edition. Oxford: Oxford University Press.

Bury, M. (1982) 'Chronic illness as biographical disruption', *Sociology of Health and Illness*, *4*(2): 167–82.

Cassileth, B. R., Lusk, E. J., Strouse, T. B., Miller, D. S., Brown, L. L., Cross, P. A. and Tenaglia, A. N. (1984) 'Psycho-social status in chronic illness: A comparative analysis of six diagnostic groups', *New England Journal of Medicine*, *311*: 506–11.

Cresswell, J. W. and Plano Clark, V. L. (2017) *Designing and Conducting Mixed Methods Research*, 3rd edition. London: Sage.

Damjanov, I. (2012) *Pathology for the Health Professions*, 4th edition. St Louis, MO: Elsevier Saunders.

Davies, A. and Newman, S. (2012) 'Systematic review of the effects of telecare provided for a person with social care needs on outcomes for their informal carers', *Health and Social Care in the Community*, *21*(6): 582–97.

De Vaus, D. (2002) *Research Design in Social Research*. London: Sage.

Denscombe, M. (2017) *The Good Research Guide: For Small-Scale Research Projects*, 6th edition. Maidenhead: Open University Press/McGraw Hill.

Dyson, S. and Brown, B. (2006) *Social Theory and Applied Health Research*. Maidenhead: Open University Press.

Evans, R. G., Barer, M. L. and Marmor, T. R. (1994) *Why Some People Are Healthy and Others Not?* New York: Aldine de Gruyter.

Foucault, M. (2003) *The Birth of the Clinic*. Abingdon: Routledge Classics.

Gabe, J., Kelleher, D. and Williams, G. (eds) (2006) *Challenging Medicine*, 2nd edition. London: Routledge.

Goffman, E. (1968) *Stigma: Notes on the Management of Spoiled Identity*. Harmondsworth: Penguin.

Greener, I., Harrington, B., Hunter, D., Mannion, R. and Powell, M. (2014) *Reforming Healthcare: What's the Evidence?* Bristol: Policy Press.

Henn, M., Weinstein, M. and Foard, N. (2006) *A Short Introduction to Social Research*. London: Sage.

Herzlich, C. (1973) *Health and Illness: A Social Psychological Analysis*. New York: Academic Press.

Hudson, N. and Culley, L. (2015) 'Cross border reproductive travel', in L. Lundt, J. Hanefeld and D. Horsfall (eds), *Handbook of Medical Tourism and Patient Mobility*. Cheltenham: Edward Elgar.

Hudson, N., Culley, L., Law, C., Mitchell, H., Denny, E. and Raine-Fenning N. (2016) 'We need to change the mission statement of marriage: Biographical disruption among couples living with endometriosis', *Sociology of Health and Illness*, 38(5): 721–35.

Ingleby, D., Krasnik, A., Lorant, V. and Razum, O. (eds) (2012) *Health Inequalities and Risk Factors among Migrants and Ethnic Minorities*. Antwerp: Garant.

John, P., Cotterill, S., Moseley, A., Richardson, L., Smith, G., Stoker, G. and Wales, C. (2011) *Nudge, Nudge, Think, Think: Experimenting with Ways to Change Civic Behaviour*. London: Bloomsbury Academic.

Kane, R. L. and Radosevich, D. M. (2011) *Conducting Health Outcomes Research*. London: Jones & Barlett Learning.

Korman N. and Glennerster, H. (1990) *Hospital Closure*. Milton Keynes: Open University Press.

Kuhlmann, E. and Annandale, E. (eds) (2012) *The Palgrave Handbook of Gender and Healthcare*, 2nd edition. Basingstoke: Palgrave.

Kuhlmann, E. and Saks, M. (eds) (2008) *Rethinking Professional Governance: International Directions in Healthcare*. Bristol: Policy Press.

Le Fanu, J. (2011) *The Rise and Fall of Modern Medicine*, 2nd edition. London: Abacus.

Lenard, P. T. and Straehle, C. (eds) (2012) *Health Inequalities and Global Justice*. Edinburgh: Edinburgh University Press.

Lovallo, W. R. (2005) *Stress and Health: Biological and Psychological Interactions*, 2nd edition. Thousand Oaks, CA: Sage.

McEvoy, R., Ballini, L., Maltoni, S., O'Donnell, C., Mair, F. and MacFarlane, A. (2013) 'A qualitative systematic review of studies using the normalisation process theory to research implementation processes', *Implementation Science, 9*(1): 1–13.

Maslow, A. (1954) *Motivation and Personality.* New York: Harper & Row.

May, C. (2009) 'Innovation and implementation in health technology: Normalizing telemedicine', in J. Gabe and M. Calnan (eds), *The New Sociology of the Health Service.* London: Routledge.

May, C. and Finch, T. (2009) 'Implementation, embedding and integraton: An outline of normalisation process theory', *Sociology, 43*(3): 535–54.

Monaghan, L. F. and Gabe, J. (2016) 'Embodying health identities: A study of young people with asthma', *Social Science and Medicine, 160*: 1–8.

Navarro, V. (1986) *Crisis, Health and Medicine: A Social Critique.* New York: Tavistock.

Neighbors, M. and Tannehill-Jones, R. (2009) *Human Diseases,* 3rd edition. New York: Delmar Cengage Learning.

Panno, J. (2010) *Gene Therapy: Treatments and Cures for Genetic Diseases,* revised edition. New York: Facts on File.

Parsons, T. (1951) *The Social System.* Glencoe, IL: Free Press; St Louis, MO: Saunders Elsevier.

Purtilo, R., Haddad, A. and Doherty, R. (2014) *Health Professional and Patient Interaction,* 8th edition. St Louis, MO: Elsevier Saunders.

Rainville, C. (2016) *Survey on Healthy Behaviors and Well-Being.* Washington, DC: AARP Research.

Realpe, A. and Wallace, L. M. (2010) *What is Co-Production?* London: The Health Foundation.

Richardson, A., Jackson, C. and Sykes, W. (1990) *Taking Research Seriously: Means of Improving and Assessing the Use and Dissemination of Research.* London: HMSO.

Saks, M. (2002) 'Empowerment, participation and the rise of orthodox biomedicine', in J. Dooher and R. Byrt (eds), *Empowerment and Participation: Power, Influence and Control in Contemporary Health Care.* Dinton: Quay Books.

Saks, M. (2006) 'The alternatives to medicine', in D. Kelleher, J. Gabe and G. Williams (eds), *Challenging Medicine,* 2nd edition. Abingdon: Routledge.

Saks, M. (2015a) 'Inequalities, marginality and the professions', *Current Sociology Review, 63*(6): 850–68.

Saks, M. (2015b) 'Power and professionalisation in CAM: A sociological approach', in N. Gale and J. McHale (eds), *The Routledge Handbook of Complementary Medicine in Social Science and Law.* Abingdon: Routledge.

Saks, M. (2015c) *The Professions, State and the Market: Medicine in Britain, the United States and Russia.* Abingdon: Routledge.

Scambler, G. (ed.) (2008) *Sociology as Applied to Medicine,* 6th edition. London: Elsevier.

Schulz, F., Chalmers, I., Hayes, R. and Airman, D. (1995) 'Empirical evidence of bias: Dimension of methodological quality associated with estimates of treatment effects in controlled trials', *Journal of the American Medical Association*, *273*: 408–12.

Smith, K. E. and Bambra, C. (2016) *Health Inequalities: Critical Perspectives*. Oxford: Oxford University Press.

Stacey, M. (1988) *The Sociology of Health and Healing*. London: Allen & Unwin.

Straub, R. O. (2011) *Health Psychology: A Biopsychosocial Approach*, 3rd edition. New York: Worth Publishers.

Török, E., Moran, E. and Cooke, F. (2009) *Oxford Handbook of Infectious Diseases and Microbiology*. Oxford: Oxford University Press.

Turner, B. S. (2003) 'The history of the changing concepts of health and illness: Outline of a general model of illness categories', in G. L. Albrecht, R. Fitzpatrick and S. C. Scrimshaw (eds), *The Handbook of Social Studies in Health and Medicine*. London: Sage.

Wadsworth, M. (1991) *The Imprint of Time: Childhood and Adult Life*. Oxford: Clarendon Press.

Yin, R. K. (2018) *Case Study Research and Applications: Design and Methods*, 6th edition. Los Angeles, CA: Sage.

3

Strategies for Health Research

JUDITH ALLSOP

Chapter objectives

- To describe the key concepts of ontology, epistemology, methodology and methods
- To outline the origins and assumptions of positivism in the clinical and social sciences
- To account for the origins of interpretivism and concerns about positivism
- To discuss the weaknesses and strengths of quantitative and qualitative methods
- To show how methods are mixed in research practice.

Introduction

In Chapter 2 we discussed the scope of health research, which covers both the natural and the social sciences and therefore uses a range of methodologies and methods. We introduced two forms of logic in the research process: collecting data on a problem and then proceeding to draw out a general proposition or theory (inductive reasoning), or beginning with a proposition and then testing this (deductive reasoning). However, we indicated that, when doing research, there is a cyclical process of moving between theory and data and then back again to assess evidence. This chapter looks at two different approaches to doing research in the health field – positivism and interpretivism. Drawn from the philosophy of knowledge, these are based on contrasting assumptions about how we know what we know, and how we can ensure that research findings add to knowledge. Positivism and interpretivism are referred to as paradigms as they draw on commonly held views about doing research.

This distinction is both helpful and unhelpful for students learning about research. It is important to understand the basis for knowledge claims and the foundation for evidence from research and also to understand the terminology used in debates in research. However, it is not helpful to suggest that certain methodologies and methods are necessarily linked with either paradigm – to link positivism with quantitative methods and interpretivism with qualitative is too simplistic.

In research practice, boundaries are fuzzy rather than rigid. In the last chapter, we showed that across the range of options for the design of a research projects, a similar range of methods are available. The choice of methods depends on various factors: the disciplinary background of the researcher; the research question posed; the kind of evidence available; and the preference of the researcher to adopt one method rather than another. It is suggested here that notions of quantity are part of all research and that the analysis of data is not only the application of a technique, but also an act of interpretation and judgement. In short, binary opposites may clarify at the level of abstraction, but are blurred when it comes to research practice (see Bryman 2016; Gorard 2010).

Approaches to knowledge in health research

Positivism and interpretivism draw on two different philosophical approaches to 'knowing' and gaining knowledge through research. Positivism follows scientific principles to produce evidence for a knowledge claim and is associated with the clinical sciences, quantitative data and statistical analysis. Interpretivism is based on the principle that all knowledge derives from human perception and, therefore, research must take into account how human subjects understand their world. A range of qualitative methods are used to collect and analyse data. However, it should not be assumed that notions of quantity are absent from qualitative studies or that clinical researchers do not use qualitative methods; rather, in practice, the research question will influence the design chosen to carry out research, but will not determine the method chosen to collect data.

These two approaches to knowledge are based on differing views of what is reality – referred to in the philosophical literature as their *ontology*. As ways of knowing, positivism and interpretivism are said to have a different *epistemology* – that is, they differ in what they define as knowledge and they also differ in what they consider as the legitimate route to acquiring knowledge. In other words, each way of knowing differs in its *methodology* or its approach to gaining that knowledge. This line of argument can be represented as a diagram, progressing from the abstract to the more concrete, as shown in Figure 3.1.

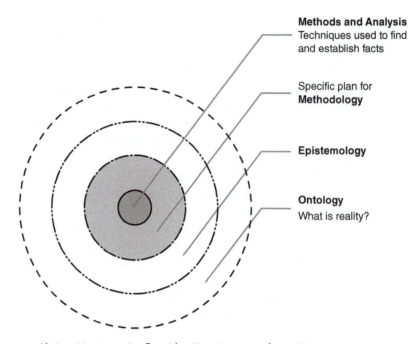

Methods and Analysis
Techniques used to find
and establish facts

Specific plan for
Methodology

Epistemology

Ontology
What is reality?

FIGURE 3.1 Abstract to concrete: Considerations in research practice

The underlying assumptions of positivism and interpretivism, commonly referred to as paradigms, represent different assumptions about how we gain knowledge about the world. They are different forms of 'truth-telling' about the social and natural world. This may become clearer through a description of their historical origins and their use in the contemporary context. In some accounts, positivism and interpretivism as research strategies are also linked to particular ideological and political views. However, we do not take this view here, as explained above.

Positivism and interpretivism: Strategies for research

How do we know that a knowledge claim is correct or true? How well founded is the claim? How much is based on belief and how much on established facts and sound evidence? Positivism aims to follow scientific principles to produce evidence for a knowledge claim. We need to know the justification for stating that something is a 'fact'.

Positivism and the scientific method

Positivism in health research rests on a number of assumptions referred to as a paradigm. This is a shorthand term for a set of taken-for-granted assumptions. The term was used by

Kuhn (1970) to describe 'normal science' – a set of rules that defined the route to solving a scientific problem or question. Thus, those within the scientific community have a set of rules that they apply when reviewing an account of a solution to a scientific problem. This is used to assess the validity of a claim based on the methodology and method employed. Examples would be the criteria used for the acceptance of an article for *Nature* or the medical journal *The Lancet*. Recently, the Medical Research Council (MRC) in the United Kingdom issued new guidelines for the management of randomized controlled trials (RCTs). These set out the revised standards to be met by researchers conducting clinical trials (Medical Research Council 2017). This will be discussed further below. However, these adjustments do not constitute a new paradigm. While the details have changed over time, the principles underlying the scientific method have a long history and are still widely shared within the scientific community.

A landmark in scientific thinking, and what is now referred to as positivism, was the establishment of the Royal Society in England in 1660. It provided an arena for a discussion of both the findings and the theories and methods for undertaking scientific inquiry into the natural world. The methods were based on observation, the recording of facts and the testing of theories. This marked a paradigm shift around how to acquire knowledge, which was reinforced during the eighteenth century in the Enlightenment, also known as the Age of Reason. As Porter (1997) shows in his history of medicine, it was not until the late nineteenth century that scientific methods began to be applied in the practice of medicine. Gradually, evidence began to replace customary practice and folk beliefs. Box 3.1 provides an early example of an experiment based on observation.

Box 3.1 Example of an early scientific experiment based on observation

In 1796 Jenner discovered the smallpox vaccine through testing a theory. He had observed that milk maids tended not to develop smallpox. He speculated that this could be because they worked with cows, which had a variant of smallpox – cowpox a less virulent strain. He tested this through an experiment. He took a sample of cowpox and injected it into the arm of a boy with smallpox which at the time was a deadly disease. The boy recovered. On the basis of this, he developed and tested a vaccine that provided sufficient immunity to control the disease in the general population.

Even in the mid-twentieth century many procedures and interventions were followed because they appeared to work well enough. The book by Cochrane (1972) entitled *Effectiveness and Efficiency: Random Reflections on Health Services* drew attention both to the lack of evidence on the outcomes of treatment procedures and to the wide variations in what doctors recommended. The book was influential in focusing health research on establishing an evidence base through RCTs. This is widely considered as the most rigorous method for carrying out research that can produce reliable findings. Later, the Cochrane Centre in Oxford, England (www.ukcc.cochrane.org), was founded to act as the hub for information on the results of systematic reviews of clinical trials worldwide. Interestingly, there is a new emphasis on the importance of both rigour and reproducibility in clinical trials. New knowledge will not become accepted as 'truthful' if the methodology and methods are not outlined in sufficient detail for a study to be reproduced by another researcher.

The aim of scientists was to discover the general laws and objective facts in the natural world. These principles were taken up by nineteenth-century philosophers and sociologists, such as Comte, Spencer and Durkheim, who aimed to follow the premises of scientific inquiry in studying society. As Giddens (1987) comments, their aim was to develop concepts and theories and, by so doing, establish a 'science of man'. They believed that the role of the researcher was to collect and interpret social facts systematically and objectively to identify the laws that governed social life to identify regularities or explain cultural differences. For example, Durkheim (1979) investigated suicide rates and how these varied across different cultures. He developed a theory to explain this, a theory that still has explanatory power today, as outlined more fully in Box 3.2.

Box 3.2 A study of the social causes of suicide

Durkheim carried out his study of suicide in 1897. This research was considered as ground-breaking as he attributed suicide to social causes, not individual characteristics. He argued that people's actions were shaped by norms, values, conventions and rules. He extracted data on suicides from official sources and showed that suicide rates varied by religious affiliation and by gender. Catholics and Jews had lower suicide rates than Protestants and women had lower rates than men. He argued that, in both of the former cases, this was due to greater integration, cohesion and social control. For the same reasons, suicide was also less prevalent among people who had children. Regulation through codes, rules and laws also acted as a form of social control. For Durkheim, the extent of integration and regulation could be either strong or weak and this led him to a classification of scenarios to explain suicides. For researchers, the important lesson to note is that Durkheim proposed objective 'truths' about the societal circumstances driving the individual decisions linked to suicide.

The various disciplines within the natural and social sciences that investigate the health field share a framework of assumptions and beliefs associated with the philosophical position known as positivism. They employ methodologies that are based on the principles of the scientific method and use methods that are quantitative.

As applied in clinical research, studies draw on a particular area of theory from the natural sciences and on relevant research findings to address a specific research question. This is typically a very narrow question as clinical science develops in small steps. Where appropriate, most trials have already been tested for effects and safety in research involving animals, then healthy volunteers, before involving patients. Clinical research is strictly regulated and must follow protocols and meet specified ethical standards, the most important criterion of which is that the researcher must obtain the informed consent of participants (see also Chapter 19 on ethics).

A key assumption made in biomedical research is that the body and body parts are taken as objects for research and assumptions are made about the similarity of the internal functioning of the body and likely course of a disease process. Typical clusters of symptoms denote the presence of a disease or malfunction. These have been named through past research and enable a diagnosis to be made and the likely course of the disease to be predicted (the prognosis). In most cases, there will be treatments available whose efficacy can also be predicted. Based on the biomedical model of disease, such studies approach the patient as a physical/mechanistic entity that can be assessed, measured, controlled and ultimately manipulated. The researcher takes a position of neutrality and is an objective observer of the intervention that is introduced as part of the research process. Participants are recruited so that findings are generalizable to a larger population. In consequence, most biomedical research methods fall squarely within the positivist paradigm.

Efforts are made to ensure that clinical researchers, who are normally also clinicians, take an objective stance in a research trial. The aim is to 'blind' the researcher as to which patient or volunteer receive the new intervention, and thus avoid bias (Altman 2000). If bias is excluded, and the study properly conducted, it can produce a clear outcome (see also Chapter 14). Data are collected through reliable methods and results are analysed using established statistical techniques. This aim is to ensure that findings have not been distorted or skewed so they can be generalized to larger populations. If methods are transparent, studies can be replicated by subsequent researchers and the validity of the research assured. This is a simplification of the real world but detachment and rigour frame working practices. If findings are replicated by other studies, then it is highly probable that treatment X will lead to outcome Y, until it is shown that there are exceptions. Clinical researchers go to some lengths to establish *causal* relationships.

The methodology and methods in the study must be transparent so that those working in the field can verify, or falsify (show to be wrong), findings by assessing the methods used to arrive at the conclusions. Transparency of working methods also allows subsequent researchers to carry out a further study to test the validity of the results. Popper (1959) recommended that scientists should aim to falsify their hypotheses rather than seek confirmation. This, he argued, is a more rigorous method for establishing new knowledge.

Social scientists also draw on the positivist paradigm in line with the scientific mode of inquiry. Again, researchers draw on a body of theory to construct ways of addressing the research question. For example, in constructing questions for a survey, the researcher will already have in mind a hypothesis to be tested (De Vaus 2014). A hypothesis states that there is a relationship between two or more variables. It decides what will be measured and predicts a relationship in the framing of questions. It is assumed that questions will elicit responses that are 'truthful' and will allow the researcher to analyse the results using techniques that are known to be reliable. It is assumed that the researcher is able to collect and interpret social facts objectively and will identify, count and measure results using statistical measures that are known to be reliable so that findings are generalizable to larger populations. By using methods that are accepted as valid within the discipline, those working in the field can verify or falsify the findings.

Social science research in the positivist paradigm follows prescribed steps and, in general, uses a deductive form of reasoning. The researcher works a theory-driven hypothesis or proposition. The proposition forms the basis for designing and planning a project to collect data that will test this (Bowling 2014; De Vaus 2014). The proposition to be tested will inform the method, say the design of a survey, and be subject to accepted forms of statistical testing. Surveys using a questionnaire aim to establish associations or correlations between independent and dependent variables in the analysis of results. This can infer cause by association, but does not establish a strong causal link, as in an RCT.

Positivist researchers claim that their research methodologies are based on scientific principles and quantitative methods that produce findings that are 'truthful' (Brown, Crawford and Hicks 2003). They also use a check of whether these methods are followed to evaluate the quality of research papers (Greenhalgh 2014). The particular strengths in contributing to knowledge are outlined in Box 3.3.

Box 3.3 The assumptions of the positivist paradigm

- Knowledge is gained by drawing on scientific and social theories to establish facts and draw causal inferences.
- Knowledge is seen as cumulative and based on previous research.
- Knowledge can be produced through the application of a rigorous methodology and quantitative methods. Data are collected, reduced to numbers and analysed using reliable statistical and mathematically based techniques.
- Researchers can take an objective stance in the research process as they are external to it.
- Phenomena exist in the natural and social world as fixed realities.

Within this framework, all knowledge is considered as contingent – that is, its claim applies for the moment until further research produces contradictory evidence. Research builds on the work of others and subsequent research will aim to confirm, modify or refute existing hypotheses through further study.

The advantages and limitations of positivism

There are many benefits of positivism and its frequently interlinked quantitative methods. These are set out in Box 3.4.

Box 3.4 The advantages of positivism

- *Reliability*: Being able to measure quantity is a powerful tool in producing data on phenomena in the natural and social world. If tested by proven statistical techniques, they provide accurate measures.
- *Rigour*: The methods adopted by quantitative researchers are logical, transparent and standardized.
- *External validity*: The methods are able to explain phenomena with independent and dependent variables. Some methods can demonstrate cause and effect, while others can make inferences through associations between variables.
- *Generalizability*: The findings of a study can be generalized to a larger population through statistical sampling.
- *Reproducibility*: By making their methods transparent, research studies can be reproduced by others. This increases the reliability and validity of findings.

Positivism and the quantitative methods associated with this paradigm have much strength but there are also limitations. The objective, hypothesis and protocol-driven stance taken by researchers misses out on a whole area of human motivation and action. The social world is different from the natural world. Social institutions and cultures are not fixed. Both stability and change are the result of human action. Even the natural world is perceived and examined through the gaze of researchers who select what to see and account for. For this reason, interpretivism developed as an alternative paradigm of research for understanding the world, and a range of qualitative methods has been developed. This strategy and associated methods are discussed further below. Meanwhile, Box 3.5 outlines some specific limitations of positivism as a research strategy.

Box 3.5   The limitations of positivism

- Critics of positivists' claim to objectivity and the existence of social laws mistake the nature of social reality and argue that the scientific method is not a route to understanding human action. The claim to 'truth-telling' occurs within a limiting set of assumptions.
- It can be argued that the measures used by positivist researchers are artificial. They measure constructs devised by the researcher and not life as it is lived by respondents. For example, patient satisfaction surveys can be said to be flawed as they measure what health service managers think is important, not patients' concerns.
- Some methods, such as questionnaires, test for associations between variables. However, we cannot be sure how a question is being interpreted by the person answering the survey.
- Surveys measure responses at a single point in time, but people have the capacity for change. Information from surveys is time limited.
- Positivist methods are less able to determine why people act as they do and how decision-making is embedded in social relations. For example, why do people delay in seeking a medical opinion? It cannot explore cultural understandings unless prior research has been undertaken already.
- In some situations, methods such as RCTs cannot be used for ethical, practical or financial reasons. An RCT requires a control group of patients, but it may not be ethical to deny treatment to people who need it.
- Many of the measures used in quantitative studies are constructs or approximate measures. What does a one-off blood test actually measure, apart from a deviation from a predetermined scale? To be meaningful, it has to be interpreted in the context of the person's particular activities and taken over a period of time to establish a norm for that person.

Interpretivism as a research strategy

We now turn to consider an alternative paradigm for doing health research – interpretivism. While this is based on some shared assumptions about acquiring knowledge, methodologies differ. Interpretivism developed in response to the perceived weaknesses of positivism, around the middle of the twentieth century, when social scientists such as Max Weber (1947) argued that knowledge depended on *verstehen*, or 'an interpretive understanding of social action'. Weber's view was that actions can only be understood in terms of their meaning for the people taking the action and this is shaped by social position and the values and culture of the time. In social life, there are no objective realities to be studied outside their social context.

The methodology and methods for researching the social world and social action had their origins in the 1920s and 1930s. Sociologists and social psychologists based at the University of Chicago began to study social problems using ethnographic methods (Blumer 1984). They collected data about communities and groups through observation and developed theories and explanations. This was an inductive form of reasoning – from observation to theory. In the late 1960s and 1970s, social scientists refocused their research on the ways in which meanings are constructed, negotiated and managed by different individuals and groups. For example, Schutz (1962: 29) commented that in order to understand social action the social scientist had to understand the 'common-sense constructs' that people use to make sense of their world and that drives their actions. From this point of view, it was argued that social order is negotiated, and cultural values and norms change through action.

Critics of positivism argue that this approach is inappropriate to researching social life. They suggest that people think and act within a particular set of cultural assumptions that provide a framework for interpretation and meaning in interaction (Glassner and Moreno 1989; Seale 2018). It is impossible to talk about, understand or communicate social phenomena without employing a particular language or conceptual scheme, as there is no such thing as a neutral stance in the research process. Moreover, it is claimed that all research instruments – such as the schedule for a survey, a clinical trial or a structured questionnaire – draw on social and cultural constructs. Researchers choose the questions and interpret the results. Ultimately, therefore, knowledge produced by positivist research methods has an element of subjectivity that may or may not be acknowledged. Some critics go so far as to argue that positivism represents an ideological and political position in the way it views the world (Rubin and Rubin 2012).

Interpretivism does not have one methodology for research. There are variations. For example, phenomenology is based on the study of how people perceive their world and make sense of it; symbolic interactionism suggests that people communicate through accepted meanings; and constructivism takes the view that meaning is constructed through interaction (see Geertz 1973; Lofland 2006; Seale 2018). Such theories have been used to study patient careers, doctor–patient interaction, institutional rules and routines.

More specialist qualitative methods include discourse analysis (Becker, Bryman and Ferguson 2012; Pope and Mays 2006). The aim is to show how social phenomena are constructed through talk and to demonstrate how the rules of discourse may differ in between settings. Narrative analysis identifies recurrent, or typical, patterns in the way that research participants account for a treatment pathway, event or process. It strives to identify commonalities and differences in a temporal sequence of events. Action research can demonstrate group collaboration or lack of it in projects to engineer social change.

Despite the different strategies, interpretivists share an assumption that the researcher looks for meaning in the talk, actions or artefacts produced by social actors in their social setting. Written documents as well as talk are an important source of information: records kept by others for bureaucratic purposes, such as hospital records; personal documents written by people themselves, such as diaries; retrospective or daily accounts structured by the researcher; and policy documents that contain implicit or explicit theories about what particular programmes aim to achieve. The methods seek to establish an understanding of people's lives and experiences through capturing the subjective meanings of social actors and understanding their world view and are often used where little is known about a research area and where there has been an absence of conceptual or theoretical development (Oakley 2000). Rather than seeking to measure attitudes or predict behaviour through standard, pre-constructed instruments, qualitative methods can assist in developing such instruments as they can identify participants' views and priorities.

As has been shown, unlike quantitative methods, there is no standard protocol for researchers using interpretivist strategies. Nevertheless, they must state how their method- ology and methods will meet the aims and objectives of their particular research question. The research designs noted in the previous chapter are open to researchers (De Vaus 2009). Analysing qualitative data presents a challenge (Silverman 2011). Concepts and theories are required to group the data into categories. These must be drawn from the data collected and should be linked to theoretical concepts and themes in order to reduce the quantity of data and to identify patterns that recur. These provide a basis for generalization.

Within interpretivism there is no standard method for data analysis. Glaser and Strauss (1967) proposed a systematic approach through grounded theory. Here, the researcher aims to develop a theoretical framework for coding data from early on in the data collection process to identify themes. Coding means labelling or categorizing chunks of data. The coding framework is refined during the later stages through a pro- cess of 'analytical induction' or 'abduction' – a reduction to themes based on theories or concepts on which to base generalizations (Bryman 2016). This strategy allows themes to be drawn from the data to provide a framework for analysis that reflects the under- standings of the social actors in the research. Ideally, themes and sub-categories can then be linked to an explanatory theory. Once the analytical framework has been constructed, data can be organized. This may be done manually but a qualitative data analysis package will aid categorization and analysis for a large data set. There are a number of packages available for this task, for example Nud*ist or NVivo. At present, there is no consensus on which tool is best. In presenting the findings from a qualitative analysis, notions of quantity are often used. Such terms as 'most', 'more', 'many' or 'few' give weight to data when presenting findings.

The advantages and limitations of interpretivism

As with positivism, there are advantages and limitations of this strategy. The benefits of interpretivism and its typically interlinked qualitative approach are set out in Box 3.6.

Box 3.6 The advantages of interpretivism

- *Flexibility in thinking*: Researchers are less likely to become stuck in conventional ways of thinking. Rather than merely testing pre-existing ideas, they can make observations that lead to the creation of new ideas and categories (Ezzy 2002; Strauss and Corbin 1998).
- *Flexibility in the research process*: Researchers can adjust their approach in their interpretation of data. They may find themes or patterns in the data that contradict their initial assumptions.
- *Rich description*: Qualitative methods provide rich, subjective experience in naturalistic settings. Findings are based on an empathetic understanding of the views of research participants, whose experiences are embedded in specific social, cultural and historical contexts.
- *Compensation*: Qualitative methods can be used to investigate areas where quantitative methods are inappropriate, where little is known, on sensitive issues (e.g. drug taking, heavy drinking, sexual practices), or observe informal decision-making (e.g. in organizational settings such as clinics or hospitals).
- *Validity*: Such methods are high on internal validity if they identify the understandings of research participants.

The disadvantages of interpretivism and its associated qualitative methods are outlined in Box 3.7.

Box 3.7 The limitations of the interpretivist paradigm

- There is a lack of consensus on best practice for data collection and analysis.
- Without an initial theory and a defined area for a literature search, the researcher is on a fishing expedition. There can be data overload and analysis is time-consuming.
- Many studies are undertaken with a small number of participants so that findings cannot be generalized to a larger population.
- Studies are difficult to replicate or reproduce. They are context and time-specific.
- There is little opportunity to assess the external validity of findings as data are interpreted by the researcher.
- Without measurement, the strength of themes cannot be assessed. Anecdotes or snippets illustrate themes, but how do we know how representative they are?
- Qualitative studies are costly in terms of time for transcribing and analysis.
- There is a problem of observer bias: researchers themselves construct categories.
- Some versions of interpretivism may ignore the structural constraints on human action, such as politics, economics and alleviating pain and disease.

TABLE 3.1   Positivism and interpretivism: Assumptions and methods

Feature	Positivism	Interpretivism
Approach to knowledge	Aim: to use existing theory to test hypotheses based on existing knowledge and to find facts, where possible, of the link between cause and effect, which is established in a narrow question.	Aim: to find meaning in social action and to develop theory by looking for patterns and regularities in talk and artefacts.
Role of the researcher	Objective and external to the research process.	Acknowledges that researchers will bring their own knowledge and sensibilities to interpret what they see and hear in the research process.
Methodology	Use well-established protocols for trials, experiments and surveys to address a specific and limited question.	Research questions explore a stated phenomenon in context. There are a number of strategies for data collection. Transparency in describing decisions in the research process is important.
Methods for data collection	The variables being investigated are stated. Instruments are developed and proven measures are chosen prior to planning data collection. Studies tend to be larger with greater numbers but smaller questions. Codes are applied to surveys prior to data collection. In experiments, data are recorded in predetermined categories. Samples are chosen to be representative and statistical techniques are used to extrapolate findings to whole populations.	Qualitative methods are used to collect data. Talk, observation, documents and artefacts and recorded. Sampling is purposive and numbers tend to be small.
Data analysis	Numbers are the unit of analysis. Initial preparation looks for trends and correlations, typically using data analysis software. Data analysis methods have been pre-planned to confirm or falsify a hypothesis and can be subject to statistical techniques.	The data collected are richer. Analysis takes place during and after data collection. Themes are identified iteratively and coded. Codes are grouped and then ordered, drawing on theory and concepts to elucidate and make an argument. The process is flexible, takes time and can be aided by the use of software.

Table 3.1 illustrates the main differences between positivism and quantitative methods compared to interpretivism and qualitative methods. An important point to note is that in the case of the former, the research protocol and all the tools used for data collection, coding and analysis must be fully outlined and prepared in advance of carrying out the data collection. If qualitative methods are used, the research protocol outlines the research objectives and method, but coding and analysis occurs during and after data collection. The process of analysis is more flexible but takes longer.

Refining methods

Some of the criticisms listed in the boxes above have been taken into account and both quantitative and qualitative methods have been refined to address criticisms. For example, when using methods such as surveys, as Chapter 13 shows, these may incorporate qualitative questions. Clinical researchers may carry out studies using observational methods or collect accounts from patients to incorporate experiential knowledge from the patient's perspective in clinical trials or in professional practice (Ledade, Shashir and Gupta 2017).

Qualitative research methods have also developed ways to check categories and to code to ensure consistency. In some small-scale studies, accounts are cross-checked with participants to make sure the account given by the researched corresponds with their own understanding. For example, Bloor (1978) undertook an observational study of ENT consultants' procedures in diagnosing whether a tonsillectomy was required for children coming to their clinic. He checked whether his account tallied with consultants' own views of the signs they looked for in making a decision. He found a high degree of agreement and then proceeded to draw conclusions from what he had found. Others have written extensively on ways to make data collection and analysis more systematic to produce accounts with greater external validity and have introduced forms of measurement into their studies. For instance, Strauss and Corbin (1998) refined their constant comparative method to identify and test dominant themes by seeking out deviant cases and to test theory by looking for alternative explanations. Silverman (2016) supports the case for counting as part of qualitative analysis, arguing that the selective use of numbers can strengthen an argument.

Research as a craft: Flexibility and mixing methods

If a purist philosophical position is taken, the positivist and interpretivist methods predominantly used represent approaches that are logically inconsistent and mutually exclusive (see Hammersley 1992). If a comparison is made between an RCT and, say, an action research project, where the shape of a project evolves and shifts and each case is unique, then there is a stark contrast between the knowledge derived from each method. However, in practice, most researchers take a realist view and align the methods chosen to answer the research question.

However, the division between positivism and interpretivism has become less relevant to research in practice. Although positivism and interpretivism produce different kinds of knowledge, and quantitative and qualitative methods have different traditions and styles, both are used across the range of research designs. Research that addresses problems for policy makers commonly uses a wide range of methods and techniques. Indeed, Gorard (2010) argues that having a variety of tools in the toolbox, and using them as appropriate, is the only sensible way to approach research. Many projects now use a range of methods, and each serves a particular purpose. In most research, the problem to be addressed will determine the research design, the research methodology and method. However, health researchers should continue to be aware of the differences between the types of knowledge produced in order to think critically about the kind of the evidence on which they base their findings and how they will integrate or not their findings in a research report.

Mixed methods is a methodological approach for conducting research that, from the start, collects data that are both qualitative and quantitative data in the same study with a particular purpose in mind. The aim is to provide a better understanding of a problem (Cresswell and Plano Clark 2017). Bryman (2016) found that researchers used mixed methods for various reasons:

- To give greater validity to a research project by seeking corroborative findings
- To offset the weaknesses of a single methodology
- To develop research instruments
- To deal with unexpected findings.

Researchers may use a mix of methods in different ways: as a qualitative element in a predominantly quantitative study; as a quantitative element in a predominantly qualitative study; or in a manner in which both were equally weighted. Methods can be used in different sequences. Where little is known about an area, focus groups, observations of action or unstructured interviews can be used provide information for designing a questionnaire, or act as a guide to sampling from a larger population. This helps to refine concepts, identify relevant theories and gain more information on the language, values and perspective of the research participants or to assess the range of views.

Alternatively, if an area has been well researched, and theories are well established, a study may begin with a questionnaire sent to the target population to collect basic descriptive data followed by a qualitative study. Baggott, Allsop and Jones (2004) used this mix of methods to collect quantitative information from groups representing the interests of patients, users and carers on membership, finances and political involvement and then, on the basis on information gathered, conducted qualitative interviews with stakeholders to assess motivations and strategies and policy networks for influencing the policy process. The case study provided towards the end of the chapter adopted a qualitative approach when the attempt to conduct a conventional survey was not feasible (Slowther et al. 2012).

There are perhaps two drivers for encouraging the use of a variety of methods in research. First, funding for research to support evidence-based clinical interventions and to address policy problems has increased – large research projects with a number of researchers have become more common. This encourages projects with more complex methodological strategies. Second, it has become more common to consider research participants as part of research production. This can encourage qualitative studies to investigate how issues are perceived by potential participants as a prelude to a subsequent quantitative study. For example, RCTs to evaluate the efficacy of cancer treatments have allowed patients to choose which arm of a trial they wish to enter in a situation where it is not known which of two treatments is likely to be the more effective. This allowed a consideration of who chose what option as well as a formal assessment of the outcome of a trial.

Another initiative is the James Lind Alliance, where patients, carers and clinicians establish research priorities jointly. This is an example of positivist researchers engaging with those who benefit from research findings to help them determine priorities. One study showed that when patients with osteoarthritis of the knee or hip were asked to prioritize, they rated trials on the outcomes of surgery and physiotherapy more highly than drug trials (Coulter 2011). The 'Chariot' research study is a long-term project to increase understanding of dementia and possible ways of treating the condition. It has developed a register of 26,000 cognitively healthy adults aged between 60 and 85 who are willing to take part in a series of trials. In this sense, studies are co-produced (dementia.prevention@imperial. ac.uk). A long-term relationship between researchers and participants can also be useful for qualitative studies. For example, a research team at De Montfort University Centre for Reproduction Research developed an ongoing programme for research on women's health. Research topics are based on priorities following discussion with members of the research group from the local Asian community. Over time, sufficient trust has been generated to investigate a range of sensitive issues (see, for example, Hudson and Culley 2015).

Doctors crossing frontiers to practise: The experiences of non-UK qualified doctors

The following is an analysis of the key tasks for researchers, based on the study by Slowther and colleagues (2012) of the experiences of non-qualified doctors working in the United Kingdom. The research was funded by the Economic and Social Research Council Public Service Programme and supported by the General Medical Council (GMC). The focus of the study is on the research process.

Context and research questions: International mobility is a feature of health care systems. In 2009 over a third of new registrations in the United Kingdom were for overseas doctors. Prior to registration, qualifications are checked as being equivalent

(Continued)

CASE STUDY 3.1

(Continued)

and language skills are tested. A literature search found evidence of social and cultural factors hindering integration and a higher incidence of complaints. There was a gap in knowledge. Which countries did doctors come from? How were doctors prepared for practice in a different culture? Were GMC guidelines for practice received and understood? What problems did doctors say they faced?

First phase: Quantitative data collection and analysis: The researchers' first task was to identify and access data. GMC data on new registrations over a period of two years was accessed and analysed to identify the main countries of origin of overseas doctors registering by year. It was decided to construct a questionnaire. Two focus groups helped to refine the research questions. One with stakeholders and a convenience sample of applicants registering at the GMC.

Questionnaire design: The focus was on doctors' receipt of GMC guidance, their understanding and perception of this, and their response to the guidelines on ethics in particular. Postal or electronic questionnaires with follow-up telephone interviews were undertaken with those who agreed to participate.

Questionnaire results: The response rate was 9 per cent. Another sample was drawn and finally 90 respondents were recruited.

Findings of this phase: The ethical dilemmas that were referred to most frequently concerned end-of-life decision-making, confidentiality when dealing with family members and relationships with colleagues.

Second phase: Qualitative data collection and analysis: A cross-sectional sample of the target population was selected for interview. Telephone or face-to-face interviews were undertaken with 26 doctors from 14 countries. NVivo was used for data analysis.

How to code and present?: Themes, grounded in the data, were agreed and coded by two researchers. These were collapsed under three headings: problems related to working in an unfamiliar world (legal and ethical differences); difficulties in communication; and participant views' on the support available.

Writing up: The themes were illustrated using quotations, the findings were discussed and the limitations of the study were stated. Recommendations were made for policy makers.

Reflection: The case study illustrates some aspects of doing mixed methods research. The researcher enters a new environment. They must negotiate entry, access and become familiar with administrative structures and, in this case, negotiate research objectives. Initial data analysis was required and the method for data collection agreed. The response to the first phase interviews was very poor, but was rescued through additional samples. Flexibility was needed to adjust to unforeseen problems. Qualitative telephone interviews added richer data, which were essential to understanding areas of uncertainty. The numbers were small but the findings were indicative of areas where further support was needed. The impact of the research will depend on dissemination.

Conclusion

In this chapter the positivist and interpretivist research strategies and their application in clinical and social science research have been considered. One strategy is not necessarily better than another. A mix of methods can provide a greater depth of understanding. The polarization between the two positions has been modified, although it is still the case that research funding is more likely to be awarded to researchers using quantitative methods. There also remain different styles of presentation. As suggested above, there is now a more eclectic approach to deciding on methodology and methods, although this does not constitute a new paradigm. At either end of the spectrum there are those that, from preference or belief, specialize in positivist or interpretivist methodologies. For most novice or jobbing researchers, it is necessary to have an understanding of the kind of knowledge that different methods produce and what constitutes good-quality research. Researchers on either side of the quantitative/qualitative divide are both concerned with the quality and rigour of their research. Ultimately, the appropriateness and usefulness of a particular paradigm is tied to the nature of the research question asked and the skills and inclinations of the researcher.

Exercise 3.1 Quantitative and qualitative data sources

Based on what you have read in this chapter, what different sorts of information are yielded by the data sources from the selected questions shown below? What does each form of knowledge contribute?

Different methodological approaches to researching the use of the internet in the case of men with prostate cancer (Broom 2005a, 2005b):

• An example of quantitative data collection from a structured questionnaire survey as set out in Table 3.2 below:

TABLE 3.2 Structured questionnaire survey

1	It would be easier to share my personal experiences in an anonymous environment such as an online (internet) support group.	1	2	3	4	5
2	In face-to-face support groups, the threat of embarrassment stops some men from sharing concerns about fears, emotional distress, symptoms or complications of treatments.	1	2	3	4	5

Where 1 = strongly disagree; 2 = disagree; 3 = neutral; 4 = agree; 5 = strongly agree.

(Continued)

(Continued)

Of the 50 men surveyed, 46 per cent agreed that it would be easier to share their experiences online. Approximately 30 per cent of respondents agreed that face-to-face support groups can deter self-expression.

- An example of qualitative data from in-depth interviews

The reasons patients gave for their decision of whether or not to use online support groups were as follows:

Andrew: 'One of the things you find is an amazing openness and frankness about these sorts of matters that I'm sure men if they were meeting face-to-face would not talk about. ... we're doing it through this medium [the internet] and we can be a lot more frank. ... There's the anonymity, there's the disembodiment ... you're able to project in a way that isn't having any comeback on you.' (Six months' post-treatment, organ-confined disease, internet user/online support, 40–50 years)

David: 'Some men don't want to be face-to-face. Maybe they're frightened of it; maybe they don't want to travel the distances. Maybe they're scared of being ridiculed or something ... all sorts of reasons like that. Maybe they're a bit anxious about having the problem [prostate cancer] and not wanting to share it with other people. I think that's men for you. Some will find it easier to talk online.' (Three years' post-treatment, organ-confined disease, internet user/online support, 61–70 years)

Recommended further reading

This book charts the way to do clinical and social research in the health field:
Greenhalgh, T. (2014) *How to Read a Paper: The Basics of Evidence-based Medicine*, 5th edition. Chichester: Wiley-Blackwell.

This is highly recommended as a comprehensive and up-to-date text on quantitative and qualitative methods written with research students in mind. It is well referenced so that readers can easily find answers to their questions:
Bryman, A. (2016) *Social Research Methods*, 5th edition. Oxford: Oxford University Press.

This is a useful book for researchers wishing to analyse and interpret quantitative and qualitative data:
Cresswell, J. and Plano Clark, V. L. (2017) *Designing and Conducting Mixed Methods Research*, 3rd edition. London: Sage.

References

Altman, D. (2000) 'Blinding in clinical trials and other studies', *British Medical Journal*, *321*: 504.

Baggott, R., Allsop, J. and Jones, K. (2004) *Speaking for Patients and Carers: Health Consumer Groups and the National Policy Process*. Basingstoke: Palgrave Macmillan.

Becker, S., Bryman, A. and Ferguson, H. (eds) (2012) *Understanding Research: Methods and Approaches for Social Work and Social Policy*. Bristol: Policy Press.

Bloor, M. (1978) 'On the analysis of observational data: A discussion of the worth and uses of inductive techniques and respondent validation', *Sociology*, *12*(3): 545–57.

Blumer, M. (1984) *The Chicago School of Sociology, Institutionalization, Diversity and the Rise of Sociological Research*. Chicago, IL: University of Chicago Press.

Bowling, A. (2014) *Research Methods in Health*, 4th edition. Maidenhead: Open University Press.

Broom, A. (2005a) 'The eMale: prostate cancer, masculinity and online support as a challenge to medical expertise', *Journal of Sociology*, *41*(1): 87–104.

Broom, A. (2005b) 'Virtually he@lthy: A study into the impact of Internet use on disease experience and the doctor/patient relationship', *Qualitative Health Research*, *15*(3): 325–45.

Brown, B., Crawford, P. and Hicks, C. (2003) *Evidence-based Research: Dilemmas and Debates in Health Care*. Maidenhead: Open University Press.

Bryman, A. (2016) *Social Research Methods*, 5th edition. Oxford: Oxford University Press.

Cochrane, A. (1972) *Effectiveness and Efficiency: Random Reflections on Health Services*. London: Nuffield Provincial Hospitals Trust.

Coulter, A. (2011) *Engaging Patients in Healthcare*. Buckingham: Open University Press.

Cresswell, J. W. and Plano Clark, V. L. (2017) *Designing and Conducting Mixed Methods Research*, 3rd edition. London: Sage.

De Vaus, D. (2009) *Research Design in Social Research*, 2nd edition. London: Sage.

De Vaus, D. (2014) *Surveys in Social Research*, 6th edition. London: Routledge.

Durkheim, E. (1979) *Suicide: A Study in Sociology*. New York: Macmillan.

Ezzy, D. (2002) *Qualitative Analysis: Practice and Innovation*. Crows Nest, NSW, Australia: Allen & Unwin.

Geertz, C. (1973) *The Interpretation of Cultures: Selected Essays*. New York: Basic Books.

Giddens, A. (1987) *Positivism and Sociology*. London: Heinemann.

Glaser, B. and Strauss, A. (1967) *The Discovery of Grounded Theory: Strategies for Qualitative Research*. London: Aldine.

Glassner, B. and Moreno, J. (1989) 'Introduction: Quantification and enlightenment', in B. Glassner and J. Moreno (eds), *The Qualitative–Quantitative Distinction in the Social Sciences*. Boston, MA: Kluwer Academic.

Gorard, S. (2010) 'Research design as independent of methods', in A. Tashakkori and C. Teddle (eds), *Handbook of Mixed Methods in Social and Behavioural Research*. London: Sage.

Greenhalgh, T. (2014) *How to Read a Paper: The Basics of Evidence-based Medicine*, 5th edition. Chichester: Wiley-Blackwell.

Hammersley, M. (1992) 'The paradigm wars: Reports from the front', *British Journal of the Sociology of Education*, *13*: 131–43.

Hudson, N. and Culley, L. (2015) 'Cross border reproductive travel', in L. Lundt, J. Hanefeld and D. Horsfall (eds) *Handbook of Medical Tourism and Patient Mobility*. Cheltenham: Edward Elgar.

Kuhn, T. (1970) *The Structure of Scientific Revolutions*. Chicago, IL: University of Chicago Press.

Ledade, S., Shashir, J. and Gupta, V. (2017) 'Narrative writing: Effective ways and best practices', *Perspectives on Clinical Research*, *8*(2): 58–62.

Lofland, J. (2006) *Analyzing Social Settings: A Guide to Qualitative Observation and Analysis*, 4th edition. Belmont, CA: Wadsworth/Learning.

Medical Research Council (2017) *Global Health Trials Involving Clinical and Public Health Interventions*. London: MRC.

Oakley, A. (2000) *Some Experiments in Knowing: Gender and Method in the Social Sciences*. Cambridge: Polity Press.

Pope, C. and Mays, N. (eds) (2006) *Qualitative Methods in Health Research*, 3rd edition. Oxford: Blackwell BMJ.

Popper, K. (1959) *The Logic of Scientific Discovery*. London: Hutchinson.

Porter, R. (1997) *The Greatest Benefit to Mankind: A History of Medicine*. London: HarperCollins.

Rubin, H. and Rubin, I. (2012) *Qualitative Interviewing: The Art of Hearing Data*, 2nd edition. London: Sage.

Schutz, A. (1962) *Collected Papers I: The Problem of Social Reality*. The Hague: Martinus Nijhof.

Seale, C. (ed.) (2018) *Researching Society and Culture*, 4th edition. London: Sage.

Silverman, D. (2011) *Interpreting Qualitative Data: Methods for Analyzing Talk, Text and Interaction*, 4th edition. London: Sage.

Silverman, D. (2016) *Qualitative Research*, 4th edition. London: Sage.

Slowther, A., Lewando Hunt, G., Purkis, J. and Taylor, R. (2012) 'Experiences of non-UK-qualified doctors working in the UK regulatory framework: A qualitative study', *Journal of the Royal Society of Medicine*, *105*: 157–85.

Strauss, A. and Corbin, J. (1998) *Basics of Qualitative Research*, 2nd edition. London: Sage.

Weber, M. (1947) *The Theory of Social and Economic Organisation*. New York: Free Press.

Doing a Literature Review in Health

KATHRYN JONES

Chapter objectives

- To outline the difference between narrative and systematic literature reviews
- To explain the importance of adopting a systematic approach to undertaking literature reviews
- To discuss the process for planning and undertaking a literature search
- To outline the process of logging and analysing literature sources
- To discuss how to structure and write literature reviews.

Introduction

The literature review aims to identify, analyse, assess and interpret a body of knowledge related to a particular topic and is normally required as part of a dissertation or thesis. In this case, it sets a context for a research study and provides a rationale for addressing a particular research question in the light of an existing body of literature. Research proposals to funding bodies also typically include a literature review. Here the purpose is to justify the proposal in terms of a gap in existing knowledge. Some literature reviews are substantive, stand-alone studies in their own right that serve to assess what is known and what is not known about an area of study. The aim is to show how a particular topic has been approached by other scholars. Within the health field, the literature review can also aim to assess existing knowledge on the efficacy of an intervention, such as the evidence base for the preferred treatment of a particular disease, or be a response to a social problem.

This chapter describes how to undertake a rigorous and thorough review of the literature and is divided into three sections. The first section examines the two main types of review: the narrative and the systematic review. The second describes some techniques for undertaking a comprehensive search, while the third gives guidance on how an analysis of the literature can be presented. The majority of sources can now be accessed electronically. In the chapter, it is assumed that those undertaking a review will have access to internet-based college or university library resources. Those who have not previously searched using an online catalogue or database are advised to seek assistance prior to starting out. Most college and university libraries offer courses, publish guidelines or make help available online. Throughout the chapter, examples are drawn from recent studies undertaken by the author and others.

Types of literature review

All reviews aim to provide an overview of what is known about a particular phenomenon and what the gaps in knowledge are. However, narrative reviews, which are used widely in social scientific research, place an emphasis on identifying the key concepts or specific terms used in the literature and the particular theoretical approaches adopted by different authors to analyse or explain a phenomenon. Concepts and theories may be employed implicitly or explicitly in an investigation of a topic. A review of the literature will identify the range of approaches and offer a critique of their contribution to understanding.

The systematic review of the literature in health and social care has a different focus. It aims to contribute to practice through an assessment of the efficacy of particular health care interventions and underpins much evidence-based practice. Initially developed as a means for synthesizing quantitative research, specific methods have since been used to review qualitative evidence (Greenhalgh 2014), and for synthesizing both qualitative and quantitative evidence within the same review (Mays, Pope and Popay 2005). A basic overview is given here, but – given the scale of the task – systematic reviews are beyond the scope of the majority of postgraduate and undergraduate dissertations (although see Boland, Cherry and Dickson 2017 for a guide for postgraduate students). This said, adopting a systematic process to logging the literature search and results is a useful approach for students undertaking narrative reviews, and Boland, Cherry and Dickson (2017) provide a more advanced guide to the systematic review.

The narrative review

The narrative review is the commonest form of literature review. It aims to show how concepts, theories and methods have developed within particular subject areas. The key differences between concepts, theories and methods are:

- *Concepts*: Terms and ideas used to describe a particular phenomenon.
- *Theories*: Ideas that have been developed to explain a specific phenomenon.
- *Empirical research*: Research that has already been undertaken to observe the phenomenon.
- *Methodology*: The philosophical approach adopted by a researcher to study a particular phenomenon and not to be confused with methods.
- *Methods*: Techniques such as questionnaires, observation or interviewing used to collect data.

In a narrative review the reviewer offers a critique in order to assess, analyse and synthesize previous research, and reframe it to fit its context. The review can take a number of forms: a chapter within a dissertation showing the context of the research; a section of a proposal justifying the work; or a stand-alone summation of thinking around a particular subject area. In each, the reviewer draws on and critiques the conceptual and theoretical approach of different authors and offers an assessment and interpretation. The narrative review should be linked to and help inform your research questions (Aveyard 2010). In essence, you are setting out an argument for the importance of your research and laying the foundation for the analysis and interpretation of your research findings.

When reading the literature, the reviewer seeks to identify the particular conceptual and theoretical approach taken by the author. This is likely to be influenced by the author's background and discipline. So, for example, a political scientist interested in public involvement in health policy making is likely to draw on theories relating to interest groups in the policy process, participation and representation. A sociologist of health and illness writing on the same topic might place their work in the context of people's experience of illness and how this may affect their ability and desire to participate in decisions and policy making. Identifying the conceptual and theoretical approaches taken by different authors is the first step to understanding the literature and, in the writing-up stage, will influence the structure of the report, which is another vital component of the narrative review, as will be seen below.

The systematic review

Over the past few decades, evidence-based practice has achieved growing recognition as a means of increasing the efficacy of health care interventions. Initiatives such as the international Cochrane Collaboration (see Chapter 21 for a fuller description) and organizations such as the National Institute for Health and Care Excellence (NICE) in England assess available evidence to inform guidelines, policy and practice. A systematic review enables the reader to appraise critically the most robust evidence available in an attempt to synthesize what is known, and not known, about the efficacy of particular interventions. According to Petticrew (2001), systematic reviews can be characterized by the following criteria:

- They aim to answer a particular question or test a hypothesis – usually in relation to a particular health care intervention on a particular population group.

- They attempt to be as exhaustive as possible, identifying all known references.
- Studies included in the review are chosen as a result of explicit inclusion and exclusion criteria.

Systematic reviews place an emphasis on judging the quality of evidence. Here, the priority is to utilize studies where the research design minimizes bias, as highlighted by the list below (Street 2001) showing the traditional hierarchy of evidence for reviews assessing the effectiveness of a particular intervention:

- *Level I*: Evidence obtained from a systematic review of all relevant randomized controlled trials.
- *Level II*: Evidence obtained from at least one properly designed randomly controlled trial.
- *Level III.1*: Evidence obtained from a well-designed controlled trial without randomization.
- *Level III.2*: Evidence obtained from a well-designed cohort or case-control analytic study, preferably from more than one centre or research group.
- *Level III.3*: Evidence obtained from multiple time series with or without the intervention, or dramatic results in an uncontrolled experiment.
- *Level IV*: Opinion of respected authorities based on clinical experience, descriptive studies or a report from an expert committee.

Clearly this hierarchy is biased towards quantitative research, but across health care and the social sciences there is a strong history of qualitative research which explores the experience and perspectives of people living with a particular medical condition or welfare intervention. If a review is attempting to understand *why* a particular intervention works, rather than *what* interventions work, then qualitative studies are likely to be of value (Dixon-Woods, Fitzpatrick and Roberts 2001). For example, Robertshaw, Dhesi and Jones (2017) used a thematic qualitative synthesis to identify the challenges and facilitators for health professionals delivering primary health care to refugee and asylum seekers in high-income countries. They argued that reviewing qualitative studies enabled them to focus on understanding health professionals' perceptions and experiences.

Both qualitative and quantitative syntheses establish an audit trail of search parameters and explicit criteria for selecting articles according to the rigour of the methodological approach employed. It should also be noted that the recognition that reviews which bring together data from both qualitative and quantitative studies, or from mixed-methods research, can strengthen the breadth and depth of evidence that policy makers base their decisions on, has meant that techniques to synthesize this evidence have also been developed (Greenhalgh 2014; Pluye and Hong 2014).

In addition, meta-analysis, the use of statistical techniques to reanalyse and reinterpret the data found in studies, has also evolved beyond a focus on quantitative data to convert and incorporate qualitative evidence (Mays, Pope and Popay 2005). The use of statistical techniques can account for differences in methods and enables the researcher to pull together the findings of numerous studies to offer a more substantive assessment of the available evidence. This is particularly useful when studies are based on a small sample. However, meta-analysis is a highly sophisticated tool and should only be undertaken by researchers with statistical skills. The Centre for Reviews and Dissemination at York (www.york.ac.uk/inst/crd) provides useful guidelines explaining the various statistical techniques that can be utilized.

The key source for identifying systematic reviews is via the Cochrane Collaboration, an international network of those working on systematic reviews (www.cochrane.co.uk). Its website includes a searchable database. The TRIP (Turning Research into Practice) Database of evidence-based articles covering medical science may also be searched (www.tripdatabase.com), alongside the Bandolier website (www.bandolier.org.uk/). In addition, it may be useful to search the EPPI-Centre database (Evidence for Policy and Practice Information) for systematic reviews in the social sciences and public policy (https://eppi.ioe.ac.uk/cms/).

Carrying out a literature search

Taking a systematic approach to planning, logging and recording the results is as valid for a narrative review as it is a systematic review (Booth, Sutton and Papaioannou 2016). This section outlines good practice in how to undertake a literature search: setting search parameters; identifying appropriate databases; writing the search strategy; and recording the results (Gash 2000). In a sense, literature searching is like detective work as the aim is to identify the most appropriate sources to answer a question within a field of study. The key sources used by information specialists are listed below:

- *Bibliographies*: A bibliography is a list of publications relating to a particular subject area.

    o *General bibliographies*: The *British National Bibliography*, published online by the British Library, provides a searchable list of all new books published in the United Kingdom (http://bnb.bl.uk).
    o *Specialist subject bibliographies*: Produced by research centres, scholars or specialist information services such as the US National Library of Medicine or the King's Fund library.
    o *Publications*: Journal articles note the works the author has quoted in a list of references at the end. Research monographs and textbooks will also provide a list of sources but will often include all items read by the author rather than just those quoted in the text.
- *Catalogues*: Most academic libraries and specialist institutions maintain a catalogue that shows the details and location of all items available electronically whether held in

the library or full-text availability of journal articles or e-books. This is the most obvious place to start any search. COPAC (http://copac.jisc.ac.uk/) is the merged catalogue of a number of university libraries and the British Library and national libraries of Scotland and Wales. Most academic libraries have reciprocal access arrangements for students via the SCONUL scheme (www.sconul.ac.uk).

- *Abstracting and indexing journals*: An abstract is a short summary of an academic journal article. This is an aid to assessing relevance without reading the full article:

  o *Abstracting journals* provide details of articles drawn from a range of journals within a particular subject area. They tend to be arranged alphabetically by author, with a subject index to locate relevant papers.

  o *Indexing journals* are usually arranged in subject order and provide basic bibliographic details of articles (title, author, journal, date, volume and page number).

Most abstracting and indexing journals are now available electronically on specialist databases.

The internet and electronic sources have made the search process quicker and broadened the range of sources that can be accessed. This can be a problem as an overwhelming number of potentially useful articles may be retrieved. It is imperative, therefore, to plan a search effectively, and to review the strategy as the search progresses.

Library catalogues typically allow searches based on author, title, subject classification and keyword. Subject codes are assigned to books and other publications using classification schemes such as the Dewey Decimal System. The majority of classifications systems are based on numeric codes. For example, in the Dewey System, books on the medical sciences are located at 610. Looking up subject classification enables you to identify books on the same/similar subject and expand your search. The classification of articles in electronic databases is more sophisticated and has a higher degree of specificity than items in library catalogues. In other words, database searching can be more precise and retrieve more items of relevance as they are coded in more depth. A number of subject headings are assigned to summarize the coverage of each article. For example, the US National Library of Medicine uses MeSH (Medical Subject Headings) in the Medline database. In addition, databases assign keywords to each item drawn from the abstract or provided by the author, and many databases make abstracts searchable. A keyword or abstract search can be a useful way to narrow down the focus of a search.

The reviewer may use various sources to identify the best database to search. Most academic libraries produce guides to the subject areas they cover which list the databases they subscribe to. It is usually possible to check where journals are abstracted and indexed on publishers' websites, although no one database will cover all journals within a subject area. Databases are generally free at the point of use for students. If a library does not subscribe to a particular database, it may be possible to gain access on a pay-as-you-go basis. Table 4.1 summarizes some of the main subject databases covering health care. In addition, there are numerous specialist databases, such as AgeInfo or PsyclNFO, which focus on particular sub-specialities in the health care field.

TABLE 4.1 Key databases in health care

Database	Scope	Content	Years
General:			
Applied Social Sciences Index and Abstracts	Health, social services, psychology, sociology, economics, politics, race relations and education. International in scope	Indexes and abstracts 500+ journals	1987–
International Bibliography of Social Sciences	Anthropology, economics, health, politics and sociology. International in scope	Bibliographic references to journal articles. Abstracts and some full-text access are provided. Includes research notes, responses and short essays, book reviews and book chapters	1951–
ScienceDirect	Science, technology and medicine full text. International in scope	Bibliographic details and abstracts from around 2,500 journals. Currently retrospectively digitizing pre-1995 journals including *The Lancet*	1995–
Health:			
Cumulative Index to Nursing and Allied Health Literature	Nursing, allied health, biomedicine, alternative/complementary medicine, consumer health and health sciences librarianship. International in scope	Bibliographic references to nearly 3,000 journals. Abstracts are also provided for about 1,000 journals. Includes a citation index from 1994. Some access to full text	1982–
Health Management Information Consortium	Clinical medicine, health policy, occupational and environmental health, health systems and services, public health, health administration and management. International in scope	Bibliographic references and abstracts from three institutions: the UK Departments of Health and Nuffield Institute for Health (Leeds University Library) and King's Fund Library	1983–
Medline	Biomedicine and health. International in scope	Bibliographic references and abstracts. Some links to full text	1950s–

How to set the search profile

While it might be tempting to start immediately entering search terms into library catalogues, internet sites and databases, an effective literature search requires careful planning.
The reviewer should begin by setting down on paper a brief title for the review; a summary
of the areas of interest, including the type of evidence and publications required; and any
parameters for the search, such as the date or language of publication. A search profile serves
two key purposes. First, it requires the researcher to clarify the scope and parameters of the
study and, second, it acts as an *aide-mémoire* throughout the search process. In this way, the
searcher is encouraged to remain focused and avoid being sidetracked down interesting but
irrelevant byways. Narrative reviews offer more temptations to the unwary researcher.

Systematic reviews usually set explicit inclusion and exclusion criteria. The search profile
in Box 4.1 for a study funded by the Office of the Deputy Prime Minister in the United
Kingdom on the effects of overcrowding on health and education (Brown et al. 2004) was
adapted from guidelines provided by Gash (2000). The profile was also used as a structure
for describing the literature search process in the final report of this project.

Box 4.1   Search profile for the effects of overcrowded housing on health and education

Scope

Health impacts: for example, mental health and infectious disease.

Educational consequences: for example, attainment and child development.

Empirical and conceptual studies: the academic literature, excluding publications
that merely report on levels of overcrowding in particular areas.

Adopt a snowball technique: read reference lists in articles and books for follow-up.
Citation search of key articles to identify other potential sources of data.

Date

1970s onwards.

Language

English.

Type

Academic literature – excluding newspaper articles and policy reports.

Sources

Academic and policy databases, websites of key research organizations, charities and government departments.

Country

OECD countries.

Keywords

'academic achievement', 'child development', 'crowding', 'deprivation', 'educational attainment', 'health', 'houses in multiple occupation', 'mental health', 'overcrowding', and 'physical health'.

Known references

Thomson, H. et al. (2001) 'Health effects of housing improvement', *British Medical Journal*, 323: 187–90.
Marsh, A. et al. (1999) *Home Sweet Home*. Bristol: Policy Press.

Source: Adapted from Gash (2000)

Writing the search strategy

While the search profile provides an overview of the scope and parameters of the search, it is the search strategy that is actually used to retrieve journal articles and books from databases. The strategy requires the identification of the terms that best describe the area of interest. These can be found in the definitions provided in subject-specific dictionaries and encyclopaedias, or from keywords cited in known articles. This list should include synonyms, abbreviations and related terms. As most databases have an international scope, researchers should allow for possible variations in language. For example, while United Kingdom authors use the word 'overcrowding' in relation to overcrowded housing, North American authors tend to use 'crowding' to describe the same phenomenon. Browsing the subject index of the database can ensure that the most appropriate words are searched for. It may also be worth checking how a key reference has been indexed in the database to see what subject terms and keywords were used to catalogue the article.

Once a list of search terms is identified, a search strategy must be written by deciding how these terms should be entered into the computer. It is rare that a search can be completed by inputting one or two words. Often the search strategy is built using Boolean operators – 'and', 'or', 'not' – which can be used to combine search terms to retrieve the most relevant articles. These three simple words can be used to broaden or narrow the search. For example, using the 'or' operator ensures that synonyms for the chosen term can be searched; the 'and' operator provides a narrower focus; and the 'not' operator ensures that records with this term are not retrieved. Prior to entering the strategy in the database, it is important to check how the Boolean operators should be entered. Some databases use symbols rather than words. Table 4.2 provides working examples of how Boolean operators were used in the overcrowding and health review. Most electronic databases provide interfaces which support Boolean searching, often under the 'advanced search' option.

TABLE 4.2   The use of 'and', 'or', 'not' in a search strategy

Search		Outcomes	Uses
Using the AND operator:			
#1		Overcrowding	
#2		Asthma	
#3	#1 and #2	Records that contain both 'overcrowding' and 'asthma'	Narrowing the focus of the search by including particular terms
Using the OR operator:			
#1		Overcrowding	
#2		Crowding	
#3	#1 or #2	Records that contain either 'overcrowding' or 'crowding' or both terms	Ensuring synonyms are included in search strategy
Using the NOT operator:			
#1		Overcrowding	
#2		Trains	
#3	#1 not #2	Records that contain 'overcrowding', but not 'overcrowding' in 'trains'	Narrowing focus of search by excluding particular variables

Refining the literature search

Always be prepared to rethink the search strategy in light of the results. The search may retrieve too many results. A useful technique is to download or print out the complete references (or a sample of them) – together with the abstract and subject classifications – and use these to identify the relevant articles. Check to see how these have been catalogued and refine the search strategy. If this does nothing to reduce the numbers, then limits such as date, language or place of publication should be applied. Most, if not all, databases offer on-screen help or prompts for this. More recent articles are likely to give a summary of previous research, and from these it should be possible to judge how far back the search needs to be taken. With luck, the search may identify an earlier review article that can be updated. If there are still too many references, then the focus of study will need rethinking in order to narrow the search further.

Conversely, searches may end with no results, or very few. This can be because little has been written on the subject, or it may be due to inconsistencies in cataloguing and indexing on different databases. Each database will have its own house style, so differences may occur in subject and keyword classification or in the logging of bibliographic details such as the author name. For example, in any database the name of the author of this chapter could be indexed as *Jones, K.; Jones, K.L.; Jones, Kathryn* or *Jones, Kathryn L.* So an author search for *Jones, K.L.* in one database may come back as having no hits, because papers are listed in the author index under *Jones, K.* Most databases offer the possibility of browsing the author index or to search for the surname alone. In the case of a common name such as Jones, this should be combined with a subject term to narrow the search focus.

Keyword searching may not retrieve results because different authors have assigned different words for the same phenomena. For example, some academics may use 'patient group', 'self-help group' or 'health consumer group' to describe similar types of organization. Or cataloguers could use the same word to describe different phenomena. For example, 'complaint' may mean an illness or an allegation that something has gone wrong. In addition, different cataloguers may code the same article under different subject headings. Most databases give the option of truncating search terms, by using a particular symbol (usually * or $) to retrieve more references. For instance, a search on 'consum$' would retrieve articles on consumers, consumerism and consumption. It is essential to browse both subject and keyword indexes in databases. Recognizing that inconsistencies can occur ensures a healthy scepticism of retrieved results. A quick way of testing the results is to look at the reference list of a relevant journal article to see if at least some of the same articles are cited.

Another technique is to search for who has quoted an important journal article as this can help to snowball the search to ensure a comprehensive coverage. The *Science* or *Social Science Citation Index* allows the researcher to identify articles and, increasingly, also books and book chapters that have cited a particular reference. This provides access to further work on the subject and gives an indication of how others view this work. In addition, many databases now include a 'cited by' function to find out who cited the article or a 'reference' function which lists the references cited in the particular article.

The literature within a particular subject area is never static, so it is essential to build in a mechanism for keeping a search up to date. Some databases will save searches that can be rerun later. Many libraries and institutions produce a current awareness service of publications. For example, the King's Fund Information and Library Service (www.kingsfund.org.uk) specializes in health policy and economics and produces reading lists and e-bulletins. The latest journal content pages are produced by zetoc Alert email service (www.zetoc.mimas.ac.uk).

Searching for grey literature

Grey literature refers to literature published independently by, for example, specialist research units rather than mainstream publishers. The *Aslib Directory of Information Sources in the UK* is a useful starting point for identifying specialist collections. Grey literature may be difficult to obtain, but can be extremely valuable as it can include cutting-edge research. Some research bodies, such as the King's Fund or the Institute of Health Services Management Research in the United Kingdom, have websites that list, and increasingly provide, their publications online. It is also worth looking at the websites of research funding bodies such as the Economic and Social Research Council (www.esrc.ac.uk), the Medical Research Council (www.mrc.ac.uk) or the Department of Health (www.dh.gov.uk). Some research reports are available electronically. In addition, they may provide an option to sign up to newsletters which provide links to reports as they are produced. There are also various specialist indexes that cover particular types of publication, such as conference papers, dissertations and official documents. These may provide access to information that has not been formally published. In the overcrowding study, grey literature was identified through hand searching specialist journals, specialist indexes and the websites of key research units and housing charities.

Although it is tempting to rely on internet search engines to locate information in relation to grey literature and other material, it is important to remember that this does not substitute for properly constructed search strategies using specialist databases. First, a search engine will not search with the same degree of rigour as an online database. Second, some literature found on the internet can look official, but it may be inaccurate and unverified by external experts.

Recording the search

The type and extent of information provided on the results of the database search will vary. Most databases provide options for how results can be viewed online. At a minimum, the bibliographic details (such as author, date, title, journal, volume/issue number and page number(s)) will be provided for each item. The majority will also provide access to the abstract, and as long as the database is accessed via the university or college library, many will also provide links to full-text articles where available. It is worth downloading or saving the bibliographic and abstract details of the search into an email account or some form of specialist software such as EndNote, RefWorks or Mendeley, so they can be reviewed at a later stage. The database will generally offer prompts to achieve this. It is vital to keep track by noting the databases searched, the years covered, the number of retrieved articles and the search strategy used, to ensure that the search is undertaken as systematically as possible. This record will also be useful if the search strategy needs to be revised. In addition, it may be good practice to put this record as an appendix in your dissertation so your tutor can see how you searched the literature.

The bibliographic details and abstract of each item retrieved should provide a good indication of whether the full article is worth reading. If a journal article or book is not available locally, it can be obtained via interlibrary loans. For each item read, the reviewer should complete a data extraction form which is used to summarize key details from the item, as set out in Table 4.3. The type of information logged will depend on the purpose of the review, but keeping a record is essential. In the example given at the end of the chapter, the bibliographic details necessary for referencing are noted as well as information on definitions of keywords; the concepts that make up the conceptual framework; the findings or results of the study; the argument put forward; and the conclusions drawn. The form also provides space for personal comment, and a prompt for a rating of the quality and relevance of the paper.

TABLE 4.3 Data extraction form

Article no:		Review date:	
Title:			
Author(s):		Publication date:	
Publisher:		Place of publication:	
Journal:		Volume: number: page no:	
Keywords/definitions:			
Conceptual framework:			
Findings/argument:			
Author conclusions:			
Own notes:			
Rating: quality of research		Rating: relevance to study	
A	High quality	1	Extremely relevant
B	Medium quality	2	Quite relevant
C	Low quality	3	Marginally relevant

For the literature review on overcrowding, a more complex form was devised that recorded details about the type of study and the methods used. It also included stricter guidelines for judging the quality of the papers (see Brown et al. 2004). Completing a form for each item may seem cumbersome, but it is essential. A number of sources are likely to be identified and it will be impossible to remember everything that has been read. In addition, most reference managing software now enables you to log this information electronically and support searches and sorting by these criteria. Some software, such as Mendeley, allow you to store and add 'e-notes' on pdf versions of articles. Recent improvements in the user-friendliness of reference managing software means it is worth spending the time to learn how to use them, especially if you are writing a dissertation at Master's or PhD level. Figure 4.1 below shows a screen print from a Mendeley library created by the author as part of a recent scoping literature review for the Arts and Humanities Research Council on argument and persuasion in policy documents on community in health, housing and local government (Hamalainen and Jones 2011).

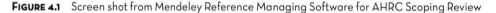

FIGURE 4.1   Screen shot from Mendeley Reference Managing Software for AHRC Scoping Review

Source: Hamalainen and Jones (2011)

Assessing relevance and quality in a literature review

A major part of the literature review will involve making a judgement on the relevance of what is being read. The significance of the findings to a project should be assessed as well as the effect of the research design on the outcome of the study. Once a number of studies have been read, it should be possible to make an accurate assessment of the importance of each item extracted.

Even within a narrative review an attempt must be made to judge the relative merits of the methods employed in each study. For example, a study rated as highly relevant may be based on only a small sample. A researcher may use this to make a case for a larger study. Alternatively, a search may identify issues that were explored using quantitative methods but there may be a benefit in further investigation using qualitative methods, and vice versa. The reviewer should comment on the reliability and validity of the methods used, and the extent to which they can be generalized to a larger population. It is also important to note whether findings support or contradict previous research.

A number of guides are available which describe approaches to evaluating different types of research in the clinical and social sciences. These have been developed for researchers wishing to undertake a systematic review. However, they raise questions pertinent for any review (see, for example, Greenhalgh 2014; NHS CRD 2009). The key questions for assessing the quality of studies in a literature review are summarized as follows:

- Conceptual framework:
  - o Are the aims clearly stated and research questions clearly identified?
  - o Does the author link the work to an existing body of knowledge?

- Study design:
  - o Are the methods appropriate and clearly described?
  - o Is the context of the study well set out? Did the research design account for possible bias?
  - o Are the limitations of research explicitly identified?

- Research analysis:
  - o Are the results clearly described, valid and reliable?
  - o Is the analysis clearly described?

- Conclusions:
  - o Are all possible influences on the observed outcomes considered?
  - o Are conclusions linked to the aims of study?
  - o Are conclusions linked to the analysis and interpretation of data?

Writing up the literature review

A literature review is not simply a regurgitation of who said what on a particular subject. A successful review is an interpretative piece of work that offers an assessment of the quality and scope of existing studies in a particular subject area. It brings together what is known in order to state what further research or analysis is required. In essence, a review acknowledges what has come before and how this can be built upon and expanded.

The review should define the key concepts to be used in the research and how these will be used within the reviewer's own work. It is good practice to draw attention to different definitions of key terms and why the researcher has decided to follow one definition rather than another. For example, the term 'consumer' is contested; different authors attach different meanings. In a study undertaken by the author and others of health consumer groups, attention was paid to explaining why this term was used rather than 'patients' group' or 'patients' association' or 'health user group' by discussing debates in the literature (Baggott, Allsop and Jones 2005).

In discussing the theoretical framework for a study, the researcher must justify why a certain theory has been adopted and spell out what research questions are raised by this approach. Some studies use a number of theories, a strategy termed by Sabatier (1999) as a 'multiple-lens' approach. For example, in the health consumer group study, the research team drew on a number of different theoretical perspectives that raised different questions to assess the influence and impact of health consumer groups on the policy process. These included theories about the configuration, and relative power, of various structural interests in health care; explanations of the power and influence of particular pressure groups; and theories about issue networks and policy communities within the policy process. Theories of representative and participative democracy were also reviewed in the context of questions about how health consumer groups represented their members, and how representatives were seen by health care stakeholders. These theories informed the questionnaire design, the semi-structured interviews with health consumer group leaders and contributed to developing a theoretical framework for subsequent analysis of the qualitative data.

A literature review should also report on previous empirical work undertaken, what methods have been adopted and relevant findings. In the study of health consumer groups, previous work on patient groups and patient and public involvement in policy making at local and national level provided the basis for identifying gaps in the research. In addition, factors that limited the validity or generalizability of previous research findings were noted.

Deciding a structure for the literature review

One challenge for the researcher is to select the most relevant articles for inclusion from a large quantity of material. The basis for inclusion in the narrative review is the relevance of the conceptual, theoretical and methodological approach taken by different authors to the study in question. A second challenge is to find a logical structure in writing the review. This will depend on its purpose. A review that seeks to assess the evidence base for a particular health care intervention will be structured differently from a review for a dissertation, thesis or project. Thus, for example, the overcrowding review took a themed approach. In the introduction, issues relating to definitions and methods were discussed. Subsequent chapters reported evidence on the impact of overcrowding on various aspects of health (such as the higher incidence of respiratory illness) and education (like the effect of overcrowding on educational attainment).

It would be unusual to follow a simple chronological arrangement in the literature review, by for instance starting a discussion with the earliest work on the subject and ending with the latest. A review is more likely to be arranged according to themes drawn from the literature or framed around certain research questions. Within a narrative review, the reviewer should take care to ensure that the structure follows the logic of their argument. In effect, the reviewer aims to establish that a gap in knowledge exists and suggests a way forward, through further research (see Hart 2018).

Effective planning is essential in order to identify the most logical structure. Before writing, an outline or plan of the review should be written. This will involve jotting down the key themes identified from the reading and making links between them to establish an appropriate order. It is helpful to identify headings and subheadings. These may not be used in the final review but can help to ensure a logical flow to the argument.

Style and referencing in a literature review

The writing style adopted in a review will depend on what is being reviewed. One benefit from reading widely around a subject area is to gain a feel for scholarly writing. Sentences commonly used to develop an argument are summarized below:

- *Where there is agreement and disagreement on particular issues*: 'While there is general agreement that this has occurred (references), there has been some debate about whether this is due to x (references) or y (references).'
- *On the criticisms levelled at particular studies*: 'Jones's work has been criticized because of a, b, c (references), but it is of relevance to this study because it suggests x, y, z.'
- *Offering suggestions of what can be surmised or understood from the literature*: 'In summary, it is possible to suggest that x is related to y; however, what is still not known is how z fits into this, which is the purpose of the study.'

A review will go through several drafts. Early drafts are likely to be more descriptive than analytical as the reviewer must first decide how the literature fits together before presenting a coherent argument. As the argument develops, the literature can be revisited. The extraction forms will be invaluable at this point to identify key findings. Articles that contradict findings or question theoretical or conceptual frameworks are also important. A good review offers a balanced perspective.

It is not necessary to cite or quote every reference retrieved, only those that are relevant to the question. The primary aim is to construct a clear narrative and to distinguish the author's argument from the works referenced. In deciding what to include, the researcher should bear in mind the intended audience. For example, a supervisor or external examiner will already have general background in the subject area. The literature should be analysed with reference to the research aims or questions. A common mistake is simply to describe the literature – the approach must be analytic and critical.

Correct attribution is also important. Failure to acknowledge a source can lead to an allegation of plagiarism. For dissertation or research students, a preferred citation style may be recommended. One common approach is the Harvard system – as used in this volume – based on an author and year system, with fuller details listed in alphabetical order at the end of the work. Another approach is the Oxford system where numbers for each source are used in the text and then full bibliographic details are given in a footnote or endnote. Legal or historical texts tend to favour page footnoting as readers may wish to see precise amplification as they read. If guidelines are provided by a book publisher or editors of a journal, they should be followed to the letter and consistently applied. Moreover, if a source is quoted directly, it should always be cited and the page number given. If particular ideas or arguments are summarized, this should also be acknowledged. Chapter 26 discusses writing style further. Two case studies now follow to illuminate the process of conducting a literature review.

The Black Report

In 1977 the Secretary of State for Health and Social Security requested a review of existing knowledge on the differences in health status between social classes, their causes, and implications for policy and future research. The review was chaired by Sir Douglas Black (then Chief Scientist at the Department of Health and Social Security, and later President of the Royal College of Physicians). This hard-hitting report on the evidence of inequalities in health (Department of Health and Social Security 1980) was finally made more widely available by Townsend and Davidson (1988) and subsequently has been updated in the light of further evidence. The aim was to provide evidence of the extent of inequality in health and offer an assessment of its implications. The report reviewed the following:

- *Concepts of health*: How is health, ill-health and inequality defined?
- *Concepts of health and inequality*: Definitions of health, indicators of health and illness, including disablement, and inequality indicators based on occupational group, income and expenditure.
- *Theoretical debates*: What theoretical approaches can explain why health inequalities occur?
- *Empirical evidence*: The sources of evidence on health inequalities, for example, the statistical returns from the General Household Survey, birth cohort studies and published reviews of data.
- *The pattern of present in equalities*: Mortality by gender, race, region, occupational class and incidence of common illnesses.

- *Trends in inequality of health; inequality in the availability and use of the health service*: A review of published studies and critique of methods.
- *International comparisons*: Comparison with developed countries, particularly European countries.
- *Towards an explanation of health inequalities*: Theoretical approaches to understanding health inequalities were assessed against the human life cycle.
- *Recommendations*: These outlined (a) the need for further primary and secondary research on particular issues and in policy terms; and (b) the need for a comprehensive anti-poverty strategy covering a range of social services based on a broader concept of inequalities in health.

Carrying out a literature review for a journal article: Health Consumer and Patients Organizations (HCPOs) and the Big Society

This review was undertaken for a journal article (Baggott and Jones 2015) examining the impact of recent policy developments and changes to the political environment of HCPOs in England. The aim of the paper was to address various developments, such as health care reform, pressures on health care budgets, including austerity, the call for a Big Society (voluntary activity to replace some of the functions of government), and the impact of devolution and the European Union. In particular, we wished to explore the various threats and opportunities these reforms posed. The avenues for exploration were identified as:

- *Conceptual issues*: How is the Big Society defined in the context of austerity? What constitutes threats and opportunities for HCPOs?
- *Theoretical debates*: How can changes in the policy environment of HCPOs be understood and explained?
- *Empirical evidence*: What are the key health reforms and changes in the policy environment which will impact the work of HCPOs? What evidence exists on the policy priorities and concerns of HCPOs in England? How do HCPOs interact with policy makers?

CASE STUDY 4.2

Conclusion

This chapter has emphasized the importance of the literature review in identifying concepts, theories and existing empirical studies on a particular phenomenon in the early stages of developing a research proposal or project. This enables a researcher to build on the basis of existing knowledge and on what other scholars have achieved, but also to identify gaps in the literature and to identify interesting new questions. While systematic reviews are a specialized form of study, narrative reviews are fundamental to any project.

The internet has brought access to a vast range of electronic sources for the researcher. A well-written review will provide enough background to bring the reader up to speed in the subject area and give them a framework within which to assess the evidence. In order to navigate a way through the quantity of sources available, two strategies may be employed. First, it is important to plan a search strategy carefully and to record sources and their content meticulously. The chapter outlines ways in which this can be done, so that, with practice, the researcher can be quick and efficient at finding the sources most likely to be relevant to their research question. Second, the expansion of the internet has led to the increase of information specialists who are employed by many organizations, and not only higher education institutions, to assist people in gaining access to information and what they need to know. This is particularly the case in the health field where a wide range of people, both professionals and the lay public, now wish to inform themselves better using both national and international sources.

Exercise 4.1   A literature search on patient and public involvement and representation in Clinical Commissioning Groups

Clinical Commissioning Groups are statutory bodies responsible for the planning and commissioning of health care services in their local area. There are currently 195 such groups in England. The following exercise provides an opportunity to think through the process of developing a search strategy and a structure for a literature review. While the subject area or context may not be one you are familiar with, the process described in this chapter should give you a framework to plan a successful search.

Think about the type of literature review that you would undertake for a dissertation entitled 'A critical analysis of patient and public involvement and representation in Clinical Commissioning Groups'.

1. What conceptual and theoretical issues will you need to consider?
    - Consider what definitional issues you will need to address.
    - How will perspectives on involvement/representation influence the analysis of the literature?

2. Which electronic databases will you need to search?
    - Consider the scope and coverage of the database. How important is it that it is international in scope?
    - Are you going to attempt to identify primary research studies, secondary policy analysis or both?

3. What search strategy will you build?
   - Consider what keywords and phrases you will need to use.
   - Consider what the most appropriate limits might be for your search – for example, language and date of publication.
   - Are there any terms that can be truncated to broaden the search?

4. What will be the most relevant sources of grey literature?
   - Which key research organizations may have an interest in Clinical Commissioning Groups?
   - What information will you need to obtain from the Department of Health website?

5. What key data will you need to log from the literature?
   - Consider how these may change according to the type of information – for example, policy documents, policy critiques and policy analyses that draw on field research.

6. How will you structure the review?
   - What information will the reader require on the Clinical Commissioning Groups?
   - What information will the reader require on the theoretical and conceptual issues underpinning your review?
   - Will you tackle the benefits/concerns relating to patient and public involvement in Clinical Commissioning Groups separately or by theme?
   - Will you discuss primary and secondary research together or separately?

Note

The author would like to thank the following for permission to draw on projects undertaken while part of a larger research team: Judith Allsop, University of Lincoln; Rob Baggott, Health Policy Research Unit, De Montfort University; and Tim Brown and Ros Hunt, Centre for Comparative Housing Research, De Montfort University.

Recommended further reading

This book provides an easy-to-understand guide on the process of planning, executing and recording a literature search. It includes more on linking the review to research questions:

Aveyard, H. (2010) *Doing a Literature Review in Health and Social Care: A Practical Guide*, 2nd edition. Maidenhead: Open University Press/McGraw-Hill.

This book provides a comprehensive guide to the process of accessing, analysing and understanding the arguments presented in academic texts, giving useful advice on how the literature review fits into undergraduate and postgraduate dissertations:

Hart, C. (2018) *Doing a Literature Review: Releasing the Social Science Research Imagination.* London: Sage.

This book provides a step-by-step guide to undertaking a literature review as part of a research project. It advocates adopting a systematic approach in the review and explores the process of scoping and managing the review in addition to discussions on analysing and synthesizing evidence:

Booth, A., Sutton, A. and Papaioannou, D. (2016) *Systematic Approaches to a Successful Literature Review,* 2nd edition. London: Sage.

References

Aveyard, H. (2010) *Doing a Literature Review in Health and Social Care: A Practical Guide,* 2nd edition. Maidenhead: Open University Press/McGraw Hill.

Baggott, R., Allsop, J. and Jones, K. (2005) *Speaking for Patients and Carers: Health Consumer Groups and the National Policy Process.* Basingstoke: Palgrave.

Baggott, R. and Jones, K. (2015) 'The Big Society in an age of austerity: Threats and opportunities for HCPOs in England', *Health Expectations.* Available at: doi: 10.1111/hex.12185.

Boland, A., Cherry, G. and Dickson, R. (2017) *Doing a Systematic Review: A Student's Guide,* 2nd edition. London: Sage.

Booth, A., Sutton, A. and Papaioannou, D. (2016) *Systematic Approaches to a Successful Literature Review,* 2nd edition. London: Sage.

Brown, T., Baggott, R., Jones, K. and Hunt, R. (2004) *The Impact of Overcrowding on Health and Education: A Review of the Research Evidence and Literature.* London: The Office of the Deputy Prime Minister.

Department of Health and Social Security (1980) *Inequalities in Health: A Report of a Research Working Group.* London: HMSO.

Dixon-Woods, M., Fitzpatrick, R. and Roberts, K. (2001) 'Including qualitative research in systematic reviews: Problems and opportunities', *Journal of Evaluative Clinical Practice,* 7: 125–33.

Gash, S. (2000) *Effective Literature Searching for Research.* Aldershot: Gower.

Greenhalgh, T. (2014) *How to Read a Paper: The Basics of Evidence-based Medicine,* 5th edition. Chichester: Wiley-Blackwell.

Hamalainen, L. and Jones, K. (2011) 'Conceptualising community as a social fix, argument and persuasion in health, housing and local governance'. Available at: https://connect-ed-communities.org/index.php/project_resources/conceptualising-community-as-a-social-fix-argument-and-persuasion-in-health-housing-and-local-governance/

Hart, C. (2018) *Doing a Literature Review: Releasing the Social Science Research Imagination.* London: Sage.

Mays, N., Pope, C. and Popay, J. (2005) 'Systematically reviewing qualitative and quantitative evidence to inform management and policy-making in the health field', *Journal of Health Services Research and Policy*, *10*(1 Supp): 6–20.

NHS CRD (2009) *Systematic Reviews: CRDs Guidelines for Undertaking Reviews in Healthcare*. York: Centre for Reviews and Dissemination.

Petticrew, M. (2001) 'Systematic reviews from astronomy to zoology: Myths and misconceptions', *British Medical Journal*, *322*: 98–101.

Pluye, P. and Hong, Q. N. (2014) 'Combining the power of stories and the power of numbers: Mixed methods research and mixed studies reviews', *Annual Review of Public Health*, *35*: 29–45.

Robertshaw, L., Dhesi, S. and Jones, L. L. (2017) 'Challenges and facilitators for health professionals providing primary healthcare for refugees and asylum seekers in high-income countries: A systematic review and thematic synthesis of qualitative research', *BMJ Open*, e015981. Available at: doi:10.1136/bmjopen-2017-015981

Sabatier, P. A. (1999) 'The need for better theories', in P. A. Sabatier (ed.), *Theories of the Policy Process*. Boulder, CO: Westview Press.

Street, A. (2001) 'How can we argue for evidence in nursing?', *Contemporary Nurse*, *11*(1): 5–9.

Townsend, P. and Davidson, N. (1988) *Inequalities in Health*. London: Penguin.

PART II
Qualitative Methods and Health

5

Methods of Sampling in Qualitative Health Research

LARA MAESTRIPIERI, ARIANNA RADIN AND ELENA SPINA

Chapter objectives

- To provide an introduction to the features of non-probabilistic sampling and how it differs from probabilistic sampling
- To discuss quota sampling and purposive sampling, how they are used and the importance of transparency in describing sampling methods
- To describe the uses of snowball and self-selective sampling and their strengths and weaknesses
- To consider the role of key informants in accessing samples.

Introduction

Sampling in qualitative research

Designing research involves making choices, one of the most important of which concerns selecting the cases to be included in a study (Merkens 2004; Merriam and Tisdell 2016). This process is known as 'sampling', and entails selecting certain cases in a controlled and rigorous manner, in order that the empirical results stemming from the sample can be applied to a wider population (Becker 1998; Flick 2014).

The most important characteristic of samples in qualitative research is that they are 'non-probabilistic'. This means that the probability that each individual in a population will constitute a part of the sample will not be known (Saunders, Lewis and Thornhill 2012). Therefore, it will not be possible to apply a statistical inference from a sample to the whole population as in the case of probabilistic sampling, which is used in quantitative research. Here random sampling is used to extrapolate findings from a group to a whole population and is discussed in Chapter 12.

The aim of non-probabilistic sampling in qualitative research is to enhance understanding of the object of a study by drawing a sample of cases for data collection that will demonstrate the diversity and complexity of the phenomenon. The data collected will be rich in detail. In the first instance, an explicit and effective research strategy must be worked out to select cases (Flick 2014). If the initial selection is insufficient, it is always possible to add new participants or objects in a second stage of the research process. Indeed, further investigation can be undertaken during a project or if it is found that an intensive study of a specific sub-population is needed (Ritchie et al. 2014).

One characteristic of non-probabilistic sampling is that individuals or items for study are selected directly by the researcher (Reybold, Lammert and Stribling 2012). This has three consequences:

- When developing sampling criteria, the researcher co-constructs the phenomenon to be studied. Sampling allows the researcher to highlight aspects that are believed to be of more relevance for answering the research questions, while eliminating those that are considered irrelevant.
- The sampling choices made enable the researcher to be explicit about the relationship between the sample of cases chosen and their particular theoretical perspective.
- The participants are usually chosen serially, which means that their selection depends on the previously sampled cases.

The robustness of a qualitative sample derives from its capacity to represent the salient characteristics of the population of cases under investigation. When developing sampling criteria, it is important to judge the appropriateness of the selection criteria in terms of the specific research questions and objectives (Ritchie et al. 2014). This will enhance the quality of the sample.

The definition of a case

The basic element of qualitative sampling is the case, which can be defined as the particular empirical entity that is, at the same time, both a part and a product of a research project (Ragin 1992a, 1992b). The case can assume different forms, depending on the specific research project. There are five main families of case that can be a unit of analysis: individuals or collectives, such as groups or territorial units; organizations or institutions; and events and cultural products, such as journal articles, discourses and pictures (Patton 1990). Behind the use of the term 'case' lies an implicit idea that the objects of investigation belong to the same broad category, but, at the same time, they are separate enough to be treated as comparable instances of the same general phenomenon (Ragin 1992a). Box 5.1 provides further detail on the case.

Box 5.1   The importance of a case

The case in qualitative sampling is both a part, and a product, of the research project. The 'case-oriented' approach is that which distinguishes qualitative analysis from quantitative analysis, which is 'variable-oriented' (Ragin 1992b). As such, it means focusing on the singularity that makes the case distinct from others and unique due to the characteristics of which it is comprised. In this sense, the main goal of the empirical inquiry is to understand its uniqueness, and its un-fragmented complexities, by assessing what is common and what is particular about the case under investigation, in comparison with the category of reference (Stake 1994).

Although several options exist for case selection, in the opinion of the authors the most effective strategy is one that aims to enhance the diversity of the cases selected. This is achieved by including as wide a range of factors and features that might be associated with the phenomenon as possible, and then by investigating all the possible interdependences between the different characteristics identified (Ritchie et al. 2014). It is also a good practice to seek out negative cases, or alternative explanations, as these can improve the theoretical breadth and the typological representativeness of the results (Becker 1998; Kuzel 1999).

Size in qualitative sampling

An important characteristic of qualitative samples is their limited size. Whereas in quantitative analysis the size of samples can include numbers in the hundreds or thousands, in qualitative analysis the usual size is generally in units or tens of cases. This means that:

- The type of information collected using qualitative techniques is usually very rich in detail, and in some extreme cases one single case can be sufficient enough to encompass all the relevant dimensions for the analysis of a phenomenon (see, for example, Maestripieri 2016).
- As statistical representation is not the aim of qualitative analysis, there is no need for the sample to be large.

In qualitative methods, in which the phases of data collection, data management and data analysis require extensive work for each single interview or observation and the number of cases in the study is necessarily limited in order to carry out affordable research (Flick 2014; Ritchie et al. 2014), the size chosen for the sample is dependent on the specific research question to be investigated. The researcher must consider what will be useful as well as credible for their specific research design (Cresswell 2002). Some authors have offered indications of the most appropriate numbers for each type of research (Guest, Bunce and Johnson 2006; Ritchie et al. 2014; Saunders, Lewis and Thornhill 2012).

In the opinion of the authors, the size of the population should be always decided on the basis of the specific design of the research project in question and time and budget constraints (Merriam and Tisdell 2016; O'Reilly and Parker 2013; Rossman and Rallis 2017). In order to decide whether interviews or observations are sufficient for the scope of the research, the principle of saturation can be applied. This is a principle that was initially formulated in the context of grounded theory (Glaser and Strauss 1967) and can be defined as 'the point of diminishing return where increasing the sample size no longer contributes new evidence' (Ritchie et al. 2014: 117). In sum, saturation is reached when no, or very little, new information would be obtained from collecting additional data. It follows from this that the number of interviews or observations likely to constitute the sample will not be foreseeable in advance (Saunders et al. 2018). In sampling, a degree of subjective judgement must be applied, and researchers may differ in the judgements they make (Flick 2014). Engaging with the analysis while gathering the data is good practice and helpful for improving the sensibility of the researcher to decide when saturation has been reached (Merriam and Tisdell 2016; Tuckett 2004).

Risks in qualitative sampling

There are further practical difficulties that can affect qualitative sampling. There may, for example, be difficulties in accessing the individuals or items under investigation (Flick 2014). Indeed, one of the most important reasons for opting for a qualitative methodology is the lack of a complete list of the population from which the researcher can derive a representative sample. The element of subjectivity in qualitative sampling can carry risks. For instance, if the selection of participants cannot be controlled, then this can affect the quality of sampling in this frame (Rossman and Rallis 2017).

Another source of risk is a bias in the selection of cases. This can occur when individuals refuse to participate in the research, and it occurs systematically. An example would be if a sample was skewed when all the women approached refused to participate in a population-wide study or when a researcher failed to recruit across social classes or missed an important sub-group. If such coverage is important to address the research question, the results of the investigation can be distorted (Merkens 2004). In non-probabilistic samples, it may not be possible to predict the likelihood of this occurrence, but researchers should be aware of possible problems (Saunders, Lewis and Thornhill 2012). Qualitative researchers need time and patience to recruit participants relevant to their research. This is particularly so with groups which are hard to reach. When accessibility cannot be improved, it is considered good practice to state clearly in a methodological note that problems of accessibility have resulted in the systematic exclusion of certain groups from the study and state that this may have had consequences for the quality of the sample (O'Reilly and Parker 2013).

In sum, one of the most serious criticisms of qualitative methods is the risk of bias due to a researcher's subjectivity in deciding who or what is to be included in the research sample (Fagnini 2013; Reybold, Lammert and Stribling 2012). In order to avoid this risk, it is important to make explicit the criteria behind the choice of cases, and to justify them on the basis of the research objectives. Defining a clear sampling procedure, and adhering to it during the research, constitutes the most effective strategy for complying with the scientific requirement for transparency. The researcher's peers can then assess the design and quality of the research and will be in a position to replicate a study if they wish (Merkens 2004; Nelson 2016). Once choices have been made, an extensive methodological note that seeks to clarify the criteria employed in the selection of cases, together with the limits of the sampling procedure, will enhance the quality and transparency of the sampling process.

Sampling in qualitative research

In non-probabilistic sampling, a distinction can be made between quota sampling and purposive sampling. In both types there is a degree of control by the researcher over who or what is sampled. Snowball sampling and sampling through the self-selection are approaches where there is less control in selecting the interviewees. The degree of control does not necessarily affect the quality of the sample and may indeed be inevitable if the aim is to attract participants who are hard to reach or there is no data available to obtain access to a population other than developing a bespoke strategy for recruitment. What is important is for the sample to match the research question being investigated and the existing data sources available to address it.

In practice, the distinction between quota sampling and purposive sampling, which exercise more control over creating a sample, and snowballing and self-selective sampling, where there is less control, is not rigid. The different types can be used separately or in conjunction with each other. For example, quota sampling may be used first to stratify cases into selected categories, for example, to get a population stratified by class or gender by region. Then, in a further stage, a purposive sample can be drawn. This will become clearer from the examples given below. Purposive sampling itself has a variety of different methods, which are shown in Box 5.2. The criteria to be employed in sampling can be developed either before, during or even after completing the data collection (Flick 2014; Merkens 2004).

To summarize:

- In both quota and purposive sampling, the researcher decides in advance the conditions by which participants are included in the study. There is sufficient information about the population of reference to decide which properties should be considered in case selection (Fagnini 2013).

- In non-purposive sampling, such as snowball and self-selection sampling, the construction of the sample is dependent on how the research develops and the construction of the sample remains flexible and open (Fagnini 2013).

As sampling techniques can be used in tandem, it is possible to adjust the non-probabilistic samples during the development of the research without affecting the quality of the sampling strategy. As a consequence, it is possible to make use of different techniques in the development of the same project. Nevertheless, it is always important to justify the choice of combining different samples in the frame of the research objectives and constraints. For example, in the same research we can use a combination of quota and purposive sampling in order to produce samples that are intuitively, if not statistically, representative.

Combining sampling strategies can offer researchers a legitimate and acceptable means for data collection, but the researcher must be aware of the possible loss of cases. In relation to more flexible sampling, for example, the researcher might simply not involve the cases proposed by others – as in snowball sampling – or those who have voluntarily proposed themselves in self-selective sampling as these are not useful for the study.

The next section will present the two main types of sampling strategy in qualitative health research. A deeper knowledge of the advantages and disadvantages of each type of strategy will assist future researchers in establishing the most appropriate approach for their research.

Types of samples: Quota and purposive sampling

Quota sampling

The quota sampling method involves dividing a sample into smaller groups that are chosen with respect to the characteristics of the population considered relevant for the study in question, such as gender, educational level and age, then building the 'quota' from individuals chosen specifically, but not randomly (Stommel and Wills 2004). This is achieved by dividing the population into strata that are as homogeneous as possible within each stratum, and as heterogeneous as possible between the strata. Then, adhering to non-probabilistic criteria, the researcher selects the participants/interviewees in order to complete the relevant quotas (Saunders, Lewis and Thornhill 2012). Quota sampling can be considered as a non-probabilistic version of stratified sampling (Bailey 1978; Tyrer and Heyman 2016). However, it is not exactly equivalent because with stratified sampling, random sampling is performed from sampling lists, while in quota sampling the selection of subjects is carried out deliberately by the researchers. They extract the data to construct the sample (Barnett 2002).

Quota sampling is more likely to be used in larger, funded projects. It can be defined as a sampling method for gathering representative data from a group (Saunders, Lewis and Thornhill 2012). The term 'representative' indicates that subjects are selected to represent the conditions to be studied, rather than to represent the wider population (Luborsky and Rubinstein 1995). All the dimensions that are considered important by the researcher must be declared beforehand in order to establish a typology that accounts for both the theoretical approach and the criteria that are considered relevant for the specific research project. Particular attention must be given to the number of cases included in each combination, even if some types may not be empirically observable (Bailey 1978; Silverman 2010). In this way, the inclusion of people who may be under-represented by convenience or purposeful sampling techniques is assured (Luborsky and Rubinstein 1995).

As Guest and Namey (2015) have noted, quota sampling can be both proportional and non-proportional. In its proportional form, the quotas available to the data collectors are set, so that the proportions of the categories in the sample are consistent with their proportions in the target population. The proportionality of the quotas aims to increase the level of the external validity of the sample. In non-proportional sampling, the quotas are not necessarily set in order that the categories will be proportional to their representation in the target population, but at the discretion of the researcher. This form of quota sampling is chosen when the proportions of the categories in the target population are not known, when a researcher wishes to compare categories of equal size to one other, or when it is necessary to over-sample a certain segment of the target population.

Quota sampling has a number of advantages. In particular, it is less costly than other types of sampling procedure as it can be established quickly (Saunders, Lewis and Thornhill 2012). It also reconciles the need for proportionality with a flexible research practice. It is not necessary for the researchers to make contact with named individuals selected in advance; instead it enlists any available individual who satisfies the specifications of an unfilled category to reach the set quota (Sim and Wright 2000). Finally, it deliberately generates variation in terms of the predetermined subject characteristics that may otherwise be absent, as in a convenience sample, for instance.

However, as Stommel and Wills (2004) highlight, quota sampling has two fundamental weaknesses:

- First, it should not involve more than a few subject characteristics since, as the quota scheme becomes more complex, it may prove challenging to locate interviewees with the desired characteristics. For example, if a researcher is seeking 40-year-old American women with diabetes covered by Medicaid, such a person may be difficult to locate.
- Second, quota sampling does not guarantee the representativeness of samples with respect to population characteristics that are not built into the quota categories. For

instance, taking the example referred to above, it may not take into account the occupational status, family responsibilities or class position of those selected.

- Third, quota sampling may favour only people who are readily available or people who can be involved easily. The diversity of the sample may thus be compromised.
- Fourth, the need to achieve a certain quota can lengthen the time involved in the search.

In market research and opinion polls, the use of quota sampling is widespread. In the medical field, it tends to be used especially in surveys that seek to find out about people's health behaviour, including their attitudes and values within a population (Bryman 2016).

In health care studies, quota sampling is not often used (Stommel and Wills 2004). However, in the case study described below, a research project commissioned in 2011 by the Italian Ministry of Labour and Social Policies, it was employed as a useful strategy to stratify focus groups. The study aimed to study the employment and organization of health and social workers in the social services within the Marche Region.

The research focused on an analysis of three professional groups: social workers, health educators and health care assistants. In the first phase, eight focus groups were organized and 15 professionals were invited to each group. These included five people from each occupational group. Individuals were selected according to the type of organization in which they practised; their field of practice in the health or social sector; their level of training; and their management and coordination role within the organization. Using quota sampling, the researchers were able to select individuals to contact easily, according to the characteristics they considered important. The technique of employing the same number of different professionals (fixed quota) by selected characteristics was useful for ensuring a similar dynamic in terms of roles and relationships within each focus group (Ministero del Lavoro e delle Politiche Sociali 2011).

The example shows that quota sampling can be adopted as 'the most cost-effective means of obtaining a representative sample …, although of course, it is not as rigorous as probability sampling', the findings of which can be extrapolated to other similar groups (Owen, McNeill and Callum 1998: 728).

Purposive sampling

Purposive sampling involves drawing a sample composed of cases that fulfil prior criteria chosen by the researcher. The main aim of this sampling strategy is to sample cases/participants in a strategic way, so that those sampled are relevant to the research questions that have been posed. Very often, the researcher will want to select in order to ensure that there is variety in the resulting sample, so that the sample members differ from each other in terms of key characteristics relevant to the research question (Bryman 2016). Information-rich cases may be chosen as they guarantee the acquisition of new knowledge or provide opportunities for further study (Patton 2002; Stake 1994).

Researchers employ their own judgement in selecting the respondents and choose only those who best match the purpose of the investigation (Bailey 1978). As Marshall (1996) notes, defining the criteria involves developing a framework based on the researcher's practical knowledge of the research area and the available literature and evidence from the study itself. This strategy requires more thought than the basic demographic stratification involved in quota sampling by age, gender and social class, as referred to above.

There are different ways of drawing a purposive sample. It may be advantageous to study a broad range of subjects (maximum variation sample), or to focus on outliers (deviant sample), or on participants who have specific experiences (critical case sample), or again on participants who have special expertise (key informant sample) to collect data (Marshall 1996). As shown in Box 5.2, many different sampling strategies have been proposed, each of which has a different intent, depending on the research problem and questions to be answered through the study, and each of the strategies has characteristics that may be appropriate for the purpose of the research project, or the particular phase of research in which they are to be used. However, a common element of the various forms of sampling is that the participants are selected according to predetermined criteria relevant to the particular research objective.

Box 5.2   The variety of purposive sampling

The different purposeful sampling strategies proposed by Creswell (2002) include the following:

- *Maximal variation sampling*: The researcher samples cases or individuals that differ with regard to some characteristic or trait. It requires that the characteristic is identified, and that sites or individuals are then located that display different dimensions of that characteristic.
- *Extreme case sampling*: Researchers study an outlier case, or one that displays extreme characteristics, identifying them by locating individuals or organizations that others have cited for their achievements or distinguishing characteristics.
- *Typical sampling*: The researcher studies a person or site that is 'typical' to those unfamiliar with the situation. What constitutes typical, of course, is open to interpretation.
- *Theory or concept sampling*: The researcher samples individuals or sites because they can assist in generating or discovering a theory, or specific concepts within it. In order to employ this method, it is necessary to possess a clear understanding of the concept or larger theory that is expected to emerge during the research.
- *Homogeneous sampling*: The researcher samples individuals or sites based on membership of a subgroup with defining characteristics. The researcher must identify the characteristics and locate individuals or sites that possess it.
- *Critical sampling*: The researcher studies a critical sample because it is an exceptional case that can explain much about the phenomenon.
- *Confirming and disconfirming sampling*: This form of sampling is employed to follow up on specific cases to test, or to explore further specific findings, and to confirm or disconfirm preliminary findings.

In purposive sampling, the sampled cases are selected based on the knowledge and judgement of the researcher. They include only those cases that possess the predetermined characteristics of the population that are considered relevant to the phenomenon under investigation. The criteria for the choice of the subjects can also be based on objective parameters, such as the resemblance of sampling cases to the target population. However, this introduces a subjective element and purposive sampling is also known as 'judgement', 'selective' or 'subjective' sampling (Dhivyadeepa 2015), since the researcher decides what kind of informant or community to involve. Sometimes cases are replaced according to the researcher's knowledge and discretionary assessments; if this introduces bias, it can be reduced if the choice of people to engage in the research is based on indications provided by key informants. The role of key informants in helping to access informants is discussed in Box 5.3. Key informants can be vital in research in assisting access, but they can also act as gatekeepers who guard entry to participants.

In summary, purposive sampling offers the opportunity to draw on a wide range of sampling techniques, and to select the best approach in relation to the research objectives posed by the specific qualitative design in which it is employed. Purposive sampling is especially useful when a piece of research involves different phases, since it allows for a different technique to be adopted for each. The main disadvantage of purposive sampling is that, irrespective of the type of technique employed, it may be subject to the researcher's bias. However, this can be reduced if their judgements are based on clear criteria that are explained and made transparent. Judgements should have a strong anchorage in relevant theory and be informed by previous research findings.

Purposive sampling is very often used in qualitative health research. It is recommended for use with relatively small samples and when a researcher wishes to select cases that are particularly informative (Neuman 2005). It is also used when the researcher wishes to add to the number of cases initially selected. As Grove, Gray and Burns (2014: 270) explain:

> In health care studies a purposive sample can be used to select participants who are of various age categories, those who have different diagnoses or illness severity, or those who received an ineffective treatment rather than an effective treatment for their illness.

Key informants can play a strategic role in qualitative research, and particularly in both purposive and quota sampling. They are individuals who possess special knowledge, status or communication skills, and who are willing to teach the researcher about a phenomenon (Creswell 1998). Interviews with key informants from a wide range of people, including community leaders, professionals or residents, who possess first-hand knowledge of the phenomenon being studied, can assist sampling. With their particular knowledge and understanding, these community experts can provide insight into the nature of problems and can recommend solutions. Box 5.3 indicates how to access key informants.

Box 5.3   The role of key informants

Rubin and Rubin (1995) suggest three guidelines for selecting key informants:

- They are knowledgeable about the cultural area, situation or experience being studied
- They are willing to talk
- They represent a range of viewpoints.

Of crucial importance is the building of strong interpersonal relationships between the researcher and the key informants, as this represents a central component of the process of 'entering the field' (Thorne 2016). As the result of their personal skills or position within a society, they can play different roles, such as:

- Helping to identify information-rich cases (Suri 2011)
- Giving more information and a deeper insight into what is occurring (Elmusharaf 2012)
- Providing the names of, and introductions to, additional key informants with specific traits, and those who represent additional segments of the population being studied (Hardcastle, Powers and Wenocur 2011)
- Reducing the necessity for the researcher to select the sample.

Purposive sampling of midwives in Italy and England

An example of purposive sampling is that employed in an Italian research project studying the professionalization process of midwives (Spina 2013). In the first phase, midwives based in hospitals had been part of an ethnography study. In the second phase, purposive sampling was employed to select midwives to be interviewed. The researcher selected expert midwives in Italy with distinct roles within the profession. These included independent midwives who worked at the homes of patients and in birthing centres, midwives who were involved in education and training, and midwives who played a formal role in their professional associations. In a parallel study, purposive sampling was also used to select English midwives to be interviewed in order to compare the two countries. In this case, the support of a key informant was fundamental. Thanks to purposive sampling, selecting the privileged witnesses and interviewing them allowed the researcher to access midwives external to the hospital context. The focus on gaining information from expert informants reduced the time and costs of the research and allowed this broader aspect of the work of midwives to be explored. Further details of the processes involved can be obtained from Spina (2013).

CASE STUDY 5.1

Finally, purposive and quota sampling can be considered similar as both seek to identify participants from selected criteria. However, the latter is more specific with respect to the size and proportion of different quotas, while purposive sampling must be employed when the number of participants is more of a target than a necessary requirement (Mack et al. 2005).

Non-purposive sampling methods: Snowball sampling and self-selection

Snowball sampling

This form of sampling technique typically proceeds after a study has commenced, and entails a researcher asking informants to recommend the names of one or more other individuals who could be involved in the study, commencing with gatekeepers or the first interviewees. The researcher may pose this request as a question during an interview or through informal conversation with individuals at a research site. As the name implies, the process of snowball sampling is cumulative and repetitive. In health care studies, this sampling method is less expensive and can be as efficient as other strategies (Sadler et al. 2010). It can be chosen at the outset of a new study as it facilitates entry into the field of study. The method is useful for overcoming the problem of access to vulnerable populations, such as people with major disabilities or with debilitating illnesses, or to people with conditions they wish to hide, such as eating disorders or cases of abortion, and populations that are hidden by choice, such as those involved in the anti-vaccine movement. It is also useful when a researcher wishes to track the connections between people in specific health subgroups or in community-based research, such as in the public health field.

This sampling method may run into particular problems. According to Biernacki and Waldorf (1981), there are a number of challenges in snowball sampling. These include finding respondents and starting a referral chain; verifying the eligibility of potential respondents; controlling the type of chain; deciding on the number of cases in any chain; and pacing and monitoring referral chains. Due to these difficulties, a major issue is maintaining data quality. Box 5.4 provides further detail.

In order to commence a referral chain efficiently, researchers must select the right time to ask their informants for contacts, for example, by asking 'Who knows a lot about...?', or 'Who should I talk to?' (Patton 1990). The researcher should verify the quality of the new informant. This can be achieved at first contact, during the search or, in the most helpful cases, when the same name is indicated by more than one informant. For this reason, a robust strategy for improving the quality of the sample is to monitor the chain by using a sampling tree (Noy 2008). This summary table that returns all the relevant data is similar to a genealogical tree and is particularly useful when working within a research team. Employing tools of this kind can facilitate the monitoring phase, especially if the researchers wish to meet to discuss and evaluate the quality of the contacts and data (Biernacki and Waldorf 1981).

Box 5.4   Resolving common problems: Recruitment issues and suggestions

Namageyo-Funa et al. (2014) propose three major categories of recruitment issues, together with suggestions for resolving them, as follows:

- *Obtaining consent*: In order to reassure some potential participants, it is important that the researcher prepares a consent form. It is possible to consider rewards and reimbursements for participation, although the best strategy is to obtain permission in the field by building a relationship of trust. For example, in a study related to children, the gatekeepers could introduce the researcher to their parents via the school administration or local associations.
- *Working with gatekeeper(s)*: Gatekeepers are not researchers and they can influence the potential participant's decision, as in the case where gatekeepers are managers or possess a coercive role. It is also important to define a clear agreement about the time the gatekeeper(s) will devote to the study because they are not paid more for this role and may not directly benefit from the research.
- *Accessing participants*: It is important that the researcher is flexible regarding recruitment times and days; that they solicit help from the gatekeepers in order to access different recruitment sites; and that they spend time in the locations. In addition, further recruitment tools may be employed, follow-up emails can be sent, telephone calls can be made, and radio and television interviews can be used. However, face-to-face interaction is sometimes more effective.

Snowball samples can be especially useful in comparative studies where the researcher is short of contacts. For example, in a study concerning obstetricians and gynaecologists in England, Italy and Belgium, the researchers recruited professionals through advertisements in a range of professional journals, invitations to particular organizations, and via telephone calls and emails, using purposive and snowball sampling (Risso-Gill et al. 2014).

In cross-national research, therefore, the researcher may be readily able to access a broad view of the systems of practice in the different contexts to be analysed. Likewise, it is valuable when a researcher wishes to study the patient community, particularly in a multicultural context. It may be preferable to use opportunistic sampling where the sample emerges during the inquiry as this strategy may divert attention away from the original aims of the research. But there are downsides. For example, too many similar potential informants may be sourced in snowball sampling, while other individuals may be excluded due to personal factors or because they are not well integrated into the relevant networks (Cresswell 1998).

Self-selection sampling

Self-selection sampling is a volunteer form of sampling (Saunders, Lewis and Thornhill 2012) in which individuals actively volunteer to be part of a study. It is an appropriate choice when the topic of study is extremely sensitive, for example in the case of sexually transmitted diseases; when the interviewees are difficult to reach, such as people with addictions; or in explorative and pilot projects, such as e-health. This form of sampling is sometimes the only alternative when dealing with risky or illegal behaviour, such as drug experimentation, or when it is required by a funding agency for ethical and privacy reasons.

However, the researcher who chooses this sampling strategy faces a variety of challenges, particularly those connected with individuals' barriers to participation (Ellard-Gray et al. 2015). First, the researcher must find a way of accessing and engaging with potential participants. Advertising the research is one solution, but the choice of language and where to advertise are critical. It is important to avoid creating a distance between researcher and the participant by using such terms as 'raped' or 'abused'. Second, the researcher must take into account the risks associated with participation both for themselves and the persons they aim to recruit. Third, ethical considerations are paramount in building a relationship, particularly if a topic is sensitive. Privacy, anonymity and safety are important even if the participation is limited to meeting with the researcher. Potential informants may mistrust the research process, especially if they do not perceive the research as interesting, relevant, or good for their community. In order to address this issue, it is important to use one or more gatekeepers. Finally, the researcher must build a trust relationship with the participants. For example, in the case of interviews, it is advisable to select the venue for the meeting in tandem with the participants, seeking to make the place as comfortable as possible, even if it is a waiting room of a clinic. In order to improve the quality of the sample, the strategy for snowball sampling can be applied along the lines described in Box 5.4. Two examples further clarify the procedure that may be used.

Women at risk

The first piece of research focused on abused rural women at risk of sexually transmitted infections. Because of the sensitivity of the topic and of the particular sample identified, the researchers defined a composite recruitment plan, as follows (Sutherland and Collins 2012):

- *Writing the flyer*: The researchers employed the term 'women and their relationships with their partners' instead of 'intimate partner violence'.
- *Winning the trust of the gatekeepers first*: The researchers discussed the study and the flyer with the clinic involved in the study. Thus, the administrative staff approved the presence of the research team in the waiting room, and the means of presenting of the study to the potential informants.
- *Winning the trust of the informants*: If the informant's information was of potential interest, the staff at the clinic requested that she 'go over and talk to the researchers'. Two months after implementing this approach, it was clear that it was not effective, so the researchers requested that the staff define them as 'the nurses doing the research', as detailed in the flyer.
- *Reducing the distance between the researchers and potential participants*: In the waiting room, the research team opted to knit instead of working at a laptop, and the women attending the clinic began to comment on the knitting with 'the nurses doing the study'. This tactic gave the researchers the opportunity to talk about the study.

Health 'All4all'

This was a pilot project to support and maintain the health of older people in a small city in Northern Italy – Health 'All4all' (Duretti et al. 2015). Applying the Living Lab approach (www.alcotra-innovation.eu) for the study, the multidisciplinary research team decided to approach individuals over the age of 65 who were not at a risk of serious health complications. They adopted the following process:

- *Involving gatekeepers*: The flyer produced by the research team was presented to the Board members of the local Retirement Unions.
- *Winning the trust of the informants*: The gatekeepers compiled a list of people who had declared an interested in the study, and these potential informants were invited by the researchers to the city's training centre to obtain details of the project, and for a question-and-answer session.

(Continued)

(Continued)

- *Becoming a reference point*: Since different researchers and stakeholders were involved in the pilot project, it was important to define *one* person as a 'mediator' to work with potential informants to explain what was expected of them and to act as a translator of the research process and the health vocabulary.

This example reflects the importance of reducing the distance between researchers and interviewees, especially when sharing the flyer with the potential informants. It was immediately apparent that the choice of the name 'All4all' for an elderly population who were not well-versed in English did not facilitate dialogue during the recruitment stage.

In the case of volunteer sampling, the researcher–participant relationship can raise different ethical concerns and dilemmas, not least if contradictory issues emerge during the study, and the researcher must choose between different methodological strategies, even if these conflict with one other (Sanjari et al. 2014). The researcher must avoid the risk of emotional exhaustion and must take responsibility for the quality of the sample, including adopting difficult solutions – for example, by excluding a participant, if necessary.

Reading health research based on qualitative sampling

In reading qualitative research, you should ask whether a sampling strategy explicitly exists for the research you are considering. This will involve the researcher:

- Being actively aware of the various forms of non-probabilistic sampling, including quota sampling, purposive and non-purposive sampling, such as snowball or self-selection sampling.
- Having a rationale for choosing one or more of these types of sampling, which should be attuned to their respective strengths and limitations and the research question.

The role of informants and their process of selection in the study should be articulated where appropriate. It is crucial that the risk of bias due to the researcher's subjectivity is minimized by explicitly setting out the sampling criteria of choice related to the research objectives.

Although smaller numbers of participants tend to be engaged in qualitative as opposed to quantitative research, usually – unless there is good reason to do otherwise – saturation should be achieved once sampling has occurred. This is based on little or no additional information being gathered by proceeding further.

Conclusion

As this overview of the sampling strategies available for qualitative health research has demonstrated, it is challenging to prescribe a valid-for-all solution. The choice of who to include in the sample, the techniques used for sampling, and the number of individuals to be recruited are always determined by the objectives of the study and the theoretical framing chosen to address the research question. Before choosing a sampling technique, it is important to be clear about the definition of the issue under investigation, and the population affected. The researcher must be mindful that selection is a complex process, and that it will have as significant an impact on the final quality of the research as any other phase of the research. The criteria for selecting certain interviewees must be defined and identified in order to study the phenomenon of interest. The interviewees selected should fit the purpose of the research and the accepted techniques for data collection must be followed.

Exercise 5.1   Health scenarios in qualitative sampling

Thinking about plausible scenarios involved in qualitative research, you are invited to consider the following three scenarios on sampling:

Scenario1

A research team promotes a survey in a big city hospital with the aim of understanding the professional behaviour of health workers involved in the birth process. Using qualitative methods, the team plans to carry out 45 in-depth interviews. There are 35 doctors (20 men and 15 women), 15 nurses (5 men and 10 women) and 40 midwives (all women) working in the maternity department. In order to reproduce the distribution of population in the different subgroups in the sample, researchers have to plan a suitable sampling strategy. What is the best strategy in your opinion?

Scenario2

As part of an investigation aimed at studying the empowerment of patients suffering from a chronic disease, the research team, after performing shadowing in some patients' homes, decides to conduct a series of interviews aimed at acquiring information about:

- The level of compliance of patients with respect to medical prescriptions
- Their membership in voluntary associations associated with that specific disease
- Their participation in social reintegration programmes
- The presence and accessibility of specially focused services in their area.

You should indicate the type of sampling you would select in this case and the participants you would include in order to collect useful information for the research project.

(Continued)

(Continued)

Scenario 3

In a study on the doctor–patient relationship during the process of decision-making care, a research group needs to respect the following sampling criteria: no minors, because they do not want to involve the parents; and no over-65s, because these subjects are more likely to suffer from multiple pathologies. Furthermore, the research team is interested in interviewing only individuals with tertiary education, because graduates are the most likely to challenge medical authority. To focus on the research objective, the research team decides to conduct interviews only with people who at least once in their life were forced to choose between different care options due to a significant health event, such as a heart attack. You should indicate which type of sampling should be adopted and how to build a potential sample, knowing that economic resources are limited and the research team does not want to involve doctors in the study, not even as gatekeepers.

Recommended further reading

If you want to answer the question of how many qualitative interviews are enough for your project, this discussion from the National Centre for Research Methods is very helpful:

Baker, S. E. and Edwards, R. (2012) 'How many qualitative interviews is enough?' Available at: http://eprints.ncrm.ac.uk/2273/4/how_many_interviews.pdf

This book positions the sampling issue in a broader context and provides an opportunity to become familiar with the practice of qualitative research:

Hesse-Biber, S. N. and Leavy, P. (2011) *The Practice of Qualitative Research*. London: Sage.

This is an article to read if you are interested in the process of recruiting interviewees and the extent of its impact on the quality of the empirical results:

Kristensen, G. K. and Ravn, M. N. (2015) 'The voices heard and the voices silenced: Recruitment processes in qualitative interview studies', *Qualitative Research*, *15*(6): 727–37.

References

Bailey, K. D. (1978) *Methods of Social Research*. New York: Free Press.

Barnett, V. (2002) *Sample Survey: Principles and Methods*, 3rd edition. London: Arnold.

Becker, H. S. (1998) *Tricks of the Trade: How to Think about Your Research while You Are Doing It*. Chicago, IL: University of Chicago Press.

Biernacki, P. and Waldorf, D. (1981) 'Snowball sampling: Problems and techniques of chain referral sampling', *Sociological Methods and Research*, *10*(2): 141–63.

Bryman, A. (2016) *Social Research Methods*, 5th edition. Oxford: Oxford University Press.

Creswell, J. W. (1998) *Qualitative Inquiry and Research Design: Choosing among Five Traditions*. London: Sage.

Creswell, J. W. (2002) *Educational Research: Planning, Conducting, and Evaluating Quantitative and Qualitative Research*. Upper Saddle River, NJ: Merrill/Prentice-Hall.

Dhivyadeepa, E. (2015) *Sampling Techniques in Educational Research*. New Delhi: Laxmi Publishers.

Duretti, S., Marchioro, C. E., Marasso, L., Vicari, C., Fiorano, L., Papas, E. G., Dimonte, V., Radin, A., Gaveglio, F. and Falda, S. (2015) 'ALL4ALL: IoT and telecare project for social inclusion', *Research and Technologies for Society and Industry: Leveraging a Better Tomorrow (RTSI), 2015 IEEE 1st International Forum*, 17–22 September.

Ellard-Gray, A., Jeffrey, N. K., Choubak, M. and Crann, S. E. (2015) 'Finding the hidden participant: Solutions for recruiting hidden, hard-to-reach, and vulnerable populations', *International Journal of Qualitative Methods*, *14*(5): 1–10.

Elmusharaf, K. (2012) 'Qualitative sampling techniques'. Paper presented at Training Course in Sexual and Reproductive Health Research, July. Available at: https://goo.gl/n6TTx5

Fagnini, L. (2013) 'Non a caso: Campionamento e scelta dei casi nella ricerca qualitativa'. PhD Thesis, XXIV cycle, University of Florence. Available at: https://goo.gl/bsnQus

Flick, U. (2014) *An Introduction to Qualitative Research*, 5th edition. Thousand Oaks, CA: Sage.

Glaser, B. G. and Strauss, A. L. (1967) *The Discovery of Grounded Theory: Strategies for Qualitative Research*. New York: Aldine.

Grove, S. K., Gray, J. R. and Burns, N. (2014) *Understanding Nursing Research: Building an Evidence-Based Practice*, 6th edition. St. Louis, MO: Elsevier Saunders.

Guest, G., Bunce, A. and Johnson, L. (2006) 'How many interviews are enough?', *Field Methods*, *18*(1): 59–82.

Guest, G. and Namey, E. (eds) (2015) *Public Health Research Methods*. Thousand Oaks, CA: Sage.

Hardcastle, D., Powers, P. and Wenocur, S. (2011) *Community Practice: Theories and Skills for Social Workers*. New York: Oxford University Press.

Kuzel, A. J. (1999) 'Sampling in qualitative inquiry', in B. F. Crabtree and W. L. Miller (eds), *Doing Qualitative Research*, 2nd edition. Thousand Oaks, CA: Sage.

Luborsky, M. R. and Rubinstein, R. L. (1995) 'Sampling in qualitative research: Rationale, issues, and methods', *Research in Aging*, *17*(1): 89–114.

Mack, N., Woodsong, C., Macqueen, K. M., Guest, G. and Namey, E. (2005) *Qualitative Research Methods: A Data Collector's Field Guide*. Research Triangle Park, NC: Family Health International.

Maestripieri, L. (2016) 'Professionalization at work: The case of Italian management consultants', *Ephemera: Theory and Politics in Organization*, *16*(2): 31–52.

Marshall, M. N. (1996) 'Sampling for qualitative research sample size', *Family Practice*, *13*(6): 522–25.

Merkens, H. (2004) 'Selection procedures, sampling, case construction', in U. Flick, E. von Kardoff and I. Steinke (eds), *A Companion to Qualitative Research*. Thousand Oaks, CA: Sage.

Merriam, S. B. and Tisdell, E. (2016) *Qualitative Research: A Guide to Design and Implementation*. San Francisco, CA: Jossey-Bass.

Ministero del Lavoro e delle Politiche Sociali (2011) 'Analisi della struttura e dell'occupazione dei servizi sociali della Regione Marche, Quaderno di Ricerca sociale 8'. Available at: http://sitiarcheologici.lavoro.gov.it/Strumenti/StudiStatistiche/Documents/Quadernodiricercasociale8.pdf

Namageyo-Funa, A., Rimando, M., Brace, A. M., Christiana, R. W., Fowles, T. L., Davis, T. L. and Sealy, D. A. (2014) 'Recruitment in qualitative public health research: Lessons learned during dissertation sample recruitment', *The Qualitative Report*, *19*(4): 1–17.

Nelson, J. (2016) 'Using conceptual depth criteria: Addressing the challenge of reaching saturation in qualitative research', *Qualitative Research*, *17*(5): 69–71.

Neuman, W. L. (2005) *Social Research Methods: Qualitative and Quantitative Approaches*, 6th edition. Boston, MA: Allyn & Bacon.

Noy, C. (2008) 'Sampling knowledge: The hermeneutics of snowball sampling in qualitative research', *International Journal of Social Research Methodology*, *11*(4): 327–44.

O'Reilly, M. and Parker, N. (2013) '"Unsatisfactory saturation": A critical exploration of the notion of saturated sample sizes in qualitative research', *Qualitative Research*, *13*(2): 190–7.

Owen, L., McNeill, A. and Callum, C. (1998) 'Trends in smoking during pregnancy, in England, 1992–7: Quota sampling surveys', *British Medical Journal*, *317*(7160): 728.

Patton, M. (1990) *Qualitative Evaluation and Research Methods*, 2nd edition. Thousand Oaks, CA: Sage.

Patton M. (2002) *Qualitative Research and Evaluation Methods*. Thousand Oaks, CA: Sage.

Ragin, C. C. (1992a) 'Introduction: Cases of "What is a case?"', in C. C. Ragin and H. S. Becker (eds), *What is a Case? Exploring the Foundations of Social Inquiry*. Cambridge: Cambridge University Press.

Ragin, C. C. (1992b) '"Casing" and the process of social inquiry', in C. C. Ragin and H. S. Becker (eds), *What is a Case? Exploring the Foundations of Social Inquiry*. Cambridge: Cambridge University Press.

Reybold, L. E., Lammert, J. D. and Stribling, S. M. (2012) 'Participant selection as a conscious research method: Thinking forward and the deliberation of "emergent" findings', *Qualitative Research*, *13*(6): 699–716.

Risso-Gill, I., Kiasuwa, R., Baeten, R., Caldarelli, I., Mitro, S., Merriel, A. and Legido-Quigley, H. (2014) 'Exploring the scope of practice and training of obstetricians and gynaecologists in England, Italy and Belgium: A qualitative study', *European Journal of Obstetrics and Gynaecology and Reproductive Biology*, *180*: 40–5.

Ritchie, J., Lewis, J., Elan, G., Tennant, R. and Rahim, N. (2014) 'Designing and selecting samples', in J. Ritchie, J. Lewis, C. McNaughton Nicholls and R. Ormston (eds),

Qualitative Research Practice: A Guide for Social Science Students and Researchers. Thousand Oaks, CA: Sage.

Rossman, G. B. and Rallis, S. F. (2017) *An Introduction to Qualitative Research: Learning in the Field*, 4th edition. Thousand Oaks, CA: Sage.

Rubin, H. and Rubin I. (1995) *Qualitative Interviewing: The Art of Hearing Data.* Thousand Oaks, CA: Sage.

Sadler, G. R., Lee, H. C., Lim, R. S. H. and Fullerton, J. (2010) 'Recruitment of hard-to-reach population subgroups via adaptations of the snowball sampling strategy', *Nursing and Health Sciences*, 12(3): 369–74.

Sanjari, M., Bahramnezhad, F., Fomani, F. K., Shoghi, M. and Cheraghi, M. A. (2014) 'Ethical challenges of researchers in qualitative studies: The necessity to develop a specific guideline', *Journal of Medical Ethics and History of Medicine*, 7: 14.

Saunders, B., Sim, J., Kingstone, T., Baker, S., Waterfield, J., Bartlam, B. and Jinks, C. (2018) 'Saturation in qualitative research: Exploring its conceptualization and operationalization', *Quality and Quantity*, 52(4): 1893–1907.

Saunders, M., Lewis, P. and Thornhill, A. (2012) *Research Methods for Business Students*, 6th edition. Harlow: Pearson.

Silverman, D. (2010) *Doing Qualitative Research*, 4th edition. London: Sage.

Sim, J. and Wright, C. (2000) *Research in Health Care: Concepts, Designs and Methods.* Cheltenham: Stanley Thornes.

Spina E. (2013) 'An evaluation of the professional status of Italian midwives', *Evidence Based Midwifery*, 11(3): 88–93.

Stake, R. E. (1994) 'Case studies', in N. K. Denzin and Y. S. Lincoln (eds), *Handbook of Qualitative Research.* Thousand Oaks, CA: Sage.

Stommel, M. and Wills, C. E. (2004) *Clinical Research: Concepts and Principles for Advanced Practice Nurses.* Philadelphia, PA: Lippincott, Williams & Wilkins.

Suri, H. (2011) 'Purposeful sampling in qualitative research synthesis', *Qualitative Research Journal*, 11(2): 63–75.

Sutherland, M. A. and Collins, F. H. (2012) 'Successful research recruitment strategies in a study focused on abused rural women at risk for sexually transmitted infections', *Journal of Midwifery and Women's Health*, 57(4): 381–5.

Thorne, S. (2016) *Interpretive Description: Qualitative Research for Applied Practice*, 2nd edition. Abingdon: Routledge.

Tuckett, A. (2004) 'Part 1: Qualitative research sampling – the very real complexities', *Nurse Researcher*, 12(1): 47–61.

Tyrer, S. and Heyman, B. (2016) 'Sampling in epidemiological research: Issues, hazards and pitfalls', *British Journal of Psychiatry Bulletin*, 40: 57–60.

6

Using Documents in Health Research

ANDY ALASZEWSKI

Chapter objectives

- To discuss documentary research and the resources required
- To consider when to use documentary sources
- To list the main forms of documentary research using unsolicited and solicited documents
- To consider how documentary data can be coded, analysed and presented
- To outline the strengths and weaknesses of the method.

Introduction

The aim of this chapter is to introduce students to the ways in which documents can be used for health research. Documents are a relatively neglected resource for health researchers. They are an economical way of accessing data, in particular data that may be difficult to obtain in other ways. Data from documents can be used in a variety of research designs, ranging from the quantitative data used in experiments and surveys to qualitative data used in ethnographic and interpretative research. In this chapter, I will examine the ways in which documents have been and can be used for health research.

Defining documentary research

A document can be defined as a human artefact that contains information. This artefact can take different forms. A document can be one or more pieces of paper (a file if loose and a book if bound) containing text, written symbols, usually words, often numbers and sometimes diagrams, drawings or illustrations. With the development of computer technology, documents increasingly take the form of computer files. *The Chambers Dictionary* (2008: 454) defines a document as: 'a paper, especially of an official character, affording information, proof or evidence of anything, a file of text produced and held on a computer'. Prior (2003: 2) expands the definition of document to include all human artefacts, such as 'paintings, tapestries, monuments, diaries, shopping lists, stage plays, adverts, rail tickets, film, photographs, videos, engineering drawings, the content of human tissue archives and World Wide Web (WWW) pages'. He argues that all such artefacts were created for a purpose and deciphering this purpose can provide insight into the individuals and groups that created them. In this chapter I will focus on a more conventional definition of documents as text, looking at how, and in what ways, the knowledge encoded in texts can used for health research.

Both the nature of technology underpinning the creation of documents and access to that technology have changed. Writing developed as a technology in the earliest states some 3000 years BCE (Scott 2017) and was used by specialist scribes to record state resources and manage state activities. Over time the range of documents expanded to include mathematical and literary texts, such as founding myths and accounts of religious beliefs and practices. In the last 400 years, the development of paper, simple writing tools and printing has increased access to education and, more recently, computer technologies have reduced the cost of creating documents, providing greater access to the skills needed to create them and making communicating and storing them easier (Alaszewski 2006a). In contemporary society, most people can create a personal document such as a diary, letter, email or blog and the internet provides a medium for global communication.

Documents can take a variety of forms. The traditional – and the one that tends to predominate and is the easiest to use for research – is written text, such as hospital records, letters and diaries. These may be stored in archives or published in collected works or as memoirs, autobiographies and institutional histories. However, with the development of other media, written text can be supplemented, or even replaced, by photographs, film, and audio and video recordings, and some archives include both types of material.

Existing documents

During their lifetime, most people living in the Global North will create a range of personal documents such as letters and diaries. However, most of these are likely to be lost or destroyed unless there are particular reasons why their creator or others consider them important enough to preserve. Alongside such personal documents are official documents, records made about individuals. These records have greater permanency as they are made and stored by organizations such as the National Health Service in Britain. The presumption is that such documents will be kept and are only destroyed by accident or to protect specific organizational secrets. As Max Weber (1978: 957) pointed out, modern society is characterized by the development of bureaucratic organizations in which management is 'based upon written documents ("the files") that are preserved'. The lives of individuals in the Global North, including their births, deaths and illnesses, are well documented. Such records form the basis for large-scale databases that are published as official statistics that can be used for epidemiological research. For example, Chapman and his colleagues (2006) undertook a statistical analysis of official statistics in Australia to examine whether the gun control introduced after the Port Arthur killings in 1996 had had a significant impact on the rate of mass killings. They found that in the 18 years prior to gun control there had been 13 mass shootings and none in the decade afterwards.

While official documents can provide evidence on the nature of health issues, they are more limited in providing insight into individuals' experience of health and illness. The best sources of such evidence are personal and family records, such as letters or diaries, that can be used as the basis for biographical case studies or life stories (Clarkson 2003; Plummer 2001). Such documents can be used to examine the ways in which individuals respond to major events in their lives, such as life-threatening illness. An example is the ways in which stroke survivors rebuild their lives (Alaszewski 2006b).

Research documents

Documentary research is not restricted to the use of pre-existing documents. Researchers can also use documents created specifically for their research. The form of such documents will reflect the purposes of the research. Researchers who are interested in experiments that measure the impact of an action in a population, or in a survey to count activities or events, can ask participants to record specific information in a structured format. For instance, researchers involved in drug trials who want to monitor the impact of a drug on illness can ask participants in the trial to monitor and record specific information in a paper or electronic diary. Stone and colleagues (2003) noted that diaries were used in approximately 25 per cent of later-phase drug trials to collect information on symptoms, especially those that 'are subjective and/or variable', such as pain. Similarly, researchers who are interested in understanding how a disease affects a specific group, or the extent to which at-risk individuals engage in risky behaviours, have used 'questionnaire-like' research diaries to access relevant data. Parkin and colleagues (2004) used them to record of the symptoms experienced by individuals who have relapsing-remitting multiple sclerosis and Coxon (1996) used them to explore the sexual activities of men who were at risk of HIV infection.

Researchers who are trying to understand how individuals interpret and communicate about experiences, such as traumatic illness or chronic illness, are likely to adopt a more open approach. One method is to encourage participants to create documents that record their experiences and reflections. For example, the researcher can invite participants in their research to maintain diaries recording their everyday life. As Plummer (2001) observes, such diaries can be seen as the 'document of life' *par excellence* and have been used in a range of health-related research.

The creation of documents such as diaries provides research participants with control of what they record and when. For example, in the study of stroke survivors, Alaszewski (2006b) recorded an unusual response from a participant. One diarist wrote to a research contact that she felt she had returned to her normal pre-stroke self and therefore her 'stroke-survivor' diaries were complete after four of the agreed 18 months. She said:

> Dear Helen [Researcher]
>
> Please find enclosed diary. I am sorry but I wish to withdraw from keeping a diary now. Life is pretty much back to normal, the hospital don't want to see me anymore and I am pleased to tell you that I really feel in control of life again. Thank you for your understanding.

However, it is important to note that when documents such as diaries are created for, and on behalf of, researchers, then the researchers will influence what is recorded as the records are shaped by the interaction between the researcher and the document creator, although in a final document this may not be apparent.

Why use documents?

Although documents are often readily available and relevant for the purposes of health research, as Scott (1990) observed, they tend to be a neglected source of data, even if they provide the only available source of information. For instance, when a researcher is interested in how specific illnesses and responses to them have changed over time, it would be virtually impossible to do so without using documents. In her study of cholera in nineteenth-century Britain, Thomas (2015) used 20 archives to access personal documents, public records and contemporary scientific articles to build a narrative matrix combining eyewitness accounts with statistics and scientific observations.

Documentary sources are particularly important where a researcher needs to minimize memory or recall problems as they are often based on records that were made shortly after the actual events. For example, in his research on the sexual activities of men who were at risk of HIV infection, Coxon (1996) compared the record that men gave of their sexual activities in diaries with those they recorded in a follow-up questionnaire. He found that in the questionnaire, participants tended to *overestimate* common and safer practices, such as masturbation and fellatio, but *underestimated* rarer but riskier practices.

Documents provide a way of collecting data that minimizes the intrusiveness associated with much social research. This is self-evident when the researcher uses pre-existing documents. Using research documents can also restrict intrusion, as the researcher specifies what sort of information is wanted. Participants are then free to decide when, and how, they record this information. Minimizing intrusion is important when a researcher wants to address sensitive issues or work in areas where groups or individuals want to avoid scrutiny of their activities.

Resources needed for documentary research

The resources required for documentary research depend on the type of document. Researchers using existing documents need to locate and access these, while researchers who create documents must locate participants and provide them with appropriate support.

Pre-existing documents

Researchers using existing documents must identify where they are held. Historic documents are likely to be stored in archives and the researcher will need the resources to identify and access these. Until relatively recently, this involved using published bibliographies and other sources to identify possible archives and then visiting each to access suitable documents (see Corti 2003; Jordanova 2000). This requires resources to cover travel costs as well as photocopying, where that is permitted, and the costs of subsequent analysis. The development of electronic and internet resources has increased access to, and reduced the costs of, using archives. Many bibliographies and other resources can be accessed online. For example, the Penn Library (2004) has produced an online research guide to finding diaries and some archives can be accessed online. In the United Kingdom, the DIPEx website (www.primarycare.ox.ac.uk/research.dipex) is an online archive of personal experiences of health and illness. The Mass-Observation archive maintains a website that provides information both on diaries and publications based on diaries. Mass-Observation recruited 500 men and women to develop an 'anthropology of [them]selves' (Sheridan 1991: 1). Most recruits kept a diary from 1939 until 1945 and some continued until 1965.

Researchers dealing with recent documents need to identify who controls access to the documents. Searching for such individuals can be a difficult and time-consuming activity and generally researchers use intermediaries. Miller (1985), in his study of Irish migrants in the United States, used personal documents, including letters and diaries, through contacting both institutions and individuals in the Irish migrant community to locate these. Researchers can also advertise through media such as newspapers and the internet. For example, the British Broadcasting Corporation used public interest in the Second World War, stimulated by sixtieth anniversary events, to promote an online archive of personal stories. Individuals were encouraged to contribute to a rapidly growing archive of personal documents by sending their stories and associated photographs electronically (WW2 People's War Team 2004).

Research documents

The resources needed by researchers who create documents for their project will depend on the aims, design and method for the study. It may be based on experimental, survey or other methods. The major resource implications are those normally associated with using such designs. For a cross-sectional survey design, resources are needed to:

- Identify the population
- Select and recruit a sample and provide instructions for the creation of the research documents
- Collect the research documents from the subjects or units in the sample
- Code and enter the data from the documents into a database
- Analyse the data statistically
- Write a report.

Traditional record-keeping requires participants to have basic competence in literacy (Corti 2003), although subjects can now use audio and video recorders as well. The chances of creating documents that are suitable for research purposes increase when there are adequate resources for the following:

- The initial recruitment process
- Training and support for document creators
- Appropriate recording equipment
- Checking the reliability of entries and providing feedback.

Some researchers have used incentives, such as the payment of modest sums of money, to compensate document creators for their time and effort, although there is some debate about the ethics of such payments (Coxon 1996; Jones and Candlin 2003).

Strengths and weaknesses of documentary sources

There are a number of strengths and weaknesses of documentary methods, which are considered in this section.

Authenticity

Documents offer an authenticity that is difficult to gain through other methods. Documents such as diaries capture the richness of everyday life as it happens. Plummer (2001: 48) notes that 'each diary entry – unlike life histories – is sedimented into a particular moment in time'. Bolger, Davis and Rafaeli (2003: 580) argue that such documents facilitate 'the examination of reported events and experiences in their natural, spontaneous context'.

The authenticity of existing documents makes them a particularly valuable resource for social or ethnographic histories. For example, MacFarlane (1970) used the diary of a seventeenth-century country vicar, Ralph Josselin, to examine the experiences of rural life, including illness and death. As MacFarlane observed, misfortune, including pain, suffering and death, were an ever-present part of daily life. For example, Josselin's wife bore ten children, of whom three died in childhood and one was stillborn, and she experienced three miscarriages. Several of Josselin's children died while he was in his 30s and several of his grandchildren died when he was over 50. The frequency of death and its distribution across the social and age spectrum shaped a relatively pragmatic approach to death, in which: 'Mourning was not to be too intense, or the memory of individuals to be retained too long, "for God would have us forget the dead"' (MacFarlane 1970: 167). Josselin's response to the death of his children was shaped by the depth of his emotional ties. For example, the death of very young babies elicited a lower key response than the death of his 8-year-old daughter. Although Josselin did discuss the practical measures he took to treat his own and his family's illnesses, he treated God as the source of all (mis)fortune and accepted that 'To stay well, to stay alive, involved placating and, in a sense, outwitting God, and at the same time it involved ever stricter uniformity to social norms' (MacFarlane 1970: 174).

If the researcher is careful to provide appropriate support, then research documents can also be used to obtain accounts of contemporary social events and experiences. Coxon (1996), in his discussion of the use of sexual diaries in Project SIGMA, noted that the diary method arose out of the researchers' experiences as sexually active gay men. Diary keeping was common and several of the researchers had kept sexual diaries for a number of years. Thus, they drew on their own experience in developing the method and encouraged the diarists to describe experiences in their own words.

Fitness for purpose

While it is tempting to treat documents such as diaries as authentic accounts, researchers should ask themselves how and why such documents were created to assess their suitability for different types of research question. Letters and diaries have a particular function and use specific structures and forms. As Clarkson (2003: 82) has noted, documents need to be treated with caution as they 'are tricky; they tell us what the author wants us to know, which is not necessarily what the researcher is really interested in'. Researchers need to consider how, and in what ways, the documents they propose to use are fit for the purposes of their research when using either personal or official documents.

In the case of personal documents, the difficulties of using them as eyewitness accounts can be seen in the case of the diary of Anne Frank. Anne Frank's diary has become a classic account of the Holocaust and, when it was first published in 1947, her father Otto Frank and the other editors asserted that it was a publication of the original text of Anne's wartime diary. As Lejeune (2009) shows in his analysis of the diary, there was no complete original text. Rather, there were two incomplete texts, and the process of creating the diary was a complex one that involved rewriting and editing by Anne herself and later editing by her father (Lejeune 2009).

Kitsuse and Cicourel (1963) have identified similar issues in the use of official documents and the statistics based on them. They observe that these sources are often treated as an accurate representation of some social or health reality. However, they argue that using these sources in this way is problematic as they reflect how official agencies categorize specific phenomena, rather than the real incidence or rates in different communities.

Flexibility

Data from letters or diaries can be used in combination with other sources of data in a range of research designs. Elliott (1997) combined research diaries with interviews in her study of illness and help-seeking behaviours. She maintained close contact with participants in the research, visiting them at least three times: once to brief them and give them their diaries; then to give them another diary and to have an initial 'conversations'; and, finally, to conduct in-depth interviews. She used both the conversations and interviews to explore themes identified in the diaries. In the interviews, participants discussed not only the actions recorded in their diaries, but also the actions they had considered but did not take, and those they intended to take at some time in the future.

So why don't health researchers make more use of documents?

Documents are relatively easy to access and contain interesting, usable data, although data protection regulations restrict access to some contemporary records. So it is puzzling that health and other researchers do not make more use of documents, as Prior (2003: 4) has noted: 'In most social science work[,] documents ... are placed at the margins of consideration.'

Prior (2003) argues that social scientists and other researchers tend to value the spoken word, accessed through interviews and other methods, more highly than the written word, the key component of most documents. However, there is a more fundamental problem. An interviewer is in direct contact with those providing the information and can directly influence the interview process. In contrast, researchers using documents, especially pre-existing ones, can exert no such influence. They have to accept and work with what is available. One response to such limitations is to focus on the ways in which documents are created and used rather than on the intrinsic information they contain. Thus, Prior and his colleagues (2002) showed that documents played a key role in a cancer genetics clinic. To identify and communicate individuals' cancer risk, clinicians used a computer program – Cyrillic – 'that draws a family tree and provides a numerical estimate for an individual' (Prior et al. 2002: 248). This was used to explain and make visible risk estimates.

Another example of the difficulties of using documents is dealing with missing data and the purpose of document creators. Garfinkel (1967: 191) tried to use routine clinical records to identify the criteria used in a psychiatric outpatient clinic to select patients and allocate treatments. He found that in most of the 661 files accessed, key data were missing. He argued that while the records were 'bad' from a research perspective, they were 'good' from the organization's perspective, as they fitted within organizational routines and were fit for organizational purposes. The main purpose of the records was not to collect accurate research data. Case files recorded and justified the decisions made by the clinic staff about the person who was the subject of the file. It was both a record and an account of the treatment the clinic agreed to provide. It was a form of therapeutic contract designed to provide a basis for the relationship between the patient and the clinic. Garfinkel (1967) argued that such documents did not have fixed meanings, but were used and interpreted in the context of interactions with patients, and professionals used them to 'make a case' and justify a course of action.

Analysing documentary material

There are a number of dimensions to analysing documentary material – including statistical analysis, content analysis and structural analysis. Each of these dimensions will now be considered in turn.

Statistical analysis

Researchers using experimental or survey methods will see the entries in such documents as recording specific forms of social reality that are reflected in recurring themes in the data. These can be coded within each case and organized into categories or variables. The data relevant to each variable for each case can then be expressed as a number (Moser and Kalton 1971). Such coding creates a data set which can be analysed using statistical techniques. The aim of the analysis is to identify relationships between variables and show that they are unlikely to be a product of chance. Parkin and his colleagues (2004) used this approach to examine the ways in which the symptoms of multiple sclerosis varied over time and asked whether such changes were more evident at an individual or group level. Using diary data on health status, through a cross-sectional time series analysis, they found that individuals' health-related quality of life scores tended to be stable and that 'greater variations in scores were observed between individuals rather than within individual cases' (Parkin et al. 2004: 351).

Content analysis

Documents that have not been created within a closely defined structure tend to produce qualitative data, which in written documents take the form of written text. Data may take other forms, such as audio or video recordings. These are usually transcribed to form written text. Researchers interested in the observations on social and health issues in documents can identify these through content analysis.

The starting point is an identification of constituent units in the text through coding. Saldaña (2009: 3) notes that a code should capture the essence of the datum and is usually 'a word or short phrase … [that is] essence-capturing'. Coding is usually an iterative process based on the reading, rereading and marking-up of texts. A researcher will read through an initial text, identifying and marking on the text each code. This process is then repeated with the remaining texts, enabling the researcher to build up a code book. Once a code book is agreed and all texts are coded, a researcher can then explore how these individual codes can be grouped together into categories or themes, and how the themes relate to each other can be explored to extract the meaning from the text. Saldaña (2009: 8) observes that this involves a search for patterns and the theories that explain them, by arranging 'things in a systematic order, to make something part of a system or classification, to categorize'.

Griffiths and Jordan (1998) used this approach in their exploratory diary/interview study of patients' experiences during recovery from a lower-limb fracture. The researchers read through the texts and identified headings and emerging categories and then coded each text. Through their analysis, they noted three major themes that were consistent with a theoretical model evident in the literature. They found that patients went through three stages during their recovery: first, feeling stressed and uncertain, then seeking control, and finally returning to normal.

Structural analysis

Content analysis provides a way of identifying and exploring the relationships between elements of the text. However, it fragments the text, treating it as a means to an end. An alternative approach is to retain the integrity of each text and explore how it works. For instance, researchers who are interested in the ways in which individuals experience danger and misfortune associated with illness can explore how such individuals use personal documents to make sense of structure and communicate their experiences.

Jones and Candlin (2003) examined the diaries that 18 gay men used to record their sexual encounters. Drawing on discourse analysis, they showed that diarists used two main devices to minimize their agency and responsibility for risk taking. The diarists presented their accounts as paired actions so that one thing led to another without explicit decision-making. Their narratives also shifted strategically between timescales, portraying risky behaviour as somehow justified, reasonable, and even 'inevitable'. For the gay men in this study, diary keeping provided a means of resolving one of the challenges of their lifestyle. It enabled them to present themselves as responsible individuals while at the same time describing risky activities, including exposing themselves to HIV infection.

By treating each text as a unit, and by considering how the narrator draws on existing conventions to create the text, it is possible both to make sense of the text and to explore its conventions. Lejeune (1996: 120) observed in his study of nearly 100 dairies of young girls in nineteenth-century France that historians tended to be 'interested in such documents only for the information they contain and neglect the history of the writing practice itself'. He gave each text equal weight as he defined his task as decoding 'the meaning of the texts within their contexts' (Lejeune 1996: 112). He noted that texts reflect dominant discourses.

Crossley (2003) also used this approach to analyse John Diamond's account of living with, and trying to make sense of, oral cancer, first published in *The Times* and then reprinted in a posthumous collection (Diamond 2001). Crossley argues that Diamond used several devices to structure and communicate his experience. In the first, early pre-cancer stage, Diamond raised the possibility of cancer, but distanced himself from this. In the second, he gave detailed descriptions of the treatment process that alternated with periods of remission. The third device was relative silence about the cancer and there is the final unspoken narrative of dying.

How documentary material can be used when presenting findings

Using numbers

If a researcher uses numbers and statistical analysis, it is important to present these in an interesting way, perhaps through visual presentations. Generally, the simpler the analysis, the easier it is to present visually. For example, the products of univariate analyses can be presented as bar charts, pie charts or histograms. Bivariate analyses can be presented as scatter diagrams. It may be more difficult to present the results of multivariate analyses visually.

Coxon (1996: 109), in his analysis of the Project SIGMA diaries, started his analysis and discussion of sexual sessions with a simple description of the number of sexual acts per session: 'The average (mean) is quite low (1.75 for most data-sets), but there is a very long tail: some sessions are quite long, and a few very long.' He then moved on to a more complex analysis to explore the structure of acts – that is, the relationship between different elements of sex acts. He used multidimensional scaling to produce a table of the co-occurrence of sex acts and a map in which each act was positioned to indicate its association with other acts. Using this analysis, Coxon was able to explore the relationship between sex acts, showing that some acts, such as oral sex, tended to be reciprocal, while others, such as penetrative sex, tended to be asymmetric or 'gendered'.

Developing themes in qualitative data

Content analysis of documents involves taking a number of written texts, breaking them into their constituent parts and reassembling these parts into a new scientific text. One way of presenting such ideas is to describe how they developed out of the analysis of the text, and then to provide illustrative sections of that text.

Developing case studies

Structural analysis focuses on the ways in which documents are created and how their creators achieve their purpose. The emphasis is on the narrative and how the narrators tell their story and how the readers understand it. One way of showing how texts are created and used is through case studies that include contextual information on the social and personal setting of each case and demonstrate how the narrator makes use of established conventions to talk or write about themselves. Simons (1996), in her study of the ways in which women used diaries in the eighteenth and nineteenth centuries, explored how women like Hester Thrale and Fanny Burney used the privacy of diary writing to subvert conventional literary forms and the gender stereotypes that excluded them from public life and achieve active agency. They used diaries to express both their grievances and create an alternative life. Case Study 6.1 sheds further light on how diaries might be used alongside other methods in contemporary health research.

Using documents to explore stroke survivors' experiences

Documents are often used alongside other sources and in our research in 2004 and 2005 on how individuals who had experienced a stroke sought to rebuild their lives, we used both interviews and documents (Alaszewski 2019). We recruited 43 younger stroke survivors. Over the 18 months of the study there was some attrition: 38 survivors completed the second interview, 34 the third and 33 all four. Of the 20 survivors who initially agreed to keep a diary for a week each month, eight changed their mind, two kept a diary but decided not to give it to the research team and ten kept and gave us their diaries. The data from the interviews and diaries followed the same pattern, but the diary data were more vivid and detailed. For example,

(Continued)

CASE STUDY 6.1

(Continued)

Mrs Jenner (all names are psuedonyms), who was 43 at the time she had her stroke, described the impact of post-stroke pain in both.

Second interview

'I've felt pretty much suicidal and what have you and wished myself dead. I wished I'd died when I had my stroke in the first place because I was failing so badly to function – to be able to function properly. It was a nightmare. It was all I could do to drag myself out of bed, but you know. And only my mum knew how much pain I was in.'

Diary entry (Sunday, 3 October):

'Laid in until 8.30 am – having had a rough night – spent in pain – I'm getting sick on the pain. It's constant and I get no relief – despite the fact that my GP increased my pain relief – I DREAD THE NIGHTS!!'

The dairies provided survivors with an opportunity to tell their own stories. The following extract is from Mrs Jarman's diary. At the time of her stroke, she was 34 years old and she lived with her husband and two children. Previously, she had been a playgroup worker, and had been setting up the business Partytime. The following extract was an entry written nine months after her stroke.

Diary entry (Tuesday, 10 August):

'I got up at 8am today as I am waiting for a new fridge to arrive as our old one has let us down (not bad for 14 years use). It is now 10:45 AM and I am typing this. My forehead is still a bit numb but I have taken my tablets this morning so hopefully should get better by tomorrow. Alice [daughter] has just come and asked if we can go to Toys R Us today – no was the answer, it won't hurt to have a day in and they have plenty to amuse them.'

'I felt very sad on Sunday afternoon, it came out of the blue but when I opened my cupboard to see all my unopened catalogues for Partytime (my new career started last September) I felt bereaved as I was so good at it and was doing so well and this year was going to be full of pride for myself and money coming in, thanks to my achievements and all of a sudden – bang it's been stopped. I know to count my blessings and maybe this is a sign to say look how far I have come. Not so long ago I would have given anything to walk, or just eat at the table without the balance in my head pulling to the right. So there you go; a moment of sadness for something that once was and maybe will again but maybe never again who knows? If Partytime had not come into my life then I would not feel anxious about it. But that is like preferring not to love so as not to feel the loss when someone dies and "if ifs and ands were pots and pans there'd be no need for tinkers!" On a more lighter note Janet (Partytime leader) had just called me and invited me along to the next launch of Christmas products – she must of known how I was feeling sad.'

Mrs Jarman used time in this extract to communicate about her situation. Not only did she date her entry (twice), but she also explicitly anchored her narrative in the present by specifying the moment she was writing the entry: 'It is now 10:45 AM and I am typing this.' Her first entry was grounded in the present, the sensations in her head and her conversations with her daughter, but she set this present within the near past, 'I got up at 8am today', and the near future, 'have a day in' and 'should be better by tomorrow'. The second entry expanded the timeframes, referring back at the start to an event a few days before and forward to an event in the near future, the launch of the Christmas products. This expansion signalled an implicit reflection on the impact of the past on the future. It referred back to the moment of the stroke – 'the bang' – and linked this metaphor to a more recent unanticipated and unpleasant event that 'came out of the blue'. Readers who share her language and culture can understand and make sense of her feelings. Underpinning her narrative is an interweaving of abstract and personal time. In terms of time past, there is an underpinning of the narrative, implicit reference to the idea of a career, progress over time that has been lost and replaced with a more immediate struggle with physical impairments.

Ethical issues

All health research must not only be ethical, it must also be seen to be ethical. When researchers ask individuals to create documents for the purposes of their research, they need to be aware of their responsibility to protect those who participate in their research. The creation of a personal document involves an investment of time and energy and, in some cases, a personal risk if the subject matter of the document challenges social norms. The researcher must be aware of participants' commitment and ensure that their investment is properly recognized and not apply undue pressure. The researcher should provide a written description of the research project and what is expected and gain their informed consent. They should also provide a 'document creator' so that the participant knows what is expected and how to contact the researcher if they need further support.

Documents contained in public archives are, unless there are specific restrictions of access and use, in the public domain. However, it is prudent to consider how, and in what ways, the researcher has a responsibility to those who created the documents and, if they are dead, their descendants. It may be appropriate to seek the views of a research ethics committee.

Researchers who want to use contemporary records need the informed consent of the patients as well as health professionals. There are regulations about the use of electronic records, to protect the interests of individuals, and some health care agencies, such as the National Health Service in the United Kingdom, treat traditional paper records in the same way. Thus, the researcher who wishes to use contemporary health records not only has to gain the approval of relevant keepers of these records, but also the approval of the subjects of those records.

Reading health research based on documents

In reading health research based on documents, you should start by considering the author's description of how and why they used documents. In particular, you should reflect on the following issues:

- Was the design of the project fit for purpose and was the use of documents necessary and appropriate?
- Which documents were selected, and how and in what ways could the selection process introduce bias?
- What was the nature of these documents, who constructed them and for what purpose? How and in what ways was the original purpose aligned with the aims and objectives of the researcher?

Having considered the appropriateness of the documents in terms of the aims and objectives of the research, you should also consider how the documents are used in the publication. In particular, you should consider whether the research is focused on the ways in which the documents are constructed and used, or whether data are being accessed by analysing the content of the documents. If it is the former, then questions should be asked as to what sort of additional information is being used to provide insight into the purpose of the document and how it has been constructed. If the researchers are drawing on the documents as a source of information, ask how relevant information is being extracted and how the analysis of the data is structured.

Conclusion

In this chapter I have examined the nature and potential of using documents in health research: to investigate the resources required, the strengths and weaknesses of the method and the way that data derived from documents can be collected, analysed and presented. The value of this comparatively neglected source of data in health research cannot be overstated, particularly given the insights it provides into areas that are otherwise often difficult or impossible to access directly. The distinctive value of the document for research is underlined in Exercise 6.1.

Exercise 6.1   Using documents in research into the experience of stroke

The following exercise is designed to make you think about the ways in which documents can be used in health research. As well as this chapter, additional material can be accessed from a library or the internet.

You want to apply to a charity for funding to undertake a study of the ways in which the experience of stroke has changed over the last 300 years in the United Kingdom.

1. **What sort of documents could you use?**
   - Consider the range of possible documents, including official records, personal documents, literature, newspapers and pamphlets, medical textbooks.
   - Consider where such documents might be retained.
   - How can you access appropriate documents?
   - How will you deal with changing terminology over time?

2. **How will you select the documents for your study?**
   - Consider what sort of design you want to use.
   - Consider whether you wish to concentrate on one type of document or compare and contrast.
   - How will you judge how 'typical' documents are?

3. **How will you analyse documents?**
   - Will you need to transcribe them?
   - Will the analysis be primarily qualitative, quantitative or both? Do you have access to appropriate support, such as statistical advice or support for qualitative software packages?
   - Will you want to use a software package to help with the analysis?

4. **What sort of resources will you need?**
   - Can you calculate an approximate time budget and identify travel and equipment costs?

5. **How will you present your findings?**
   - Who do you see as the main users of your findings and what are their needs?
   - How will you structure publications, such as reports, articles and presentations?
   - How will you present the evidence supporting your findings?

Recommended further reading

This is a flagship entry in the new Sage methods encyclopaedia that provides a comprehensive overview of the different ways in which one type of document, the diary, can be used for social and health research:

Alaszewski, A. (2020, forthcoming) 'Diaries', in P. A. Atkinson, S. Delamont, M. A. Hardy and M. Williams (eds), *The SAGE Encyclopaedia of Research Methods*. London: Sage. Available at: https://kar.kent.ac.uk/id/eprint/66620

Having made major contributions to the study of autobiography, Philip Lejeune decided to explore the reasons why, and the ways in which, 'ordinary' people write a diary. This text provides a summary of his findings, including reflections on the origins, theory and practice of diary keeping:
Popkin, J. and Rak, J. (eds) (2009) *Philip Lejeune: On Diary*. Honolulu: University of Hawaii Press.

This collection brings together critical analyses of the use of documents from a wide range of sources. Volume I examines documents as a source of data and evidence, Volume II reflects on the social construction of documents, Volume III considers how people use and do things with documents, and Volume IV explores the ways in which documents shape actions and networks:
Prior, L. F. (ed.) (2011) *Using Documents and Records in Social Research*, Volumes I–IV. Los Angeles: Sage.

This is an overview of the strategies and debates surrounding the diverse range of documents that can be employed in research, giving examples of their use. Prior adopts a broad definition of documents and is particularly interested in how they are created and used:
Prior, L. F. (2003) *Using Documents in Social Research*. London: Sage.

References

Alaszewski, A. (2006a) *Using Diaries for Social Research*. London: Sage.

Alaszewski, A. (2006b) 'Diaries as a source of suffering narratives: A critical commentary', *Health, Risk and Society*, 8(1): 43–58.

Alaszewski, A. (2019) 'Using repeat interviewing and diary keeping to research the impact of life-threatening events: The example of stroke survivors' narratives', in A. Olofsson and J. O. Zinn (eds), *Researching Risk and Uncertainty: Methodologies, Methods and Research Strategies*. Basingstoke: Palgrave Macmillan.

Bolger, N., Davis, A. and Rafaeli, E. (2003) 'Diary methods: capturing life as it is lived', *Annual Review of Psychology*, 54: 579–616.

The Chambers Dictionary (2008) 11th edition. Edinburgh: Chambers Harrap Publishers.

Chapman, S., Alpers, P., Agho, K. and Jones, M. (2006) 'Australia's 1996 gun law reforms: Faster falls in firearm deaths, firearm suicides, and a decade without mass shootings', *Injury Prevention*, 12(6): 365–72. Available at: doi: 10.1136/ip.2006.013714

Clarkson, L. (2003) 'Documentary sources', in R. L. Miller and J. D. Brewer (eds), *The A–Z of Social Research*. London: Sage.

Corti, L. (2003) 'Documentary sources', in R. L. Miller and J. D. Brewer (eds), *The A–Z of Social Research*. London: Sage.

Coxon, A. P. M. (1996) *Between the Sheets: Sexual Diaries and Gay Men's Sex in the Era of AIDS*. London: Cassell.

Crossley, M. L. (2003) '"Let me explain": Narrative employment and one patient's experience of oral cancer', *Social Science and Medicine*, 56: 439–48.

Diamond, J. (2001) *Snake Oil and Other Preoccupations*. London: Vintage.

Elliott, H. (1997) 'The use of diaries in sociological research on health experience', *Sociological Research Online*, 2(2). Available at: www.socresonline.org.uk/socresonline/2/2/7.html

Garfinkel, H. (1967) 'Good organizational reasons for "bad" clinical records', in H. Garfinkel, *Studies in Ethnomethodology*. Englewoods Cliffs, NJ: Prenctice-Hall.

Griffiths, H. and Jordan, S. (1998) 'Thinking of the future and walking back to normal: An exploratory study of patients' experiences during recovery from lower limb fracture', *Journal of Advanced Nursing*, 28: 1276–88.

Jones, R. H. and Candlin, C. N. (2003) 'Constructing risk across timescales and trajectories: gay men's stories of sexual encounters', *Health, Risk and Society*, 5: 199–213.

Jordanova, L. (2000) *History in Practice*. London: Arnold.

Kitsuse, J. L. and Cicourel, A. V. (1963) 'A note on the uses of official statistics', *Social Problems*, 11(2): 131–9.

Lejeune, P. (1996) 'The "Journal de Jeune Fille" in nineteenth century France', in S. L. Bunkers and C. A. Huff (eds), *Inscribing the Daily: Critical Essays on Women's Diaries*. Amherst, MA: University of Massachusetts Press.

Lejeune, P. (2009) 'How Anne Frank rewrote the diary of Anne Frank', in J. Popkin and J. Rak (eds), *Philip Lejeune: On Diary*. Honolulu: University of Hawaii Press.

MacFarlane, A. (1970) *The Family Life of Ralph Josselin: A Seventeenth-Century Clergyman: An Essay in Historical Anthropology*. Cambridge: Cambridge University Press.

Miller, K. A. (1985) *Emigrants and Exiles: Ireland and the Irish Exodus to North America*. New York: Oxford University Press.

Moser, C. A. and Kalton, C. (1971) *Survey Methods in Social Investigation*. London: Heinemann.

Parkin, D., Rice, N., Jacoby, A. and Doughty, J. (2004) 'Use of a visual analogue scale in a daily patient diary: Modelling cross-sectional time-series data on health-related quality of life', *Social Science and Medicine*, 59: 351–60.

Penn Library (2004) *Finding Diaries: Research Guide*. Available at: http://gethelp.library.upenn.edu/guides/general/diaries.html

Plummer, K. (2001) *Documents of Life 2: An Invitation to Critical Humanism*. London: Sage.

Prior, L. F. (2003) Using Documents in Social Research. London: Sage

Prior, L. F., Wood, F., Gray, J., Pill, R. and Hughes, D. (2002) 'Making risk visible: The role of images in the assessment of (cancer) genetic risk', *Health, Risk and Society*, 4(3): 241–58.

Saldaña, J. (2009) *The Coding Manual for Qualitative Researchers*. London: Sage.

Scott, J. C. (1990) *A Matter of Record: Documentary Sources in Social Research*. Cambridge: Polity Press; Oxford: Basil Blackwell.

Scott, J. C. (2017) *Against the Grain: A Deep History of the Earliest States*. New Haven, CT: Yale University Press.

Sheridan, D. (ed.) (1991) *The Mass-Observation Diaries: An Introduction*. The Mass-Observation Archive (University of Sussex Library) and the Centre for Continuing Education, Falmer: University of Sussex. Available at: www.sussex.ac.uk/library/massobs/diaries

Simons, J. (1996) 'Invented lives: Textuality and power in early women's diaries', in S. L. Bunkers and C. A. Huff (eds), *Inscribing the Daily: Critical Essays on Women's Diaries*. Amherst, MA: University of Massachusetts Press.

Stone, A. A., Shiffman, S., Schwartz, J. E., Broderick, J. E. and Hufford, M. R. (2003) 'Patient compliance with paper and electronic diaries', *Controlled Clinical Trials, 24*: 182–99.

Thomas, A. J. (2015) *Cholera: The Victorian Plague*. Barnsley: Pen and Sword History.

Weber, M. (1978) *Economy and Society*. Berkeley, CA: University of California Press.

WW2 People's War Team (2004) *About WW2 People's War*. Available at: www.bbc.co.uk/dna/ww2/About

7

Unstructured and Semi-structured Interviews in Health Research

JACQUELINE LOW

Chapter objectives

- To explore the advantages of unstructured and semi-structured interviews
- To give an account of the stages of a project using these methods
- To consider issues of data collection and techniques for data analysis
- To discuss issues of validity, reliability and generalizability and techniques for enhancing rigour
- To show how to present research findings and how to read research in this area.

Introduction

Unstructured and semi-structured interviews are a favoured method of data collection in qualitative research in the social sciences (Silverman 2014), as well as in studies of health and health care (Chafe 2017). They are also used in nursing studies (Gelling 2014) and in other evidence-based clinical research (Curry 2016) where 'lay knowledge' has contributed to health policy and practice. They are essential tools, especially where there are sensitive issues, vulnerable informants, or the researcher faces particular challenges in obtaining information (Dempsey et al. 2016). The unstructured interview – also referred to as the in-depth, open-ended, narrative or the long interview – is useful in these contexts. Semi-structured interviews are of particular relevance where researchers have narrower and specific research questions. Almost all of the methodological techniques employed in these interviews are standard, irrespective of substantive context.

The advantages of using unstructured and semi-structured interviews

Unstructured and semi-structured interviews differ from survey research and the structured questionnaire. As discussed in Chapter 3, quantitative methods set out with specific questions in mind to test a particular hypothesis. In contrast, research from an interpretivist theoretical perspective uses qualitative methods and takes an inductive approach that provides access to the subjective perceptions of individuals and the meaning they give to their experiences. In this case, hypotheses emerge and are tested throughout the process of data collection and analysis. While quantitative data provides invaluable contexts for qualitative findings by furnishing data concerning the number and demographic characteristics of people with a chronic illness (Silverman 1998), it can tell us less about the lived experiences of these individuals. Thus, many argue that the best way to gain access to experiences of health and illness, where people already feel disempowered, is the unstructured interview. An example is the study by Engström and colleagues (2013) of the successful use of unstructured interviews with people on mechanical ventilation.

Corbin and Morse (2003) and others have discussed with clarity the advantages of the unstructured interview, which also apply to the semi-structured interview. These have been summarized in Box 7.1.

Box 7.1   The advantages of unstructured and semi-structured interviews

As Corbin and Morse (2003) note, there are many advantages of unstructured and semi-structured interviews:

- They are a cost-effective way of collecting a great deal of data in a relatively short timeframe.
- They are useful when exploring research areas that are complex or about which little is known.
- They can address how and why questions – that is, they allow researchers to explore the perceptions of individuals and how they interpret their experiences.

- They are flexible, allowing the researcher to pursue emergent themes and follow the lead of the interviewee about how they construct a particular phenomenon, thus gaining new insights.
- The pace of unstructured and semi-structured interviews can be adjusted throughout. This is particularly useful in dealing with people who are ill, may tire easily, or who begin to feel pain.

In addition, others have noted that unstructured and semi-structured interviews:

- Allow the researcher the opportunity to seek ongoing informed consent. This is important when dealing with sensitive issues (Smythe and Murray 2000).
- Give informants more control over what gets discussed, and how it is discussed (Johnson and Rowlands 2012).
- Allow researchers the opportunity to reflect on, and distance themselves from, their tacit knowledge of the topic under study (Tracy 2010).

Stages of research using unstructured or semi-structured interview techniques

The first step in carrying out a qualitative study is to decide on your research question(s) and then carry out a literature review. The questions you wish to address will inform the choice of an unstructured or semi-structured method for data collection. The next task is to recruit informants.

Recruiting research participants

Most commonly, 'purposeful' sampling is used where informants are selected who have specific knowledge about the research question (Silverman 2014). This is made easier if informants are members of a pre-existing group or if they congregate in particular places (Johnson and Rowlands 2012). Alternatively, organizations such as physicians' professional associations or health consumer groups like the Multiple Sclerosis Society can be approached in order to make contact with potential informants. Hospital administrators can also be asked for help in recruiting participants. This is known as the 'health system' model of recruitment, where health service providers or agencies may provide help in contacting patients and/or recruit on behalf of the research team (Vat, Ryan and Etchegary 2017). However, there are ethical issues to consider. In the United Kingdom, issues related to the confidentiality of records may preclude this form of access, although if the research is considered a high priority, a service provider may agree to publicize a study and ask for participants to contact the researcher directly if they would like to take part in a two-stage process. Only when permission has been received should details be given to a researcher. Chapter 19 discusses this and other ethical issues in research further.

In many cases, there is no specific setting in which to recruit people. For example, when I first began researching the lay use of alternative therapies in Canada, there were few holistic health centres and, as I did not want to limit my analysis to the clients of any one type of alternative practitioner, there was no one setting in which to recruit informants (Low 2004). Therefore, I had to use a combination of snowball sampling (that is, asking one informant to suggest another) and convenience sampling (that is, contacting known, rather than randomly selected, informants) in making contact (Silverman 2014). Using 'insider awareness' (Chavez 2008), where the researcher has personal experience of the substantive topic or social world under study, I began convenience sampling by approaching an acquaintance who had used alternative health care. Snowball sampling occurred at the end of each interview when I asked informants if they knew of anyone else who would be interested in taking part in the study. Researchers should keep track in field notes of how they have made contact with informants, as well as noting the nature of any relationships between informants. They can then differentiate in their analysis between patterns that reflect friendship or other related networks from more general patterns in the data (Low 2004). Snowball sampling is discussed further in Chapters 5 and 11.

Decisions must also be made about how many informants to recruit, as well as how many interviews to conduct. For instance, in research using grounded theory, it is the concept, not the informant, which is the unit of analysis (Corbin and Strauss 1990). Theoretically, therefore, one interview is sufficient provided it is adequate in terms of conceptual richness. However, a commonly used guideline is 20–30 informants (Charmaz 2014). In narrative analysis, and some types of linguistic or discourse analyses, the number of interviews is typically very small. Enough data must be collected to enable the researcher to reach 'theoretic saturation' (Glaser and Strauss 1967). Theoretic saturation is satisfied when the data reflect a conceptual richness that both accounts for 'variations' in the data and allows for a detailed description of the 'processes' informants experience (Low 2019, forthcoming).

The unstructured and semi-structured technique

It would be a mistake to conclude that the central difference between the unstructured and semi-structured interview is the absence or presence of structure as, in practice, there is no interview technique that is totally devoid of structure. At the very least, an unstructured interview must be informed by a research question or questions and researchers should have some idea of how they will begin and end the interview. As the name suggests, unstructured interviews do not follow a set path and may vary in length and/or richness. The questions employed in the unstructured interview should be open-ended and as non-directive as possible. This means that the researcher should say as little as possible, allowing informants to tell their stories in their own fashion. The unstructured interview typically opens with a 'grand tour' question (Leech 2002). These are questions that encourage informants to begin speaking without directing the content or substance of their discourse. For instance, a researcher might begin by saying something like: 'Tell me about your experiences in communicating with your physician.' In contrast, when using the semi-structured interview, several questions that are prepared in advance will be asked of all informants. However, unlike a survey questionnaire, which features consistently worded, close-ended and strictly ordered questions, there is no epistemological imperative to ask questions in exactly the same way or in the same order in each individual unstructured or semi-structured interview. Indeed, questions may need to be modified to fit the biographical and socio-cultural contexts that shape informants' lives.

In both semi-structured and unstructured interviewing, subsequent questions are based on what the informant says, and prompts are used to assist informants in telling their story, and to solicit further information, clarification or explanation. According to Leech (2002), floating prompts such as looking for and noting features of everyday speech – such as eyebrow raises or the repetition of a keyword – maintain the flow of responses without undue interruption of the informant's narrative. Planned prompts, or probes, are used when further explanation is required, or when the researcher wishes to delve deeper. Recapitulation probes are also used where informants are asked to 'retell parts of stories'. In so doing, they may add new details (Laylor, Begley and Galavan 2009). Some researchers choose to wait until the interview is complete before probing, as they believe that any type of interruption of the informant's speech will affect the meaning of the findings. Others choose to prompt as the interview progresses, which is often a better strategy as themes can be pursued in the context in which they emerge. Any potentially sensitive question, including those related to age, gender, class, income and ethnic background, should be asked at the conclusion of the interview after trust and rapport between the researcher and informant have been established.

Researchers must also be aware of the implications of silence in unstructured and semi-structured interviews. Periods of silence may indicate that an informant is becoming tired, that illness or disability is compromising their ability to speak, or that they are in pain. Silence may also indicate a breach of communication norms. For example, something the researcher says may literally 'silence' the informant. Informants may silence the researcher as well when they decline to answer a question (Charmaz 2002). The researcher must therefore listen carefully and prompt judiciously in response to what informants say, or do not say. Silence should be noted and accounted for in the analysis. Also important for researchers using an unstructured or semi-structured interview technique is that they practise reflexivity. This means that they must be aware of their 'tacit' or assumed knowledge about the topic they are researching, and they should be able to distance themselves from it so that they do not make unwarranted assumptions about their informants' views. Thus, they must remember to ask informants to explain what they mean (Tracy 2010).

Resourcing the unstructured and semi-structured interview

In addition to technical skills, unstructured and semi-structured interviews require important interpersonal skills, as well as access to resources. One such resource is willing and informed research participants. Not all potential informants are sufficiently motivated to participate in an unstructured interview as a greater commitment in terms of time and emotional energy is required (Johnson and Rowlands 2012). Furthermore, not all informants are articulate and not all interviews result in an equally high degree of conceptual richness. However, it would be a mistake for the researcher to equate succinct responses with a lack of richness of the data, especially in cases where illness or disability constrain the informant's speech. As Booth and Booth (1996: 66) argue, 'it is possible for people to communicate a story in one word answers. Even single words can leave a big wash.'

Another significant resource required using unstructured and semi-structured interviewing is time. Setting up and conducting interviews, and particularly transcribing and analysing data, are time-greedy activities. Time is required to recruit informants, schedule interviews and allow the scope for re-interviews. In health research, more time may be required as, for example, informants with a chronic illness may tire easily and several short interviews may be necessary. Analysis of the vast amount of data that results from unstructured and semi-structured interviews is also time-consuming. Unstructured and semi-structured interviews are typically long, and transcription of one audio-taped interview can take up to ten hours and can 'generate 20–40 pages of single-spaced text' (Pope, Ziebland and Mays 2000: 114). Thematic or comparative coding, where transcripts are read, and re-read, several times throughout the analysis, can take even longer.

If unstructured and semi-structured qualitative interviews require more of informants, they also require more from the researcher. Glaser and Strauss (1967) argue that researchers must develop 'theoretic sensitivity' so that they can judge when theoretic saturation and conceptual richness have been reached. Furthermore, locating and contacting informants, especially in medical settings, can be difficult and requires reserves of energy and ingenuity. Unstructured and semi-structured interviews also mean that researchers need to invest much of themselves and their emotions in the interview process (Charmaz 2014). Corbin and Morse (2003: 344) argue that interviewers can 'become involved in the story and reach out with empathy to participants'. Consequently, the unstructured and semi-structured interview method is always demanding and can often be exhausting for the researcher.

Collecting and analysing unstructured and semi-structured interview data

There are several aspects to collecting and analysing unstructured and semi-structured interview data – principally, recording data, methods of data analysis and data coding.

Recording data

It is important to record unstructured and semi-structured interviews as an informant's words must be presented verbatim in the analysis to preserve meaning (Johnson and Rowlands 2012). Silverman (2014) advocates the use of video recording to better record the interactive aspects of the semi-structured or unstructured interview. However, this may be felt to be too intrusive and may jeopardize confidentiality. Digital audio-recorders are currently the best means of audio-recording interviews. They are typically very small and even the least expensive have sharp sound and little if any interference in playback. Digital audio files can be imported into qualitative analysis software and synchronized with the corresponding transcript. NVivo 11 also has a function that allows direct coding of audio files. The advent of digital technology in qualitative methodology means that researchers need to use encryption protocols and secure password-protected storage of all digital data. See Chapter 19 for a wider discussion of ethical protocols in qualitative research.

The setting chosen for the interview should be one in which the informant feels comfortable and affords a degree of privacy. For instance, if the interviews are with hospital nurses and focus on workplace stress, interviewing them in the hospital where they work would not engender trust and, thus, their workplace would not be a suitable setting for the interview. In all cases, the researcher should ask the informant where he or she would like the interview to take place and efforts must be made to accommodate the informant's wishes.

In addition, there are situations where audio-recording is difficult. An informant may refuse to give permission for the interview to be recorded or the interview might take place in noisy or crowded locations were recording is impossible. In such cases, researchers must use their note-taking skills during, and after, the interview to preserve as much of the informant's actual words as possible. Even when audio or video recording the interview, field notes should be taken that include non-verbal aspects of the interview, such as facial expressions, body language, the setting and informant/researcher interaction, as these may affect interpretation (Oltmann 2016).

Methods for data analysis

Discussions about how to analyse, such as making decisions about how to collect data, are informed by the epistemological assumptions held by the researcher. For instance, if the researcher is aiming to develop a grounded theory, analytic induction is a technique for deriving theory from empirical research, in contrast to a deductive approach, where data are collected to support or refute an existing theory (see also Chapter 3). In the case of grounded theory, theoretic sampling and comparative coding are the forms of analysis most employed. According to Glaser and Strauss (1967: 45), theoretic sampling is a method by which 'the analyst jointly collects, codes, and analyses data and decides what data to collect next and where to find them, in order to develop theory as it emerges'. Open coding is 'the process of breaking down, examining, comparing, conceptualizing, and categorizing data' (Corbin and Strauss 1990: 61) – a technique also covered in Chapter 6 of this book.

Other theoretical approaches dictate different types of coding. For instance, Baker (2002: 778) asserts that within ethnomethodology, informants' stories are understood 'as accounts rather than reports'. Such analysis therefore involves coding for individuals' explanations for their beliefs and behaviour. Depending on the mode of analysis followed, the style of transcription will also vary. Thus, in the case of narrative analysis transcription, this will include recording pauses, hesitations, the timing of responses and other linguistic devices, in addition to the words spoken by the informant. The analyst will then be able to discern how a text is structured and organized in order to bring out its meaning.

Data coding

Regardless of the particular mode of analysis chosen, coding of unstructured interviews involves thematic analysis (Ryan and Bernard 2003). More specifically, the rigorous and systematic analysis of data results in the development of concepts and categories that emerges from the words of informants, culminating in the development of conceptual and explanatory models (Silverman 2014). This kind of analysis means more than merely count-ing occurrences of key terms, and while qualitative researchers should note repetition of themes in the data (Ryan and Bernard 2003), the researcher analysing unstructured or semi-structured interviews more often codes for similarity of meaning rather than for repetition of words or phrases, as people hardly ever express themselves in exactly the same way. This does not indicate that they are inconsistent in terms of the conceptual meaning intended. For example, in my analysis of the lay model of alternative health and healing, one infor-mant used the words 'inner self', while another spoke about her 'higher self', but what they were both talking about was the importance of drawing on their own spiritual power to heal themselves (Low 2004).

It is important to pay attention to discordant elements or seeming contradictions within the discourse of informants as they can give insight into its deeper meaning. In addition, attention must be paid in the analysis to divergent themes: what some researchers call 'devi-ant cases' (Silverman 1998). This is essential for capturing conceptual richness and enhanc-ing the validity of unstructured and semi-structured interview findings. For instance, in my study of the lay use of alternative therapies, I found that only *one* out of 21 informants said that they had a desire for control over their health and their process of healing. This enabled me to argue that the generic social process of problem solving, not individual motivating factors, better explained informants' health-seeking behaviour (Low 2004).

In analysing qualitative data, it is also useful to look for the use of metaphors and analogies that people rely on in explaining their experiences (Ryan and Bernard 2003). For example, in my research on alternative and complementary health care, the people I interviewed who told me that an attribute of the person engaged in alternative healing was being grounded or centred would use analogies in trying to explain to me what they meant. One person said it is like 'being in the middle and being able to see all the sides around one as opposed to being on the edge … and you're just having to exercise all this energy just to stop from falling off'. Important, too, are indigenous categories embedded in speech, such as the shared language and slang that people use in talking with each other (Ryan and Bernard 2003). For example, Goldman (2014: 3) found that Canadian doctors use the slang term 'Hollywood Code' to refer to doing 'a pretend resuscitation in which it looks like [they were] trying to save [but were not]' in a situation where the patient's heart had stopped but the patient's family were not ready to agree to a 'do not resuscitate' order. Ryan and Bernard (2003: 90) also point out that 'naturally occurring shifts in content', such as a new paragraph in a transcript or 'pauses [or] changes in voice tone' in an audio recording, may indicate themes to explore. The themes that the researcher discerns in the data must then be examined to assess the conceptual relationships they have together. For example, the themes Lawton (1998) found in her analysis of hospice care in the United Kingdom were that there were many references by participants to 'how the body broke down' in serious diseases such as cancers. These could be connected together and allowed her to develop a conceptual model of the 'unbounded body'.

How the researcher goes about the practical task of coding and categorizing is a matter of preference. Some highlight transcripts; others use word-processing search, copy and paste functions; and still others photocopy and physically cut up the transcripts to categorize data. Increasingly, qualitative researchers make use of qualitative analysis software as a tool to aid in categorizing data from unstructured and semi-structured interviews. It is important to be aware that qualitative analysis software does not do the conceptual or analytic work for the researcher, who must still discern themes and develop concepts and categories by reading and rereading the transcripts as well as making analytic notes. Software merely helps in storing, moving and collating large amounts of data. However, the current generation of qualitative analysis software has some very useful functions.

What is most valuable about using qualitative analysis software is the time that it can save in analysing interview transcripts. For example, in an interview project with 30 informants, it would not be uncommon to have almost 1,000 pages of single-spaced interview transcript. If one wished to see if there was a relationship between gender and a particular emergent theme, qualitative analysis software can search for, and collate, all the places in those thousand pages of transcript where such a relationship exists in a matter of minutes. This is a task that would take hours if it was done through reading the transcripts and manually noting instances of the relationship. In addition, qualitative analysis software like NVivo 11 can facilitate 'inter-rater reliability'. This is where more than one researcher can code the same transcript as the program keeps track of, and displays, the coding of different researchers. Audio and video files, photographs and other images, as well as social media data such as Twitter feeds, can also be coded in using quality analysis software by more than one researcher.

There is at least one task in qualitative analysis that is accomplished better by qualitative analysis software than can be done manually. This is the development of conceptual models.

Here NVivo 11's automated mapping features are invaluable. Once data are coded into concepts and categories, they can be loaded onto one of three mapping screens where they appear as labelled shapes. These can be easily highlighted and dragged to different positions on the screen as the researcher makes decisions about the hierarchical arrangements within their emergent conceptual model. This kind of diagramming can be done by hand, but it cannot be modified as quickly as is possible when using the software. The critical point here is that thinking conceptually often happens very quickly and the software can keep up with the researcher's thought processes in a way that drawing by hand can never do. Finally, NVivo 11 comes with online help functions and tutorial videos to help new users make the most of what is valuable about qualitative analysis software.

Enhancing rigour

Rigour is an important term that is used to assess the 'quality' of qualitative analysis. There are two approaches in assessing the appropriate terms to use. One, represented by researchers such as Lincoln, Lynham and Guba (2011), argues that qualitative analysis needs its own language. They use terms like 'credibility' and 'trustworthiness', referring to the confidence one can have in the findings. They also use the term 'transferability': that is, the ability to apply the findings from one study or setting to another social context. In contrast, the other camp advocates that, as social scientists, the terms 'validity', 'reliability' and 'generalizability' should be used as they are part of the shared language of all social scientists. However, these terms have specific meanings in the context of qualitative research.

Validity

The validity of unstructured and semi-structured interview findings centres on the richness of the data that are generated by this method. This richness derives, in part, from the fact that the researcher allows the informant to direct the flow of conversation, saying as little as possible. This bolsters the validity of the finding as statements volunteered by informants and the non-directive nature of open-ended questions enhance validity as informants are able to articulate their experiences, rather than having to conform to predetermined answer categories imposed by the researcher (Silverman 2014). Informants can also be asked to review the analysis and provide feedback on whether or not concepts and categories reflect their understanding of their experience, enhancing the validity of findings.

In the case of qualitative research, validity can be understood as 'theoretic' or alternatively 'construct' validity: that is, findings are valid because they correspond to the data collected. For instance, I had occasion to review an article on Dr Spock's breast-feeding manuals from the 1950s and 1960s, prior to its publication. The study was excellent in the sense that the researcher provided a detailed textual analysis of the manuals and contextualized her findings in the appropriate socio-cultural and historical contexts. However, at the end of the article the researcher made statements about how women at the time *felt* after reading these manuals. In terms of 'construct validity', the article was rated as 'poor'. No interviews had been undertaken with women readers, so the researcher would not have had any idea how they felt. Rather, her comments are likely to have reflected her own views.

Reliability

The quantitative notion of reliability, that research instruments continually yield an unvarying measurement, is not only inappropriate to research using unstructured or semi-structured interviews, it is also impossible to achieve using this method of data collection (Kirk and Miller 1986). This is because the social world is dynamic, not static. Consequently, two researchers who interview the same informant at different times using the same questions will invariably collect different data (Becker 1970). However, this should not be taken as an indication that the unstructured or semi-structured interview method is unreliable. Rather, it is that the social context and the informant's perspective have changed over time. Instead, the unstructured or semi-structured interview must satisfy the standards of synchronic reliability; that is, achieve a similarity of observations made within the same time period. They must also achieve consistent observations in line with the researcher's conceptual concerns (Kirk and Miller 1986). More simply, the words that informants use will rarely be the same, yet they can still be conceptually consistent. Concepts and categories must be clearly defined and criteria for including or excluding data as representing a concept or category should be documented. This will help to demonstrate the reliability of the data analysis. Furthermore, any subsequent reader should be able to follow the logic of a project. This must flow from the research questions through the research procedures used in all phases of the research cycle, from recruitment, data collection and analysis to the presentation of findings and the conclusions reached by the researcher.

Generalizability

The researcher must pay particular attention to the nature of the generalizations that can be made from their findings as well as being concerned with validity and reliability. Specifically, they can make what Williams (2000) refers to as 'moderatum generalisation' or 'generalisations about everyday life'. Such generalizations are appropriate to research where the intention is theoretic or conceptual generalization, rather than statistical generalization. This is where an informant's individual perceptions, beliefs and experiences can be seen as indicators of larger socio-cultural features or generic social processes (Blumer 1969). Williams (2000: 215) illustrates what he means by 'moderatum generalisation' by invoking the classic ethnographic analysis by Geertz of the Balinese cockfight, in writing:

> Geertz's claim … 'that every people loves its own form of violence' is an example of such a general feature, which is then reworked and enriched through the specific inferences about the [particular] – the 'cockfight'.

In order to generalize the findings from research using semi-structured or unstructured interviews, the findings must be situated in the relevant historical, socio-cultural, political and biographical context in which they occur (Silverman 1998). For example, Lupton and Chapman (1995) ground their analysis of media coverage of the role played by cholesterol in heart disease in the socio-cultural context of contemporary discourses about food – as being 'healthy' or 'unhealthy'. Biographical context refers to how the social identities of the people who take part in your research shape their actions and experiences. For instance, health status, such as living with chronic illness, may be one biographical factor that shapes experience, perceptions and action. And in doing research with people living with HIV and AIDS in the United States, it really matters whether or not your research is focused before or after the 1980s, when major political and cultural changes regarding LGBTQI (lesbian, gay, bisexual, transgender, queer or questioning, and intersex) rights began to change (Wagaman 2016).

Selected techniques to enhance validity and reliability so that the overall integrity of the findings can be assessed are set out in Box 7.2.

Box 7.2   Techniques to enhance validity, reliability and generalizability

Techniques to enhance validity, reliability and generalizability include:

- Audio-taping interviews and taking comprehensive field notes.
- Systematic transcription and analysis, allowing others to assess how researchers have analysed their data and developed theoretic constructs.
- Using a combination of methods or sources of data, such as observation or documentary analysis (see Chapter 24 for a discussion of triangulation).
- Employing inter-judge or inter-rater techniques – here, more than one researcher codes the transcripts. Comparing coding can increase consistency, reliability and validity in both coding and the subsequent analysis.
- Using a 'member test' or informant validation – here, analysis and early findings are assessed through the informant's confirmation that these reflect accurately their perspectives and experiences.
- Discussing the socio-cultural, historical, political and biographical contexts in which your findings are situated.

Presenting unstructured and semi-structured interview findings

How findings from unstructured and semi-structured interview analysis are presented orally, or in publications, makes an impact on how the rigour of the research will be perceived. For example, when presenting findings from semi-structured or unstructured interviews, informants' speech should be used verbatim as rewording or summarizing inevitably reduces validity by changing the meaning of their words. It also detracts from the reliability of the findings as readers cannot assess the validity of the data for themselves. Ideally, research questions and informant responses should be presented together as answers are inextricably linked to the questions to which they are a response. Furthermore, in order to allow the reader to assess validity, the researcher needs to indicate whether or not the labels applied to concepts and categories presented in the findings emerge from the actual words of the informants or are researcher constructs (Silverman 1998).

It is also important for researchers to indicate whether the quotations selected are representative of some, many or all of the participants in the research. Researchers must make it plain how deviant cases have been accounted for. To this end, Silverman (2014) argues that counting events should be included in presentations. However, presenting findings in the form of percentages may be misleading when the findings are derived from a small number of interviews (Pope, Ziebland and Mays 2000). Finally, by failing to provide discussion of the context that frames the findings, the researcher prevents the reader from assessing the generalizability of the research.

In presenting their findings, researchers should provide detailed descriptions of how reliability and validity have been ensured. They should include excerpts from field notes that describe how data were collected, transcribed and analysed to provide a paper trail to demonstrate the reliability of the findings. Including all of these important aspects of the unstructured and semi-structured interview method can fill several pages of an article or report. Researchers must be aware that many journals, especially those in medicine and nursing, typically publish only very short articles. Editors of such journals may object to lengthy methodology sections or to the inclusion of the large amount of data that is necessary to present the findings adequately. It may therefore be wise for health researchers using this method to include, in the covering letter accompanying their submission, the argument that such information is essential so that both referees and readers can assess the rigour of their study. Another strategy is to publish a separate methodological appendix as a companion to published presentations of the research findings.

Limitations of the unstructured and semi-structured interview method

While conducting unstructured and semi-structured interviewing can be more cost-effective than survey research, a corresponding weakness of the method is the amount of time invested in the analysis of unstructured interview data compared with statistical analysis. In addition, Silverman (2014) concludes that the unstructured interview should never be used as a substitute for observation. He calls into question its usefulness as a stand-alone method and asserts that while unstructured interviews are an effective method of gathering data about what people say, they are less useful as a means of capturing what they do. However, what people say about what they do can provide valid and useful information. It is an account of their experience of what they do. Observation and interview are different methods. They measure different things. Thus, one is not inherently better than the other (Seale 2004). It is also the case that when more than one method of data collection is used, the findings from each can enhance the rigour of the study.

Another weakness of the unstructured interview method is that the data collected are retrospective. It is an informant's description of event(s) that happened in the past, and therefore cannot be an accurate account of their experience at the actual time the event(s) occurred. However, the moment we experience something, it becomes part of our past, thus we always make sense of our lives retrospectively. In the end, all methods have strengths and weaknesses. Good researchers are aware of them and use their informed judgement to select the method appropriate to the research question at hand. This applies no less to the use of unstructured or semi-structured interviews in health research than for other methods. This brings us to an illustrative case study.

CASE STUDY 7.1

The use of semi-structured interviews in research with seniors who rely on domiciliary care services

I conducted a government-partnered study to develop evidence-based policy on sustainable domiciliary care services for seniors in New Brunswick, Canada (Low et al. 2011). It illustrates many of the methodological issues already discussed in this chapter. In this government-partnered study, we used semi-structured interviewing to collect data from people over the age of 65 (over half of whom were between the ages of 80 and 94), who received some form of domiciliary care for activities such as preparing meals, home maintenance or personal care. Semi-structured interviewing was chosen rather than unstructured interviewing because our research question had a specific focus on what support services seniors needed to remain living at home. We needed to know what they wanted.

Recruiting informants

One issue was that recruiting seniors takes time (Jancey et al. 2006). In our research it took four months to recruit the 24 seniors who took part in the interviews. Many seniors opted out as they had serious health problems or were worried that participation might compromise the services they depended on. This was despite the fact that we used the health system model, where the recruitment letter in my name was sent out by the government service providers to all their clients. The letter was sent out on my university letter head and in my name. Clients replied directly to me, so that our government partners had no knowledge of who was taking part in the project, something we explained in the recruitment letter. We also found that some care-givers had dissuaded seniors from participating and, late in the project, we learned that several seniors discarded our recruitment letter because when they saw my academic title 'Dr' on the letterhead, they thought we were offering medical services.

Conducting interviews

This research demonstrated the benefits of semi-structured interviews in terms of their flexibility in data collection. Many participants were very frail and lived with chronic illness and disability. The semi-structured interview allowed us to start and stop interviews when this was necessary when people became tired or were in pain. This gave more scope for probing or seeking clarification by repeating questions or keywords and checking and rechecking that we had understood each other.

Contextualizing findings

One aspect of socio-cultural context that framed our analysis is that New Brunswick is an officially bilingual province, yet is linguistically divided with most French speakers living in the north of the province. Thus, an important aspect of biographical context was that most of our Francophone informants were Catholic and consequently had large families making them less dependent on government support services. About half of our informants were Francophones from birth yet as adults had opted to speak English as that is the dominant language of service providers in the province, making bilingual research team members a necessity.

Reading health research based on unstructured/ semi-structured interviews

As will be apparent from the foregoing, in reading health research based on unstructured and semi-structured interviews, it is important to consider how far:

- The type of the interviews is appropriate in addressing the research question(s)
- Relevant data are being gathered, with suitable richness
- Interviews are properly recorded and coded, in appropriate settings

- Explicit consent has been obtained from the participants
- There are sufficient, well-selected participants
- The interview findings are appropriately contextualized
- The analysis links back to the theoretical approach of the researcher
- Due attention is paid to validity, reliability and generalizability
- Sufficient quotations are given to enable evaluation of the findings
- Suitable consideration is given to the triangulation of the results if more than one method is used.

The complexities of using this method are thrown further into relief by recent efforts to innovate by gathering material using mobile and smart phones (Garcia, Wellford and Smith 2016) and social media platforms (Lunnay et al. 2014) rather than through face-to-face interviewing. The reader should reflect on the implications for conducting the kind of research described in Case Study 7.1 using new methods for data collection as well as how articles on the findings of research using new technologies can be appraised.

Conclusion

The strengths and weaknesses of unstructured and semi-structured interviews in health research have been covered in this chapter – along with the issues that they raise in practice in the various stages of research, from recruiting research participants and resourcing interviews, to analysing data and presenting research findings. These highlight that unstructured and semi-structured interviews can be extremely helpful as a qualitative research method but are not as straightforward to carry out as first meets the eye. A contrast with structured questionnaires can be made by referring to Chapter 13, which covers quantitative survey methods.

Exercise 7.1   The use of unstructured and semi-structured interviews to conduct research into the experience of burns

Using unstructured or semi-structured interviews, you intend to conduct research focused on how individuals who have suffered serious burns experience coping with pain. The burns have left those concerned with severe scarring over large portions of their bodies. Address the following questions:

- How would you go about purposeful sampling in this research?
- What problems would you anticipate in recruiting informants for your study?
- How many informants would you need to participate in the interviews?

- What kind of probing questions do you anticipate would be useful in interviews with these informants?
- What aspects of informant biographies must you be aware of?
- Of what particular socio-cultural, historical and political contexts should you be aware to ground your analysis?
- How might class, gender, stigma and cultural notions of beauty, among other contextual factors, shape the experiences of your informants?
- In addition to unstructured or semi-structured interviews, are there other sources of data you could draw on to increase the validity, reliability and generalizability of your analysis?

Recommended further reading

This is an excellent article that provides a framework for evaluating rigour relevant across a diversity of qualitative research:

Brynjulf, S., Malterud, K. and Midtgarden, T. (2009) 'Toward an agenda for evaluation of qualitative research', *Qualitative Health Research*, *19*(10): 1504–16.

This is an accessible and comprehensive text covering the unstructured interview method in general:

Gubrium, J. F. and Holstein, J. A. (eds) (2012) *Handbook of Interview Research: The Complexity of Craft*. Thousand Oaks, CA: Sage.

This is a comprehensive text that can be recommended on qualitative data analysis:

Silverman, D. (2014) *Interpreting Qualitative Data*, 5th edition. Thousand Oaks, CA: Sage.

References

Baker, C. D. (2002) 'Ethnomethodological analyses of interviews', in J. F. Gubrium and J. A. Holstein (eds), *Handbook of Interview Research: Context and Method*. Thousand Oaks, CA: Sage.

Becker, H. S. (1970) *Sociological Work: Method and Substance*. Chicago, IL: Aldine.

Blumer, H. (1969) *Symbolic Interactionism: Perspective and Method*. Englewood Cliffs, NJ: Prentice-Hall.

Booth, T. and Booth, W. (1996) 'Sounds of silence: Narrative research with inarticulate subjects', *Disability and Society*, *11*: 55–69.

Chafe, R. (2017) 'The value of qualitative description in health services and policy research', *Health Policy*, *12*(3): 12–18.

Charmaz, K. (2002) 'Stories and silences: Disclosures and self in chronic illness', *Qualitative Inquiry*, *8*(3): 302–28.

Charmaz, K. (2014) *Constructing Grounded Theory*. Thousand Oaks, CA: Sage.

Chavez, C. (2008) 'Conceptualizing from the inside: Advantages, complications and demands of insider positionality', *The Qualitative Report*, *13*(3): 474–94.

Corbin, J. M. and Morse, J. M. (2003) 'The unstructured interactive interview: issues of reciprocity and risks when dealing with sensitive topics', *Qualitative Inquiry*, *9*(3): 335–54.

Corbin, J. M. and Strauss, A. L. (1990) 'Grounded theory research: Procedures, canons, and evaluative criteria', *Qualitative Sociology*, *13*(1): 3–21.

Curry, L. A. (2016) 'An open letter to The BMJ editors on qualitative research', *British Medical Journal*, *3*(52): 563.

Dempsey, L., Dowling, M., Larkin, P. and Murphy, K. (2016). 'Sensitive interviewing in qualitative research', *Research in Nursing and Health*, *39*(6): 480–90.

Engström, A., Nyström, N., Sundelin, G. and Rattray, J. (2013) 'People's experiences of being mechanically ventilated in an ICU: A qualitative study', *Intensive and Critical Care Nursing*, *29*(2): 88–95.

Garcia, B., Welford, J. and Smith, B. (2016) 'Using a smartphone app in qualitative research: The good, the bad and the ugly', *Qualitative Research*, *16*(5): 508–25.

Gelling, L. (2014) 'Qualitative research', *Nursing Standard*, *29*(30): 43–7.

Glaser, B. G. and Strauss, A. L. (1967) *The Discovery of Grounded Theory: Strategies for Qualitative Research*. Chicago, IL: Aldine.

Goldman, B. (2014) *The Secret Language of Doctors: Cracking the Code of Hospital Slang*. Toronto: HarperCollins.

Jancey, J., Howat, P., Lee, A., Clarke, A., Shilton, T., Fisher, J. and Iredell, H. (2006) 'Effective recruitment and retention of older adults in physical activity research: PALS study', *American Journal of Health Behavior*, *30*(6): 626–35.

Johnson, J. M. and Rowlands, T. (2012) 'The personal dynamics of in-depth interviewing', in J. F. Gubrium and J. A. Holstein (eds), *Handbook of Interview Research: The Complexity of Craft*. Thousand Oaks, CA: Sage.

Kirk, J. and Miller, M. L. (1986) *Reliability and Validity in Qualitative Research*. Newbury Park, CA: Sage.

Lawton, J. (1998) 'Contemporary hospice care: The sequestration of the unbounded body and "dirty dying"', *Sociology of Health and Illness*, *20*(2): 121–43.

Laylor, J., Begley, C. M. and Galavan, E. (2009) 'Recasting hope: A process of adaptation following fetal anomaly diagnosis', *Social Science and Medicine*, *68*: 462–72.

Leech, B. (2002) 'Asking questions: Techniques for semi-structured interviews', *Political Science and Politics*, *35*(4): 665–8.

Lincoln, Y. S., Lynham, S. A. and Guba, E. G. (2011) 'Paradigmatic controversies, contradictions, and emerging confluences, revisited', in N. K. Denzin and Y. S. Lincoln (eds), *The Sage Handbook of Qualitative Research*, 4th edition. Thousand Oaks, CA: Sage.

Low, J. (2004) *Using Alternative Therapies: A Qualitative Analysis*. Toronto: Canadian Scholars' Press.

Low, J. (2019, forthcoming) 'A pragmatic definition of the concept of theoretical saturation', *Sociological Focus*.

Low, J., Thériault, L., Luke, A., Hollander, M. and van den Hoonaard, D. (2011) *Sustainable Home Support for Seniors in New Brunswick: Insights from Seniors and Social Workers*. Department of Sociology, University of New Brunswick. Report for the Department of Social Development, Government of New Brunswick, Canada.

Lunnay, B., Borlagdan, J., McNaughton, I. D. and Ward, P. (2015) 'Ethical use of social media to facilitate qualitative research', *Qualitative Health Research*, *25*(1): 99–109.

Lupton, D. and Chapman, S. (1995) '"A healthy lifestyle might be the death of you": Discourses on diet, cholesterol control and heart disease in the press and among the lay public', *Sociology of Health and Illness*, *17*(4): 477–94.

Oltmann, S. M. (2016) 'Qualitative interviews: A methodological discussion of the interviewer and respondent contexts', *Forum Qualitative Sozialforschung / Forum: Qualitative Social Research*, *17*(2). Available at: www.qualitative-research.net/index.php/fqs/article/view/2551/3998

Pope, C., Ziebland, S. and Mays, N. (2000) 'Qualitative research in health care: Analysing qualitative data', *British Medical Journal*, *320*: 114–16.

Ryan, G. W. and Bernard, H. R. (2003) 'Techniques to identify themes', *Field Methods*, *15*(1): 85–109.

Seale, C. (2004) *Social Research Methods: A Reader*. London: Routledge.

Silverman, D. (1998) 'The quality of qualitative health research: The open-ended interview and its alternative', *Social Sciences in Health*, *4*(2): 104–18.

Silverman, D. (2014) *Interpreting Qualitative Data*, 5th edition. Thousand Oaks, CA: Sage.

Smythe, W. E. and Murray, M. J. (2000) 'Owning the story: Ethical considerations in narrative research', *Ethics and Behaviour*, *10*(4): 311–36.

Tracy, S. J. (2010) 'Qualitative quality: Eight "big-tent" criteria for excellent qualitative research', *Qualitative Inquiry*, *16*: 837–51.

Vat, L. E., Ryan, D. and Etchegary, H. (2017) 'Recruiting patients as partners in health research: A qualitative descriptive study', *Research Involvement and Engagement*, *3*(15): 1–14.

Wagaman, M. A. (2016) 'Self-definition as resistance: Understanding identities among LGBTQ emerging adults', *Journal of LGBT Youth*, *13*(3): 207–30.

Williams, M. (2000) 'Interpretivism and generalisation', *Sociology*, *34*(2): 209–24.

8

Participant Observation in Health Research

DAVID HUGHES

Chapter objectives

- To introduce readers to the method of Participant Observation (PO)
- To examine its application in the health care field with reference to classic and contemporary research studies
- To outline the rationale for selecting PO rather than other methods, and its strengths and challenges
- To describe the ethical issues raised by PO
- To explain how PO researchers analyse data
- To discuss how PO is evolving and developing.

Introduction

This chapter discusses the method of Participant Observation (PO) in health research. The term PO is sometimes used interchangeably with 'sociological ethnography', but traditionally ethnography is a broader category that includes methods such as the ethnographic interview and the analysis of cultural artefacts, as well as observation. PO is one of the oldest and least 'high tech' research methods, emphasizing as it does the importance of gathering data through observing, interacting with and listening to the human subjects under study. The participant observer typically spends an extended period of time in a natural setting, such as a hospital ward or an intensive care unit, following the activities of staff members, observing particular classes of activities, or generally 'hanging out' with a view to understanding what is going on. It is this requirement for the researcher to participate in social interaction as part of the research process that separates PO from the systematic observational methods used in psychology and organizational studies, where the observer looks on and records, but does not interact (Emerson 1981; McCall 1984). In consequence, there is an extensive literature on field relations and the participant observer role. Although naturalistic observation takes many forms and involves varying degrees of participation, all PO methods share the need to manage social interaction with subjects in the field (Gold 1958).

This chapter examines the characteristics of PO and the types of study that have been carried out in health care settings. It looks at the problems of access and ethics raised by PO studies, the strengths and weaknesses of the approach, the methods and techniques for collecting, coding and analysing data, and identifying and writing up findings. It presents a case study to illustrate how the method is used in practice and reflects on how far the nature of PO research has changed in recent years.

The characteristics of Participant Observation

Almost all recent PO research takes the form of a case study where there is intense observation in a specific setting. PO would not, for example, undertake an investigation of the ecology of a city, nor would it be the method of choice to examine the characteristics of a geographically dispersed social group. In the health field, most PO studies examine a patient or staff group or particular social processes associated with selected settings, such as the emergency ambulance service, the accident and emergency department, the outpatient clinic, a hospital ward, hospice or nursing home. A typical study might last between six months and two years, with the researcher completing several observation periods per week. Usually, a period of relatively unfocused fieldwork, where the researcher 'feels out' the setting and attempts to develop an appropriate field role, will be followed by a strategy to spread observations between different categories of subject and the aspects of activity that need to be covered.

Typically, access will be negotiated first with senior staff, who act as formal gatekeepers to the setting, and then with the various levels of actors who will be the subjects of study. Usually, access will need to be maintained or renewed on an ongoing basis, so that it will remain a preoccupation throughout the period of fieldwork. A handful of studies in settings such as mental hospitals or acute wards (Caudill et al. 1952; Porter 1995) have been carried out covertly, without the knowledge of people in the setting, but for ethical reasons most studies now depend on explicit access agreements, with researchers operating in an open researcher role.

The origins of PO are often traced back to anthropology (Hume and Mulcock 2004) and the Chicago School of Sociology, with the method as we know it today deriving directly from the work of later 'neo-Chicagoan' sociologists, particularly in the sociology of deviance and medical sociology (Fine 1995). Classic health studies focused on the process aspects of health care, such as:

- Professional socialization in medical school (Becker et al. 1961)
- The temporal experience of polio (Davis 1963) and TB care (Roth 1963)
- The management of death in hospital (Sudnow 1968) and the organization of terminal care (Glaser and Strauss 1965)
- The professional socialization of nurses (Olesen and Whittaker 1968).

All these studies involved long periods of fieldwork spent observing and talking with research subjects in natural settings: charting the various stages, transitions or attitudinal shifts associated with professional education, patient 'careers' or illness trajectories.

There is some evidence that changes in the nature of health care systems have resulted in a change in the focus of research. Zussman (1993) has pointed out that the once flourishing tradition of studies of hospitalized patients' social worlds has all but disappeared, as patient throughput speeds up and specialized units replace traditional wards. He contends that the focus of hospital research has shifted from ward culture and felt experience to detailed studies of professional work in specialized settings. Certainly, a series of well-regarded studies deal with professionals and their regulation, such as:

- The research by Dawn Goodwin (2009) on anaesthetic and intensive care practices and the associated technologies.
- The study by Katherine Kellogg (2011) of how surgeons resisted a new regulation limiting the number of hours that residents should work.
- The insider research by Ruth Horowitz (2013) on state medical boards and their deliberations about the licensing, investigation and sanctioning of physicians.

Outside the hospital there has also been interest in patient experience in community settings, including those suffering mental health issues or problems of cultural adjustment. Examples are:

- The study by Anne Fadiman (1998) of the cultural misunderstandings between the Hmong refugee parents who understand their child's fits as a manifestation of spirit disturbance and American paediatricians who diagnose epilepsy.
- The study by Neely Laurenzo Myers (2016) of mental health care and the possibility that patients can exercise agency to bring about service change.

Partly because of major public funding programmes for research in areas such as the National Health Service (NHS) and the delivery and innovative medical technologies, a series of British ethnographies have been undertaken in these areas, such as:

- Studies of how NHS panels ration funding for high-cost treatments (Hughes and Doheny 2011; Russell and Greenhalgh 2012, 2015).
- The investigation by Davina Allen (2014) of how the 'invisible work of nurses' supports and sustains the delivery and organization of health services.
- The study by Alexandra Hillman (2014) of the triage process in a hospital emergency department.
- The paper by Graham Martin and colleagues (2017) on care pathways and quality improvement.

The rationale for employing Participant Observation as a research method

The rationale for using the PO method is bound up with its instrumental effectiveness in answering certain kinds of research question. Qualitative methods have traditionally been concerned with questions of explanation and understanding, rather than with questions about frequency or quantity. These methods may be used at the exploratory stage of research to map out variables in a field and generate hypotheses for testing in later quantitative studies. They can also have a role in making sense of observed correlations or patterns in quantitative data by elucidating the social processes that produce these patterns.

Qualitative studies can provide a snapshot of the behaviour or perspectives of a hard-to-reach or stigmatized group inaccessible via other methods (Wight and Barnard 1993). They have shed light on seemingly illogical aspects of illness behaviour: such as poor compliance with drug prescribing, unsafe sex practices and teenage smoking behaviour. In any situation where the context of a health care intervention or programme or policy is likely to affect outcomes, qualitative studies can help identify real-world factors that may slip below the gaze of experimental or survey research.

In an early and influential paper, Becker and Geer (1957) suggested that PO has clear advantages over interview studies where special in-group languages (such as medical argot) are used; in situations where informants are unwilling to talk or find it difficult to describe an unfolding or complex social process; or where group myths and stereotypes feature centrally in accounts. Other writers have emphasized the importance of obtaining accounts that give an authentic representation of the social world by 'being there' and 'telling it as it is'. However, while PO undoubtedly provides data that could not be obtained via other methods, it is important to avoid a naive realism that overlooks the role of the observer in 'interpreting' or making sense of observational data (Hammersley 1992).

The resources required for Participant Observation

PO is resource-intensive in terms of human resources rather than technology. It makes heavy time demands, but usually involves individuals or small teams rather than the large team characteristic of survey research. The need to build up field relationships over time militates against the kind of 'hired-hand' research common in quantitative projects (Roth 1999). In recent times, many researchers have supplemented the classic tool of the research notebook with the audio recorder to collect and record data, and the computer to analyse data using qualitative data analysis applications, as discussed below.

Audio recording permits more rigorous recording of organizational discourse and is particularly useful when focused interactions, such as patient consultations, case conferences, ward rounds or management meetings occur at key junctures of organizational processes. Several contemporary ethnographies combine elements of field note-based data collection with recording conversation or discourse so that a general description of organizational processes may be illustrated through a series of detailed exemplars. However, the decision to audio-record has significant implications for costs and the nature of data analysis.

Transcribing and analysing recordings are expensive and time-consuming processes – much slower than the reading of conventional field notes – and will probably be beyond the capabilities of a lone researcher who cannot afford secretarial support. Making sense of recorded interactions typically involves forms of sequential or discourse analysis that will represent a steep learning curve for many qualitative researchers.

A number of qualitative data analysis (QDA) packages, such as NVivo, ATLAS.ti, QDA Miner, HyperRESEARCH and MAXQDA, have been developed to assist with the management of field note and interview data (Bazeley and Jackson 2013; Lee and Esterhuizen 2000). Most of these applications are essentially 'chunkers and coders', which attach electronic labels to passages of text and allow the retrieval of extracts coded under a chosen index term. Most packages permit more complex operations, such as Boolean searches, using the three logical operators 'or', 'and' and 'not' for search terms, searches for co-occurring categories and the merging of codes. However, they are no substitute for the time-consuming processes of interpretation, synthesis and theory generation that researchers have traditionally performed on field data. Such programs are useful as a support tool for conventional thematic content, but can create problems with forms of process analysis where change over a series of sequential data entries or the narrative structure of a text are important.

Ethics and Participant Observation

Although PO studies raise much the same ethical concerns that come up in other research (see Chapter 19), some issues arise in accentuated or changed form. Among the features of PO that give rise to special problems are:

- The close relationships between researchers and subjects developed during fieldwork
- The 'emergent' nature of most research designs
- The fact that PO characteristically involves 'thick description' of natural settings and subjects.

These characteristics of PO affect the way researchers think about notions of informed consent, anonymity and confidentiality.

Informed consent implies that a participant freely agrees to participate, and fully understands the consequences of this agreement. The difficulty is that formal agreement in advance is more difficult to arrange in a PO study than, for example, in a social survey. There is rarely a single, initial stage where subjects are given full information about the research and the demands to be made on them, so they can agree or decline to take part. The research design at the time of the initial access approach may not be the same as the design three months later. Often access will involve multiple gatekeepers, and it may be obtained step by step as the research moves through different sites and encounters new actors, or as research plans change. Moreover, the classic PO studies generally negotiated access in relation to settings rather than specific individuals, partly because the settings were populated by individuals who were not regular participants and could not be approached in advance.

The period of agreeing access thus overlaps with the period during which the researcher seeks to cultivate the good relations needed to stay in the field. Research relationships may be embedded in social relationships with associated emotions: likes and dislikes, and so on. Consequently, informed consent may be sought against the background of personal pressures arising from the etiquette of social relationships. Lower participants may be asked for consent *after* superiors have agreed access minimizing their scope for choice. Issues of power and hierarchy are always present.

These are difficult problems where issues of ethics and practicality are intertwined. Any requirement that a PO study can only go ahead when all subjects within the field of observation have given informed consent in advance would limit the types of research that could be done. The extent to which an initial research design could be varied at a later stage would also curb changes. Some researchers draw a distinction between focused interactions, such as closed meetings or restricted settings that will be attended and perhaps audio-recorded, and observation of more 'open' settings such as accident and emergency departments, where the researcher cannot know which individuals will attend on a given day. They conclude that while it is viable to obtain advance consent (perhaps on prepared consent forms) in respect of focused interactions, they will not seek formal consent from occasional actors in open settings. In consequence, they may opt not to describe such individuals and their actions in great detail in research field notes and research reports. The approach to access adopted in many of the classic PO studies would clearly not meet the requirements of today's research ethics committees. Murphy and Dingwall (2007) discuss the problems that arise when what they term the 'anticipatory regulation' approach of conventional ethical review is imposed on observational studies. These may involve extended periods of time in the field, may evolve in focus and design because of the emergent nature of findings, lead to extended relationships between researchers and participants, and often take place in public or semi-public settings. The extent to which Participant Observation studies should conform to the conventional model of ethical review remains a subject for debate, as is discussed further in Chapter 19.

Researchers usually seek to manage any problems arising from thick description by promising to take special measures to safeguard anonymity and confidentiality. With regard to anonymity, they undertake to ensure that no uniquely identifying information is attached to the data, so that readers of research reports cannot trace the data back to the individual participant. Confidentiality is addressed by promising that the data will be handled and managed in such a way as to secure storage, use password-protected data files and remove real names from files, so that individuals are protected from the consequences of information leaks to third parties. But these guarantees may not be absolute (see the example in Case Study 8.1 below), and PO researchers should be careful not to make promises they cannot keep.

Strengths of Participant Observation

The strengths of PO studies lie in their ability to shed light on issues that other methods are less effective in investigating. Becker and Geer (1957) spell out the advantages of PO as a tool for exploring local cultures and the unfolding of social processes over time. However, in practice, there are different sets of arguments about the strength of PO in illuminating culture and subjective experience and its strength in examining social organization and organizational practices.

The argument that PO is a naturalistic method concerned with immersion in the culture and authentic representation of what the famous anthropologist Malinowski (1922: 25) termed 'the native's point of view … his vision of his world', still holds sway – even if it has become increasingly controversial. It is clear that observation does not in itself provide the researcher with access to the inner mental states of research participants, and research which claims to provide a window into the social worlds of staff or patient groups must back this up with supporting evidence that goes beyond inferences about what outward appearances indicate about subjective perceptions. Some naturalistic studies have made a convincing case about the value of examining previously neglected user perspectives, and strongly support this with data (for instance, Daly, McDonald and Willis 1992). However, several influential commentators argue that observational research should be about documenting practices, rather than ascribing meanings to participants' action or talk, and advocate a refocusing of analysis to centre on propositions that can be plausibly derived from observational data (see Dingwall and Strong 1985; Silverman 1998).

Indeed, for observational researchers with an interest in policy making, organizational processes and practices have been of greater interest than meanings. They have viewed PO as a promising alternative to interviews for seeing inside the 'black box' of health care organizations and understanding service delivery and change. PO can be viewed as a pragmatic way of 'reaching the parts other methods cannot reach' (Pope and Mays 1995). It can reveal routines of which participants are unaware, probe the micro-level behaviours that lie between known differences in outcomes and shed light on how policies or programmes may be subtly reshaped in the course of implementation. For instance, the following studies in the United Kingdom have documented:

- The implementation of the new general practitioner contract (McDonald, Harrison and Checkland 2009)
- The impact of the Quality and Outcomes Framework in general practice (Checkland and Harrison 2010)
- How emergency ambulance call handlers deploy a computer decision support system (Pope et al. 2013)
- How risk management strategies to minimize harm to older people were implemented in four acute hospitals (Hillman et al. 2013)
- The reframing of national policies on rationalizing hospital services as a local clinical issue linked to patient safety (Jones and Exworthy 2015)
- How clinician-managers and clinicians seek to build a bottom-up dimension to health improvement campaigns (Waring and Crompton 2017).

Many of these studies explore the process of implementing complex clinical interventions or organizational changes that require considerable bottom-up cooperation and commitment if they are to be integrated into practice. This is an area where ethnographic studies of the introduction of new medical technologies and the utilization of evidence for practice have contributed to theory building. Several prominent British researchers have been involved in the development of Normalization Process Theory (May et al. 2007) that maps out how actors at different levels invest in and contribute to service innovations and put together the assemblages of actions needed to embed them in accepted organizational procedures and practices.

The challenges of Participant Observation

The challenges of PO appear at several junctures as outlined below.

In the fieldwork phase

Some major disadvantages of PO, particularly in a contemporary British context preoccupied with research outputs as an institutional indicator of the quality of research, are the time-consuming nature of fieldwork and the strain of sustained contact with subjects. While some accounts of the research experience may have overdramatized the emotional trauma of fieldwork (see Punch 1986), researchers undoubtedly face taxing challenges in terms of managing their identity in the research setting, mediating between different actors and interest groups, deciding just how much participation is appropriate, and determining when, and how, to put information into the public domain. There are also well-documented ethical dilemmas concerning trust and disclosure which arise when researchers build up social relationships for research purposes.

Furthermore, given that research funding bodies are often seeking a review of a whole service or population, there may be a temptation to tack a limited observational component on to an interview study covering multiple settings, and to come away with very limited data that are hard to contextualize. Malinowski (1922: 7) emphasized the importance of 'close contact' and cautioned that: 'There is all the difference between a sporadic plunging into the company of natives, and being really in contact with them.' One of the risks associated with contemporary mixed-method studies is that the PO element is so episodic and dispersed across settings that it cannot examine the process aspects of social organization that the method has traditionally coped with so well. This same trend has also affected case studies which in recent times are often of limited scale and of an episodic and truncated nature (Marinetto 2011).

Methodological problems and solutions

The fact that some studies trade wider coverage against some loss of depth often reflects a quest for increased representativeness and generalizability. PO has traditionally been seen to be weak in these areas, but this is a topic about which more than a few misconceptions exist. There are undoubtedly situations where PO studies can illuminate general social patterns affecting a wide range of settings and where sampling may be appropriate (Bryman 1988). Yet the model of statistical inference from sample to population seems unsustainable in real-world situations where the 'population' of organizations from which a researcher might select the sample is itself small and diverse.

As a consequence, examples of conventional sampling in PO studies are thin on the ground. Instead, some PO researchers have opted for purposive samples, intended to facilitate observations and comparisons that will help to build theory. Case studies may permit theoretical generalization rather than statistical generalization (Mitchell 1983), so the issue is not whether the events observed in the case study site precisely represent events elsewhere, but whether the analysis of social processes produced by the research has more general applicability. For Yin (2018) and other exponents of case analysis, the path towards generalizability is not about filling in the gaps by progressively achieving more complete population coverage, but about replication studies that could disconfirm or affirm the theoretical propositions generated by earlier case studies.

The problem of researcher influence

A problem that features prominently in many textbook accounts of PO is 'reactivity' – the possibility that the researcher's presence influences the behaviour observed. This phenomenon, also known as the 'Hawthorne effect', featured centrally in the classic study by Roethlisberger and Dickson (1939) of human relations in the Hawthorne plant of the Western Electric Company in Chicago. Here, a series of 'experiments' carried out by production engineers on a small group of telephone relay assembly workers appeared to show that almost any change in the factory environment led to improved productivity, including both increasing and reducing the lighting (although the data have subsequently been questioned). Clearly, research subjects may very well modify aspects of their behaviour under observation, but arguably this is usually more of a problem in the early stages of a research project than when field relations are well established. Certainly, it is not unknown for a study to be prematurely terminated because of non-cooperation or resistance from subjects (for example, Clarke 1996).

However, even where attempts are made to conceal things from the researcher, many features of social organization are difficult to change without disrupting the work of the setting. In my own experience, the kinds of data that subjects do not want recorded are more likely to involve individual mistakes or indiscretions, such as negative comments about colleagues, than routine work practices. Once the researcher has become familiar to them, subjects may be surprisingly open in discussing sensitive and potentially problematic issues.

Data coding, analysis and interpretation in Participant Observation

Most PO studies rely on some form of thematic content analysis. In line with the neo-Chicagoan influences on PO, many observational researchers base their approach to analysis on analytic induction (Znaniecki 1952) or grounded theory (Glaser and Strauss 1967). In contemporary research, both approaches typically start with a general orientation to an issue, rather than a definitive hypothesis for testing, and move through a process where problems and concepts relevant to an organization are identified, and theoretical propositions for further investigation formulated. Analysis goes on as data are collected and further data collection takes its direction from the provisional analysis. At this stage, the analysis must necessarily remain provisional because of the exigencies of fieldwork, and the final comprehensive analysis will only take place when the fieldwork is completed.

Analytic induction and grounded theory

Analytical induction, as originally conceived by early Chicago researchers, was an approach concerned with the systematic search for falsifying evidence and the progressive refinement of theory until no disconfirming evidence could be found. In the work by Lindesmith (1947), this involved the progressive modification of a hypothesis, set out as a formal proposition at the start of the study. For Znaniecki (1952), analytical induction offered the prospect of producing universal propositions that could then be used to predict future patterns of behaviour. Later writers built on the core notions of inductive inference of theory from data and deviant case analysis, but abandoned the quest for empirical prediction and often avoided any initial hypothesis.

The approach by Glaser and Strauss (1967) to grounded theory emerged out of this period of reappraisal and represented an extension and elaboration of analytic induction. Grounded theory studies start with a general area of concern, rather than a hypothesis, and move to identify the concepts and theoretical connections emerging from the data. Where some contemporaneous qualitative studies (as well as almost all quantitative studies) were concerned mainly with verifying theories, Glaser and Strauss placed primary emphasis on generating theory by discovering relevant concepts and hypotheses through fieldwork. The core ideas of the constant comparative method and theoretical sampling have over time been supplemented by guidelines for a complex system of coding (Strauss and Corbin 1990).

The increasing formalization of grounded theory has led to considerable controversy among its exponents (Melia 1996) and may have made the approach less attractive to pragmatically inclined health service researchers. Many contemporary health researchers utilize modified versions of analytic induction or grounded theory. These make use of techniques like thematic coding, constant comparison and deviant case analysis, but do not adhere strictly to the original models (Murphy et al. 1998).

The growth of interest in the use of language has led to the emergence of more sophisticated approaches to the analysis of spoken interaction, such as the ethnography of communication, conversation analysis and discourse analysis. This has led many PO researchers to question whether their field notes adequately represent the interactions they have observed. *The Social Organization of Juvenile Justice* by Cicourel (1968) marked an important step because it encouraged researchers to pay greater attention to language and to produce field notes that were as near verbatim as possible. The emergence of linguistically sensitive forms of PO has changed the way many PO researchers present data (Dingwall and Strong 1985). It has led some to supplement observations recorded in field notes with audio recordings of key events or meetings, and to combine thematic content analysis with sequential analysis of transcribed talk based on conversation analysis or discourse analysis techniques.

Data selection

The process by which a researcher observes and records events, and then analyses them to build descriptions and theories in published form, has led to a good deal of soul searching for several generations of participant observers. There are difficult issues concerning the selection and representation of observations that are not easy to resolve, even when data are presented in considerable detail. There are questions of trust and also about just how ethnographic accounts might be said to represent reality. This quickly leads into the deep waters of epistemology and ontology, which are beyond the scope of this chapter.

Many pragmatically inclined researchers have opted for a position of 'subtle realism' (Mays and Pope 2000; Murphy et al. 1998), which accepts that research reports can never encapsulate a single 'truth' but rejects the relativism of postmodern ethnography. They argue that a researcher's aim is to produce a credible account of social processes, which are acknowledged to be representations, rather than reproductions of, social reality. This may be used to build theories that can be developed in the light of findings from later studies.

Writing up and presenting findings

Different PO studies address different aspects of social organization and rest on different theoretical foundations, and this is reflected in striking differences in how findings are written up and presented. A classic interactionist ethnography like *Boys in White* (Becker et al. 1961) takes a very different form from an anthropology-influenced study like *The Cloak of Competence* by Edgerton (1967), just as the linguistically sensitive study *Medical Talk and Medical Work* by Atkinson (1995) is presented in a different style from the policy ethnography of Strong and Robinson (1990). In recent years, styles of writing have come under increasing scrutiny (Hammersley 1993). For example, there is extensive debate about issues such as the viability of realist ethnography (including representational devices such as the invisibility of the author), and the use of alternative forms of textual organization such as chronology, narrative and analytic themes. From a practical perspective, researchers are often required to produce output for multiple readerships, and which need to meet the stylistic requirements of different journals.

Health care reform in England and Wales and the importance of informal social organization

Many of the dilemmas and trade-offs discussed above were evident in a study of the changing landscape of NHS contracting undertaken by myself and associates (see Allen et al. 2016; Hughes, Allen et al. 2011; Hughes, Petoulas et al. 2011; Hughes et al. 2013; Petsoulas et al. 2011). The research investigated contracting behaviour in two English and two Welsh NHS purchasers and their provider hospitals, taking account of the influence of the overseeing English strategic health authority or Welsh government regional office. Fieldwork extended over two contracting rounds

CASE STUDY 8.1

(Continued)

(Continued)

at a time of considerable organizational turbulence. The study was conceived as a 'policy ethnography' and utilized a combination of observations, in-depth interviews and documentary analysis to examine NHS management processes. We observed a variety of meetings linked to the commissioning process and interviewed relevant participants, varying the interview content according to context. Most meetings and all interviews were tape recorded and fully transcribed, something that was possible with a large study funded by the National Institute of Health Research.

By the late 2000s NHS policy in England was taking a market turn that distinguished it from the other three home countries. At face value, England was introducing harder-edged service contracts incorporating financial penalties and incentives, while Wales was retreating from the 1990s internal market and emphasizing cooperation and flex-ibility in the contracting process. But there were also cross-border spill-overs involving common contracting technologies and management cultures that meant the differences on the ground were less pronounced than might have been expected.

Wider policy differences between the two NHS systems were reflected in differing contracting frameworks, involving regional commissioning in Wales and commis-sioning by primary care trusts (PCTs) in England. However, one development that appeared to run counter to the logic of a market system was that both systems used standard template contracts from 2007 onwards. Despite efforts to introduce a comprehensive ('complete') contract, we found that, in practice, purchasers and providers often reverted to a more relational style of contracting. Indeed, in a period of financial constraint and uncertainty, it was informal social organization and long-term relationships rather than the new framework of rules, penalties and incentives that kept the systems functioning in a period of rapid change. In England, we found examples where PCTs relaxed contractual requirements to assist partners faced with financial deficits. For instance, there were cases where hospitals accepted payment for unplanned additional treatments at rates beneath the official NHS tariff, and where a PCT allowed a hospital that had delivered fewer treatments than planned to sign a block contract (again, not based on national tariffs) that maintained its expected income. In Wales, news of plans to end the purchaser/provider split meant a return to less precisely specified block contracts and a renewed concern to build cooperation between managers in the health boards and hospitals.

Such informal compromises and bending of rules would have been less visible in a study that did not engage with participants in the field on an at least weekly basis over a period of many months. Compared with the original version of policy ethnography, as outlined by Strong and Robinson (1990), our work incorporated a larger observational component and paid more attention to the specifics of discourse by making extensive use of verbatim transcriptions of meetings. Our interviews were focused on a limited number of case study settings rather than replicating Strong and Robinson's more synoptic scan of a large num-ber of organizations. We observed and audio-recorded 36 contracting-related meetings in

England and 41 in Wales, and completed 24 English and 43 Welsh qualitative interviews. In both countries a lead investigator and a research officer shared the workload of fieldwork. A policy ethnography of this type centres mainly on a series of timetabled events and appointments, and thus falls short of the full 'immersion' in the field described in classic PO studies. However, it did typically involve visiting various research sites in each country three or four times in an average week. The maintenance of good field relations was crucial, particularly with key post holders, such as commissioner organization chief executives or contracts managers, who could facilitate introductions to other actors.

Securing informed consent in a study of this type can be quite challenging. Regular members of health board and hospital contracts teams can be approached in advance, but the researcher is faced with an ever-changing cast of peripheral actors who appear when meetings touch on their areas of interest, and typically need to be approached as participants assemble for a meeting. Often the key players who have acted as informal sponsors of the study can make introductions and smooth the way for agreement to research before meetings begin, but sometimes the researchers needed to make their own introductions. Broaching the subject of permission to audio-record meetings was the trickiest thing to negotiate with one-off participants, but I am unaware of any occasions when subjects declined. There were a few instances where meeting chairs asked us to pause our recording when discussions entered a sensitive area. In the case of interviews, a handful of informants declined tape recording, so that we instead made notes by hand.

Maintaining access and cooperation were more challenging in this study than in my previous research on NHS contracting in Wales (see previous editions of this publication), and the flexibility of the qualitative design was critical in overcoming these problems. The controversy surrounding the NHS market in England meant that two PCTs that had given in-principle agreement to participate subsequently reversed their decision, leading to a scramble for late replacements. This meant that one English case study started later than the other and could only cover the first contract round and used interviews rather than observation. In Wales, too, there were unexpected changes in plans. A shift to regional commissioning early in the fieldwork meant negotiating cooperation with partner health boards alongside the original two case study health boards that had already agreed access. Later, the announcement by the Welsh government that the internal market would end quickly changed the nature of contracting meetings as health board and hospital managers digested the implications. Fortunately, the flexibility of the observational design meant that the study could adapt. This would not have been possible with a survey study. As the market lost momentum in Wales, we switched from the now infrequent contract team meetings to new meetings that discussed the channelling of funding via a new planning framework. With fewer secondary-care contracting meetings in one health board we took the opportunity to add a case study of an individual patient commissioning (IPC) panel that decided funding for high-cost referrals not covered by existing contracts (Hughes and Doheny 2011).

Quite unexpectedly, our observations in the IPC panel brought about one of the most challenging situations we encountered in this study. Problems emerged when a patient started judicial review proceedings against the health board after the IPC panel declined to fund a high-cost cancer drug. The health board requested copies of the audio recordings we had made of meetings concerning this patient so that these were available if demanded by the court. Disclosure of research data, even to the host health board, posed complicated issues. We had to gain permission from the Department of Health as funder, inform the NHS research ethics committee that had oversight of the project and the individual study participants, as well as cooperating with the university administration to safeguard its and our position (see Hughes 2017). In the event, the case did not proceed to a full hearing, but it highlighted the importance of properly completed consent forms and ethical clearance, and also alerted the author to a risk of legal proceedings that is rarely considered by qualitative researchers. Fortunately, the team's positive relationship with the health board meant that we were allowed to continue attendance at our usual meetings, despite the complications that had arisen because of our audio-taping.

This project generated a large corpus of recorded and textual data. Our preference in this project, based on our previous experience of using qualitative database applications, was to analyse our data using a version of thematic analysis based on manual coding. Essentially, we opted to gather together themed extracts under various categories, and order and re-order those relating to a theme of interest in ordinary text files prepared with Microsoft Word, before selecting extracts to use in published outputs. Policy ethnographies usually need to tell a policy story, so that the chronology and sequencing of data extracts is important. We found it easier to analyse events in successive meetings via the manual analysis described above, as opposed to using a QDA application package. Our worry was that an over-preoccupation with generating themes and hierarchically organized codes would risk breaking our data into de-contextualized chunks that would be damaging to a study of this kind. Our approach was to limit our coding to a fairly basic taxonomy of key themes and subthemes and not to attempt the complex hierarchical codes developed by some grounded theory researchers who wish to build theoretical constructs or models.

Policy ethnographies that examine the implementation of health care reforms or programmes rarely start with the blank slate that some grounded theory writers advocate. Such studies usually need to be contextualized within the existing policy process and implementation study literatures, which are already heavy with theory. Our work, with its focus on contracting as a social process, built on such sources as that of the idea of Marc Granovetter (1985) about 'the smoothing role of social relations in the market', the notion by Michael Polanyi (1944) of a 'double movement', whereby swings towards unrestrained markets spark corrective attempts to re-build social cohesion, and the claim by the socio-legal theorist Ian Macneil (2000) that exchange transactions necessarily occur within a 'social matrix'. Hence our analysis was more about re-combining elements from these existing theories in a way that fitted the behaviour we were observing than building an entirely new theory.

Indeed, we found that our findings converged with those of other contemporary work that highlighted 'social embedding' and the persistence of relational contracting in the wake of market reforms (Jones, Exworthy and Frosini 2013; Porter et al. 2013; Shaw et al. 2013).

Reading health research based on Participant Observation

Not all PO studies are carried out in the same way. To assess the quality of a particular study, the reader should ask the following pertinent questions:

- Does the author provide sufficient information on fieldwork and data analysis for the reader to be able to construct the main steps in the research process?
- Is the description of the setting presented in a way that is detailed, plausible and internally consistent?
- Are the data presented sufficiently rich to give a sense of life in the setting and do they support the wider analysis put forward?
- Are the conclusions of the study supported by sufficient corroborating evidence, preferably from more than one data source?
- Are the chosen approaches to data collection and analysis appropriate to the research question?
- Are there indications that disconfirming evidence has been given as much attention as evidence that supports the conclusions presented, perhaps through deviant case analysis?
- Do the theoretical conclusions of the study emerge from the data, or is there a suspicion that the findings have been presented selectively so as to support the theory?

For further discussion of how to assess quality in PO specifically, and in qualitative research more generally, see Mays and Pope (2000) and Seale (1999).

Is Participant Observation changing?

The classic Chicago School studies of the 1920s involved only episodic field observations, often employing hired-hand observers rather than the principal investigators, and the method of PO has evolved considerably since those early days. One innovation in recent years has been netnography (Kozinets 1998), which is discussed more fully in Chapter 25. Advocates claim that net ethnography can allow the same deep immersion in cyber-communities and online cultures that PO can achieve in conventional field research, but it poses distinctive ethical and methodological issues that are outside the scope of this chapter (see Gatson 2011). Another new departure is global ethnography. Burawoy and colleagues

(2000) argue that globalization changes ethnographic sites by creating transnational connections, spaces and imaginations that transform the dynamics of interaction but again pose difficult questions about the nature of fieldwork.

The theoretical landscape of PO research is also changing as actor-network theory (see, for instance, Allen 2014; Moreira 2004), Bourdieu-influenced scholarship (for example, Angus et al. 2005; Holmes 2006) and other innovative perspectives jostle for space alongside more familiar interactionist or negotiated order approaches. Yet arguably, PO studies should emphasize their family resemblance and shared challenges rather than their differences. Howard Becker (2017), a leading exponent of PO research since the 1950s, returns in his latest book to the craft of fieldwork and, in what can be seen as a reassertion of the virtues of the neo-Chicagoan School, redirects our attention to the need to do the best we can in terms of rigour and evidence.

Conclusion

The argument put forward in this chapter is that PO has a number of strengths in addressing particular kinds of research question. In health research, PO can help researchers penetrate social processes and, handled with care, the perspectives of social actors, in particular settings. Most recently, it has been used to penetrate the 'black box' of health care organizations, probe gaps between public accounts and informal behaviour, and offer a better understanding of organizational change and the implementation of complex interventions. Moreover, most PO studies incorporate flexible research designs, which are not derailed by rapid and unpredictable organizational change. Thus, PO studies have a place within a multifaceted research programme in which appropriate methods are selected to match the research questions at hand. To shed further light on PO as a health research method, we have included a practical exercise based on the use of the method in a health contracting meeting.

Exercise 8.1 Participant Observation and a health contracting meeting

The following exchange occurred in a health authority contracting team meeting. The first speaker, the finance director (FD), is the team leader. The other speaker, the contracts manager (CM), is the team member with hands-on responsibility for managing provider contracts. Caerbrook is a regional specialist hospital providing children's cancer services – indeed, the only hospital offering some treatments in this geographical area. Metro is a regional hospital providing a wider range of tertiary services. The tape recording was made openly with the team's permission. No special assurances were requested after this meeting. Like many Welsh NHS purchasers, this health authority inserted a clause in service contracts with hospital providers that imposed a cash penalty if they breached maximum waiting times for surgery. This was based on the Patient's Charter (Department of Health 1991), a high-profile government initiative that offered a commitment to the maximum surgical waiting times for different categories of patients.

FD You'll have to be careful how you minute this. What we've agreed with Caerbrook ... is that the penalties for Patient's Charter will only be a thousand pounds this year, not five thousand or ten thousand. The reason for that is that they weren't prepared to sign a contract if we insisted on the other penalties. Their contract is a quarter of a million and they have never incurred a penalty with us.

CM We need to be careful, George.

FD I got a personal assurance from their chief executive, Neil Hayward, that the deal is strictly confidential and not to be leaked to any other East county provider, and that they will not incur any penalties. If they do, we will review. But given that they were only a quarter of a million; given that, well, my figures say, and certainly his were, that they haven't incurred any penalties – that seemed to be confirmed by the budget reports – that we wouldn't ... it's not in our interest not to sign a contract. But we wouldn't want the same to apply to Metro, because Metro is a completely different provider. They have incurred fifty penalties in the last year, and ...

CM It's vital that information doesn't get out. Once that gets out we haven't got much of a contract there.

FD We've got to hold the line here. Nobody has heard that.

We were already aware from other observed meetings that three local providers had been arguing hard against the inclusion of penalty clauses but had been told that they would be applied in all contracts, and that another regional specialist hospital was also said to be unhappy with penalties.

Answer the following questions:

- What does this extract show about the use of penalty clauses in the NHS quasi-market?
- What, if anything, does the extract show about the problem of 'reactivity'?
- What weight can be attached to a single observation, without corroborating information? How could such corroboration be obtained?
- What questions does this data extract suggest should be explored in later interviews?
- What practical problems does knowledge of this arrangement pose, if any, for the research team in managing field relations?

The researchers decided to use this extract, but not until after this health authority was reorganized and the people concerned had moved to new jobs. What ethical problems does this raise, if any?

Recommended further reading

This is a British PO study that blends a classic negotiated order perspective with more recent theory:
Allen, D. (2014) *The Invisible Work of Nurses: Hospitals, Organisation and Healthcare.* Abingdon: Routledge.

This is a fascinating reflection on contemporary research practices by a prominent member of the neo-Chicagoan School:
Becker, H. S. (2017) *Evidence.* Chicago, IL: University of Chicago Press.

This is a journal special issue featuring ethnographic papers on the spatial organization of hospitals that combine anthropological and Foucauldian perspectives:
Street, A. and Coleman, S. (eds) (2012) 'Hospital heterotopias: Ethnographies of biomedical and non-biomedical spaces', Special issue, *Space and Culture, 15*(1): 4–17.

References

Allen, D. (2014) *The Invisible Work of Nurses: Hospitals, Organisation and Healthcare.* Abingdon: Routledge.

Allen, P., Hughes, D., Vincent-Jones, P., Petsoulas, C., Doheny, S. and Roberts, J. (2016) 'Contracts as accountability mechanisms: Assuring quality of care in public healthcare in England and Wales', *Public Management Review, 18*(1): 20–39.

Angus, J., Kontos, P., Dyck, I., McKeever, P. and Poland, B. (2005) 'The personal significance of home: Habitus and the experience of receiving long-term home care', *Sociology of Health and Illness, 27*(2): 161–87.

Atkinson, P. (1995) *Medical Talk and Medical Work: The Liturgy of the Clinic.* London: Sage.

Bazeley, P. and Jackson, K. (2013) *Qualitative Data Analysis with NVivo,* 2nd edition. London: Sage.

Becker, H. S. (2017) *Evidence.* Chicago, IL: University of Chicago Press.

Becker, H. S. and Geer, B. (1957) 'Participant observation and interviewing: A comparison', *Human Organization, 16*: 28–32.

Becker, H. S., Geer, B., Hughes, E. C. and Strauss, A. (1961) *Boys in White: Student Culture in Medical School.* Chicago, IL: University of Chicago Press.

Bryman, A. (1988) *Quantity and Quality in Social Research.* London: Unwin Hyman.

Burawoy, M., Blum, J. A., George, S., Gille, Z. and Gowan, T. (2000) *Global Ethnography: Forces, Connections and Imaginations in a Postmodern World.* Berkeley, CA: University of California Press.

Caudill, W., Redlich, F. C., Gilmore, H. R. and Brody, E. B. (1952) 'Social structure and interaction processes on a psychiatric ward', *American Journal of Orthopsychiatry, 22*: 314–34.

Checkland, K. and Harrison, S. (2010) 'The impact of the Quality and Outcomes Framework on practice organisation and service delivery: Summary of evidence from two qualitative studies', *Quality in Primary Care*, *18*: 139–46.

Cicourel, A. (1968) *The Social Organization of Juvenile Justice*. New York: Wiley.

Clarke, L. (1996) 'Participant observation in a secure unit: Care, conflict and control', *Nursing Times Research*, *1*: 431–40.

Daly, J., McDonald, I. and Willis, E. (1992) *Researching Health Care: Designs, Dilemmas, Disciplines*. London: Routledge.

Davis, F. (1963) *Passage Through Crisis: Polio Victims and their Families*. Indianapolis, IN: Bobbs Merrill.

Department of Health (1991) *The Patients' Charter*. London: HMSO.

Dingwall, R. and Strong, P. M. (1985) 'The interactional study of organisations', *Urban Life*, *14*: 205–31.

Edgerton, R. (1967) *The Cloak of Competence*. Berkeley, CA: University of California Press.

Emerson, R. (1981) 'Observational fieldwork', *Annual Review of Sociology*, *7*: 351–78.

Fadiman, A. (1998) *The Spirit Catches You and You Fall Down: A Hmong Child, Her American Doctors, and the Collision of Two Cultures*. New York: Farrar, Straus and Giroux.

Fine, G. A. (ed.) (1995) *A Second Chicago School? The Development of Postwar American Sociology*. Chicago, IL: University of Chicago Press.

Gatson, S. N. (2011) 'The methods, politics, and ethics of representation in online ethnography', in N. K. Denzin and Y. S. Lincoln (eds), *Collecting and Interpreting Qualitative Materials*, 4th edition. New York: Sage.

Glaser, B. G. and Strauss, A. L. (1965) *Awareness of Dying*. Chicago, IL: Aldine.

Glaser, B. G. and Strauss, A. L. (1967) *The Discovery of Grounded Theory: Strategies for Qualitative Research*. New York: Aldine.

Gold, R. L. (1958) 'Roles in sociological field observations', *Social Forces*, *36*: 217–23.

Goodwin, D. (2009) *Acting in Anaesthesia: Ethnographic Encounters with Patients, Practitioners and Medical Technologies*. Cambridge: Cambridge University Press.

Granovetter, M. (1985) 'Economic action and social structure: The problem of embeddedness', *American Journal of Sociology*, *91*: 481–510.

Hammersley, M. (1992) *What's Wrong with Ethnography?* London: Routledge.

Hammersley, M. (1993) 'Ethnographic writing', *Social Research Update*, 5.

Hillman, A. (2014) '"Why must I wait": The process of legitimacy in a hospital emergency department', *Sociology of Health and Illness*, *36*(4): 485–99.

Hillman, A., Tadd, W., Calnan, S., Calnan, M., Bayer, A. and Read, S. (2013) 'Risk, governance and the experience of care', *Sociology of Health and Illness*, *35*(6): 939–55.

Holmes, S. M. (2006) 'An ethnographic study of the social context of migrant health in the United States', *PLoS Medicine 3*(10): e448. Available at: https://doi.org/10.1371/journal.pmed.0030448.

Horowitz, R. (2013) *In the Public Interest: Medical Licensing and the Disciplinary Process*. New Brunswick, NJ: Rutgers University Press.

Hughes, D. (2017) 'Informed consent, judicial review and the uncertainties of ethnographic research in sensitive NHS settings', SAGE Research Methods Cases (Online Collection). Available at: doi: http://dx.doi.org/10.4135/9781526431561 http://methods.sagepub.com/case/informed-consent-judicial-review-and-uncertainties-sensitive-nhs-settings

Hughes, D., Allen, P., Doheny, S., Petsoulas, C., Roberts, J. and Vincent-Jones, P. (2011) *NHS Contracts in England and Wales: Changing Contexts and Relationships*. Final report. NIHR Service Delivery and Organisation Programme. London: HMSO.

Hughes, D., Allen, P., Doheny, S., Petsoulas, C. and Vincent-Jones, P. (2013) 'Co-operation and conflict under hard and soft contracting regimes: Case studies from England and Wales', *BMC Heath Services Research*, 13 (Suppl 1): S7. Available at: doi: https://10.1186/1472-6963-13-S1-S7.

Hughes, D. and Doheny, S. (2011) 'Deliberating Tarceva: A case study of how British NHS managers decide whether to purchase a high-cost drug in the shadow of NICE guidance', *Social Science and Medicine*, 73(10): 1460–8.

Hughes, D., Petsoulas, C., Allen, P., Doheny, S. and Vincent-Jones, P. (2011) 'Contracts in the English NHS: Market levers and social embeddedness', *Health Sociology Review*, 20(3): 321–37.

Hume, L. and Mulcock, J. (2004) *Anthropologists in the Field: Cases in Participant Observation*. New York: Columbia University Press.

Jones, L. and Exworthy, M. (2015) 'Framing in policy processes: A case study from hospital planning in the National Health Service in England', *Social Science and Medicine*, 124: 196–204.

Jones, L., Exworthy, M. and Frosini, F. (2013) 'Implementing market-based reforms in the English NHS: Bureaucratic coping strategies and social embeddedness', *Health Policy*, 111(1): 52–9.

Kellogg, K. C. (2011) *Challenging Operations: Medical Reform and Resistance in Surgery*. Chicago, IL: University of Chicago Press.

Kozinets, R. V. (1998) 'On netnography: Initial reflections on consumer research investigations of cyberculture', in J. W. Alba and J. W. Hutchinson (eds), *NA – Advances in Consumer Research*, Volume 25. Provo, UT: Association for Consumer Research.

Lee, R. M. and Esterhuizen, L. (2000) 'Computer software and qualitative analysis: Trends, issues, and responses', *International Journal of Social Research Methodology*, 3: 231–43.

Lindesmith, A. (1947) *Opiate Addiction*. Bloomington, IN: Principia Press.

Macneil, I. R. (2000) 'Relational contract theory: Challenges and queries', *Northwestern University Law Review*, 94: 877–907.

Malinowski, B. (1922) *Argonauts of the Western Pacific*. London: Routledge & Kegan Paul.

Marinetto, M. (2011) 'Case studies of the health policy process: A methodological introduction', in M. Exworthy, S. Peckham, M. Powell and A. Hann (eds), *Shaping Health Policy: Case Study Methods and Analysis*. Bristol: Policy Press.

Martin, G., Kocman, D., Stephens, T., Peden, C. and Pearse, R. (2017) 'Pathways to professionalism? Quality improvement, care pathways, and the interplay of standardisation and clinical autonomy', *Sociology of Health and Illness*, *39*(8): 1314–29.

May, C., Finch, T., Mair, F., Ballini, L., Dowrick, C., Eccles, M., Gask, L., MacFarlane, A., Murray, E. and Rapley, T. (2007) 'Understanding the implementation of complex interventions in health care: The normalization process model', *BMC Health Services Research*, 7. Available at: doi: 142-10.1186/1472-6963-7-148.

Mays, N. and Pope, C. (2000) 'Qualitative research in health care: Assessing quality in qualitative research', *British Medical Journal*, *320*: 50–2.

McCall, G. J. (1984) 'Systematic field observation', *Annual Review of Sociology*, *10*: 263–310.

McDonald, R., Harrison, S. and Checkland, K. (2009) 'The new GP contract in English primary health care: An ethnographic study', *International Journal of Public Sector Management*, *22*: 21–34.

Melia, K. M. (1996) 'Re-discovering Glaser', *Qualitative Health Research*, *6*: 368–78.

Mitchell, J. C. (1983) 'Case and situation analysis', *Sociological Review*, *31*: 187–211.

Moreira, T. (2004) 'Coordination and embodiment in the operating room', *Body and Society*, *10*(1): 109–29.

Murphy, E. and Dingwall, R. (2007) 'Informed consent, anticipatory regulation and ethnographic practice', *Social Science and Medicine*, *65*(11): 2223–34.

Murphy, E., Dingwall, R., Greatbatch, D., Parker, S. and Watson, P. (1998) 'Qualitative methods in health technology assessment: A review of the literature' (whole issue), *Health Technology Assessment*, *2*: 16.

Myers, N. L. (2016) *Recovery's Edge: An Ethnography of Mental Health Care and Moral Agency*. Nashville, TN: Vanderbilt University Press.

Olesen, V. L. and Whittaker, E. W. (1968) *The Silent Dialogue: A Study in the Social Psychology of Professional Socialization*. San Francisco, CA: Jossey-Bass.

Petsoulas, C., Allen, P., Hughes, D., Vincent-Jones, P. and Roberts, J. (2011) 'The use of standard contracts in the English National Health Service: a case study analysis', *Social Science and Medicine*, *73*: 185–92.

Polanyi, K. (1944) *The Great Transformation: The Political and Economic Origins of Our Time*. Boston, MA: Beacon Press.

Pope, C., Halford, S., Turnbull, J., Prichard, J. S., Calestani, M. and May, C. (2013) 'Using computer decision support systems in NHS emergency and urgent care: ethnographic study using normalisation process theory', *BMC Health Services Research*, *13*(111): 1–13.

Pope, C. and Mays, N. (1995) 'Qualitative research: Reaching the parts other methods cannot reach – an introduction to qualitative methods in health and health services research', *British Medical Journal*, *311*: 42–5.

Porter, A., Mays, N., Shaw, S., Rosen, R. and Smith, J. (2013) 'Commissioning healthcare for people with long term conditions: The persistence of relational contracting in England's NHS quasi-market', *BMC Health Services Research*, *13*(Suppl 1): S2. Available at: https://doi.org/10.1186/1472-6963-13-S1-S2

Porter, S. (1995) *Nursing's Relationship with Medicine: A Critical Realist Ethnography.* Aldershot: Avebury.

Punch, M. (1986) *The Politics and Ethics of Fieldwork.* London: Sage.

Roethlisberger, F. J. and Dickson, W. J. (1939) *Management and the Worker: An Account of a Research Program Conducted by the Western Electric Company, Hawthorne Works, Chicago.* Cambridge, MA: Harvard University Press.

Roth, J. A. (1963) *Timetables.* New York: Bobbs Merrill.

Roth, J. A. (1999) 'Hired-hand research', in A. Bryman and R. G. Burgess (eds), *Qualitative Research.* Volume *One*: *Fundamental Issues in Qualitative Research.* London: Sage.

Russell J. and Greenhalgh T. (2012) 'Affordability as a discursive accomplishment in a changing National Health Service', *Social Science and Medicine*, 75(12): 2463–71.

Russell, J. and Greenhalgh, T. (2015) 'Being "rational" and being "human": How National Health Service rationing decisions are constructed as rational by resource allocation panels', *Health*, 18(5): 441–57.

Seale, C. (1999) 'Quality in qualitative research', *Qualitative Inquiry*, 5(4): 465–78.

Shaw, S. E., Smith, J. A., Porter, A., Rosen, R. and Mays, N. (2013) 'The work of commissioning: A multisite case study of healthcare commissioning in England's NHS', *BMJ Open*, 3: e003341.

Silverman, D. (1998) 'Qualitative research: Meanings or practices?', *Information Systems*, 8: 3–20.

Strauss, A. L. and Corbin, J. (1990) *Basics of Qualitative Research: Grounded Theory Procedures and Techniques.* Newbury Park, CA: Sage.

Strong, P. and Robinson, J. (1990) *The NHS: Under New Management.* Milton Keynes: Open University Press.

Sudnow, D. (1968) *Passing On: The Social Organization of Dying.* New York: Prentice-Hall.

Waring, J. and Crompton, J. (2017) 'A "movement for improvement"? A qualitative study of the adoption of social movement strategies in the implementation of a quality improvement campaign', *Sociology of Health and Illness*, 39(7): 1083–99.

Wight, D. and Barnard, M. (1993) 'The limits to participant observation in HIV/AIDS research', *Practicing Anthropology*, 15(4): 66–9.

Yin, R. (2018) *Case Study Research and Applications: Design and Methods*, 6th edition. Los Angeles, CA: Sage.

Znaniecki, F. (1952) *Cultural Sciences.* Urbana, IL: University of Illinois Press.

Zussman, R. (1993) 'Life in the hospital – a review', *Milbank Quarterly*, 71(1): 167–85.

9

The Use of Focus Groups in Health Research

JUDITH GREEN

Chapter objectives

- To describe some typical uses of focus groups in health research
- To outline the main stages of a focus group discussion
- To identify when to use a focus group in preference to, or as well as, other qualitative methods
- To introduce key issues in analysis of focus group data
- To consider the main ethical issues raised by focus group research.

Introduction

Focus groups have become a widely used qualitative research method of data generation. They include a number of different approaches for bringing together either strangers or 'natural groups' of participants who already know each other to discuss a topic in a 'focused' way. Typical uses in health research include needs assessments, gathering health service users' views of interventions or service provision, and exploring public or professionals' understanding of health topics. They have some methodological advantages over individual interviews and other methods of qualitative research, but also some disadvantages:

group interviews are most appropriately chosen when interaction between participants is needed to address the research question, or when the topic of research is the property of social groups, not individuals. An example might be group norms in relation to the topic in question.

This chapter examines the typical structure of a focus group and the kinds of questions that can be explored in a focus group setting. It examines the pragmatic issues to consider in running focus groups, methodological strengths and weaknesses, and ethical considerations. Questions of data management, analysis and presentation are a particularly challenging issue when using focus groups and the researcher must keep in mind that it is the group, rather than individuals within it, that is the focus of the analysis. A case study example demonstrates the various stages of a project using a focus group method in practice.

What is a focus group?

Although there are many variations, a focus group typically consists of 6–10 people brought together to discuss a topic, with one or more facilitators (sometimes called 'moderators') who introduce and guide the discussion and record it in some way. Sometimes the group is also asked to carry out exercises together, such as sorting a set of cards with statements on them or ranking a list of priorities. A typical focus group might include the stages set out in Box 9.1.

Box 9.1   The stages of a typical focus group discussion

- *Welcome*: the facilitator welcomes the participants, asks for consent forms to be completed, and perhaps provides refreshments.
- *Ice breaking and/or introductory exercises*: once the group is together and seated, and the aims of the group outlined, an introductory exercise is used to introduce the participants to each other and establish a relaxed, informal atmosphere. This might be an invitation for each participant to say their name and one thing about themselves (such as their favourite food), or could be a task to get participants thinking about and discussing the topic, such as an invitation to sort or rank pictures or phrases.
- *Group discussion*: a series of questions (the topic guide) is used to 'focus' the discussion. These usually move from the general to the more specific. For instance, here are some possible prompts for a study to explore the experiences and understanding of older adults offered statins by their doctor:
  - Let's start by talking about health in general: how would you describe your own health now?
  - Thinking about the future, what do you do to keep healthy?

---

o Who has been offered statins? Can you tell us how you decided to take them? How did the doctor explain what they were for?
o What other sources of information do you have about statins?
o Look at this diagram about the risks of a future stroke or coronary heart disease [show decision aid with graphic indicating how many people might not have stroke or coronary heart disease if they take a statin]. Do you remember your doctor showing you something like this, or any other diagrams, when discussing whether you might want to take statins? What does it mean to you?

- *Summing up*: the facilitator summarizes the key issues raised and asks for any additional comments.

Focus group studies can either bring together strangers, such as patients from a clinic who have never met, or can include what are called 'natural groups', who know each other already. These can be, for instance, members of a household, or groups of friends or work colleagues.

Why use focus groups?

Focus groups provide an opportunity to research not only people's knowledge, experiences and attitudes, but also how these are communicated within social interaction. As health topics are often readily discussed in everyday contexts, such as workplaces and social environments, a group setting often works well for generating talk about health and health services. In the example in Box 9.1, for instance, knowledge about statins is something that people typically share with their partners and friends (Polak and Green 2016). This might therefore be a topic that could generate discussion within a focus group. Like most qualitative methods, focus groups have the advantage over more quantitative approaches of allowing participants to frame their concerns in their own terms rather than that of the researcher, and to bring issues to the agenda that researchers might not otherwise have considered. Bringing together people with something in common, such as using the same hospital services or having similar health problems, can be a direct way for service providers and commissioners to find out what users think about services.

Health researchers have made extensive use of focus groups, either on their own or in combination with individual interviews or other methods, to explore the public understanding of health and how accounts of health and illness are used in everyday talk. One example is from Evans and colleagues (2001), who explored parents' decisions about accepting the combined measles, mumps and rubella (MMR) immunization for their children. In the wake of considerable media coverage of controversy about the safety of the MMR vaccine in the United Kingdom, there was concern that rates of immunization were falling to dangerously low levels. The researchers used group interviews to explore in detail how parents made decisions and asked about the sources of knowledge they drew on. They found that most parents considered the decision of whether to immunize their children or not very stressful, and that they were dissatisfied with the information available. Parents wanted more open and informed discussion with health professionals about the risks and benefits. By bringing together groups that included only parents who had immunized or only those who had not, Evans and her colleagues provided a safe environment in which parents could discuss their views.

Focus groups are particularly appropriate for topics relating to groups, rather than individuals, such as social norms or group practices. For instance, in a study of the links between cars and public health in Northern Ireland (Christie et al. 2017), we used focus groups composed of young adults to explore the roles of being a driver and being a passenger. Interaction within the groups provided access to data on how cars are essential in rural areas for accessing some determinants of health (employment, social life, goods and services), but also on how social groups have their own 'norms' that might make it difficult to avoid risky behaviour. For example, they might have to accept lifts from those who drove dangerously.

Finally, focus group discussions are widely used in preparatory work within larger health research projects. They may be used to map out key domains of interest to include in a survey questionnaire, or to identify the main issues that are likely to affect people's willingness to participate in research.

Focus groups in practice: Issues to consider

Focus groups are often selected because they appear to be a relatively efficient data generation method compared with alternatives, such as individual interviews or participant observation. A small number of groups can certainly generate a large data set, without the labour-intensive commitment of long-term ethnographic fieldwork. However, identifying participants and organizing the groups can be resource-intensive. Key issues to consider when thinking about the resources required for a focus group study include:

- Deciding how participants will be recruited
- Identifying a suitable location
- Assessing the skills required from the facilitators to manage discussion.

Recruitment

Possibilities for recruitment are: advertising for volunteers; 'snowballing' (asking for referrals) from personal contacts; working with established gatekeepers, such as community leaders, school heads or trade unions; or paying for professional recruitment. These methods have advantages and disadvantages, and a combination may be required to recruit sufficient numbers. Advertising is relatively cheap, but generic calls often elicit few responses unless there are financial or other incentives. Targeted approaches work better, such as using social media platforms utilized by the community of interest. Working with gatekeepers is often more effective, but it does take time to establish good relationships, and the researcher may have little control over the selection of participants. Professional recruitment agencies, such as market research companies, can be efficient recruiters, especially for participants from very specific sub-populations, but they are expensive, as they include both their own charges and those for paying participants. There is some debate about both the ethical and methodological implications of paying participants. Offering an incentive may make it difficult for low-income people to refuse to take part and paying people may make them more likely to say what they think the researcher wants to hear. It is difficult to judge these concerns empirically, but there is some justification for paying focus group participants. They will usually turn up at a time and place of the researcher's choosing, devoting several hours to a study. There are ways of minimizing any potential impact of payment on the quality of data by not advertising the payment but offering store vouchers at the end of the group as a 'thank you'.

Location

A relatively neutral location with good facilities for refreshments, seating and transport access will maximize attendance and goodwill. In practical terms, choosing an appropriate location is crucial. Barbour and colleagues (2011) report poor attendance from those invited to attend a focus group at a hospital, but better attendance from those invited from pre-existing mother-and-toddler groups. The specific location also has an impact on the kind of data collected. People's accounts are context-dependent and if you talk to them in the workplace, for example, they are more likely to be in work roles and their accounts will reflect this. In their study of children's views of risk around accidental injury, Green and Hart (1999) found children gave very different accounts depending on whether the group was held at school or in youth club premises. Those in the school-based groups were more likely to take 'sensible' views, whereas the youth club groups were more likely to tell stories in which they had taken risks.

The skills of the facilitators

Facilitating a focus group discussion requires the ability to establish rapport with a group of people, set the tone for a productive exchange, and manage group dynamics. For most groups, two people will be needed: one to lead the discussion, making sure the topic guide is covered, and the other to take responsibility for practical issues, such as meeting and greeting participants, organizing refreshments, checking that audio-recording equipment is working and perhaps taking notes or summarizing at key points. Additional help may be needed for specialized support, such as interpreting or childcare.

Focus groups differ from interviews in that the facilitator has less control over the flow of conversation. When there is lively interaction between participants, discussions can be unpredictable. The facilitator may need to manage issues arising from group dynamics, such as: overly dominant participants taking all the time or inhibiting other members from speaking; groups or participants who say little or do not interact with each other; groups which veer off-topic; or conflicts between participants with different views. How far these are problems depends on the research aims and type of data needed. In a focus group that brings together strangers with the aim of accessing a range of opinions, the facilitator will need strategies for ensuring that all members can contribute and that dominance is minimized. In natural groups, the facilitator may be more willing to let discussion depart from the topic guide, or to let particular individuals dominate a bit, as they are more interested in accessing something akin to informal 'everyday' conversation rather than formal discussion. However, all facilitators need skills in both eliciting useful discussion for the research question and in managing potential problems arising from interaction between participants. When planning the study, the introduction, questions, prompts and probes should all be carefully considered (and practised on a pilot group) to ensure that participants will feel at ease and be encouraged to participate. Facilitators might need the following strategies at their disposal:

- To break off eye contact or tactfully interrupt overly talkative participants
- To make sure their body language does not signal agreement with particular speakers or suggest their personal opinions
- To remind participants that all their views are important – and include prompts that deliberatively elicit alternative viewpoints (for instance, 'That is one view: does anyone around the table have a different experience?')
- To use pauses, rather than rushing to the next prompt, to allow participants time to consider responses to the contributions of others
- To try to ensure that a wide range of participants can contribute by using alternatives to verbal prompts. Drawing maps or posters, or ranking and sorting objects or pictures, can be effective.

Focus groups in health research: Methodology

A key advantage of focus groups over individual interviews is that they provide access to *how* topics are discussed as well as the content of views. The decision to use focus groups should be based primarily on whether this is relevant to the aims of the study. Bloor and colleagues (2001: 90) suggest that focus groups are the method of choice when:

researching topics relating to group norms, the group meanings that underpin those norms and the group processes whereby those meanings are constructed. … Focus groups are a particularly advantageous method where these group norms, meanings and processes are hidden or counter-cultural.

If access to discussion between participants is a methodological advantage for some topics and groups, it can be a disadvantage for others. Focus groups are not usually a good way to generate detailed, personal narratives or marginal views, or experiences of stigma or discomfort. If the aim is to access these, individual interviews, where stories can be shared privately, may be a more appropriate choice of data generation method. Two particular issues illustrate the methodological and ethical considerations of choosing focus groups: how interaction will be used and whether the topic is a sensitive one for the participants.

Using interaction

Access to interaction between participants, rather than just to answers to an interviewer's questions, potentially generates rather more 'naturalistic' talk about the topic of interest. This, it is assumed, might reflect the ways in which people discuss issues in everyday life. The advantage is maximized in natural groups that consist of people who might ordinarily interact in work, domestic or other settings. Household interviews are one particular kind of 'natural group' that utilizes this interaction between people who might be making shared health care decisions in everyday life. The smallest is the couple interview: Polak and Green (2016) note that interviewing couples has many advantages over individual interviews when the topic is one that the couple have some shared ownership over, such as managing chronic illness, or making decisions about health practices. Dew and colleagues (2015) used household interviews with 55 households in New Zealand to find out more about health practices. In this case, they were interested in what happened to medications once they were in the home. Their study used a variety of methods, including discussions between all members of the household, to investigate how they used and stored medications, and what sources of knowledge they drew on to make decisions about medication.

The general methodological advantages of access to interaction within natural groups are well described by Kitzinger (1994) in her study of how media messages about HIV/AIDS were understood by various audiences in a United Kingdom context. She comments:

We chose to work with pre-existing groups – clusters of people who already knew each other through living, working or socialising together. We did this in order to explore how people might talk about AIDS within the various and overlapping groupings within which they actually operate. Flatmates, colleagues and friends – these are precisely the people with whom one might 'naturally' discuss such topics. The fact that research participants already knew each other had the additional advantage that [they] could relate each other's comments to actual incidents in their daily shared lives. They often challenged each other on contradictions between what they were professing to believe and how they actually behaved. (Kitzinger 1994: 105)

This kind of interaction has advantages for many of the kinds of questions health researchers wish to address. We are often interested not just in the content of knowledge, but in how decisions come to be made, or how information about health is transferred between people within social networks. Individual interviews are often criticized for providing information on what people say, but not on what people do. In interaction between people who know each other, stories about how people say they behave are challenged, corroborated or under-cut, giving some information on the relationship between behaviour and how people talk about it (Kitzinger 1994; Polak and Green 2016). For instance, in a European study on attitudes to food risk, discussed below (Green, Draper and Dowler 2003), adolescents talked during the discussions about how they avoided 'fast food' as 'unsafe'. However, as the group discussion progressed, friends challenged each other, with reminders of how they had eaten burgers from street stalls, especially when they were returning late from clubs or concerts. In analysing focus group data, the researcher can contrast what might be called a 'public' account, such as 'we don't eat fast food', with stories drawn from everyday experience. This can provide data on normative ideas about health – that is, what people think they should do – as well as accounts of situations in which these normative ideas do not necessarily impact on behaviour.

Talking about sensitive issues

A group setting can offer a more supportive environment for participants to discuss sensitive issues. One example is dissatisfaction with health services. In a one-to-one interview, it may be difficult to express dissatisfaction, especially if the interviewer is known to be a health professional or associated with the provider service. In a group, other participants can legitimate negative views, and one participant's story about their experiences can trigger other participants' recollections. However, this has the potential disadvantage of over-emphasizing negative experiences.

There are also some topics for which a focus group might not be an appropriate setting. Using focus groups to explore deviant behaviour, or socially stigmatizing experiences, may be inappropriate if some participants are likely to feel uncomfortable. Interviews may be a more appropriate choice for marginalized participants or sensitive topics. Some studies combine both. Carter, Green and Thorogood (2013), for instance, used household interviews and individual interviews in their study of how electric toothbrushes were used. The household interviews covered issues related to all the members (how decisions were taken to buy a toothbrush, where everyone kept theirs) and individual interviews asked about more sensitive topics (bad breath and hygiene practices).

The growth of digital methods for bringing people together to discuss an issue online, rather than in the same physical location, provides one choice for some sensitive issues (Stewart and Williams 2005). Reisner and colleagues (2019, forthcoming) discuss one example of the advantages of the relative anonymity of online posting. They were interested in the issue of disparities in health screening between transgender and cisgender populations (respectively, those whose personal gender identity does not, or does, correspond with their birth sex). This is a topic about which some transgender individuals were uncomfortable discussing in one-to-one interviews. However, as transgender populations are relatively dispersed, it was difficult to recruit enough volunteers for a physical focus group. The researchers therefore recruited a national sample of female-to-male trans masculine participants for an online focus group, using a variety of targeted advertisements, outreach and snowballing to contact volunteers. They used an asynchronous online bulletin board to conduct their discussion. This was a website which enabled participants to address (in text) a series of posted questions, and respond to the posts of other participants, when they chose to, over a three-day period. Moderators encouraged interaction but discouraged participants from sharing personal details. Reisner and colleagues (2019, forthcoming) conclude that as well as having methodological advantages for accessing marginalized voices from dispersed geographical communities, asynchronous online methods also provide a forum for eliciting considered responses from all participants.

Sampling groups and participants

Sampling in focus group studies entails considering both the selection of groups and the selection of individual participants. As in most qualitative research, the sampling strategy is usually purposeful. That is, it does not aim to be statistically representative of a larger population, but rather to include those groups, and range of groups, most likely to furnish the data needed to address the research question. Pragmatic concerns are also likely to influence both the sample size and who is included. For instance, when focus group research is done with an aim of influencing policy, the sample has to be credible in its coverage of all the constituencies in which policy makers are likely to be interested.

The number of groups needed depends largely on how many constituencies there are within this population of interest. In a local study of health care users, it may be enough to convene two groups of patients, perhaps segregated by gender, as men and women tend to talk very differently in mixed as opposed to single-gender groups. In a study with a broad research question, such as the case study reported at the end of this chapter on how consumers in four European countries choose safe food, there might be a larger number of population segments, and groups can be selected across a sampling grid, as illustrated in Table 9.1 towards the end of the chapter.

Within each group, a key decision is whether to sample participants for homogeneity, where some characteristics are shared, or heterogeneity. Heterogeneity can be an advantage for fostering a range of views within each group, or data on how such views are defended or changed in interaction. Including a range of participants can also be a useful way to trigger participants' accounts of issues that they may consider too 'common sense' to mention, unless prompted by someone who does not share their perspective. Homogeneity, particularly around shared experiences, can provide a more supportive environment for discussing a difficult or sensitive issue, as in the example of transgender participants given earlier.

Ethical considerations

In a focus group, participants outnumber researchers, and this can help shift the balance of power towards participants. In projects that aim to listen to communities, or to access the voice of groups that are traditionally marginalized in the public arena, this can be an important ethical advantage. In work with young people, for instance, using group, as opposed to individual, interviews can be a very useful way of redressing the power imbalance between interviewer and interviewee. However, bringing together strangers with opposing views, or inadvertently eliciting conflict within natural groups can have significant ethical implications. Farnsworth and Boon (2010), for instance, in reporting their experiences with groups brought together to discuss the impact of deprivation, discuss the often under-reported issues of conflict between participants – either between those who had pre-existing relationships or who disagreed vehemently on topics. This can generate considerable anxiety and hostility.

Focus groups differ from individual interviews in that the researcher is not in a position to guarantee the confidentiality of what is said. Participants are reliant on other members to treat them with respect and keep their contributions confidential. The facilitator should set ground rules at the beginning of the discussion, but researchers should be aware that the supportive environment of a group can lead people to 'over-disclose' and perhaps talk about issues in a way that they regret later. This is a particular risk for natural groups. Vissandjee, Abdool and Dupere (2002), in their report of how they used focus groups in a study of women's health behaviour in rural Gujarat in India, discuss this as a particular problem in doing research in small communities. People have to interact with each other long after the research team has gone home. There is an ethical obligation, therefore, to deflect over-disclosure and to make sure that participants do not reveal information they had not intended to and which might make them vulnerable in their everyday lives.

Discussions of ethics tend to focus on informed consent and ensuring that participants have not been cajoled or bullied into taking part. This is of course crucial, particularly if working with gatekeepers who may have put pressure on people. However, there are also ethical concerns about those who do not get the opportunity to contribute. For young people, the need to secure parents' consent may mean that some children are disenfranchised (Green and Hart 1999). Similarly, if using community leaders to aid recruitment, it is worth considering who is not being invited to participate as well as ensuring that those who do have given their genuine consent.

Finally, researchers have an ethical duty to consider what happens to the data from focus groups. Those invited to a group to discuss an issue may have more investment in the research than those who fill in a survey or take part in a brief interview. Where possible, it is good practice to feed back summaries of the findings to those who took part and to let them know what will happen to the findings.

Analysing and presenting focus group data

Managing focus group data can be challenging. In particular, 'naturalistic' data can take time to transcribe and the transcripts may be difficult to comprehend, as participants interrupt, talk over each other and use non-verbal modes of communication. In social research, it is usual to transcribe fully audio-recordings of all group discussions and use these as a basis for analysis. However, in many projects it may be enough to use notes of the discussion, transcribing only those sections of the recording that are most relevant. This is justifiable if only a summary of key concerns is needed or if the aim is to access a group's consensus view on a particular topic, rather than to identify how they came to that decision. If it is not possible to record and transcribe the discussion for practical or political reasons, facilitators should ensure that detailed notes are taken and that the group's views are summarized at key points during the process, perhaps on a white board or flip chart.

Strategies for analysis are similar to techniques for analysing any other qualitative data set, with the approach depending on the aims of the study (see Green and Thorogood 2018). If the focus groups were convened to provide a broad-brush overview of community views or to identify some common issues to feed into later studies, then a fairly simple content analysis of transcripts or notes will suffice. When there is a need to understand public views or health practices, then a more analytical approach, such as grounded theory or some kind of discourse analysis, can be used (Green and Thorogood 2018).

Thematic content analysis

A thematic analysis involves identifying recurring themes within the data, exploring typologies of these themes, and looking at variations in relationships between, and within, themes. Analysis is an iterative process that begins with the first data collected and continues into the writing up of the project. It involves moving between the data and theory in a way that helps to make sense of the data and aids discussion within the research team about 'what is going on here'. This is not just a technical exercise in coding extracts of talk, but one that involves some analytical imagination. However, there are some steps that can help with a simple thematic analysis, which are set out in Box 9.2.

Box 9.2 Steps for thematic analysis

- *Familiarization with the transcripts*: reading and rereading the transcripts and listening to the recordings to get an overall sense of key issues for participants. For example, what made participants angry, enthusiastic or nervous? A summary can be written of each group discussion.
- *Developing a coding frame*: it is worth doing this in a group, with either a team of researchers or colleagues. Read early transcripts in detail, identifying in each segment the key concept. Ask: what is the participant 'talking about'? Try to label these concepts in as abstract a way as possible. Rather than merely summarizing the content, think about what the extracts are an example of and then build these into a coding frame. A coding frame is a list of concepts and their labels (the 'codes').
- *Coding*: when you have a coding framework, the entire set of transcripts can be 'coded' by identifying each segment as an instance of a code. This can be modified as more data are analysed.
- *'Cut and paste'*: all the instances of the same code can now be gathered together, either manually by literally cutting up the transcripts or by using a word processor or specialized software. Then look at the list of extracts under each code to identify the range of talk about each topic.

Thematic content analysis is suitable for mapping out the range and strength of views and comparing the kinds of issues that arise across the group. To exploit the strengths of focus group data and maximize the chance of producing useful policy-relevant findings, a more detailed analysis will probably be needed, which takes interaction into account.

Discourse analysis and social interaction

A common criticism of much focus group research is that researchers often stress the advantage of interaction, but rarely show in published papers how this has been used in the analysis. One exception is Wilkinson and Kitzinger (2000), who studied women's talk about 'thinking positive' in the context of cancer. They provide a good illustration of how analysing interaction can generate a much more sophisticated understanding of health knowledge than merely identifying common content themes. They note that their data could have furnished a number of quotes, such as 'You just have to think positive', stripped out as single utterances reflecting women's views. In a superficial content analysis, these could be identified as 'evidence' of the importance of 'thinking positive' in cancer patients' lives. However, analysis of this talk as discourse enabled Wilkinson and Kitzinger to reflect on how and why such comments are used in interaction. First, they argue that a comment such as 'thinking positive' is a common idiom in English: a taken-for-granted summary of common-sense knowledge. It is used as a general-purpose statement within everyday talk to move the conversation along and to take it from a personal to a general frame. Participants used such idioms when they wanted to cite a shared norm, something with which the audience could agree, and turn a conversation from a potentially difficult one about personal difference into an inclusive one about affiliation. Thus, through paying attention in the analysis to the content of what was said in the context of a discussion, Wilkinson and Kitzinger could identify how interaction works discursively. They were able to specify much more precisely what participants were doing when they invoked such phrases as 'thinking positive'. By so doing, they uncovered the social context in which such statements might be made. In this case, a broad cultural norm was expressed in a setting where 'thinking positive' was the expected and morally required response.

The group as the unit of analysis

Given that focus group studies often include a large number of individual participants, it can be tempting to treat any data as derived from individuals, rather than from groups, and to quantify views expressed by those individuals. This is a mistake. Individuals are not selected as representatives of a broader population, but as a group, and the group should properly be the unit of analysis. Sufficient context should be given about group composition, setting and how data were elicited (for instance, what prompts were used), to enable the reader to judge how the data were generated. This might include details of how the groups and participants were recruited, what social characteristics they shared and which issues they were asked to discuss. A description of the discursive context should also be provided, to indicate how particular utterances were used within the discussion, rather than merely using individuals' statements as indicators of their beliefs. This might include details of which issues elicited agreement or disagreement, which topics were difficult to discuss or joked about and how persuasive particular kinds of accounts were in interaction.

Exploring accounts of food risk using focus groups

As part of a European study of the public perception of risk associated with bovine spongiform encephalopathy (BSE), we wanted to explore public concerns about food risk in general, and to identify what kinds of information on food safety were trusted (Green, Draper and Dowler 2003; Green et al. 2005). The aim was to include

(Continued)

CASE STUDY 9.1

(Continued)

people from four European countries, which had been chosen to represent a range of 'food cultures' (Germany, Italy, the United Kingdom and Finland), and to include people from different stages in the life cycle theoretically associated with different approaches to food choice – adolescents, young adults, those responsible for shopping for young children and older citizens.

In addition to providing detailed data on how people talked about their food choices, we also aimed to compare findings across the four countries and the four life-cycle stage groups. We therefore wanted a similar range of groups in each of the four countries. However, within each country, the meaning of the life-cycle stages and other demographic factors differed. For instance, young men in Italy had rather less experience of choosing their own food than those of a similar age in other countries; and in some countries, regional or rural/urban differences were more pronounced than in others. To include sufficient ranges of groups across life-cycle stages, demographic and geographical differences, we created a sampling grid, which aimed to include a total of 36 groups sampled across the factors, as illustrated in Table 9.1.

TABLE 9.1   Sampling grid for the food risks study focus groups

Country and location	Adolescents	Young adults	Family food purchasers	Older citizens
Finland:				
Kuopio	X	XX	XX	XX
Germany:				
Kiel	X	X	XX	X
Eckernförde	X	X	X	X
Italy:				
Bologna	X	X		X
Naples		X	X	
Trento	XX		X	X
United Kingdom:				
London and environs	X	X	XX	X
Midlands	XXX	X	X	X

Note: X = one focus group

Source: Green et al. (2005)

We recruited natural groups wherever possible, to maximize the methodological advantages discussed above, using a mixture of recruitment methods, including contacting community groups such as church-based or local associations and working with schools to recruit friendship groups of adolescents. However, to recruit 'young adult' groups, which may consist of relatively mobile individuals with few obvious community allegiances, we relied on market research companies.

The protocols for running the groups had to balance comparability with flexibility. We used icebreaking exercises, asking participants to rank pictures of foodstuffs in terms of their 'riskiness', to generate discussion in all groups, with the pictures reflecting the kinds of food eaten locally. The list of topics to cover in each group was the same, but facilitators worded prompts appropriately for local participants.

To analyse a data set in four different languages, we first took pilot data from each country, and transcribed and translated the data into English, so all the project teams could collaborate on initial thematic analysis and generate a combined coding scheme to aid comparative analysis. This was used within each country to generate a country report and provide a more detailed analysis. These reports were then subject to a 'meta-analysis' to produce integrated results across the study.

Access to interaction in the groups provided useful accounts of choosing, preparing and eating safe food. In the transcripts, we could see to which sources of knowledge people referred and how effective these sources were in persuading others. For instance, personal anecdotes about food risk were observed as more effective for convincing others than media reports. Interaction provided evidence of consequences of talk about risk. For instance, talk about 'differences', such as ethnicity and religion, was reframed in many group discussions into talk about risk, illustrating some of the social uses of the rhetoric of risk in a multicultural society. This example is from a group of women in the United Kingdom, who quickly reframed one participant's religious rationale for avoiding pork into a frame of 'hygiene':

A: We don't eat pork in any case ... for religious reasons.

B: A lot of the religious things to do with meat come from the hygiene aspect anyway, like Jewish people, they won't store meat in the same fridge as dairy produce – a lot of that is down to hygiene.

C: They are dirty, pigs.

D: Absolutely, it has been proved apparently, many years ago.

E: So it all comes down to hygiene.

Source: Green, Draper and Dowler (2003: 42)

Reading health research based on focus groups

The criteria used to judge the usefulness or quality of published focus group research will depend on the reader's needs. For instance, readers may want an insight into the views of a population or to understand in greater depth the barriers to service uptake. Journal editors, particularly for biomedical journals, now often require authors to conform to guidelines for reporting on focus group and other qualitative methods (see Tong, Sainsbury and Craig

2007). Although there is debate about the appropriateness of such formal quality criteria, they do suggest some questions to ask when assessing the quality of focus group studies. These questions include:

- Is the rationale for the use of focus groups (rather than, say, individual interviews) made clear?
- Have the authors explained their sampling strategy? Is there a rationale for the selection of particular focus groups, the range, or the homogeneity of the groups?
- Have the author(s) said how participants were recruited? Is there some evidence of reflexivity about the role of the research team and the choice of setting?
- Is there enough evidence for the reader to judge how the context may have shaped the data generated?
- Are interactive data extracts reported, rather than just utterances from single participants?
- Does the analysis take interaction into account?

Conclusion

Focus groups have a number of advantages as a method of data generation, as they can provide access to the way in which people discuss issues and deal with problems related to health in everyday life. These advantages are particularly pertinent where people share a common background or already know each other. Interaction within the group enables the researcher to understand frameworks of meaning, what resources people use and how they draw on social networks to deal with matters that arise on a day-to-day basis. Focus groups that bring together a group of people from different backgrounds to discuss a particular topic can also serve to demonstrate the range of views about a specific issue. However, using focus groups can be challenging in terms of management, resources, process, data recording and analysis, particularly for the lone researcher. It is also important for researchers using focus groups to remember that they have generated data on groups, not on individuals within those groups. Case Study 9.1 demonstrates how focus groups can be used to explore people's understanding of food risk. Exercise 9.1 provides the opportunity for readers to consider employing the method to find out about people's experience of maternity services and their priorities in any reorganization.

Exercise 9.1   Planning a focus group study of maternity services

There are plans to reorganize local maternity services, and a research programme has been commissioned to find out the views of staff and users on what could be improved in the new system. You have been asked to carry out some focus groups, with professionals and users, to explore their views of current service provision and their priorities for change. Write a brief (500-word) proposal for a focus group study. This should cover the following issues:

- Sampling:
    - Which groups of users and professionals should be included?
    - How many will be needed to cover the main constituencies of interest?
    - Are there particular subgroups of the population that should be included?
    - Will the groups be homogeneous or heterogeneous, and what is the rationale for your decision?

- A protocol for running the groups:
    - Think of an introductory exercise that would be appropriate for the groups of professionals and users.
    - List 5–6 prompts for a topic guide.

- Resources:
    - What resources are needed to conduct your study?

- Ethical issues:
    - What particular ethical issues are raised by conducting your proposed study?
    - How will these ethical issues be addressed?
    - What issues might be raised in disseminating the findings?

- Assessment:
    - What are the main advantages and disadvantages of using focus groups for this study?

Recommended further reading

This book is a practical guide to using focus groups, taking the reader through the whole process from design to writing up, with many examples from health research:
Barbour, R. (2018) *Doing Focus Groups*, 3rd edition. London: Sage.

This book usefully discusses the more methodological issues raised by employing focus groups in social research in health and is particularly strong on issues of analysis and interpretation:
Bloor, M., Frankland, J., Thomas, M. and Robson, K. (2001) *Focus Groups in Social Research*. London: Sage.

The authors of this text use their experience of a range of studies/participants to provide excellent practical advice on all stages of an applied focus group study – planning and recruiting, moderating, coping with problems and managing and reporting data:

Kreuger, R. and Casey, M. A. (2015) *Focus Groups: A Practical Guide for Applied Research*, 5th edition. London: Sage.

References

Barbour, R. S., Macleod, M., Mires, G. and Anderson, A. S. (2011) 'Uptake of folic acid supplements before and during pregnancy: Focus group analysis of women's views and experiences', *Journal of Human Nutrition and Dietetics*, *25*: 140–7.

Bloor, M., Frankland, J., Thomas, M. and Robson, K. (2001) *Focus Groups in Social Research*. London: Sage.

Carter, S., Green, J. and Thorogood, N. (2013) 'The domestication of an everyday health technology: A case study of electric toothbrushes', *Social Theory and Health*, *11*(4): 344–67.

Christie, N., Steinbach, R., Green, J., Mullan, M. P. and Prior, L. (2017) 'Pathways linking car transport for young adults and the public health in Northern Ireland: A qualitative study to inform the evaluation of graduated driver licensing', *BMC Public Health*, *17*(1): 551.

Dew, K., Norris, P., Gabe, J., Chamberlain, K. and Hodgetts, D. (2015) 'Moral discourses and pharmaceuticalised governance in households', *Social Science and Medicine*, *131*: 272–9.

Evans, M., Stoddart, H., Condon, L., Freeman, E., Grizzell, M. and Mullen, R. (2001) 'Parents' perspectives on the MMR immunisation: A focus group study', *British Journal of General Practice*, *51*: 904–10.

Farnsworth, J. and Boon, B. (2010) 'Analysing group dynamics within the focus group', *Qualitative Research*, *10*(5): 605–24.

Green, J., Draper, A. and Dowler, E. (2003) 'Short cuts to safety: Risk and "rules of thumb" in accounts of food choice', *Health, Risk and Society*, *5*: 33–52.

Green, J., Draper, A., Dowler, E., Fele, G., Hagenhoff, V., Rusanen, M. and Rusanen, T. (2005) 'Public understanding of food risks in four European countries: A qualitative study', *European Journal of Public Health*, *15*: 523–7.

Green, J. and Hart, L. (1999) 'The impact of context on data', in R. Barbour and J. Kitzinger (eds), *Developing Focus Group Research*. London: Sage.

Green, J. and Thorogood, N. (2018) *Qualitative Methods for Health Research*, 4th edition. London: Sage

Kitzinger, J. (1994) 'The methodology of focus groups: The importance of interaction between research participants', *Sociology of Health and Illness*, *16*: 103–21.

Polak, L. and Green, J. (2016) 'Using joint interviews to add analytic value', *Qualitative Health Research*, *26*(12): 1638–48.

Reisner, S. L., Randazzo, R. K., White Hughto, J. M., Peitzmeier, S., DuBois, L. Z., Pardee, D. J., Marrow, E., McLean, S. and Potter, J. (2019, forthcoming) 'Sensitive health topics with underserved patient populations: Methodological considerations for online focus group discussions', *Qualitative Health Research*.

Stewart, K. and Williams, M. (2005) 'Researching online populations: The use of online focus groups for social research', *Qualitative Research*, *5*(4): 395–416.

Tong, A., Sainsbury, P. and Craig, J. (2007) 'Consolidated criteria for reporting qualitative research (COREQ): A 32-item checklist for interviews and focus groups', *International Journal for Quality in Health Care*, *19*: 349–57.

Vissandjee, B., Abdool, S. and Dupere, S. (2002) 'Focus groups in rural Gujarat, India: A modified approach', *Qualitative Health Research*, *12*: 826–43.

Wilkinson, S. and Kitzinger, C. (2000) 'Thinking differently about thinking positive', *Social Science and Medicine*, *50*: 797–811.

10

Action Research and Health

HEATHER WATERMAN

Chapter objectives

- To outline the main features of action research
- To highlight the challenges of action research
- To indicate how these challenges can be overcome
- To demonstrate how action research can positively transform health.

Introduction

Action research is a participative method of research that seeks to gain knowledge and to change people's circumstances for the better by engaging them in the research process. The process of action research is therefore complex and requires participants to develop skills in research, practice, education and change management. This chapter outlines some of the challenges of action research and how difficulties can be overcome. Despite the pitfalls, the literature on action research shows that this approach can have a positive impact on people's health and health services.

From a personal perspective as an action researcher, I have shifted from a position of viewing action research as a technical approach to solving problems in health care to seeing the method as one that aspires towards empowerment and democracy. In this case, empowerment refers to enabling research participants to take action, often in difficult situations, and democracy, to encouraging people from diverse backgrounds to debate freely and work towards improving their circumstances through research. As a practitioner, a ward manager, I was enthusiastic about the immediacy of action research and challenged by the idea of studying a situation and changing practice at the same time. Later, after participating in several action research projects, I came to appreciate the significance of critical reflection within groups and joint decisions on action, thus empowering participants, both practitioners and patients, in health care settings. The increased knowledge and confidence that occurs enables changes to be made by those who are experiencing a problem, whether they are patients or staff, in areas related to direct patient care, management, administration or education. Action research, by its nature, is an exercise of democracy as it encourages a group of people who normally may not be heard to change their lives, to work together actively and take responsibility for changing their situation.

However, over time, I have become more realistic and critical of the method. In this chapter, I will expand on these issues by:

- Examining the main characteristics and rationale for action research in health care settings and the resources required to apply it in practice
- Considering the strengths and weaknesses of action research and the challenges of data analysis and report writing
- Providing an example of action research and an exercise to help the reader understand the interrelationships between theory, method and data.

Action research: Background rationale

The definition, methods and history of action research are now explored.

Definition and methods

Action research is defined by Kemmis and McTaggart (1988: 5) as:

> simply a form of collective self-reflective enquiry undertaken by participants in social situations in order to improve the rationality and justice of their own situations, their understandings of these practices and the situations in which these practices are carried out.

This definition captures the essence of action research in highlighting its participatory and action-oriented goals. It also underlines that learning is an important part of the process. In practice, action research has been variously interpreted and applied depending on the research paradigm and discipline base of the researcher (Jagosh et al. 2012). For example, action research in a health education setting will tend to play out differently from that found in commercial organizations (Hart and Bond 1995). The former is likely to focus on a single teacher who has chosen to improve the quality of their teaching, and the latter will tend to concentrate on institution-wide problems as identified by senior managers.

History of action research

Action research emerged from a branch of social psychology in the early-mid part of the twentieth century. Kurt Lewin has been identified as the originator of action research. He fled Nazi Germany and settled in the United States (Adelman 1993). There, he was influenced by John Dewey, who was critical of approaches to science that divorced knowledge from action and preferred a form of science that tested theories in practice (Dewey 1929). Lewin was also interested in improving the situation of minority groups through reflection, research and collective responsibility. Lewin believed that to tackle issues of inequality there needed to be practical 'experiments' undertaken through democratic participation of all participants (Adelman 1993). He outlined the participatory cycle of action research that incorporated fact finding (also known as reflection or reconnaissance), planning, action and evaluation, reflection, planning, and action (Lewin 1947). Each phase is the foundation for the next. Readers from a nursing or quality assurance background will find the outline of this process similar to the nursing process and the audit cycle. However, as Figure 10.1 shows, it is fundamentally different from both as there is iteration between reflection, action and research, and an ethos of empowerment and democracy that is fundamental to action research.

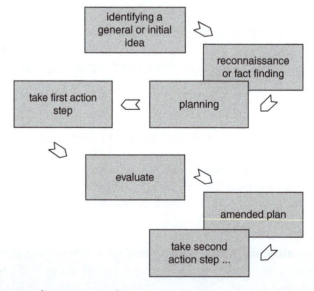

FIGURE 10.1   Diagram of action research

Source: Lewin (1947), adapted from Smith (2007)

Research may be undertaken using a range of methods: surveys, interviews with patients and practitioners, focus group interviews, observation of practice and the secondary analysis of previous research. Qualitative and quantitative research methods are employed, depending on the nature of the problem and the scope of the project (van Buul et al. 2014). The research should aim to provide insight into different perspectives on a problem and may be undertaken throughout the process of action research in order to help assess what needs to be done and to monitor and evaluate any changes introduced. In the study to be discussed, patients' perspectives were sought through letters and focus group interviews; staff views were gathered via interviews; clinical nursing care was observed; and the effect of different post-operative 'posturing regimes' was measured (Waterman et al. 2005a, 2005b).

The principles of action research: Improving practice, critical reflection, participation and implementation

In discussing the principles of action research, and its strengths and weaknesses, illustrative examples will be drawn mainly from this one study, referred to throughout the chapter as the 'Posturing Study.' This action research study was undertaken at a regional eye hospital in the United Kingdom. The study aimed to encourage patients to maintain a regime of 'face-down posturing' following retinal surgery. This had been recommended as a regime to maintain healing, but there was uncertainty about how best to support patients in following the regime at home. The first phase of the action research project consisted of interviews with nurses and doctors from both inpatient and outpatient settings to learn about current practice and how this could be improved. This led to a consensus among staff that the best way forward was to make 'take-home' specialist equipment available for patients to help them to 'posture' for longer and, in consequence, achieve more cost-effective treatment. This study illustrates a number of principles of action research.

Principles to improve practice

The first principle of action research in health care is to improve practice and patient outcome. Action research aims to assist both practitioners and patients to understand their problems better and to enlighten and inform them so that they can decide on action (Ericson-Lidman and Strandberg 2015). The research moves beyond describing the 'status quo' as in traditional research, to speculating on what 'might or ought to be', then by introducing changes and assessing the results. Thus, the research is about producing knowledge for action (Winter and Munn-Giddings 2001).

Critical reflection

A second principle is critical reflection. While presented for the purposes of explanation as separate from research method, in practice critical reflection has an interdependent relationship to it. It binds together all activities associated with the research process and leads to empowerment and action. In practice, critical reflection in a group setting refers to the process of identifying and examining the assumptions that underpin daily activity and asks whether the ideologies and attitudes that influence practice are those that best serve the interests of patients and staff. It means examining critically professional values and assumptions and assessing whether these are carried into practice.

Professionals will have their own views of what actually happens in practice. A further test is to investigate the views of patients. Critical reflection aims to examine the (power) relationships between practitioners and patients as well as between, and within, professional groups. Different perspectives on a problem are deliberately sought to help illuminate an issue and prevent one viewpoint from taking precedence. Some techniques aim to enable patients and practitioners to discuss issues together and for professionals from different disciplines to share their experiences with one another (Norbye 2016). An example of this process is described by Waterman and colleagues (2005a, 2005b) in the Posturing Study. Here, the key stakeholders in the project on post-retinal surgery – namely, nurses, a specialist registrar and managers – watched a number of videos of patient focus group interviews. These showed that patients were critical of the lack of warning about, and information on, posturing. This provoked discussion that was critical of the ethos, practicalities and effects of existing forms of nursing and medical care.

A synthesis of different perspectives occurs over time, both in the group and individually. By drawing on experiences and integrating these with other types of evidence, conclusions can be drawn about how, and why, practice should be changed. The main result of this critical reflection led to the setting up of nurse-led, pre-operative clinics so that patients could be provided with detailed information about 'posturing' two weeks in advance of their surgery. The process of critical reflection is challenging. It takes time and, as indicated later, may not always be successful.

Participation

A third principle in action research is participation. This is linked to ideas of democracy and the belief that people should be able to inform providers of health care and participate in, or be consulted about, decisions (Jagosh et al. 2012). Compared with traditional approaches to research, where participants may play a passive role where they do not determine research questions or affect practice, participants in action research tend to be active. Cornwall and Jewkes (1995) argue that action research was born out of methodological critiques of conventional research that ignored issues of power and subjugated the research subject. A partnership between researchers and participants is seen as equitable and liberating. Action research can therefore address the contemporary NHS agenda for patient and public involvement (INVOLVE 2017a). However, resources are required to achieve participation by a range of people and this is discussed below.

The level of participation may vary within a project and between projects. Cornwall (1996) identifies six types of participation, ranging from co-option and token representation with no real input, to collective action where local people set, and carry out, the research agenda without assistance from professional researchers. In many action research projects in health, participants have been practitioners – that is, mainly nurses and doctors (Waterman et al. 2001). In health and social care, clients and carers, and students are consulted and may cooperate with a project, but they tend not to be placed in an equal position with health care practitioners (Norbye 2016). As Cornwall and Jewkes (1995) describe, they are 'participants in a process' over which they have no real control.

Research by Bradburn and Mackie (2001) is an exception. In their project, clients with cancer jointly led an action research project. The aim was to raise awareness of the needs of cancer service users in cancer service planning meetings of the local health authority. The clients were directly involved in determining the course of the project. One hazard of research with patients who have a particular illness is that some patients may be, or become, too ill to participate actively. Researchers in these circumstances must take care to respect the wishes of participants.

Box 10.1   Forms of Action

There are several forms of action research:

- *Innovation*: an instance was a study that developed and introduced individual performance review in hospital practice for doctors (Trebble et al. 2013).
- *Improvements*: an example is the project to provide an individualized meal schedule in residential care for older people that overcame shortcomings in a rigidly organized meal regime (Ericson-Lidman and Strandberg 2015).
- *Development of knowledge and theory*: for instance, nurse educators formed an action research group to develop peer reflective supervision and report on seven themes of a practical tool box that could be used by others in a similar situation (Bulman et al. 2016).
- *Involvement of users and health care staff*: for example, action research was employed to involve end-users, health care staff, in the improvement of electronic health record systems (Vabo, Slettebo and Fossum 2016).

These examples do not take account of the subtler actions that can occur through critical reflection.

Change intervention

A fourth principle of action research is the inclusion of a change intervention. A systematic review identifies areas where action research may be useful (Waterman et al. 2001). Examples are shown in Box 10.1 above.

When to choose action research

Action research may be an appropriate choice of research methodology when a problem is complex, poorly understood, culture-bound, raises ethical issues or where there are conflicts that require resolution. It is particularly useful where one occupational group dominates another. Koshy, Koshy and Waterman (2011) suggest that meetings and other fora allow for critical reflection and help to empower all participants. For example, the Posturing Study and the iterative action research process demonstrated differences in perception between staff. Nurses felt they were doing their best to encourage patients to posture, but patients found it difficult to carry out the instructions given by doctors, while doctors themselves thought that their post-operative instructions were being ignored. Through the research process, nurses and doctors came to see that their consultations in the outpatients' clinic had been too superficial to convey to patients the importance of following a face-down posturing regime and patients had not been given sufficient information to follow advice at home.

Resources: Human, technical and support staff

Action research is resource intensive and costly. For instance, the Posturing Study involved eight members of staff in the core team as well as the author as research director. There were also on-costs for implementing changes in practice. While a systematic review on action research projects showed that a majority did not secure external funding (Waterman et al. 2001), more recent action research studies report having attracted financial support (Ericson-Lidman and Strandberg 2015; Marshall et al. 2006; van Buul et al. 2014). Funding is essential, in part because participants must be released from their day-to-day activities and this may be gained from health authorities, charities and research funding agencies, or governmental bodies. However, action researchers face certain barriers as their proposals may not fit the conventional research template. They should ensure that there is a match between what they want to do and the objectives of the funding organization.

Table 10.1 outlines the main tasks and resources needed to carry out an action research project. The budget should be worked out between participants so that all their costs are accounted for. Sometimes full economic costing is required, including overheads and costs of supervision. Action researchers should seek advice on what they need to cost from research accountants, business managers and experienced action researchers.

TABLE 10.1 Resources typically required for an action research project

Item	Purpose
Research assistant	To facilitate the research and the process of critical reflection; to work closely with the clinical team
Time for all stakeholders	To pay for staff replacements so staff can attend meetings
Travel expenses including accommodation	To pay for travel costs incurred – for example, by clients to attend meetings and to pay for a hotel
Tape recorder and transcribing machines	To record meetings/interviews and to speed up the process of transcribing
Transcribing costs	To pay for a typist to undertake transcription of interview recordings
Costs for educational qualification	To pay for MSc, MPhil or PhD fees, where necessary/ permitted
Miscellaneous costs	To pay for unforeseen costs that may occur in action research, including implementation costs and dissemination costs

The strengths of action research

Action research has three main strengths. First, it can lead to contextually relevant changes or innovations in practice, education or management that will have a positive effect on the outcome of a health care interventions and the patient experience. Second, the knowledge and theory gained are directly relevant for action. Third, participants are empowered to find solutions to their problems. Each of these strengths will now be explored in turn.

Action research: Change and innovation

The rhetoric of action research focuses on how it can improve people's situations. There are many examples of action research where this ultimate goal has been achieved. These include the reorganization of inpatient and outpatient services; the identification and development of new professional roles for nurses and allied health professionals; new care planning documentation; better assessment and management of patients; and the development of educational packages for students and educational videos for patients. However, not all projects bring about successful changes (Waterman et al. 2001).

There is no single cause for a lack of success, but bear in mind the following factors: over-ambition; the imposition of researchers' goals upon participants; a high staff turnover so group cohesion is lost; power relations where one professional group dominates another; poor external supervision; a lack of research skills; poor interpersonal skills on the part of the researcher; a lack of, or withdrawal of, organizational support; and, lastly, deliberate sabotage. Action research is more likely to succeed when realistic expectations are set; where there are good collaborative relationships; the research is supervised; and the lead researcher is familiar with action research and has good people-management skills. Finally, organizational support is vital.

It has been argued that action research can promote professional development as staff can reflect critically on their situation and participate in various activities. As Norbye (2016) indicates, this is thought to lead to:

- Greater self-confidence as the process is self-validating
- Enhanced competence as it is a learning exercise
- Reassessment and consolidation of professional values as these are dissected and reconstructed.

However, it is not easy to demonstrate whether and how these changes in practice have taken place, let alone attribute them to action research. A self-reflective diary and interviews may record personal views of changes in understanding, or observations of nursing care in practice may demonstrate that changes have taken place.

Action research, knowledge and theory development

Another of the main advantages of action research is that it produces knowledge and theory that are relevant to a particular context (Coghlan and Casey 2001). Typically, knowledge and theoretical ideas are identified in the first phase of a project and then tried out and evaluated. Findings are reflected upon and action plans amended. In other words, practice is studied in order to change it and then to change it again in the light of this assessment (Winter and Munn-Giddings 2001). The interaction between reflection, research and action broadens the developing theory and makes it more applicable to the particular research setting. As Hope and Waterman (2003) argue, the dialectical process of action research prevents premature closure and provides opportunities for further study to enhance the depth and breadth of analysis. The Posturing Study illustrates this process of change and reassessment. While initially research participants thought that the purchase and use of specialist equipment would facilitate adherence to post-operative posturing instructions, as the equipment was utilized it became apparent that there were other issues. An analysis suggested that both better communication with patients and further education were also necessary.

Informal 'theory' is locally bound, unwritten, practical and experiential. It takes place within individuals and helps to develop personal explanatory frameworks for action. In the Posturing Study, discussions among nurses showed they felt competent in what they were doing to help patients and the reasons that underlay their practice (Waterman et al. 2005a, 2005b). Theory may also be formal, communicable and generalizable beyond the specific setting. Within action research, there is a tension between undertaking rigorous research to develop theory that is generalizable and the pragmatic concerns of the staff group or institution to improve practice. In the Posturing Study, managers wanted changes to be made before we had completed the research into patient experiences of face-down posturing. We carried on with the research and documented the parallel changes and their effect, but this led to some loss of rigour and reduced the possibilities for generalizability. Coghlan and Casey (2001) underline the importance of understanding the institutional context in action research to identify potential hazards early on in a project.

Action research and empowering participants

A common justification for action research is the empowerment of those who are oppressed or marginalized. Empowerment is a subtle process that occurs as participants gain in confidence, knowledge and understanding but it takes time. An example can be drawn from the Posturing Study. It took a number of phases in the project before nurse-led instruction could be introduced in outpatient pre-operative clinics.

Limitations and dilemmas in action research

As well as strengths, there are a number of limitations and dilemmas in action research: empowerment and management issues; the challenge of data collection and analysis; ethical issues; and writing up and presenting findings.

Empowerment and management issues

Empowerment is not always achieved in action research. For example, Sturt (1997) attempted to carry out action research in a primary health care trust in a study to improve health promotion practices for smoking cessation. She reports that the practice nurses were effectively disempowered by the doctors, who took a decision to halt the project without negotiation. This led to frustration and dissatisfaction for all concerned. Ironically, although empowerment is thought to be useful in conflict resolution, when hitherto hidden power relations are revealed, this may lead to surprise, shock or even explicit conflict. Cornwall and Jewkes (1995) suggest that while action researchers may be enthusiastic about empowerment, participants may prefer the status quo of hierarchical relationships. Inevitably, empowerment means going outside one's 'comfort zone', provoking anxiety and uncertainty. It is important also for the researcher to be wary of raising expectations at the beginning of the study by discussing possibilities of empowerment. The starting point of any project is a careful analysis of the original problem and an assessment of how the project fits into the wider organization (Coghlan and Casey 2001).

Closely connected to the issue of empowerment is the question of whether a project should be managed by an insider or outsider. Action researchers may be insiders holding a formal position of employment in the research institution, or they may be outsiders who are facilitating a project in an organization where they have no formal position. In practice, the two positions are often blurred. For example, a researcher may be an employee – that is, an insider – but at the same time an outsider to the group taking part in the research. Both situations have advantages and disadvantages. An insider will have knowledge of the organizational structure and this is useful in getting support and approval for the project. On the other hand, they may be constrained by unwritten organizational rules and may have to live with the consequences of the action research process (Coghlan and Casey 2001). In contrast, an outsider will have to spend time getting to know formal organizational structures and informal social relationships. However, they may be in a better position to see the opportunities for change.

The challenge of data collection and analysis

A further challenge in action research is how to collect and analyse data. Winter and Munn-Giddings (2001) identify three reasons for undertaking data analysis in action research:

- Data may be analysed to provide insights into what changes can be made in the future
- Data interpretation helps to make findings generalizable
- Data can be used to provide a baseline to explore what learning has taken place.

If participants discuss and plan their approach to data analysis in advance, then any tension between these objectives will be reduced.

In a conventional research project, the researcher is 'detached' from the research setting and has sole responsibility for data collection and analysis. In action research, not only are there difficult and possibly conflicting purposes for data collection, but priorities may shift over time. Moreover, there may be various sources of data that will be available at different points in the life of a project. How data are to be analysed, by whom and for what purpose, will require active management in a participative manner (Christensen and Atweh 1998). In the Posturing Study, for example, a staff nurse and I undertook most of the detailed analysis of patient focus group interviews. Then, the team as a whole participated in reflective discussions based on the results. In a subsequent randomized controlled trial, a research student undertook all the statistical analysis so that the results could be presented for discussion.

As indicated, action researchers may collect both qualitative and quantitative data over the course of an action research project. Using a mixed-methods approach is advantageous as it provides multiple perspectives of the issue under consideration but, on the other hand, it can be challenging. Westhues and colleagues (2008) aimed to improve practice in a community mental health organization. They carried out an extensive literature review, set up focus group interviews (a qualitative method) and undertook an online survey (a quantitative method). The research took place in two geographic locations, had four sub-projects and a multidisciplinary team, and provided multiple perspectives. The data collection in the different arms of the study was conducted in parallel, which was useful in terms of a timely triangulation of data. However, had the researchers carried out a sequential form of data collection, they would have had the opportunity to explore unexpected issues that emerged more thoroughly. They report that the process of reaching a shared understanding within the team of the findings from the different data sets was time-consuming and intellectually challenging. Moreover, engagement with practitioners and patients in the study was not constant, so their interest waned, particularly when the researchers were undertaking the analysis and synthesis of data. In summary, participants, including researchers, also found it difficult to fully grasp all the research findings.

Ethical issues

Ethical issues arise in the course of action research both before and during a study. These require discussion and negotiation with participants. Participating in action research may lead to additional burdens for participants who may be ill, or who face difficulties in their daily lives, and the commitment of professionals may fluctuate due to work and external life events during a project (Salmon, Browne and Pederson 2010). In the course of the Posturing Study, family commitments affected staff participation. Issues of confidentiality and maintaining the anonymity of participants were issues. It should not be assumed that identities are hidden by using anonymous quotes (Williamson and Prosser 2002). Acknowledgements and contact details can give away information that can lead to the identification of participants. On the other hand, in an action research project that took place in Kenya, project participants wanted their contributions acknowledged, as this gave recognition and status, but did not want to be individually cited in quotations (Waterman et al. 2007). Guidance on these matters is provided on websites for INVOLVE (2017b), a United Kingdom national advisory group.

Writing up and presenting findings

Christensen and Atweh (1998) rightly suggest that writing a report is an essential stage in action research. This represents the final and formal end of reflective activities in which all strands of the study should be pulled together. The submission of a report to a funding agency is a significant act of closure. The public distribution of a report and papers are also important in the external validation of the work and usually involves external peer review. Yet there may be different interests in what kind of report should be written and for what audience.

In preparing to write their report, McNiff, Lomax and Whitehead (1996: 134) identified four different audiences for a research project: 'your boss, your colleagues, your tutor, and your academic peers'. These may require different kinds of report. Most reports are presented chronologically to tell a 'story' of the different cycles of the project (van Buul et al. 2014), or focus on one part of it (O'Brien, Butler and Casey 2017), or discuss methodological issues (Mayan and Daum 2016).

In keeping with the rest of the process of action research, writing up should be participative. However, as Christensen and Atweh (1998) identify, this is not always straightforward. If a number of researchers undertake different parts of the research, deadlines will have to be coordinated. Some participants may not have the experience or confidence to write, but nevertheless may feel excluded if they are not included in some way. To maintain the integrity of the project and to prevent conflict, writing up and authorship should be discussed openly in the early stages of the project and revisited often. Christensen and Atweh (1998) present three strategies for participative writing:

- One person takes responsibility to write the full first draft, which is then passed around other participants for comment. This is progressive writing.
- Accounts may be written by different groups and placed together in a final report.
- A small group of people plan and write together. This is 'shared writing' (Wagaman and Sanchez 2017).

In all of these situations, agreement must be reached on whose 'voice' is given priority. This is tied into issues of power and the importance of retaining a sense of shared ownership. Sharing and learning skills requires time and patience, but they can be rewarding. This leads neatly on to Case Study 10.1.

CASE STUDY 10.1

A participatory action research project: Health care professionals plan, take and evaluate action to prevent maternal mortality in rural Nigeria

The following provides an example of how action research can be applied in resource-limited countries (Esienumoh, Allotey and Waterman 2018).

Context

A third of the 300,000 maternal deaths that occur globally are in Nigeria and India (WHO et al. 2015). Most of these deaths could be prevented if community support was mobilized and if maternity care was accessible and delivered by trained staff (United Nations 2007).

Participatory action research was set up with members of a rural Nigerian community and health care professionals to plan, take action and evaluate to reduce maternal mortality. Twelve people from across the community volunteered to be part of a Participatory Action Research Group (PARG). The PARG included women of child-bearing age, menopausal women, husbands, community elders, a woman's leader, clergymen, midwives, a doctor and a traditional birth attendant (TBA). This group became co-researchers with the primary researcher in undertaking the project.

PARG members and the primary researcher carried out and analysed 29 semi-structured interviews with community members, observations of the practice of five TBAs and eight focus groups to understand the perceptions and behaviour about the causes of maternal mortality and how it could be prevented. It was found that maternal deaths were often attributed to certain folk beliefs, although some respondents referred to biological reasons, including post-partum haemorrhage. Some saw the practices of TBAs with inadequate facilities as contributing to infection and others considered that decisions to refer to hospital were left too late. These factors were exacerbated by poor transport and a lack of trained staff.

The PARG and the primary researcher considered a course of action to raise awareness of the biological causes of maternal mortality, ways to improve transportation to hospital and to make the health services more accessible. Education workshops were set up for TBAs to establish a link with qualified midwives and provide them with basic birthing kits.

Subsequently, a further eight focus groups were held with participants to assess the impact of the actions taken on the knowledge, attitudes and practices. As before, the data were co-analysed. The interview data demonstrate some improvements with, for example, efforts to provide better transportation, earlier referrals to hospital and better attendance at the local health facility for antenatal care.

In conclusion, the project has empowered a group of people into becoming an important resource in itself in the fight against maternal mortality and enabled a critical approach to the prevention of maternal mortality and led to findings that will be of interest and use to settings beyond this particular context.

Reading health research based on an action approach

Action research can be appraised like any other research methodology but should be carried out from the perspective of its characteristics. Waterman and colleagues (2001) suggest the following criteria for assessing the quality of the action research:

- Were the phases of action research clearly outlined? This question helps reviewers to assess whether the process of action research was shown: fact-finding, planning, action, evaluation and reassessment.
- Were the inclusion criteria for participants and stakeholders described and justified? How were they selected?

- Was the local context described together with the plan for change and cultural factors to be taken into account?
- Was the relationship between the researchers and participants adequately considered? Was the level and extent of participation appropriate? Is there critical reflection on changing perspectives and roles?

Conclusion

The argument underlying this chapter is that the action research method is an appropriate tool where the aim is to change practice or behaviour. A key aspect of achieving this change is to include the range of professionals who provide a service; those who are the clients or patients using a service; people in groups or communities who stand to benefit from improved practice; and researchers with relevant skills. Depending on the nature of the project, all members of such groups or their representatives should be included. The role of the lead researcher in an action research project is a challenging one; not only are research skills required, but also the ability to play a number of roles as an educator, facilitator and mediator. Furthermore, unlike other forms of research where the researcher tends to act as a detached observer, in action research they should be committed to achieving the outcomes of the research while not allowing this commitment to cloud their judgement in evaluating data and findings. Case Study 10.1 on action research and maternal mortality in resource-limited countries shows that action research is a flexible method that may be used in a variety of settings. Exercise 10.1 focuses on applying action research to a health-related work setting with which you are familiar.

Exercise 10.1   The use of action research in a health-related work setting

This exercise is intended to help readers critically explore the issues raised in this chapter, and particularly to explore the interrelationship between theory, method and data in action research. On the basis of the practical advice provided in this chapter, draw up a proposal for an action research project based on your own experience in a work setting in which you either operate, or of which you have some knowledge. First, identify an area of practice that you think causes problems. This may, for example, give rise to conflict among professional groups or relate to an aspect of practice that is not up to standard. You should then answer the following questions:

- Where would you obtain funding to carry out the project?
- What methods could be used to understand the problem better?
- Who will be the key participants in the action research team and what is the rationale for inclusion?

- How will you promote and maintain participation in the project?
- How will you apply the action research process to your issue and context?
- What process of critical reflection might be implemented and what part will it play in moving the research project forward?
- Will you be an insider or outsider to the research setting and what effect will your position have on the project?
- What ethical issues will be encountered in the course of the project and how will they be addressed?
- What knowledge and theory will be generated for participants and service users planning to improve the care of patients in your area of interest?
- What will be the limitations of your project?

Recommended further reading

This book offers a good introduction to action research, containing a useful typology and history of the methodology involved:

Hart, E. and Bond, M. (1995) *Action Research for Health and Social Care: A Guide for Practice.* Milton Keynes: Open University Press.

The latest version of this classic book provides a detailed framework for the first phase of action research, giving much helpful advice:

Kemmis, S., McTaggart, R. and Nixon R. (2013) *The Action Research Planner*, 4th edition. Singapore: Springer Verlag.

This text is a handbook for action researchers, describing and exploring the theoretical issues underpinning action research:

Winter, R. and Munn-Giddings, C. (2001) *A Handbook for Action Research in Health and Social Care.* London: Routledge.

References

Adelman, C. (1993) 'Kurt Lewin and the origins of action research', *Educational Action Research*, *1*(1): 7–24.

Bradburn, J. and Mackie, C. (2001) 'A foot in the door: A collaborative action research project with cancer service users', in R. Winter and C. Munn-Giddings (eds), *A Handbook for Action Research in Health and Social Care.* London: Routledge.

Bulman, C., Forde-Johnson, C., Griffiths, A., Hallworth, S., Kerry, A., Khan, S., Mills, K. and Sharp, P. (2016) 'The development of peer reflective supervision amongst nurse educator colleagues: An action research project', *Nurse Education Today*, *45*: 148–55.

Christensen, C. and Atweh, B. (1998) 'Collaborative writing in participatory action research', in B. Atweh, S. Kemmis and P. Weeks (eds), *Action Research in Practice: Partnerships for Social Justice in Education*. London: Routledge.

Coghlan, D. and Casey, M. (2001) 'Action research from the inside: Issues and challenges in doing action research in your own organization', *Journal of Advanced Nursing*, *35*(5): 674–82.

Cornwall, A. (1996) 'Towards participatory practice: Participatory rural appraisal and the participatory process', in K. De Koning and M. Martin (eds), *Participatory Research in Health: Issues and Experiences*. London: Zed Books.

Cornwall, A. and Jewkes, R. (1995) 'What is participatory action research?', *Social Science and Medicine*, *41*: 1667–76.

Dewey, J. (1929) *The Quest for Certainty: A Study of the Relation of Knowledge and Action*. New York: Minton, Balch & Company.

Ericson-Lidman, E. and Strandberg, G. (2015) 'Troubled conscience related to deficiencies in providing individualised meal schedule in residential care for older people: A participatory action research study', *Scandinavian Journal of Caring Sciences*, *29*: 688–96.

Esienumoh, E., Allotey, J. and Waterman, H. (2018) 'Empowering members of a rural southern community in Nigeria to plan to take action to prevent maternal mortality: A participatory action research study', *Journal of Clinical Nursing*, *27*(7–8): e1600–e1611. Available at: https://doi.org/10.1111/jocn. 14244

Hart, E. and Bond, M. (1995) *Action Research for Health and Social Care: A Guide for Practice*. Milton Keynes: Open University Press.

Hope, K. W. and Waterman, H. (2003) 'Praiseworthy pragmatism? Validity and action research: Methodological issues in nursing research', *Journal of Advanced Nursing*, *44*(2): 120–7.

INVOLVE (2017a) Available at: www.invo.org.uk/

INVOLVE (2017b) Available at: www.invo.org.uk/resource-centre/payment-and-recognition-for-public-involvement/

Jagosh, J., Macaulay, A. C., Pluye, P., Salsberg, J., Bush, P. L., Henderson, J., Sirett, E., Wong, G., Cargo, M., Herbert, C. P., Seifer, S. D., Green, L. W. and Greenhalgh, T. (2014) 'Uncovering the benefits of participatory research: Implications of a realist review for health research and practice', *Milbank Quarterly*, *90*(2): 311–46.

Kemmis, S. and McTaggart, R. (1988) *The Action Research Planner*, 3rd edition. Geelong: Deakin University.

Koshy, E., Koshy, V. and Waterman, H. (2011) *Action Research for Healthcare: A Practical Guide*. London: Sage.

Lewin, K. (1947) 'Frontiers in group dynamics: Social planning and action research', *Human Relations*, *1*: 143–53.

Marshall, M., Noble, J., Davies, H., Waterman, H., Walshe, K., Sheaff, R. and Elwyn, G. (2006) 'Development of an information source for patients and the public about general practice services: An action research study', *Health Expectations, 9*(3): 265–74.

Mayan, M. J. and Daum, C. H. (2016) 'Worth the risk? Muddled relationships in community-based participatory research', *Qualitative Health Research, 26*(1): 69–76.

McNiff, J., Lomax, P. and Whitehead, J. (1996) *You and Your Action Research Practice.* London: Routledge.

Norbye, B. (2016) 'Healthcare students as innovative partners in the development of future healthcare services: An action research approach', *Nurse Education Today, 46*: 4–9.

O'Brien, D., Butler, M. M. and Casey, M. (2017) 'A participatory action research study exploring women's understandings of the concept of informed choice during pregnancy and childbirth in Ireland', *Midwifery, 46*: 1–7.

Salmon, A., Browne, A. J. and Pederson A. (2010) '"Now we call it research": Participatory health research involving marginalized women who use drugs', *Nursing Inquiry, 17*(4): 336–45.

Smith, M. K. (2007) 'Action research'. Available at: www.infed.org/research/b-actres.htm

Sturt, J. (1997) 'Placing empowerment research within an action research typology', *Journal of Advanced Nursing, 30*(5): 1057–63.

Trebble, T. M., Cruickshank, L., Hockey, P. M., Heyworth, N., Powell, T. and Clarke, N. (2013) 'Individual performance review in hospital practice: The development of a framework and evaluation of doctors' attitudes to its value and implementation', *BMJ Quality and Safety, 22*: 948–55.

United Nations (2007) *Millennium Development Goals Report.* Geneva: UN.

Vabo, G., Slettebo, A. and Fossum, M. (2016) 'Participants' perceptions of an intervention implemented in an action research nursing documentation project', *Journal of Clinical Nursing, 26*: 983–93.

van Buul, L. W., Sikkens, J. J., van Agtmael, M. A., Kramer, M. H, van der Steen, J. T. and Hertogh, C. M. (2014) 'Participatory action research in antimicrobial stewardship: A novel approach to improving antimicrobial prescribing in hospitals and long-term care facilities', *Journal of Antimicrobial Chemotherapy, 69*(7): 1734–41.

Wagaman, M. A. and Sanchez, I. (2017) 'Looking through the magnifying glass: A duoethnographic approach to understanding the value and process of participatory action research with LGBTQ youth', *Qualitative Social Work, 16*(1): 78–95.

Waterman, H., Griffiths, J., Gellard, L., O'Keefe, C., Olang, G., Obwanda, E., Ayuyo, J., Ogwethe, V. and Ondiege, J. (2007) 'Power brokering, empowering, and educating: The role of home-based care professionals in the reduction of HIV-related stigma in Kenya', *Qualitative Health Research, 17*(8): 1028–39.

Waterman, H., Harker, R., MacDonald, H., McLaughlan, R. and Waterman, C. (2005a) 'Advancing ophthalmic nursing practice through action research', *Journal of Advanced Nursing, 52*(3): 281–90.

Waterman, H., Harker, R., MacDonald, H., McLaughlan, R. and Waterman, C. (2005b) 'Evaluation of an action research project in ophthalmic nursing practice', *Journal of Advanced Nursing*, *52*(4): 389–98.

Waterman, H., Tillen, D., Dickson, R. and De Koning, K. (2001) 'Action research: A systematic review and assessment for guidance', *Health Technology Assessment*, *5*(23): iii–157.

Westhues, A., Ochocka, J., Jacobson, N., Simich, L., Maiter, S., Janzen, R. and Fleras, A. (2008) 'Developing theory from complexity: Reflections on a collaborative mixed method participatory action research study', *Qualitative Health Research*, *18*(5): 701–17.

WHO, UNICEF, UNFPA, World Bank Group and United Nations Population Division (2015) *Trends in Maternal Mortality 1990 to 2015*. Geneva: World Health Organization.

Williamson, G. R. and Prosser, S. (2002) 'Action research: Politics, ethics and participation', *Journal of Advanced Nursing*, *40*(5): 587–93.

Winter, R. and Munn-Giddings, C. (2001) *A Handbook for Action Research in Health and Social Care*. London: Routledge.

11

Qualitative Data Analysis and Health Research

MIWAKO HOSODA

Chapter objectives

- To discuss the challenge of qualitative fieldwork in health research
- To describe how to collect and record qualitative data
- To explain how to identify patterns in the data
- To discuss category analysis, coding the cycle of analysis and refining codes
- To describe context analysis and how it is used with some qualitative methods.

Introduction

This chapter introduces the process of qualitative analysis in health and health care, with some pointers to deepen our understanding of data and the process of data analysis. Two key methods for analysis are explained: category analysis and context analysis. The chapter also suggests how to draw out findings from the data using each of these forms of analysis. Readers of this chapter will acquire the method for analysing qualitative data that will enable them to identify and understand the patterns within the data and present them in a scientific way.

In doing qualitative research, health researchers face a number of challenges. In some cases, they may have begun with a hypothesis related to their question. However, once data collection begins, unexpected findings may emerge, and some may even contradict the initial hypothesis. This may seem overwhelming, but it is part of the research process – not all data will align with the findings that were expected. The researcher may also encounter social norms, values and situations with which they are not familiar. They may face obstacles or barriers to access and can even experience culture shock. It is important to be aware of these reactions, to take notes on what they see, feel, and hear when in the field and to jot these down in a notebook at the time, making sure to record the date. Of course, interviews should be recorded, and transcripts of these recordings created. With all this information, how can field workers manage to analyse everything?

When researchers come to the point of analysis, they will have a sizeable amount of data from the methods they have chosen to address their research questions. These may be in the form of documents, individual interviews, focus group interviews, or notes from observations. The next step in the process is to analyse all the information collected. The aim of this chapter is to introduce the process and techniques of analysis with reference to health research.

The process of qualitative data analysis

The chapter begins by providing an overview of the qualitative data analysis process. The questions to ask are: What is the nature of the qualitative data collected and how can they be analysed? There may be various sources of data: observations that the researcher has written down before, during and after their fieldwork. These may be fragmentary and in the form of notes and diaries that relate to reflections on the research process, the topic under investigation, or include the researcher's impressions of the environment in which participants live.

These materials are called field notes, in the tradition of cultural anthropology (Sanjek 1990), and form a record of the research process and impressions of the data collected. The notes should be filed and dated even if, at the time, they do not appear to be significant. If more formal interviews have been undertaken, the contents should be recorded on a tape or an IC digital recorder or written up immediately afterwards. If the former, transcripts should be made of these recordings.

The challenges of carrying out fieldwork are provided by an example of my own research. My research focused on 27 stroke survivors. I conducted interviews and made observations at rehabilitation hospitals, at patient associations meetings as well as at meetings held for patients. The initial experience was overwhelming. I found that people who had suffered from stroke were in despair and many were considering suicide. Nevertheless, I found that over time, through various strategies and for different reasons, each patient overcame the limitations of their condition. In my research, I wanted to investigate this process of transition and how patients managed to prevail over their pain and suffering (Hosoda 2006).

My encounter with those affected by stroke was my initial exposure to such problems and later I had the opportunity to work as a volunteer for four years with a Patients' Association for people who suffered from aphasia after a stroke. Aphasia is defined as an inability to comprehend and formulate language because of damage to specific brain regions. This may range from occasional difficulty in finding words to losing the ability to speak, read and write (www.nhs.uk/conditions/Aphasia).

I found that the stroke survivors I talked to maintained their caring and gentle attitude towards others and valued their personal relationships, even though they experienced pain and had suffered a loss of function. Through them, I became curious and believed that if I persevered, I would find out something important about their determination to continue to live.

I had taken notes of my early observations at the rehabilitation hospital and at the Patients' Association and then decided to interview patients and families individually using snowball sampling or chain referral sampling (see Chapter 5). I recorded conversations with and between patients and observed their interactions. All of this was collected as data relevant to my research. Box 11.1 summarizes the different methods for data collection in qualitative research.

Box 11.1   Ways of collecting qualitative data

- *Memos*: You should take notes of what you see and hear on memo pads, notebooks or notecards during interviews and observations. You will refer back to them multiple times while analysing your data.
- *Field notes*: These are a summary of observations and thoughts of one or several days of observation. Taking field notes is a way to turn visual and auditory input into text. By creating field notes, you will have already completed the first stage of analysis (Emerson, Fretz and Shaw 1995).
- *Transcripts*: These are written versions of audio or video recordings. It may take up to 5–6 hours to create a transcript for an hour-long interview. If there are a large number of subjects to be surveyed, sometimes the researcher can outsource the transcription, but this is costly. As part of the learning process, it is better for researchers to transcribe recordings themselves as they may notice tone of voice, pauses and silences when creating a transcript that may be missed by others.

All the records gathered qualify as important data and can be subject to analysis. By looking back over the data, the researcher will notice patterns and repetitions of certain events or keywords and this helps them to narrow down their focus. Early interviews can be analysed to provide clues about emerging themes deemed to be significant and then further interviews can be conducted to test for patterns or hypotheses relevant to the research questions.

This is called iteration in qualitative research, and it describes the back-and-forth process between data collection and data analysis. Through this process, new research findings will be discovered to provide the substance for writing a report on findings of general interest (Patton 2002; Teddlie and Tashakkori 2009).

In the interviews I conducted with stroke survivors, I noticed some important key words that many participants used repeatedly. They said they had felt 'despair' when they were told by their doctors that they would not recover from their stroke. They felt they were forced to accept the label of being disabled and they therefore had to find some way to internalize what they saw as their new identity.

I noticed this pattern and I began to ask the participants how they understood the concepts of 'despair' and 'the acceptance of disability', and what they understood by the 'internalization of a new self'. In some cases, I undertook multiple interviews with the same patient in order to understand exactly what they wanted to express. All these interviews were recorded and later transcribed.

Some studies have used conversational analysis as a methodology for understanding communication and this has been used to explore what happens in everyday interaction between people with intellectual disabilities and others, including support workers, with whom they interact. For example, Williams (2010) undertook a detailed study to show how this group living in a sheltered environment could be supported and gradually given opportunities to manage their own affairs. Video data alongside textual data can also be used in qualitative research. However, for the purpose of this chapter, I will be focusing primarily on written data.

Reading between the lines

So, how can written text data be analysed? Saussure (1972), a linguist, pointed out that symbols or signifiers, such as words and phrases used in speech or text, do not make sense by themselves. He insisted that words, including languages, have meanings when in context and in relation to the situations in which they are spoken. He argued that between 'signifier' (*signifiant*) and 'signified' (*signifié*) there exists a certain kind of relationship as meaning depends on the context of the situation. Therefore, the same words may have different meanings depending on the situation in which a word is used or who says the word.

For example, the term 'an acceptance of disability' can carry different meanings for the patient and the medical professional. While medical professionals want to persuade patients to 'accept their disabilities', patients tend to resist this. Even a word as simple as 'acceptance' can be ambiguous, and its interpretation differs depending on the context. If faced with the task of interpreting or reading meaning into words in a text, we can begin to understand the complexity and multi-layeredness of words. Thus, according to cultural anthropologist Geertz (1973), well-written qualitative research is said to have 'thick description'. The meaning of words and phrases, if repeated across transcripts and filled out in a descriptive context, provides rich data by describing situations in detail. The precise words spoken should be given.

Points to keep in mind when reading data

When researchers examine the data they have collected, it is necessary to read the material thoroughly and deeply. It is important to stop and think when something catches your attention. It is not only important to read into the meaning of the words, but also to focus on the manner in which words are spoken and the attitude or behaviour displayed by the interviewees when they are speaking. Even silences should be noticed and can be subjected to analysis. They can be taken up by the interviewer, questioned and interpreted. I offer some tips on how to pinpoint areas to focus on in Box 11.2.

Box 11.2   What to look for and record in qualitative data

- *Iteration*: Words, sentences, topics and motifs that are repeatedly used. These may hold an important meaning to the interviewee.
- *Rephrasing*: When something is rephrased, that is repeated using different words, the researcher should pay attention to the content of the text before and after the rephrasing to interpret the meaning.
- *Avoidance of terms or phases*: When participants choose to avoid using a specific name or common description of groups, people, places or disease names, this may be an indication that this is purposeful and carries a special meaning. In some cases, they may want to conceal personal information, but there is also the possibility that the individual is trying to suppress a memory or thought. For example, patients refrain from saying the name of their disease and instead refer to it as 'this illness, disease or other euphemism'.
- *A stutter, pause or the use of a filler word*: These may also carry meaning. When an interviewee interrupts their speech by saying 'um', 'well', 'what to say', and so on, you should think about the timing in which this occurs and consider what it may mean.
- *Facial expressions*: Laughter, tears, a bitter smile and so on may also have meaning.
- *Body language*: For example, pointing, nodding and shaking the head can all offer significant types of data.
- *Silence*: There are multiple possible explanations for silence. It may mean that the interviewee is trying to remember words, is at a loss as to what to say, or is just tired or in pain.

Other relevant characteristics may occur. As previously noted, when interviewing stroke patients, for instance, I heard multiple mentions of 'the new self'. One particular individual used this phrase excessively. Therefore, I added 'new self' to my list of keywords.

My 27 interviews were conducted with people who had suffered from stroke and were aged between 40 and 60. They had been living with stroke for a period of between two months and up to 10 years. I undertook multiple interviews with each individual and these lasted for a period from one to three hours. The term 'new self' was mentioned many times during the interviews. People talked about their initial feeling of loss due to the stroke and described their feeling of being cut off from their daily routines. They said they could not face the reality of what had happened and most described a period of denial when they had thoughts of committing suicide. Some of the interviewees said they had tried to kill themselves.

From such a dire situation, they had then resolved to turn their thoughts to living again. In doing so, they greatly altered their values. Before their stroke their view was that only those who are capable of working and maintaining their health could be valued. After their stroke, they had come to believe that life is worth living even if they were unable to work or live as they had before.

Based on this series of interviews, I created a hypothesis using the concept 'reality of everyday life', first described by Berger and Luckmann (1966). These authors comment that: 'The world of everyday life is not only taken for granted as reality by the ordinary members of society in the subjectively meaningful conduct of their lives. It is a world that originates in their thoughts and actions, and is maintained as real by these' (Berger and Luckmann 1966: 33). So, it can be said that all subjective reality can be rebuilt. Through the interviews with stroke survivors, I found that they had discovered a 'new self' and created a renewed sense of value and a new reality for themselves from a position of weakness.

The analysis of qualitative data

The word 'analysis' is derived from the Greek word meaning 'to unravel tangles' or 'to reduce'. Thus, in qualitative research, it is about researchers referring back to their field notes and transcripts as well as to the literature to make sense of their data. They should also bear in mind the tips mentioned in Box 11.2.

Qualitative data analysis is an attempt to interpret the mass of data and make sense of the complicated and often miscellaneous contents, drawing on knowledge of concepts or theories and reading the literature to find ways of identifying patterns and interpreting meaning. Analysis does not happen at once, and reinterpretation will occur throughout the whole research cycle. Even if some data are left untouched initially, they may become important at a later stage. The process of qualitative analysis is shown in Figure 11.1 and in the three easy steps that follow.

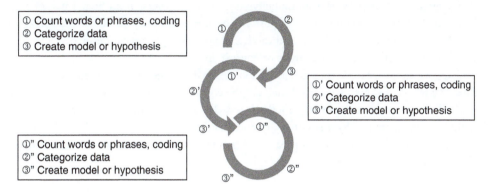

① Count words or phrases, coding
② Categorize data
③ Create model or hypothesis

①' Count words or phrases, coding
②' Categorize data
③' Create model or hypothesis

①" Count words or phrases, coding
②" Categorize data
③" Create model or hypothesis

FIGURE 11.1   The process of data analysis

Step One

- In the mass of data, you will notice certain things from your perspective and think about their meaning.
- Try to create a collection of things you noticed and find connections between them. Then, look at the connection and also try to think about what you cannot connect.
- Organize the results of the comparison and integrate them. Think about what you can say from the data. You can then formulate models and hypotheses.

Step Two

- With the model and hypothesis in mind, think about what you noticed by reviewing the data.
- Make connections.
- Consolidate.

Step Three

- Find more areas of further investigation and think about the data.
- Make more connections.
- Consolidate further.

As shown in Chapter 2, the idea of induction is to derive rules and theories from multiple cases, facts or observations. On the other hand, the deductive method is used to test general theories against a conclusion based on general and universal facts and theories. The flow from Step One to Step Three is an inductive task, and the reverse from Step Three to Step One is deductive. The combined use of both has been referred to by Teddlie and Tashakkori (2009) as eclecticism. There are several methodologies that have been developed and they are classified as either category analysis or context analysis.

Category analysis can be regarded as an analysis that focuses on the conceptualization of data. The terms used are various and include: the conceptualizing method, the categorizing method, the constant comparative method and the grounded theory approach. Context analysis is characterized by analysing sequences and includes: phenomenological analysis, discourse analysis, the narrative approach, ethnomethodology, and conversational analysis. These features are highlighted in Table 11.1.

TABLE 11.1   Types of qualitative data analysis

Categorical strategy	Conceptualizing method
	Categorizing method
	Constant comparative method
	Grounded theory approach
Contextualizing strategy	Phenomenological analysis
	Discourse analysis
	Narrative approach
	Ethnomethodology
	Conversational analysis

Analysis through the categorization of data

Category analysis is a conceptualizing method in which data are systematically classified according to a certain characteristic and are conceptualized by generality or commonality. Fox's classic publications on medical sociology are good examples of a conceptual approach (Fox 1959, 2011, 2014; Fox and Swazey 1992). When Fox wrote her initial publication in 1959, *Experiment Perilous*, she used intensive and prolonged participant observation among the patients and physicians at a hospital in the Metabolic Group on Ward F-Second, and carried out focused interviews. She conducted content analyses of several data sources: the charts of patients on the ward relating to their case; articles published in medical journals by the physicians on their cases; reports on research studies on the ward; and articles published in various media. In addition, she had access to verbatim copies of interviews with patients on the ward conducted by the hospital's Psychiatric Group as part of an ongoing research project.

From this wide range of sources, Fox (1959) used the term 'experiment perilous' as a meta-theme or key category to analyse the risks and challenges in medical practice where the outcomes of interventions are uncertain. She drew on Hippocrates' first aphorism for a medical professional: 'Life is short, and Art is long; a crisis fleeting; experience perilous and the decision difficult'. This category allowed Fox to analyse subsets of patient and physician perspectives through stages in the trajectory of the treatment process to manage uncertainty and risk. This served to reduce the huge and varied quantity of 'thick' descriptive data into a number of more limited themes.

The grounded theory approach is also well known as a categorization method. Glaser and Strauss (1967) criticized sociological research that had an excessive focus on verifying facts having first accepted these as true – that is, *a priori*. As a replacement, they suggested the grounded theory approach, which is developing theories based on data. They would generate hypotheses and theories as the research progressed, rather than formulating hypotheses and theories in advance and verifying them with data.

When Glaser and Strauss (1965) wrote their early publication, *Awareness of Dying*, they conducted intensive fieldwork at six hospitals for six years, using combinations of observations and interviews. They observed nurses and physicians at work and found that there were different aspects of dying, as perceived by nurses and physicians, and concluded that patient care was affected by these different perceptions.

Subsequently, Glaser and Strauss (1967) wrote *The Discovery of Grounded Theory*, which outlined their new research method. They argued that grounded theory 'fills the gap between theory and empirical investigation' (Glaser and Strauss 1967: 4) and that new insights into the social and human aspects of the medical domain will thereby be revealed. They showed that the hypotheses and theories that a researcher believes will be applicable before collecting data may, or may not, be verified by the data collected in the field. With qualitative analysis there are times when our preconceptions of reality are found to be too simple. People and things are more complex.

Coding data

These studies highlight that by examining the collected data closely, the researcher will come across certain key concepts. Grouping them together and giving names to these categories is a process called 'coding'. Initially, there will be a large number of codes from your data. As you continue the coding work and review your categories more carefully, you will gradually notice some of the codes can be fitted into a more general category with subsets. Certain groups can be put together.

You may think that all data must be fitted into a code, but this is not necessary. You will have an extremely large amount of field notes and transcripts, so it is not realistic to code every piece of information. In addition, as you are conducting analyses to deepen your research, you do not need to code data that seem to be irrelevant. Of course, data that originally appear unrelated may turn out to be related later. In this case, add a new code and reanalyse your data.

At the beginning of the analysis, you should use the exact phrases that the informants have used. The perspectives of informants are often reflected in specific wording. Glaser and Strauss (1967) encouraged researchers to use the constant comparative method to make systematic comparisons by linking like with like, and also to merge codes into more general categories. Sometimes multiple codes are given to the same data or multiple data can be grouped together under the same code. By developing coding, the data are classified or categorized, and therefore can be manipulated. This organization allows the researcher to get a better overall view of an entire data set.

Managing a pile of qualitative data is usually time-consuming and challenging. As noted in Chapter 7, for example, in an interview project with 30 informants, the transcript may be almost 1,000 pages. This volume of data is very large so it takes a long time to develop a thematic coding scheme.

Qualitative analysis software provides a useful tool for selecting data and applying codes. Therefore, if you wish to find the valuable and significant keywords quickly, software which is designed for qualitative data analysis, such as NVivo, ATLAS. Ti, and NUDIST, may be helpful. The primary merit of using this software is that it is faster and easier to carry out the analysis than it being done manually. It both saves time and offers greater flexibility by arranging keywords accurately from the data. In addition, the software helps the researcher to create comprehensive analytic modelling by positioning concepts and categories in hierarchical arrangements. Despite the many positive reasons for using software, great attention must still be paid to the categories identified when data are collected through interviews or other methods. In the first instance, researchers are advised to try out codes manually with 'pen and paper'. It is also important to note cases that fall outside codes and represent a deviant or minor opinion.

The comparison of data and composition of categories

As noted above, when looking over the collected data, the researcher will find the repetition of certain words, topics, action patterns and events. In noticing something that appears repeatedly, is stressed by the informant, or leaves an impression, you should try to create connections between it and other keywords. The next step will be to organize the data into categories, as shown in Figure 11.2.

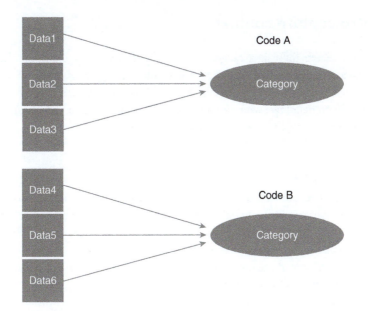

FIGURE 11.2   Data coding: Organizing data into categories

The decision to categorize is based on the individual researcher's judgement. While classifying in this manner, you are constantly naming each category and comparing them, thereby using what is referred to as the 'constant comparative method'. This gives a provisional order to diverse and miscellaneous qualitative data, ensuring that the overall data are easier to comprehend – comparing each item of acquired data with other related data, making them into a group. Not all codes can be grouped together with other codes and some codes can belong in multiple categories. Based on categories, the final theory and model will be created.

In my interviews with stroke patients, many described themselves as having become a 'new self'. I came to interpret this expression as meaning that the informant changed their way of thinking and came to value themselves again. Therefore, I made a provisional hypothesis that 'finding a new self' and 'finding hope from despair' indicate a key turning point in life after illness.

As the interviews progressed, I tried to focus more on what aspect of their 'self' was 'new' to these patients. As a result, other keywords became significant, such as 'encounter' and 'transformation'. What did these indicate? I found that to transfer from despair to hope, the subjects had often met new people, such as medical professionals or care-givers, who had encouraged a change. They also commented sometimes on a drastic event that had acted as a trigger to enable people to reflect and change. In this way, I was able to elaborate on my original hypotheses and theory. There is a continuous cyclical process of repetition in the examination of data.

Analysis to capture context

In qualitative research there is a range of methods of analysis to interpret the research context from various perspectives. This process is called sequence analysis and some examples are discourse analysis, conversation analysis and narrative analysis. These analyses are derived from phenomenology, which emphasizes the importance of the researchers' interpretation of events related to human action and to society.

Discourse analysis

Discourse analysis is conducted on the premise that what an individual verbalizes during the course of an interview not only reflects their inner thoughts, but also reveals something about the society and culture in which they live. A narrative or an account will have a different meaning depending on the socio-cultural situation.

Let us take the analysis of the response to a stroke and to the process of rehabilitation and retraining as an example. One response to a post-stroke patient who refuses to go through rehabilitation could be: 'They do not accept their disability' or 'They are just lazy'. A patient may then say in response: 'It cannot be helped' or, as I have heard one patient comment, 'I am able to walk because of rehabilitation even though I hated the training'. What is the reality? Why is there such a stark contrast between the patients? Even the same person may change their story when they reflect on an episode during their illness. The after-effects of stroke and rehabilitation training depend on a number of factors: the culture of the society in which they are living, their position within that society, and their way of thinking. In discourse analysis, the researcher tries to capture the context in which changes in attitude have come about. In other words, they try to establish the context of, or the background to, such narratives.

Narrative analysis

Narrative analysis is an approach taken when researchers or professionals seek to 'read and understand the life stories of individuals'. The main feature of this method lies in analysing the parts of people's speeches that focus on what they cherish most in their lives. Narrative analysis 'zeroes in' on one episode in someone's life story and undertakes a close analysis of their account (Andrews, Squire and Tamboukou 2013). For example, in my research, I paid attention to how the stroke survivors overcame their problems and the meaning they attached to their experience rather than simply listening to the facts.

From the 1980s, pioneers in the sociology of health and illness and qualitative analysis introduced the concept of life history or biography. Rather than thinking solely of patients with illnesses whose end goal is to recover, they tried to understand how people came to understand and live with their illness or disability (see Bury 1991; Charmaz 1983; Corbin and Strauss 1990).

Even in cases where there is no cure, when patients must live with chronic illness or disability, they found that it was individuals themselves who took the initiative. They made the decision (or not) to take advantage of the techniques and the services available. The narrative approach, which values individuals' direct voices, is probably the most appropriate method when trying to understand people's adjustment to illness or disability (see Williams 2010, for an account of empowerment). In my study of stroke patients' lives following their diagnoses, even if people try to deny their experience, the fact that they had suffered a stroke is undeniable. While relying on help from others, they must find a balance between being self-sufficient and dependent through trial and error. They may be unable to perform certain tasks with the same efficiency as they had previously, and they must look for other things that they can do – and it is through this process that they become more self-aware and discover their 'new selves'. Difficulties in communication may not be resolved just by changing the method of communication through the use of hand gestures or the provision of wheelchairs, but rather by a willingness to experiment.

Ethnomethodology and conversational analysis

Conversation analysis focuses on the interaction between the narrator (interviewer) and the listener (interviewee). This form of analysis is developed through a careful examination of the structure of conversations rather than their content. Factors such as the talk order, who is taking the initiative, and who was interrupted at what part of the conversations are the targets of analysis. For example, the conventional rule that 'the listener always speaks after a silence, after which the speaker speaks' is particularly intriguing and deserves further investigation.

The basic idea of conversation analysis is described at length by Garfinkel (1967) in *Studies in Ethnomethodology*. He had been influenced by the lectures of Harvey Sacks, given at the University of Berkeley, California. These early lectures were published much later (see Sacks 1992). Both Sacks and Garfinkel focused on how ethnomethodological methods in talk help to create order and sustain consistency in daily life. Ethnomethodology investigates how people manage experiences in different aspects of their social life, such as work, study, quarrels and going for a walk. In studying these ordinary activities, the researcher draws conclusions from observations. An example of this would be understanding what people think of ordinary phenomenon such as 'standing in a line' and 'talking'. Later, Sidnell (2010) stressed that the best way to obtain data was to go out and video-record face-to-face interaction. He commented that video 'provides an extremely rich source of data that allows the conversation analyst to examine not just talk, but also the use of the body and especially the gaze and gesture in the organization of interaction' (Sidnell 2010: 22).

When undertaking conversational analytical procedures, the first step is to create transcripts using unique symbols and rules. In conversation analysis, there is no need to summarize the contents of the conversation, but you must transcribe all 'sound' as accurately as possible. You will listen to tapes or watch audio-visual data to familiarize yourself with the situation and assess the emotions expressed by participants when they talk and show their feelings. You need to assess whether they are happy, angry, sad, nervous, enthusiastic and so on.

Various symbols and system codes used for the transcription of sounds have been established by Jefferson (2004) and are commonly used by conversational analysts worldwide. These symbols and system codes allow a transcription to describe the details of performance: the acts, texts, movements and the interaction between actors in terms of content and context. This provides researchers with data so they can analyse the complex nature of interactions.

In the analysis, attention must be paid to 'turn-taking', a type of organization in conversation and discourse where participants speak one at a time in alternating turns. For example, during a medical interview at a hospital, when a doctor is looking at the computer screen, they tend not to interact with the patient. It has been observed that the patient does not start speaking until the doctor turns towards them, and they wait for this moment. Conversational analysis of talk shows that participants in a conversation constantly monitor each other's situation. They construct interaction collaboratively. Investigations into the correlation between social status, gender and age difference between actors help to show how these factors can shape interaction.

Case studies: Analysing the role of support groups for patients

I have been conducting both qualitative and quantitative research targeting the patients' support groups and their role as social movements. Government agencies, associations of health care professionals and lawyers have worked to solve problems of access and provide appropriate services and undertake research. I have undertaken research on stroke survivors, people recovering from Hansen's Disease and people with Myalgic Encephalomyelitis (ME)/Chronic Fatigue Syndrome (CFS). In my view, when undertaking research, listening to patients' voices and the role of collective action are particularly important. Brown and Zavestoski (2005) called these activities a health social movement.

My strategy prior to starting the research was to get to know a range of people with disabilities and their families. I identified individuals through support groups or group meetings to discuss the project in person, on the phone or via email. Through this interaction, I identified problems and issues from their perspective and came to be aware of the complexity of their world in navigating services, legal regulations and day-to-day frustrations in a world designed for the well and the able-bodied. I will now present three case studies of my research on these topics.

Hansen's Disease: How survivor recoverers helped to repeal discriminatory laws

People with Hansen's Disease, commonly known as leprosy, are represented in Japan through a support group called the Zen-Ryo-Kyo, the National Hansen's Disease Sanatoria Residents' Association. Since the 1950s, their work has made a major contribution to changing attitudes and laws that were discriminatory (Hosoda 2010).

My research aimed to investigate why and how Zen-Ryo-Kyo's activities as a support and pressure group were carried out, not just to investigate what, where and when events happened. It was a qualitative sociological study that used a mixture of methods, including archival and historical research method, collecting oral life histories and conducting in-depth interviews. Hence, focused examples are presented descriptively to identify the reasons for the activities and their meaning.

The study used published and unpublished documents as data. These included monthly newsletters published by Zen-Ryo-Kyo since 1952, memorial books edited by Zen-Ryo-Kyo and autobiographies and biographies of people living in the sanatoria. I carried out the fieldwork through in-depth interviews with key members of the Zen-Ryo-Kyo organization and long-time activists Mr H, Mr and Mrs M, and Mr and Mrs S between May 2004 and June 2008. I used snowball sampling as one key person, including the director of the Hansen's Disease support organization in Japan, introduced me to another to access both activists and people who had recovered from the disease. The interviews were written up as author's field notes and recorded by digital recorder with textual transcriptions.

I conceptualized the activities of people with Hansen's Disease as a social movement that aimed to bring about social change through efforts to 'normalize' the condition. The research gave an explanatory description of the activities of Zen-Ryo-Kyo in achieving change through addressing issues related to social stigma and discrimination. I found that the objective of the group was to reduce stigma, with a focus on respecting human rights and needs, not on highlighting difference.

The most remarkable achievement was the repeal of the 1931 Leprosy Prevention Law. This had established a policy of absolute isolation and was repealed in 1996. I undertook a number of intensive interviews with those who had lobbied for the repeal of the law and looked in detail at the role of Zen-Ryo-Kyo: their activities and the part played by supporters. I found that Zen-Ryo-Kyo was able to bring together a broad coalition of interest groups. These included the medical profession, central government officials and other support groups speaking for those who felt discriminated against due to disability or illness, as well as members of the general public. The analysis of political movements in health illustrated how social movements can shift the stigma associated with illness and disability and design social support systems.

CASE STUDY 11.1

Stroke survivors changing the regulation of a range of health insurance rehabilitation services

This study focuses on stroke patients who opposed the revision of the 2006 Social Health Insurance Fee Schedule for rehabilitation therapy. It illustrates the social process of the movement for change and examines the feasibility of the movement to create 'medical governance', or public participation and collaboration among various actors in health policy making (Hosoda 2013b).

In this study, I tracked and analysed the activities of the Association for Rehabilitation Therapy (ATFR) and their response to the new Social Health Insurance Fee Schedule (SHIFS). The new system was announced in March 2006 and modified in April 2007. The research questions addressed were:

- Why did ATFR emerge as a pressure group against the new insurance schedule and who were the actors?
- What were the activities of ATFR and how was it seen by other actors?
- How did ATFR interact with other actors to form a coalition?
- What were the consequences of ATFR's activities?

The objective of the research was to identify the factors that advanced and hindered the movement. Data were collected through a literature search and in-depth interviews to investigate why and how ATFR activities were carried out – not just the what, where and when. Hence, this focused case study was conducted to identify the reasons for the activities and their significance.

As for interviews, I used snowball sampling to interview six selected members of ATFR. Mr T was a stroke survivor and a symbol of the movement; Dr A was a rehabilitation doctor and a secretary of ATFR; Mrs B and Mr C were from the Polio Association; Mrs D was from the Japan Traumatic Brain Injury Association and Dr E was a rehabilitation doctor. I also identified one government officer (Mr F) in the department dealing with the Social Health Insurance Schedule in 2006–07 and interviewed him by email. The face-to-face interviews were conducted from December 2007 to July 2010 with the meetings and email communications before and after the interviews.

Written materials were collected from various sources, such as websites and newsletters of ATFR and other patients' groups, governmental documents, and media coverage such as newspaper articles and editorials, TV programmes, and weekly and monthly magazine articles.

The issue was as follows: in early 2006, the Central Social Health Insurance Council (CSHIC), which is located in the Ministry of Health, Labor and Welfare (MHLW), conducted a review of the fees for rehabilitation services. A subsequent report recommended limits on the number of insurance-covered days of rehabilitation, depending on the original disease or injury – such as stroke, heart disease, trauma or respiratory disease. Reflecting this report, on 6 March 2006, the central ministry informed all medical facilities that the maximum number of days of insurance-covered rehabilitation would be 180 in total from 1 April 2006. This announcement caused great concern among many people in different domains. Prior to 2006, the number of days of insurance-covered rehabilitation was determined by physicians, depending on the medical needs of the patients. Patients in need complained that they would no longer have sufficient rehabilitation therapy. Medical professionals argued that large numbers of patients would be denied the necessary rehabilitation allowable under this policy and did not take the cause of the illness into account. Subsequently, individual patients, patients' associations and medical professionals formed the coalition referred to above. They made a request backed by petitions to the ministry to withdraw the revision.

Such action relating to a central component of national health care policy was unprecedented (Hosoda 2010). As a result of these efforts, on 25 December 2006, the MHLW released a new version of the SHIFS for rehabilitation. This increased coverage for patients with specific conditions and was implemented beginning in March 2007.

Using the theory related to social movements and professions, this study described the social process of the movement to assert the rights of patients and maintain some professional autonomy in decision-making, and investigated the factors that advanced or hindered resistance to central government. After analysis of the qualitative and other data, the study concluded that the movement can be understood not only as a manifestation of the patients' rights to health and professionals' autonomy against institutionalized authority, but as a challenge in creating a new platform for health care reform.

This type of research was difficult because the movement was campaigning against government policy, so the people who participated in the movement were stigmatized by others. The doctor who supported this movement was especially criticized by an association of doctors and decided to withdraw from these kinds of activities. Since I had established a good level of communication with this doctor, I was able to conduct an interview, although the doctor did not want to talk to other people, such as journalists. This highlighted that researchers should be sensitive to informants' social status when they conduct research related with political issues.

Myalgic Encephalomyelitis/Chronic Fatigue Syndrome: Advocacy activities

The aim of this study was to examine how patients' support groups change and create the health care service by reviewing the activities of organizations for people with Myalgic Encephalomyelitis/Chronic Fatigue Syndrome (ME/CFS) and focusing on their advocacy activities (Hosoda 2013a). The advocacy activities of the groups can be called health social movements.

It is said that there are 340,000 people suffering from ME/CFS in Japan, and 17 million sufferers in the world. Despite the great number of people affected by the

(Continued)

(Continued)

disease, there are still uncertainties surrounding ME/CFS. As of today, the causes of ME/CFS have not been identified and no specific diagnostic tests are available. However, according to the international criteria, it is known that people with ME/CFS are so run-down that the syndrome interferes with their lives and can make them dysfunctional. Furthermore, they are not just dealing with extreme fatigue, but with a wide range of other symptoms, including sudden severe fatigue, sleep without feeling refreshed, muscle and joint pain without swelling, intense or changing patterns of headaches, sore throats, swollen lymph glands in the neck or armpits, memory problems, and an inability to concentrate.

I explored the real-life difficulties of people with ME/CFS by conducting a questionnaire survey and interviews. Participants were collected through the Japan ME/CFS Association and other ME/CFS patients. Two hundred and fifty-six questionnaires were distributed from March 2012 to October 2012 and 135 were returned (a response rate of 53 per cent). Half of the participants were in their 40s and 50s, while 7 per cent were teenagers. Most of the participants were female.

I also conducted semi-structured interviews with four ME/CFS patients in the same period in 2012. Most of them were members of the Japan ME/CFS Association. They had difficulties with transport from their home, so I visited these participants to conduct interviews in their home. Based on the transcript of the interviews, I found that ME/CFS sufferers have not only physical pain, but also social pain. The social pain that the ME/CFS patients are suffering is stigma and social discrimination caused by their disease.

As a result of my analysis, the sense of total isolation was found to sometimes make them feel that their lives are useless (Hosoda 2010). They can be said to experience 'structural isolation'. They cannot work, so they lose their friends at their workplace. They cannot go out, so they lose their private friends. They can sometimes move, so their family does not understand their terrible physical condition. Even worse, when their physical condition does allow them to try to have fun, they are blamed for dishonesty. Once they contribute to support group activities, people outside the group expect them to work instead.

I also found that the support group encouraged medical professionals to conduct scientific research on the condition and lobbied for government workers to provide acceptable social services. Patients' activities became a connector among many stakeholders, such as government officials, medical professionals, clinical practitioners and laboratory researchers (Hosoda 2010).

This research used a qualitative method to gain an understanding of peoples' motivations in taking action to support change. It suggests that the advocacy activity of patients' groups can become increasingly important for both the patients themselves and health care providers. It is a sign that a wider social transformation is occurring. The health care system is moving from a top-down bureaucratically driven service to one where citizens can organize and make their voice heard. Such patient and public involvement could be a key factor in designing a more sustainable and supportive health care system.

Reading health research based on qualitative data analysis

When reading health research based on qualitative data analysis, the following questions should be borne in mind:

- Is there a clear and cogent account of how the qualitative data were collected and recorded?
- What patterns were apparent in the data – including not just the use of words, but also facial expressions, body language and silences?
- What methodologies were employed in the data analysis – how far, in particular, did they draw on types of category or context analysis?
- How did the methodologies and methods used in the study relate to the research question?

Analysing qualitative data is not an easy task and a key question to be asked is how the researchers' subjectivity was addressed in analysing the data.

Conclusion

As Weber (1949: 81) commented: 'All knowledge of cultural reality, as may be seen, is always knowledge from particular points of view.' He pointed out that when researchers observe and analyse, they select things that are subjectively important and ignore other elements. In consequence, there is no absolutely objective scientific analysis of 'social phenomena' that is independent of a special and 'one-sided' viewpoint. Data may be selected either consciously or unconsciously and are then analysed and organized for expository purposes.

Following this line, Berger and Luckmann (1966) argue that reality affects researchers themselves. The circumstances in which researchers are placed reflect the qualitative data that they collect. Thus, it becomes necessary to reconsider the subjectivity of researchers. Various factors can impede objectivity: personal circumstances, such as the researchers' own interests, the institutions to which they belong, and their own values may influence their perceptions and their research. Research may also be constrained by the samples they collect and material factors such as geography, time and financial resources.

Qualitative researchers are criticized when they are subjective, so it is important in analysing data and in the other stages of qualitative research to take care to explain your decisions and methods, to 'reflect' on findings and to demonstrate as far as possible the objectivity of your analysis. In addition, it is important for qualitative researchers to demonstrate that they have 'insider awareness'. They should show that their findings reflect the views of participants and how they see the world and the topics under study.

In order to ensure that dialogues are expanded, there should be continuous interaction with participants in the field. It is important to go back and forth between collecting data and thinking and reflecting on your findings and their meaning in their wider context. Dialogue with research participants and interviewees is important, but so is conversing with colleagues and others within the wider society who may be affected by, or interested in, your research.

It is important, too, to know when to stop collecting data, when to stop coding and analysing that data and when to turn to writing up your report or thesis. A good indicator of this is when you reach the stage where you cannot find a new perspective. The writing process also necessitates careful analysis and internal dialogue. It is through this dialogue that new ideas can be are generated, leading to deeper, richer content in researching health and other areas.

Exercise 11.1   The experience of illness

Using unstructured or semi-structured questions, ask an individual to describe their experience of an episode of illness. Transcribe their account. Identify key words and expressions in your analysis of their depiction of their experience. What does the qualitative data that you gather tell you about their interpretation of their condition at the time of their illness?

Recommended further reading

This book is an excellent piece of qualitative research with a cross-cultural dimension based upon the author's participant/observer involvement for almost two decades:
Fox, R. C. (2014) *Doctors without Borders: Humanitarian Quests, Impossible Dreams of Médecins Sans Frontières*. Baltimore, MD: Johns Hopkins University Press.

This introductory book covers a wide range of qualitative research for both undergraduate and postgraduate students. It indicates the big picture of qualitative research and shows how to conduct a research project and analyse data:
Silverman, D. (2016) *Qualitative Research*, 4th edition. London: Sage.

This is a comprehensive text that can be recommended on both qualitative data analysis and mixed methods research:
Teddlie, C. and Tashakkori, A. (2009) *Foundations of Mixed Methods Research: Integrating Quantitative and Qualitative Approaches in the Social and Behavioural Sciences*. London: Sage.

References

Andrews, M., Squire, C. and Tamboukou, M. (eds) (2013) *Doing Narrative Research*, 2nd edition. London: Sage.

Berger, P. L. and Luckmann, T. (1966) *The Social Construction of Reality: A Treatise in the Sociology of Knowledge*. Garden City, NY: Anchor Books.

Brown, P. and Zavestoski, S. (2005) 'Social movements in health: An introduction', in P. Brown and S. Zavestoski (eds), *Social Movements in Health*. Oxford: Blackwell.

Bury, M. (1991) 'The sociology of chronic illness: A review of research and prospects', *Sociology of Health and Illness, 13*(4): 451–68.

Charmaz, K. (1983) 'The grounded theory method: An explication and interpretation', in R. M. Emerson (ed.), *Contemporary Field Research*. Prospect Heights, IL: Waveland Press.

Corbin, J. M. and Strauss, A. (1990) 'Grounded theory research: Procedures, canons, and evaluative criteria', *Qualitative Sociology, 13*(1): 3–21.

Emerson, R. M., Fretz, R. I. and Shaw, L. L. (1995) *Writing Ethnographic Fieldnotes*. Chicago, IL: University of Chicago Press.

Fox, R. C. (1959) *Experiment Perilous: Physicians and Patients Facing the Unknown*. Glencoe, IL: Free Press.

Fox, R. C. (2011) *In the Field: A Sociologist's Journey*. New Brunswick, NJ: Transaction.

Fox, R. C. (2014) *Doctors without Borders: Humanitarian Quests, Impossible Dreams of Médecins Sans Frontières*. Baltimore, MD: Johns Hopkins University Press.

Fox, R. C. and Swazey, J. (1992) *Spare Parts: Organ Replacement in American Society and Observing Bioethics*. New York: Oxford University Press.

Garfinkel, H. (1967) *Studies in Ethnomethodology*. Englewood Cliffs, NJ: Prentice-Hall.

Geertz, C. (1973) *The Interpretation of Cultures: Selected Essays*. New York: Basic Books.

Glaser, B. G. and Strauss, A. L. (1965) *Awareness of Dying*. Chicago, IL: Aldine.

Glaser, B. G. and Strauss, A. L. (1967) *The Discovery of Grounded Theory: Strategies for Qualitative Research*. Chicago, IL: Aldine.

Hosoda, M. (2006) *The Meaning of Living with Stroke*. Tokyo: Seikaisha Publisher (in Japanese).

Hosoda, M. (2010) 'Hansen's disease recoverers as agents of change', *Leprosy Review, 81*(1): 5–16.

Hosoda, M. (2013a) 'Living with a misunderstood disease: Myalgic Encephalomyelitis/ Chronic Fatigue Syndrome in Japan', *Eubios Journal of Asian and International Bioethics, 23*(3): 70–2.

Hosoda, M. (2013b) 'Feasibility of "medical governance": A case study of the social movement against the limitation of the Social Health Insurance Fee Schedule for rehabilitation therapy in Japan', *Journal of Kyosei Sciences, Seisa University Research Bulletin, 8*: 45–54.

Jefferson, G. (2004) 'Glossary of transcript symbols with an introduction', in G. H. Lerner (ed.), *Conversation Analysis: Studies from the First Generation*. Philadelphia, PA: John Benjamins.

Patton, M. Q. (2002) *Qualitative Research and Evaluation Methods*, 3rd edition. Thousand Oaks, CA: Sage.

Sacks, H. (ed.) (1992) *Lectures on Conversation*, 2 Volumes. Oxford: Basil Blackwell.

Sanjek, R. (ed.) (1990) *Fieldnotes: The Making of Anthropology*. Ithaca, NY: Cornell University Press.

Saussure, F. (1972) *Cours de Linguistique Générale*. Paris: Payot.

Sidnell, J. (2010) *Conversation Analysis: An Introduction*. Oxford: Wiley-Blackwell.

Teddlie, C. and Tashakkori, A. (2009) *Foundations of Mixed Methods Research: Integrating Quantitative and Qualitative Approaches in the Social and Behavioural Sciences*. London: Sage.

Weber, M. (1949) '"Objectivity" in social science and social policy', in E. Shils (ed.), *The Methodology of the Social Sciences*. New York: Free Press.

Williams, V. (2010) *Disability and Discourse: Analysing Inclusive Conversation with People with Intellectual Disabilities*. Chichester: Wiley-Blackwell.

PART III
Quantitative Methods and Health

12

Methods of Sampling in Quantitative Health Research

NICHOLA SHACKLETON, MARTIN VON RANDOW
AND LARA GREAVES

Chapter objectives

- To discuss the rationale of sampling and describe techniques employed in probability sampling and issues that can arise
- To cover the theory behind inferential statistics and sources of error in research, as well as how to reduce their impact
- To consider forms of non-probability sampling and where they can be useful
- To provide several case studies relevant to health research to illustrate important concepts.

Introduction

Sampling is an important concept to master for the health researcher carrying out a quantitative study. Whether conducting your own survey or using a secondary data source, understanding sampling methodology is vital for resolving potential issues with collected data, implementing appropriate analyses and drawing sensible conclusions. With a properly constructed sample, time and financial costs can be kept to a minimum without losing generalizability (the ability to make accurate statements about a group in which the researcher is interested). In reading this chapter on quantitative sampling you may find it particularly helpful to cross-reference to Chapter 5 on qualitative sampling and Chapter 17 on quantitative data analysis.

What is a sample?

Sampling is the process of selecting units from a population of interest, or 'target population', to learn something about it. A target population can be general, and include all humans, or it can be narrow, such as people with a specific condition or illness. It does not necessarily consist of people, but rather can refer to any unit of analysis – institutions such as hospitals/schools, households or geographical areas.

As researchers, we rarely have access to every member of the target population, so we collect information from a subset of it – a sample – and use data from that subset to infer things about the population as a whole. When drawing a sample, we need to consider its representativeness. There are many factors that will impact on how well a sample reflects the target population, and thus how accurate insights gained from it are. The process of making generalizations from a sample to a population is called inference, and it is the basis of many statistical procedures. Crucially, sampling is the science and practice of selecting information from populations in a manner that allows defensible inferences to be drawn.

How big should my sample be?

The appropriate size for a sample from a target population can be determined by several pieces of information: the degree of accuracy you require, the 'power' you require, the rate of non-response you expect, and of course the budget and timeframe for the research.

Accuracy

A smaller sample size will result in a lower likelihood that estimates from the sample are the same as actual values in the population (the possibility of 'sampling error'). Larger sample sizes are recommended, but the relationship between accuracy and sample size is non-linear. The general rule is that to halve the sampling error (to reduce the uncertainty in estimates by half) we must quadruple the sample size (De Vaus 2014). There are large gains in accuracy from increasing the sample size from 100 to 200, but there is little gain from increasing it from 2,000 to 2,100. Many survey companies limit their sample size to 2,000, as beyond this point the additional cost of increasing the sample size is not worth the small gains in accuracy (De Vaus 2014).

Power

An alternative way to determine sample size is to consider how big a sample needs to be in order to find a relationship, or detect an effect in the population. This could be something like the relationship between poverty and hospital admissions related to infectious diseases (which may be expressed as a correlation), or the effect of an intervention for improving mental health (which may be expressed by the difference in mean values of those receiving and those not receiving the intervention). Power is determined by three things:

1. The hypothesized effect size (for example, the strength of a relationship such as a correlation coefficient or the difference in the mean between two groups).
2. The alpha value: the significance level of the test. This refers to the chance that we observe a relationship or effect due to sampling error.
3. The sample size.

Effect sizes are estimated based on pilot studies or previously published research. An alpha value of 0.05, meaning there is a 5 per cent chance that a relationship observed in a sample does not exist in the population, is standard in quantitative research. The stronger the relationship – or the larger the effect – the smaller the sample size required to detect it. Power analysis calculates a power statistic that ranges between 0 and 1. The most common power statistic criterion used is 0.8 or higher (80 per cent power), meaning that 80 per cent of the time, if there is a true relationship in the population we will observe it in our sample. Conversely, there is a 20 per cent chance of accepting a false negative – that is, we will not observe a relationship or an effect in our sample even though such a relationship or effect exists in the population.

Non-response

For a variety of reasons, people selected into a sample may choose not to participate. Therefore, even if we select 2,000 people to participate in a study, only 1,000 may actually participate. This would be a response rate of 50 per cent. Response rates can vary dramatically in survey research depending on the mode of the survey (face-to-face interview, telephone interview, mail survey, online survey), and its topic and length (Dillman, Smyth and Christian 2009). There are a number of ways to improve response rates with careful preparation, such as interviewer training (De Vaus 2014; Groves et al. 2009).

We can also use response rates from similar surveys to guide us on sample size. Imagine we want to survey 2,000 adolescents about alcohol use, and two previous studies on adolescent alcohol use had response rates of 60 per cent. This means we could expect about 1,200 adolescents to respond. We could initially draw a larger sample to take account of this expected non-response, by dividing the required sample size (2,000) by the proportion expected to respond (0.6), and thus sample 3,333 adolescents to hopefully achieve a sample size of 2,000. Boosting sample size in this way does not deal with bias, as those who respond to surveys differ from those who do not.

How do we draw a sample?

There are two main types of sampling:

- *Probability sampling*: every unit in the target population has a known probability of being selected into the sample.
- *Non-probability sampling*: units are selected into a sample on an unknown, non-random basis – for instance, based on the presence of some specific characteristic.

We shall now consider each of these in turn.

Probability sampling

In probability sampling, each unit has a specifiable chance of being selected. Knowing the probability for selection enables us to apply statistical techniques of estimation and make inferences about the population.

Sampling frame

Probability sampling is the most widely used approach in quantitative health research, and there is a well-established body of theory and practice on sampling design and inference (Laake and Fagerland 2015; Shapiro 2008). The process of probability sampling begins with a sampling frame. This lists the units – such as people, households or hospitals – in the population from which the sample will be selected. Ideally, it includes all such units in the target population, and only those units.

The target population does not always have a sampling frame that matches it perfectly. When a sampling frame includes units that are not eligible for inclusion, this is referred to as over coverage. Imagine we used a business directory that contained the mailing address of every business in a given city, but it was compiled a year ago, as our sampling frame. Some of these businesses would have closed down or moved in the interim, and some addresses might now be residential. Therefore, the sampling frame would contain ineligible units. Over coverage can be remedied if the proportion of ineligible units included in the sampling frame is known. We could then select additional units from the sampling frame up front, to account for the proportion of ineligible units in much the same way as we described for non-response earlier. This way we would still hope to achieve the desired number of responses from our sampling frame.

When the sampling frame does not cover the entire target population, this is referred to as under coverage. Some units in the target population thus have zero chance of being included. Following the business directory example above, under coverage would occur if new businesses had opened between when the business directory was compiled and when we drew our sample. They could not be selected into our sample from that sampling frame. Under coverage can be alleviated by using more than one sampling frame – that is, multiple-frame sampling (Wu 2008).

Simple random sampling

The most straightforward type of probability sample is the simple random sample: every unit in the target population has an equal chance of selection. For example, imagine we want to survey 2,000 students within a university with a population of 50,000 students – our sample equates to 4 per cent of our target population. The university has a list of all its students – our sampling frame. The probability of inclusion into the sample is 2,000/50,000 = 0.04 or 1 in 25 – that is the sampling fraction.

To ensure equal probabilities of selection, we could assign the students a number from 1 to 50,000. Then using a random number generator, which is often built into statistical software, we could select 2,000 different numbers in that range. This is the same as putting all 50,000 names on folded pieces of paper in a hat and selecting 2,000 names, but much more practical.

Systematic random sampling

Systematic sampling selects units from the sampling frame based on a *constant interval*. Every unit in the sampling frame is given a number, typically consecutive numbers in ascending order. Sorting is important – for instance, this method can be useful for ensuring coverage of the whole age range where the sampling frame is sorted by age. However, this can also lead to bias if there is a certain feature that occurs in the list at the same frequency as the interval, or if certain features are clustered at points in the list (Bernard 2013).

The sampling interval is set based on the sampling fraction, and a start point is randomly selected, between 1 and the sampling interval. If we use the university example, we know that we need to select 1 in every 25 students to obtain a sample of 2,000. Using systematic sampling, we would select every 25th student in the sampling frame. For the starting point, say our random number generator came up with 3. We would start by selecting the 3rd student in the sampling frame, and would then select students 28, 53, 78, 103, 128, and so on, until we had selected 2,000 students.

It is typical for administrative lists (such as the above) to be sorted in alphabetical order of surnames. This can lead to poor coverage of different ethnic groups due to surnames clustering at certain points in the alphabet. Therefore, we might generate random numbers next to each record and sort these in ascending order, to ensure that the ordering of students on the list is random, and that characteristics of the students, such as their ethnicity, do not influence their probability of being included in the sample.

Stratified random sampling

Stratified random sampling involves dividing the population into smaller distinct groups, known as 'strata'. One of the main reasons to do this is an interest in specific subgroups within the population. This is the case for both of the main types: proportionate stratification and disproportionate stratification.

Proportionate stratification ensures that units are sampled in proportion to their representation in the population. This involves calculating the required sample size for each of the strata, and then applying either simple or systematic random sampling to select the required number of units from them.

Extending the university example, let us say there are six faculties within the university, each with a different percentage of the population of students: Arts (10 per cent), Business (5 per cent), Education (40 per cent), Law (5 per cent), Medicine (20 per cent) and Science (20 per cent). We would calculate the number of students in each faculty and multiply that by the sampling fraction of 0.04 (4 per cent). Table 12.1 shows the results of this: the Faculty of Education has 20,000 students, of which 4 per cent or 800 students would be sampled. We would repeat this for the other faculties.

Table 12.1   University example with proportionate stratified sampling

Faculty	Percentage of students	N(population)	n(sample)=N* sampling fraction(0.04)
Arts	10	5,000	200
Business	5	2,500	100
Education	40	20,000	800
Law	5	2,500	100
Medicine	20	10,000	400
Science	20	10,000	400
Total	**100**	**50,000**	**2,000**

Disproportionate stratification is often referred to as oversampling of one or more subgroups. This is when different sampling fractions are applied to different strata, such that we include a higher number of units from some strata than would be required for proportionate stratification. A key reason to stratify is to obtain adequate numbers from smaller groups within a population so that separate analyses can be conducted by subgroup.

When we oversample, the sample is no longer representative of the population as subgroups have been intentionally overrepresented. To obtain unbiased estimates at the population level, surveys employing disproportionate sampling have to be weighted, so that groups that were 'oversampled' are brought back in line with their actual share of the population. This essentially means that, for analytical purposes, certain respondents will be treated as worth a bit more or a bit less than *one* respondent each (Lavallée and Beaumont 2016).

The New Zealand Attitudes and Values Study (NZAVS)

CASE STUDY 12.1

The NZAVS is a 20-year longitudinal survey of New Zealanders' social attitudes, personalities and health outcomes. It was started in 2009 by Professor Chris Sibley at the University of Auckland (Sibley 2014). The NZAVS has a longitudinal panel design, meaning that the same people are surveyed each year. The initial study was based on a national probability sample of New Zealand registered voters aged 18 and over. Participants were selected from the national electoral rolls, which are available by application for scientific researchers in New Zealand.

The electoral rolls contain both permanent residents and citizens, but while it is compulsory to enrol to vote in New Zealand, it is estimated that only 89 per cent of the eligible population are on the rolls. Researchers can ascertain people's age, area of residence, Māori (indigenous) ancestry and occupation from the rolls, so stratified sampling frames can be created if desired.

For the first NZAVS sample, a survey was posted to 40,500 people or approximately 1.36 per cent of registered voters in New Zealand – 35,000 randomly selected from the electoral rolls and 5,500 randomly selected from areas of the country with high proportions of Māori, Pacific and Asian participants (the largest minority ethnic groups in New Zealand). Researchers in New Zealand can find out the characteristics of geographical areas from national census data. The final data set from that first wave of the NZAVS had 6,518 respondents, an overall response rate of 16.6 per cent.

Retention is a key challenge in longitudinal designs – that is, managing to get the same people to fill out the survey every year. Participants may lose interest, move house, or simply decline to take part. In the NZAVS, researchers have found that demographic and social characteristics affect retention. Satherley et al. (2015) showed that over the first four years of the survey, men, immigrants, Māori and Asian participants, younger people, those with less education and those of lower socioeconomic status were the most likely to stop responding. Therefore, several booster samples were drawn to target people with certain characteristics. For the survey's fourth wave (2012) researchers conducted a booster with four sampling frames, as follows:

(Continued)

(Continued)

1. A random sample of 20,000 people from the electoral rolls
2. A random sample of 10,000 people in the Auckland region (the largest city of New Zealand)
3. 3,000 people from the Canterbury region, as a number had dropped out following a series of large earthquakes there
4. 9,000 people from areas that were in the most economically deprived 40 per cent of the country.

The NZAVS publishes detailed information on their post-stratification weighting to correct for sampling complications. It is an example of good sampling practice in a longitudinal study.

Cluster sampling

In cluster sampling, the target population is first divided into a number of groups, which then become the sampling units – that is, we randomly select groups rather than individuals. This method is useful when there are natural groups in the target population: patients in hospitals, people in households, employees in companies, or children in schools. Then we are often interested in the characteristics of the groups and group-level effects. For example, we would use cluster sampling if we were interested in the influence of hospital characteristics (such as number of staff, policies, size) on patients' length of stay. The higher-level units here (hospitals, households, companies, or schools) would be selected into the sample, rather than the individual patients, people, employees or children.

Cluster sampling can be useful when there is no full list of individual units, but there is information about the clusters. For example, a sampling frame of all university students in the country may not be accurate, or even exist at all, but a list of all universities in the country would be relatively simple to compile. We would randomly sample from the list of universities and then select all students within those universities.

Multi-stage cluster sampling adds an additional step by taking a random sample of units within each chosen cluster, rather than sampling all of them. With the university example, we would first randomly sample from the list of universities, and then randomly select a subset of students within the selected universities.

While cluster sampling is a cost-effective means of sampling a large number of units, units within clusters tend to be more similar than units selected from different clusters (Shackleton et al. 2016). This can be measured using the intra-class correlation coefficient (ICC), which gives the average amount of within-cluster correlation for a particular variable of interest. In consequence, a larger sample size is required with cluster sampling to achieve the same 'statistical power' as a simple random sample. To estimate the required sample size for a given level of statistical power in cluster sampling, we first estimate the design effect, which is a function of the average number of subjects sampled per cluster and the ICC.

Design effect = 1 + (m-1) × ICC, where m is the average number of units per cluster.

Based on this we see that the more similar units are within clusters than between clusters (the larger the ICC), the larger will be the design effect. Also, the larger the clusters are on average, the larger will be the design effect. This means that with a cluster sample you need to sample the design effect times as many individuals (patients, people, employees or children, to use our earlier example) overall as you would with a simple random sample of the same population, in order to have the same amount of statistical power.

You can also calculate the effective sample size, an estimate of the sample size that a simple random sample would have required to achieve the same level of sampling error. This is the sample size in the cluster sample divided by the design effect. It should be clear that the effects of clustering need to be accounted for in analysis with these departures from simple random sampling. This manifests itself in the estimation of standard errors, which affects the precision of results and ensures appropriate statistical inference.

Another important issue in cluster sampling is deciding the number of clusters to sample. Selecting only a few clusters can lead to reductions in the representativeness of samples – say, just three clusters with a large number of units in each. It is recommended that a larger number of clusters is sampled with a smaller number of units per cluster.

Thinking of the university student example, imagine that we want to interview 2,000 students from the whole population, rather than from a single university. If we employ only simple or stratified random sampling, we might end up selecting students (units) from every university (cluster) in the country. Travelling to every university would require substantial amounts of time and money. Multi-stage cluster sampling would provide an efficient alternative: we could randomly select five universities and then select 400 students from each by simple or stratified random sampling. Now imagine we are primarily interested in wellbeing scores and have estimated the ICC for wellbeing scores at 0.10. In this scenario, our design effect would be:

$$\text{Design effect} = 1 + (400\text{-}1) \times 0.10 = 40.9$$

This is an incredibly large design effect, meaning that we would need to sample 40.9 times as many students to have the same power as a simple random sample of this population. The effective sample size would be 2,000/40.9 = 49, so our sample of 2,000 students would have the same power as a simple random sample of just 49 students.

To reduce the risk of ending up with a sample that is not representative of the population and has low power, we could increase the number of universities sampled to 40, and randomly select 50 students from each university. This would reduce the design effect to 5.9, and increase the effective sample size to 339, but it would increase the travelling costs and time needed to be spent in the field. There is always a trade-off.

Initiating change locally in bullying and aggression through the school environment (INCLUSIVE)

The INCLUSIVE study is a three-year cluster randomized controlled trial (RCT) with the primary aim of reducing bullying and violence within schools. The secondary aims are to reduce risky behaviours to health, such as substance use and sexual activity, and to increase psychological function and wellbeing (Bonell et al. 2014). The intervention is universal and combines changes in policy in the school environment with the promotion of social and emotional skills, and restorative practices. It has an impact on every student in the school.

In RCTs, those who receive the treatment are compared to those not receiving the treatment. Assignment to receive the treatment (the intervention) or not (the control) is random. In a well-designed RCT there is no difference between the two groups except for the intervention. This allows us to isolate its effect.

Initially, 500 eligible secondary schools (students aged 11–18) within a one-hour travel time from central London were contacted to participate in the study. Power and sample size were key considerations given the clustered nature of the sample. The researchers worked out that the average English school has approximately 190 students per year level. They used evidence from published systematic reviews to estimate the likely effect size for the intervention (0.3–0.4) and used information from published sources to estimate the ICC values for aggression and bullying in schools (0.01–0.03).

The researchers decided they would base their power calculation on more conservative estimates, so that they would have the power to detect changes in behaviour even if the effect size was smaller (0.25); the ICC was slightly larger (0.04); and the number of students per school was lower than the average (150).

As discussed above, the ICC and the number of units selected per cluster determine the design effect, which describes the statistical power of a sample. The power calculations demonstrated that 20 schools in the intervention and 20 control groups each was sufficient, and that even if two schools per group (10 per cent) opted out of the study, they would still have 80 per cent power to detect an effect size of 0.25. The final sample was 6,700 students across 40 schools, with 20 in the intervention and 20 in the control group.

Eligible schools whose head teacher gave informed written consent to participate were allocated on a 1:1 ratio between intervention and control groups. To ensure that the two groups were as similar as possible at baseline, schools were stratified by school-level determinants of violence. Schools were then allocated to the intervention or control group within each of these strata to ensure equal numbers of schools from each stratum in the intervention and control groups.

At baseline and at annual follow-ups, surveys of students and school staff were administered in both the intervention and control schools. Retaining participation from schools in the control group was difficult. To encourage continuing participation, these schools were given a financial incentive of £500.

This case study highlights several key issues for sampling and how it applies in real-world situations. The intervention, by nature, required a cluster sampling design, as it took place at the school level and influenced every student within the school. It would have been impossible to run this RCT by selecting a simple random sample of pupils. The school environment could not have been changed just for them.

Drawing inferences

The central strength of probability sampling is the ability to draw inferences about a population from the data produced by a sample. This is due to our knowledge of the probabilities of selection and established statistical theory, in this case distribution theory and the central limit theorem. We know how a normal distribution (you may know it as a bell curve) behaves and that, given a large enough sample size, we may use its properties to describe our data set. We want to infer summary measures from the sample to the population and approximation to normality allows us to do this, albeit with some uncertainty.

The basis of this is that 95 per cent of the values in a normal distribution lie within ±1.96 standard deviations of the mean. This is complicated by sampling design, but at its core it is what leads to 'confidence intervals' – that is, ranges around sample estimates within which we can say that the true population value lies. You may have heard of the 'with 95 per cent confidence' reporting standard.

With good sampling design, we should be in a position to draw inferences that are both precise (with a narrow range around the sample estimates) and accurate (close to the true values of parameters in the population). The base case is one in which a simple random sample has been drawn and a single parameter – for example, the mean of a single variable – has been estimated. These are the conditions for a typical 'test of significance' in statistical terms.

The variable in question needs to be a 'scale' variable for the most straightforward tests, so that a mathematical mean makes sense. The traditional first step is to have a research question, which drives you to draw a sample and collect data in the first place, and thereby a 'null hypothesis' about the value of the true population mean value. The test of significance, which in this case would be a 'one-sample t-test', looks for evidence against that null hypothesis. There is usually an alternative hypothesis in place, often simply that the true value is different from what the null claims. The t-test examines the properties of the sample, as in the actual observations on the variable, and returns a value from the t-distribution. This is mathematically linked to a 'p-value', which, again, you may have heard reported.

The p-value can be interpreted as follows. If the population mean were indeed the hypothesized value, how often would we observe, in an equivalent simple random sample, a mean that was as far from that value as the one we *did* observe? For this to be useful there needs to be a cut-off where we decide that that is *too often* – the cut-off for 'statistical significance'. The most common is the value 0.05, so effectively once in 20 random samples. If the p-value is lower than that, we say that we can reject the null hypothesis; otherwise, we cannot reject it with the sample we took. If we want to be more certain, we can reduce the cut-off, say to 0.01.

Sources of error

Whatever sampling design you employ, the process will generate 'error' in terms of how the sample reflects the target population. Some types of error can be controlled for within the design. At the highest level, there are two types of error: random and systematic. There are also two sources: sampling and non-sampling. A main aim of sampling is to minimize error. Effort is usually focused on sampling error, and particularly the random element, which is easy to estimate and control for. Systematic error, or bias, is harder to identify, and the theory and practice for non-sampling error are less developed than those for sampling error.

Sampling error is one of two reasons for the difference between the estimate from a sample and the true population value, and is due, as the name suggests, to the fact that we sample from the population. Multiple probability samples of the same size from the same population would result in different estimates so values obtained from probability samples are unlikely to match the true value.

Larger sample sizes improve the precision of sample estimates, but a large sample size alone will not ensure the accuracy of estimates from samples. An estimate can be highly precise but inaccurate. For example, if we have a sample of 10,000 adults and measure weight, we might end up with a reasonably precise estimate of weight – let's say the sample mean is 74.1kg, with a standard error of 0.3, giving us a 95 per cent confidence interval of 73.5–74.7kg. If some sampled adults refuse to be weighed and they happen to be heavier on average than those who are weighed, or if those who are heavier are simply less likely to be included in the sampling frame, then we would underestimate weight in the population based on that sample. These are sources of non-sampling error. Others include coverage errors, measurement errors, non-response errors, processing errors and adjustment errors (Groves et al. 2009).

We introduced coverage errors when we discussed sampling frames, which do not always cover the entire target population. Certain subgroups, such as the homeless, highly mobile, and those living in rest homes, prisons and other such institutions, are not well captured in administrative records, and we can only make generalizations to the population in the sampling frame(s). Sampling frames can also have biases in their coverage of the population. For example, electoral rolls tend to cover a very high percentage of the population aged 70+, but a lower percentage of those aged 18–24. Stratifying a sample by age can help to ensure that the age composition reflects that of the population as a whole. However, those who are enrolled to vote differ in important ways from those who are not, even within age groups. A sample can only ever give as good a representation of the population as its sampling frame.

Measurement errors are differences between response values and true values. Respondents may not be able to answer certain questions accurately, such as the overall income of their household. Sometimes, time periods may be given to help jog the memory: health surveys may ask about doctors' visits: the number of visits in the last year, or when the most recent visit was. Errors can be alleviated by using well-trained, experienced interviewers, tried-and-tested questions, and scales that have been shown to be reliable.

Non-response errors occur when the people sampled are not interviewed or do not respond because they are unable, unavailable or unwilling to do so. Certain segments of any population will be less likely to respond to surveys: those in poverty, the young, the very old, minority ethnic group members and recent immigrants, and those with lower levels of education. These are all systematic biases, meaning that those who do respond tend to be moderately wealthy, well-educated, middle-aged people.

Non-response can be minimized by sending reminders during the data collection period and/or offering incentives to respond. As stated above, oversampling can be used to increase the response rate. This can be expensive and can be limited by information from the sampling frame. Non-response bias can also be addressed if we know who has not responded.

The sampling frame can often provide useful information such as age, sex, ethnicity, occupation and area of residence. Knowing how the characteristics of the responders and non-responders differ allows us to calculate the extent to which our sample is underrepresenting some groups (such as young males from minority ethnic groups who live in deprived areas) and overrepresenting others (such as affluent, middle-aged, white females). Adjustments such as weighting can be made during the analysis phase to account for this bias. Weighting means that people who were less likely to respond are given more weight, or are worth more, in the analysis than those who were more likely to respond based on the characteristics available in the sampling frame.

Non-probability sampling

A key element of probability sampling is that the sample is selected at random – the researcher defines the target population and specifies the rules for selection into the sample. Beyond that, neither the researcher nor anyone in the sample has any influence on whether or not other people are selected to join. There is minimal potential for researcher bias. Non-probability sampling does not involve random selection; it is a form of sampling where either the researcher, people in the population, or both, decide who is included in the sample. We do not know the extent to which estimates from non-probability samples reflect the population, so we cannot estimate the level of error or use statistical methods to make inferences.

Why, then, do researchers use non-probability samples? There are instances in applied health research where it is not feasible or practical to conduct probability sampling, for instance if a sampling frame is not available or the population is widely dispersed. It would be difficult to obtain a random sample of people with bipolar disorder or cystic fibrosis. Non-probability sampling can also be useful in the initial stages of probability-based research, for example to pilot a questionnaire. Representativeness is less important than identifying the range and variety of responses in that stage of a study.

Key non-probability sampling techniques include:

- *Convenience sampling* that involves selecting units into the sample based on ease of recruitment. For instance, psychological studies, both experiments and surveys, are often based on convenience samples of undergraduate students. Usually these are pre-liminary studies for developing theories and refining ideas prior to testing them with a probabilistic sample. There are two advantages to this practice: first, psychology students gain first-hand experience of being a research participant and, second, potential problems can be identified quickly and at a relatively low cost.
- *Call for volunteers* is where members self-select into the sample. Experimental research often relies on volunteers and incentives to encourage participation. Websites showcase studies, such as the aptly named www.callforparticipants.com.
- *Snowball sampling* may also be used in studies where access is difficult. The researcher starts out with a known group or individual, say people with a particular health condition, and increases the sample size mainly through word of mouth.

CASE STUDY 12.3

Pacific surveys for those bereaved by suicide

A recent real-world example of a non-probability sample of a hard-to-reach population is this project led by Dr Jemaima Tiatia-Seath of Hibiscus Research and the University of Auckland, New Zealand (Tiatia-Seath, Lay-Yee and von Randow 2017). The researchers wanted to find out more about the experiences of Pacific people in New Zealand who had suffered through the suicide of a loved one.

New Zealand has a population of 4.5 million, around 100,000 of which are people of Pacific ethnicity. There is no available sampling frame that identifies this group in terms of ethnicity, let alone the tiny fraction who met the criteria for inclusion. In this exploratory study, the researchers' only option was to use their own networks to build the sample through snowball sampling. SurveyMonkey was used to administer the survey online once contact was made, which simplified delivery and reduced costs.

The questions related to the support that people had received, who had given it, in what context and over what period. Participants were provided with a list of formal organizations that provided community support and were invited to attend focus groups, to discuss their experiences further and to try to address common obstacles encountered in getting support.

The study also carried out a non-probabilistic sample survey of people employed to provide support to those bereaved by suicide – an easier group to identify in the population, but still not possible to sample randomly. To provide the broader context, a statistical analysis of hospital administrative data was undertaken. This looked at the mortality and morbidity of Pacific peoples with self-harm given as one of the causes of death (Tiatia-Seath, Lay-Yee and von Randow 2017). Non-probability sampling can be very useful when combined with other components in a study.

Online panels

A major area of growth in survey methodology recently has been the online panel market. Research is an expensive and time-consuming endeavour. There are high costs in employing interviewers for phone or face-to-face samples, and in mail studies there are the costs of printing and postage. As response rates decrease over the years, these costs continue to increase. In consequence, researchers have turned to online samples and, recently, online panels. Many online panel samples have been recruited through non-probability, convenience sampling methods. Internet or social media advertisements recruit through click and register adverts offering cash incentives. Others recruit through customer lists from corporations. Both sources produce biased non-probabilistic samples.

One way in which panels try to avoid bias is through quota sampling. Panel members are invited to complete a survey until a number of people from certain demographic groups have been recruited. For example, a researcher may want 1,000 participants. They recruit members until 500 women and 500 men have responded, to keep the sample representative in terms of gender, and then stop recruiting participants. This creates bias as those who respond early may differ from those who respond later. For example, those who respond early may be less likely to be employed because they have more time to spare.

Some researchers have started to combine the convenience of online panels with the rigour of probability sampling.

The NatCen online panel

Combining the convenience of having an online panel with the versatility of probability sampling allows researchers to obtain data efficiently and without compromising sample quality. Previously, many online panels were opt-in, so they were biased across many demographics and attitudinal measures. Now there is a growing market of national probability online panels, such as the NatCen panel (http://natcen. ac.uk/taking-part/studies-in-field/natcen-panel). NatCen aims to provide a representative sample of adults aged 18 and over from England, Scotland and Wales.

(Continued)

CASE STUDY 12.4

(Continued)

Participants were recruited to the NatCen panel from the 2015 and 2016 British and Scottish Social Attitudes Surveys, using a 'piggy-back' approach. That is, after a survey interview, participants were asked if they wished to join the NatCen panel. This allowed the panel to recruit participants using face-to-face methods, which normally lead to higher response rates, while avoiding the financial cost associated with obtaining a fresh face-to-face sample.

The Social Attitudes Surveys use face-to-face interviews with individuals from randomly selected households. The sampling frame is the British Postcode Address File, a list of addresses created and maintained by the Post Office. Once a household is selected at random, the interviewer uses a computer-generated random selection procedure to choose the individual household member to interview. The interviewer then visits the household multiple times to try to achieve an interview with that person.

At the end of the Social Attitudes Survey interview, participants were asked if they wanted to join the NatCen panel, and 4,205 (58 per cent) opted to do so. Panel participants were asked for complete contact details and were sent an information leaflet and a confirmation letter.

Although the panel aims to be nationally representative, there are still small biases that the researchers correct for with sample weighting. These include a higher proportion of women than men, lower proportions of young people and a lower proportion of people living in London, compared to the whole population.

NatCen panel participants are sent a survey every one to two months. Most participants have access to the internet and complete the surveys online, but 11 per cent are surveyed by phone. The surveys vary on topic: for example, the Mental Health Foundation used the NatCen panel to investigate mental health in the British population, and surveys have been conducted on political attitudes. Around 60 per cent of the panel participants complete each survey. Non-response is due to a variety of factors, and participants tend to become non-responsive over time through illness, migration, and other factors. Around 13 per cent opt out after a year on the panel. Nevertheless, it is a great resource as it allows researchers to access a representative sample without the financial and time costs of obtaining one from scratch.

Reading health research based on quantitative sampling

Questions to ask in critically appraising sampling design in reading quantitative research studies include:

- Is the sampling design appropriate/useful for providing answers to the research question(s)?
- Is the sampling frame reported and is it open to scrutiny?
- If cluster sampling was used, are intra-class correlations and design effects provided?

- Is the sampling design structured so as to ensure adequate coverage of any sub-populations of interest, such as minority ethnic groups?
- Is the sample size large enough to permit precise estimates of key parameters?
- Is the response rate high enough to have confidence about sample representativeness?
- Is there information about non-responders and the level of non-response?
- Do non-responders differ from responders?
- Is there information about how the investigators tackled non-sampling error?
- Is there information about measurement error and its estimation and control?

Conclusion

This chapter has outlined the basic principles of probability and non-probability sampling related to health research. Probability sampling is the more reliable in statistical terms, as it is based on the theory of random numbers. However, the decision of how to sample depends on a number of factors: cost, convenience, whether a reliable sampling frame exists and the research question itself. Sometimes probability sampling is inappropriate given the nature of the research. Researchers should also be mindful of ethical issues: consent, appropriate use of data, confidentiality and respect for the participants of the research – whatever the choice of method. When disseminating findings, researchers should explain clearly why they chose their approach, how the sample was drawn and any limitations on inferences drawn.

Exercise 12.1   Scenarios for developing effective sample designs

Below are two health research scenarios where a social scientist might be involved in helping to formulate a plan. An essential part of this would be the development of an effective sampling design. These scenarios were selected because they require engagement with communities and target populations that might be seen as outside the standard range for orthodox sampling theory and practice. Therefore, aside from the more conventional considerations of sample design, frame and coverage, sample size and distribution, and sampling and non-sampling error, you will also need to think about how to engage with key stakeholders and keep them supportive of your research goals.

Scenario 1

An industrial area has recently seen a spate of cancers among residents in a nearby neighbourhood. Most of those affected had worked at a timber treatment plant

(Continued)

(Continued)

that had recently closed. Those living in the community are concerned that the cancers may be the result of chemical poisoning from the timber plant. They have approached you as a researcher for help in investigating a possible association between the chemicals and the recently diagnosed cancers.

Scenario 2

You are a member of a research team that has developed a new type of follow-up and self-management plan for managing diabetes symptoms, aimed at those diagnosed as having chronic diabetes. This system has generally proved effective, but you are interested in implementing it in deprived rural communities where diabetes is rife. Your research team is interested in improving the management of diabetes in this group.

For each scenario, develop a written plan, proposing an appropriate sampling design and outlining the key considerations.

Note

This chapter is written in memory of the late Professor Alastair Scott who was the co-author of this chapter in previous editions of the book.

Recommended further reading

Appropriate sampling design is vital for making accurate inferences as one piece of a larger puzzle. For researchers planning on running a survey, this textbook on survey methodology provides readers with an extensive overview of the many potential sources of error within survey research:

Groves, R., Fowler Jr, F., Couper, M., Lepkowsi, J., Singer, E. and Tourangeau, R. (2009) *Survey Methodology*, 2nd edition. Hoboken, NJ: Wiley.

For practical advice on how to plan, conduct and analyse survey data, this book is recommended. It assumes no prior knowledge of survey methodology or statistical concepts, making it highly accessible:

De Vaus, D. (2014) *Surveys in Social Research*, 6th edition. London: Routledge.

For further information on how sampling methodology relates to research design, this book provides further guidance on sampling in qualitative research, giving detailed accounts and examples of purposive sampling methodologies:

Bryman, A. (2016) *Social Research Methods*, 5th edition. Oxford: Oxford University Press.

References

Bernard, H. (2013) *Social Research Methods: Qualitative and Quantitative Approaches*, 2nd edition. Los Angeles, CA: Sage.

Bonell, C., Allen, E., Christie, D., Elbourne, D., Fletcher, A., Grieve, R., LeGood, R., Mathiot, A., Scott, S. and Wiggins, M. (2014). 'Initiating change locally in bullying and aggression through the school environment (INCLUSIVE): Study protocol for a cluster randomised controlled trial', *Trials*, *15*(1): 381.

De Vaus, D. (2014) *Surveys in Social Research*, 6th edition. London: Routledge.

Dillman, D., Smyth, J. and Christian, L. (2009) *Internet, Mail, and Mixed-Mode Surveys: The Tailored Design Method*. New York: Wiley.

Groves, R., Fowler Jr, F., Couper, M., Lepkowsi, J., Singer, E. and Tourangeau, R. (2009) *Survey Methodology*, 2nd edition. Hoboken, NJ: Wiley.

Laake, P. and Fagerland, M. (2015) 'Statistical inference', in P. Laake, H. Benestad and B. Olsen (eds), *Research in Medical and Biological Sciences: From Planning and Preparation to Grant Application and Publication*, 2nd edition. London: Academic Press.

Lavallée, P. and Beaumont, J. (2016) 'Weighting: Principles and practicalities', in C. Wolf, D. Joye, T. Smith and Y. Fu (eds), *The Sage Handbook of Survey Methodology*. London: Sage.

Satherley, N., Milojev, P., Greaves, L., Huang, Y., Osborne, D., Bulbulia, J. and Sibley, C. (2015) 'Demographic and psychological predictors of panel attrition: Evidence from the New Zealand attitudes and values study', *PLoS One*, *10*(3): e0121950.

Shackleton, N., Hale, D., Bonell, C. and Viner, R. (2016) 'Intra-class correlation values for adolescent health outcomes in secondary schools in 21 European countries', *SSM – Population Health*, *2*: 217–25.

Shapiro, G. (2008) 'Sample design', in P. Lavrakas (ed.), *Encyclopedia of Survey Research Methods*. Thousand Oaks, CA: Sage.

Sibley, C. (2014) 'Sampling procedure and sample details for the New Zealand attitudes and values study', *NZAVS Technical Documents*. Available at: www.psych.auckland.ac.nz/en/about/our-research/research-groups/new-zealand-attitudes-and-values-study/nza-vs-tech-docs.html.

Tiatia-Seath, J., Lay-Yee, R. and von Randow, M. (2017) 'Supporting the bereavement needs of Pacific communities in Aotearoa, New Zealand, following a suicide', *Journal of Indigenous Wellbeing Te Mauri – Pimatisiwin*, *2*(2): 129–41.

Wu, C. (2008) 'Multiple-frame sampling', in P. Lavrakas (ed.), *Encyclopedia of Survey Research Methods*. Thousand Oaks, CA: Sage.

13

Quantitative Survey Methods in Health Research

MICHAEL CALNAN

Chapter objectives

- To explore the use of survey methods in research into health and health care which are widely used in this and other fields of research
- To define and explain what quantitative survey methodology is – including the techniques and resources required for carrying out a survey
- To outline the role of theory and the process of translating concepts into indicators
- To assess the strengths and weaknesses of different techniques for collecting data
- To identify the major issues in managing a survey and analysing and presenting data.

Introduction

Survey methods can be defined in a number of different ways but the most cogent is provided by De Vaus (2014), who argues that the two defining characteristics of a survey are: how data are collected and the method of analysis used. In a survey, data should be collected on the basis of the same characteristics – such as social position, beliefs, attitudes, health-related behaviours and biomarkers – from a number of cases or units of analysis to provide a structured data set. Analysis in survey methods involves a comparison of cases.

This can be descriptive, for example, by identifying the level of satisfaction with health care by group, or it can be taken further analytically to locate cause. For instance, the level of public satisfaction with health has been systematically associated with age: older people have higher levels of satisfaction than younger people. Causal inferences may then be drawn by a careful comparison of the characteristics of cases to explain why age may affect levels of satisfaction. It is important to avoid the mistake of attributing a *causal* link between age and satisfaction. Showing that two variables are associated does not, in itself, provide sufficient evidence to prove a causal link. There are other techniques to establish causation through survey experiments and matching (see Murnane and Willett 2010).

Types of survey

Surveys can be of different types (Czaja and Blair 2005). An *ad hoc* survey is carried out for a one-off purpose, such as a local survey of health care users to find out the level of satisfaction with a particular organization or service. Cross-sectional surveys are regular surveys that monitor trends over time, such as the British Social Attitudes Survey (Clery, Curtice and Harding 2016; Park et al. 2003). This national survey is annual and consists of a set of core questions with new questions added to cover current problems. Regular surveys are used to monitor general trends.

Another example of a regular national survey is the Health Survey for England (HSE). This has a focus on public health questions. It is an annual cross-sectional survey designed to collect information from a nationally representative sample of those aged 16 years and over who live in private households (Mindell et al. 2012). The HSE collects a variety of demographic, socioeconomic and health data using questionnaires and objective biomarker measures of health. A two-stage stratified random sampling process is used with the Postcode Address File as the primary sampling unit. Individuals selected for inclusion in one survey are excluded from selection for the following three years. Adult interview response rates have declined since the survey was introduced from around 70 per cent in the 1990s to 60 per cent in the 2000s (Mindell et al. 2012). The HSE is particularly useful for exploring questions such as: Can the widening gap in social inequalities in health in England be explained by changes over time in the prevalence of health-related behaviours between different socioeconomic groups? For this analysis, the data set for selected survey years consisted of 76,628 respondents (Stait and Calnan 2016).

There are also international surveys that collect data on health and related questions. For example, the Survey of Health, Ageing and Retirement in Europe (SHARE) is led by a multidisciplinary and cross-national panel. It has a database on health covering socioeconomic status and social and family networks for more than 120,000 individuals aged 50 or older based on more than 297,000 interviews. SHARE covers 27 European countries and Israel and is currently in its seventh wave (Dragano, Siegrist and Wahrendorf 2011).

It should be stressed, though, that national surveys may not be able to identify certain aspects of change. For example, the British Social Attitudes Survey can show people's attitudes to private health care, the level of coverage and number of subscriptions to private health insurance, and how these change over time. During the 1980s, this survey showed a gradual increase in the proportion of the population covered by private insurance. However, as the overall figure did not identify the proportion of lapsed subscribers, which in the case of private health insurance was high, the data could not show whether the increase reflected a large or small increase in new subscriptions (Calnan, Cant and Gabe 1993).

Surveys carried out on a regular basis can be useful for measuring gross change but longitudinal designs, using cohort or panel studies, are more appropriate for understanding individual and within-group net change. A longitudinal study, that is a survey repeated with the same cohort or population at different points of time, would show the proportion of those over time who took out a new subscription to private health insurance, the proportion who maintained their subscription to private health insurance, and the proportion who let their subscription lapse.

In the United Kingdom, although there is no longitudinal study of health as such, a number of longitudinal studies collect data on health-related questions. One of these is the 1970 British Cohort Study (BCS70), which follows the lives of more than 17,000 people born in England, Scotland and Wales in a single week of 1970. The BCS70 has collected information on health, physical, educational and social development, and economic circumstances, among other factors (www.cls.ioe.ac.uk/Default.aspx).

Survey methods are often associated with the use of a questionnaire, where data are collected through interview (face-to-face or by telephone) or are self-completed through postal or other means. However, surveys can draw on a wide range of techniques. One common format for dealing with responses to closed-choice questions is through numerical rating scales where responses are ordered from low to high. Four common scaling types, according to De Vaus (2014), are:

- Likert scales where respondents are given the five alternatives: strongly disagreeing, disagreeing, agreeing and strongly agreeing with the neutral point in the middle of neither agreeing nor disagreeing.
- Horizontal rating scales where the respondent is given opposite attitude positions. They are asked to indicate numerically where their own belief falls.
- Semantic differential scales where respondents are provided with opposite adjectives at each end of the scale and a numerical scale between the items, and the respondents are asked to rate their response numerically.
- Vertical rating ladder scale where respondents are asked on a 10-point scale from high to low where they might rate something or someone.

These scales can be used as alternatives or in combination. There may also be a qualitative element when the interview schedule includes both open-ended and semi-structured questions. Some surveys include structured observation where specific activities are recorded. For example, if the aim is to explore practitioner–patient encounters, activities may be recorded in a hospital ward or general practice. Another technique for data collection is the structured record review where the researcher uses a specially created form to elicit information from, for example, patients' medical records. Qualitative data in a survey may be organized and analysed quantitatively, using a content analysis method (Fink 2003). The frequency with which topics occur in respondents' narratives could be counted, as discussed in Chapter 5. In sum, a survey is not synonymous with using a questionnaire. Various methods can be used to collect and analyse data, just as it can in case study and experimental designs.

The rationale for employing survey methods

When is it appropriate to use quantitative survey methods? The sample survey using different data collection techniques can be used to address descriptive questions, such as: What? Who? When? How? A survey can also identify variation in the characteristics of different groups. It is also possible, as suggested above, to use a survey for explanatory research to explore 'Why?' questions, where the aim is to impute cause or consequence. In cross-sectional surveys, information is collected at one point in time to take a 'snapshot'. This approach lacks a time dimension that can hinder the exploration of causal influences. Surveys that are repeated, or repeated at intervals, can explore changes in relationships and the strength of interrelationships between variables and can also identify naturally occurring variation. Nonetheless, as stated above, it is generally difficult to pinpoint a specific cause and impossible to eliminate a range of confounding or contaminating factors. In summary, survey methods are distinguishable from other research methods in terms of the form of data collection and methods of analysis adopted. However, surveys are not necessarily distinguished by the techniques of data collection that may also be used in other methods. Survey methods tend to address questions that are both descriptive and analytical, although they have limitations in relation to exploring specific causal influences.

The techniques and resources required for the survey method in practice

What resources are required in terms of time and money to carry out the survey method? Fink (2003) suggests that the researcher should address the following questions:

* What are the major tasks of the survey?

- What skills are needed to complete each task?
- How much time does each task take?
- How much time is available to complete the survey?
- Who can be recruited to perform each task?
- What are the costs of each task?
- What additional resources are needed?

These questions may be addressed by quantifying and listing basic information on the direct and indirect costs and expenses incurred by the survey. See a tool for project planning in Chapter 26, but these questions specifically include:

- Decide on the number of days (or hours) that constitute a working year.
- Formulate survey tasks or activities in terms of the number of months it will take to complete each task.
- Estimate how long, in a number of days (or hours), you will need for each person to complete their assigned task.
- Decide on the daily (hourly) rate for each person who will need to be paid.
- Agree on the cost of benefits (such as superannuation).
- Decide on other expenses that will be specifically incurred in the study, such as questionnaire piloting or focus groups.
- Decide on the indirect costs that will be incurred to keep the survey team going, such as overheads and accommodation.

Translating concepts into indicators

Operationalizing concepts

Survey research should be informed by theory, and the impact of theory, as with most other research methods, helps to focus questions and enhance the value of findings. Once a theoretical framework is constructed, an important issue is deciding how concepts should be translated into questions or indicators – in other words, how theory can be operationalized in the survey. De Vaus (2014) sees concepts as abstract summaries of sets of behaviours, attitudes and characteristics that share something in common and concludes that the operationalization of a concept involves three essential steps: clarifying the concept, developing an indicator and evaluating the indicator.

These are set out in Figure 13.1, which uses 'deprivation' to illustrate the different elements involved in operationalizing a concept. First, obtain a range of definitions. In the case of deprivation, five different definitions are identified: physical, economic, social, political and psychic. Second, decide upon a particular definition, which in the case of deprivation might be the 'social' aspect. Third, the dimensions of the concept must be delineated.

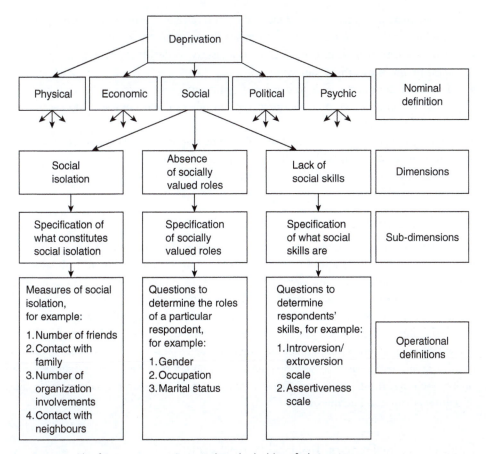

FIGURE 13.1 Clarifying concepts: Descending the ladder of abstraction

For deprivation, three dimensions have been identified: social isolation, the absence of socially valued roles and a lack of social skills. The process of moving from abstract concepts to the point where they can be operationalized via a specific questionnaire item is called 'descending the ladder of abstraction'. Clarifying concepts involves descending this ladder.

How many indicators should be used?

There is no definite or clear-cut answer to the question, but the following points provide a guideline for indicator development:

- Where there is no agreed way of measuring the concept, it is helpful to develop indicators for a range of definitions in order to see the effect on the results.
- If the concept is multidimensional, it is necessary to decide if there is interest in all, some or any one of these dimensions.
- The researcher must be able to develop measures of key concepts.
- Complex concepts are best measured via a number of questions so as to capture the scope of the concept.
- Piloting indicators is an essential way of eliminating unnecessary questions.
- The number of items will be affected by pragmatic considerations (for example, the length of the questionnaire and the method of administration).

How should indicators be developed?

For certain concepts, it is simple to identify indicators as they are well established, as is the case with age or marital status. Other more abstract concepts are more difficult, although there are a number of different ways of approaching the problem. First, a well-established measure from previous research may be used. This allows a direct comparison to be made between the results of your research and previous research findings. The danger with using an 'off-the-shelf' instrument is that it may not be tailored to measure the specific concept one wishes to explore. Second, a qualitative method such as informal face-to-face interviews or focus groups can be used to develop questions, although this is less convenient and more time consuming. Third, interviews with key informants or interest groups can provide clues or pointers to appropriate questions.

Evaluating indicators: Reliability and validity

How should indicators be evaluated to ensure that they are reliable and valid before the survey is conducted? Reliability occurs when a similar result is obtained in response to a particular question or indicator on repeated occasions. Questions can be unreliable if they are poorly worded or ambiguous or influenced by the style or characteristics of the interviewer. Reliability can be tested for single items by the method of test–retest and by item-to-item correlation for multiple-item scales. This means examining the strength of the statistical relationship between items. Using multi-item indicators and removing the unreliable item after testing should increase reliability. Other ways of improving reliability are through using well-tested questions, training interviewers prior to data collection and reading, and re-reading questions, preferably with colleagues to find wording that is unambiguous.

The question of validity is more complex. The aim is to find an indicator that is operationalized in a way that measures the concept it is intended to measure, and whether this in turn is a valid empirical indicator of the theoretical concept. There are various methods of judging validity, but the four outlined in Box 13.1 are the most common (see also Fink 2003; Litwin 1995).

Box 13.1   Methods for judging validity

- *Content validity*: This refers to the extent to which a measure thoroughly and appropriately assesses the characteristics or skills it is intended to measure. A concept should be derived from a conceptual framework or set of theoretical ideas and the indicator should closely match the concept.
- *Face validity*: This refers to how a measure appears on the surface and whether all the required questions are framed in the appropriate language. In this case, it may not necessarily have been informed, at least explicitly, by theory.
- *Criterion validity*: This refers to the degree of convergence or divergence with a tried-and-tested indicator of the concept. Criterion validity may be concurrent or predictive. Concurrent validity refers to the validity of a measure (for example, for current health status), while predictive validity is the extent to which a measure forecasts future health status. A general health examination, may, for instance, predict health status over the coming years.
- *Construct validity*: This refers to examining whether or not a proposition that is assumed to exist is actually confirmed when the new indicator is tested. For example, there is strong evidence of a positive relationship between health status and affluence/deprivation. Thus, the development of an indicator of deprivation could have its validity tested by examining its relationship with a robust measure of health status.

Strengths and weaknesses of the survey method

There are specific techniques used in surveys to elicit information. As suggested above, survey methods are valuable in examining comparisons and variations between groups, particularly in large populations. The standardization of the data collected is also seen as another distinctive strength (Babbie 2008). Surveys can provide a broad overview of a social phenomenon. What are the weaknesses? One weakness is that surveys are incapable of effectively capturing the meanings and perceptions of social actors and the context in which action is taking place. Qualitative methods, such as informal interviews and observation, are more appropriate in addressing this type of research question as they provide greater flexibility. Surveys have also been seen to be tied to a more positivistic school of thought (see Chapter 3), which emphasizes the importance of structural forces or 'causes' and neglects the importance of human action and agency. Certainly, survey methodology is associated with measurement and not all social phenomena are measurable. As Babbie (2008: 309) comments, 'survey research is comparatively weak on validity and strong on reliability'. It also must be remembered that unreliable measures cannot be valid.

Box 13.2 shows the shortfalls of the most common forms of data collection through questionnaires administered by postal, telephone, face-to-face and web-based methods.

Box 13.2   Shortfalls of common methods of data collection

These limitations are as follows:

- Postal questionnaires are poor in avoiding response bias. They do not often use open-ended questions or control question sequence. They cannot motivate people to answer 'boring' questions and may not produce high-quality entries.
- Telephone interviews are more costly than postal surveys, more difficult to implement and tend not to be useful for exploring sensitive topics.
- Face-to-face questionnaires are difficult to implement. They are costly, slow and involve recruiting suitable staff. It is difficult to ensure the quality of responses due to interviewer characteristics. They may be intrusive, and it is difficult to protect anonymity. Some surveys use a mix of face-to-face interviews with a self-completion element for more sensitive topics.
- Web and internet-based questionnaires have become more common using email and websites. Email and internet questionnaires are particularly useful for eliciting sensitive data – the quality of answers is higher than found in face-to-face interviews (De Vaus 2014). However, there are problems in sampling representative populations as the internet is still not available and accessible to all. This is particularly the case in low to middle-income countries. It is also difficult to know in internet surveys if there is implicit bias in the sampling frame since access may be linked to age, socioeconomic position and other social characteristics.
- Survey techniques can achieve good response rates. Telephone surveys con-sistently produce significantly higher response rates than postal surveys, but lower response rates than face-to-face interview surveys (Bourque and Fielder 2003). Web-based surveys are popular (Couper 2008), but response rates are rarely above 50 per cent (Wilson et al. 2010), which is lower than other methods of data collection (Lozar Manfreda et al. 2007; Shih and Fan 2008). Low levels of response can lead to an unacceptable reduction of sample size and also possible bias as non-responders may differ from responders.

Management of the survey and survey data

Data collection and fieldwork

The management of the survey and the fieldwork are important for the quality of the data collection and adherence to the study method. The tasks involved with a telephone interview survey will include ensuring that: all questions are asked; the response rate at each follow-up is recorded; the interviewer stays within the time limit set; and the interests of the respondents are respected. Ethical guidelines must be agreed prior to interview. Computer-assisted questionnaire administration can be used irrespective of the mode of the questionnaire delivery. De Vaus (2014) provides an extensive list of the advantages of the use of such software that includes enhancement of feedback, error-checking, consistency checks and sample controls.

The design and layout of the questionnaire is important. There should be a general introduction and clear instructions throughout, with section introductions that relate to how many of the responses the respondent can choose from and instructions with signage for the use of contingency questions. Contingency or filter questions are used to steer respondents to questions that are relevant to them, skipping those that are not applicable (De Vaus 2014). Does the length of a questionnaire have an effect on completion and response rates? There is little research evidence available to support this. De Vaus (2014: 112) concludes: 'As a general rule the experience of participating in the survey should be made as pleasant and rewarding as possible. Pay attention to the other aspects of survey design and ensure that they minimize respondents' burden and length will probably become a relatively unimportant factor in determining response rates.'

Managing a postal survey places responsibility on survey coordinators who must develop identifiers and package questionnaires to include self-addressed, pre-paid envelopes for respondents to return. Evidence suggests that follow-ups are important for boosting response rates. Thus, there needs to be a method for identifying and sending out follow-up letters or reminders to those who did not respond by the due date. Non-response to questionnaires can affect the validity of surveys and introduce bias. Survey coordinators should record the reasons for non-response so that a distinction can be made between those who refused to take part and those who did not do so because, for instance, they moved away or were too ill. In the United Kingdom, it is becoming difficult to gain a high response rate to a survey and researchers use rewards and incentives to try to encourage respondent participation. The distribution of incentives such as prizes or shopping vouchers will have to be managed. A crucial element in organizing an interview survey is ensuring that interviewers are well trained and that training is standardized. This is generally the responsibility of the researcher or project manager.

Financial incentives have been widely used to increase response rates to postal questionnaires. A Cochrane systematic review evaluated different ways to do this for a wide range of populations. It found that the odds of response can be doubled through offering a monetary incentive (Edwards et al. 2009). Other factors included pre-notification, follow-up contact, unconditional incentives, shorter questionnaires, providing a second copy at follow-up, mentioning an obligation to respond and university sponsorship. However, the relationship between incentives and participation is not straightforward, as illustrated by evidence from a study which used a randomized control design to test whether knowledge of a financial incentive would increase the response rate to an online questionnaire (Wilson et al. 2010). The randomized controlled trial included 485 principal investigators of publicly funded health services and population health research based in the United Kingdom. Participants were randomly allocated to receive either 'knowledge of' or 'no knowledge of' a financial incentive (a £10 gift voucher) to be provided on completion of the survey. At the end of the study, gift vouchers were given to all participants who completed the questionnaire, regardless of initial randomization status. Reminder emails were sent out to non-respondents at one-, two-, three- and four-week intervals; a fifth postal reminder was also undertaken. The primary outcome measure for the trial was the response rate one week after the second reminder. At the third reminder, the 'no knowledge' group members were informed about the incentive, ending the randomized element of the study. However, all respondents were followed up from reminder three onwards and no significant differences were observed in responses between the two groups. The authors concluded that knowledge of a financial incentive did not significantly increase the response rate to an online questionnaire, suggesting that other factors, such as the salience of the topic, may be more important. The data are presented graphically in Figure 13.2.

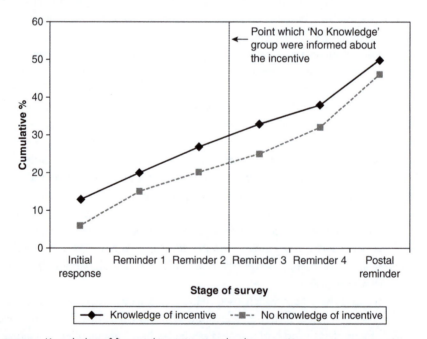

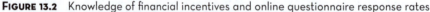

FIGURE 13.2 Knowledge of financial incentives and online questionnaire response rates

Key: Intervention = knowledge of incentive; Control = no knowledge of incentive; vertical dotted line signifies point at which control group were informed about incentive.

Source: Wilson et al. (2010). Reproduced with permission under the terms of the Attribution 2.0 Generic (CC BY 2.0) license.

Ethics and survey research

Social inquiry can result in a range of ethical dilemmas that should be considered before research is undertaken and during the course of a project (Babbie 2008; Bryman 2016). Social surveys are no different. Formal ethical approval is required if human subjects are involved, which they will be if a survey is being used as a primary data source (see Chapter 19 on ethics in health research). Researchers need to note a number of issues, including:

- The right to autonomy and self-determination, which involves the right to agree or not agree to take part in the survey.
- The right to be informed about the study, encompassing the right to informed consent.

A balance has to be made between encouraging and persuading respondents to participate in the study and the unethical practice of coercing or harassing the respondent to take part. Informed consent usually involves a prospective respondent being supplied with information about the purpose of the research, how it is funded and whether participants will be identified by name. Researchers must also give potential participants an information sheet about the research and ask them to sign a consent form. This must state that they can withdraw from the study at any time.

A further ethical question relates to the concern to protect privacy and the right for people to limit access to themselves by others. A social survey may breach privacy by asking personal and intrusive questions. This is related to issues of confidentiality and the right to control information about oneself. Data should be anonymized, so they are 'non-attributable' to specific persons, and stored carefully to follow the requirements of the Data Protection Act. This and related questions are usually addressed in the decision to grant ethical approval or not.

Coding and management of survey data

Data management begins when the first batch of survey questionnaires is returned, and a key task is to develop a coding frame. The coding frame contains the definition of *all* the variables with categories for each. Using the example of age: this can be divided into 10-year intervals (10 years or younger, 11–20 years, 21–30 years and so on) or other breakdown; and the location of the variables and their values (often expressed as numbers in columns). The development of the coding frame, as well as its operationalization, is the method whereby the data are translated from the respondent's answer to the survey questions to a database where aggregate data can be analysed. The development of the coding frame is based on the questions asked. The complexity of the coder's task will depend on the extent to which the questions are pre-coded, that is codes have been allocated already in the questionnaire, or are open-ended, with no pre-codes attached.

For some variables, such as marital status, educational qualifications and socioeconomic status, there are pre-existing sets of codes. Where possible, these can be used. They have been well tested and enable comparison with other studies. Open questions require the development of specific codes to accommodate the range of answers. This can be done by coding a sample of responses to identify the answers most frequently reported. Provisional coding categories can be refined if new categories emerge as the main body of the questionnaires are coded.

Data entry is a major activity in data management. There can be variation in how items are coded, particularly for open-ended questions. It is very important that those coding the questionnaires are well trained and directed. The codes entered will represent data. Entries can be checked by double-coding the data, or at least a sample of them, to test for reliability and consistency. This can identify questions that are ambiguous or where there may be variations in interpretation.

Survey data can be entered into a computer spreadsheet or statistical program. Statistical programs can verify accuracy, although it is important, once again, that those entering data are well trained and directed during the project. Data entry tends to be automatic with computer-assisted, online or scanned surveys that have used pre-coded, closed questions.

A common problem in surveys is that some questions are better answered than others. There may be marked variations in the response rate to specific questions. Thus, the overall response rate to a questionnaire may not be applicable to all questions and will not always reflect usable questions. There are a number of computer programs available but one of the most popular and widely used is SPSS (originally Statistical Package for the Social Sciences), now in its 25th version (IBM SPSS Statistics 25.0 2015). It aids data management, data documentation and statistical analysis. The latter include: descriptive statistics (frequency), bivariate (correlation), linear regression and predictions for identifying groups such as factor analysis (see Bryman (2016) on how to get started with SPSS).

Issues of data analysis and presentation

The approach to data analysis will depend upon the specific research questions or objectives being examined. For example, the five objectives outlined in Box 13.3 have different implications for data analysis.

Box 13.3   Satisfaction with health survey: Objectives of data analysis and their implications

The main objectives considered here are to examine use and levels of satisfaction with general practitioners (GPs), how that might vary by certain variables measuring social position, gender, age and income, and how these data could be analysed.

- *Background data*: Respondents who took part in a 'satisfaction with health care' survey: here, a frequency count may be appropriate or percentages calculated of the proportion of respondents who were men or women or who owned or did not own a car. The latter could be used as a possible indicator of deprivation.
- *Consultation rates*: Describe responses to specific questions: for example, on average how many times did respondents consult their GP in the past year? The average might have been four with the range between zero and 20. Average refers to the measure of central tendency and range to the measure of dispersion.
- *The relationship between recent use of the GP and satisfaction*: This would involve estimating the relationship between the level of use of GPs and the level of satisfaction. One way of estimating the relationship between the two would be through correlation. The expected result would be a positive relationship or correlation, with levels of satisfaction increasing with higher use.
- *Satisfaction – differences between men and women in GP care*: This would involve comparing the average satisfaction scores for men and women and using a test of statistical significance to see if any differences observed are statistically meaningful, rather than simply due to chance. The type of statistical test used will depend on whether the survey data being analysed are nominal (that is, with no numerical preferential values), ordinal (the rate or order of a list of items) or numerical (numbers, such as age in years or height in metres).
- *Does gender,age or income predict the level of satisfaction?* To answer this question, a distinction needs to be made between independent and dependent variables. Independent variables are usually applied to explain or predict a result or outcome – in contrast to the dependent variable. In the case of a patient satisfaction survey, the independent variables are gender, age or income and the dependent variable is level of satisfaction. However, to choose an appropriate statistical method of analysis, it is necessary to specify the purpose of the analysis and identify the number of independent and dependent variables and whether the data being analysed are nominal, ordinal or numerical. Once these questions have been addressed, then a choice of statistical method can be made. The appropriateness of choice depends on the extent to which the assumption about the characteristics and quality of data associated with the method can be met (Fink 2003).

Presenting survey findings

Pie, bar and line charts provide different kinds of figures:

- Pie charts are useful for describing proportions or slices that make up the whole.
- Bar charts are common because they are relatively easy to read and interpret and useful for purposes of comparison.
- Line charts are helpful when plotting trends and changes over time.

Tables can complement charts and are particularly useful for providing detailed information and the results of statistical analyses and findings. The number of tables presented will depend on the purpose and are more commonly used in research reports. Charts, on the other hand, are useful in oral presentations for maximizing visual impact. In terms of writing up, it is important for the discussion and conclusion to be based on the results presented. The limitations of the methods and design should be identified and explained, followed by an interpretation of the findings and their significance.

Case studies: Examples of the use of different survey methods in practice

Examples of survey methods in the area of health and health care are numerous. The following examples illustrate different types of survey methods based primarily on the author's own research.

Postal survey of trust in health care

Calnan and Sanford (2004) aimed to assess levels of trust in health care in England and Wales. This formed part of an international study including the Netherlands and Germany that compared levels of trust across health care systems (van der Schee et al. 2007). A postal survey was used as the most efficient means for eliciting information. It contained a common core of structured questions derived from a survey instrument developed in the Netherlands. One of the problems with carrying out national surveys is finding an easily accessible, comprehensive and up-to-date sampling frame. The Electoral Register provides an accessible and up-to-date source of information but is biased towards those who are more likely to register and underrepresents those who do not. Registers may also be out of date.

Pilot work indicated that allowance should be made for at least 10 per cent inaccuracy when estimating sample size. No information was available about non-respondents, so estimates could not be made of the representativeness of the respondents. A comparison with the respondents to the National Census data showed that our survey underrepresented the younger age groups and healthy people. This was particularly important, as the overall response rate was low at 48 per cent (n = 1,187) (there was a 49 per cent non-response rate and a refusal of 3 per cent). The original sample of 2,777 was reduced to 2,489 as 288 had died or moved away. Respondents had been sent three follow-up mailings in addition to the first mailing.

This study illustrated a common problem in international studies using survey methods. Comparison requires the same core questions. Yet language differences sometimes create a barrier. For example, in the English survey, the two terms 'confidence' (in the doctor's competence) and 'trust' (that the doctor worked in the patient's interest) could be distinguished. No such semantic distinction is made in Dutch or German. To deal with this difference, confidence was used as equivalent to trust in the core questions, but when undertaking the survey in England and Wales additional questions were asked about other aspects of trust (for example, whether respondents thought the practitioner worked primarily in the interests of the patient or the organization) to see if they were associated with confidence in competence. This is depicted in Figure 13.3. The statistical analysis showed that correlation between the two indicators was strong. Coupled with evidence from qualitative, informal, face-to-face interviews, this suggested that confidence was embedded in, and formed part of, trust (Calnan and Rowe 2008).

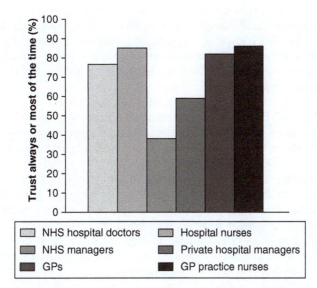

FIGURE 13.3 Public levels of trust in health services staff: Putting the interests of patients above the convenience of organizations

Source: Calnan and Rowe (2008)

Using a mixture of methods in upper-limb pain

A study using a postal survey may combine various methods. For example, a survey can be preceded by a qualitative method, such as using focus groups, as an antecedent. Focus groups may be used to identify the salient themes and help to refine the questions for a postal survey. Alternatively, postal surveys are sometimes used as precursors to qualitative methods to identify cases for follow-up with in-depth interviews.

An example where survey methods acted as a precursor to qualitative methods may be found in a study of sufferers with upper-limb pain using both orthodox and complementary care (Calnan et al. 2005). The study aimed to find out why people sought help and how symptoms were presented; how the problem was managed and treated; and the implications for the outcome of a treatment regime. There were several design options considered, each with strengths and weaknesses. However, the study aimed to obtain information from a broad range of informants, some of whom did not consult orthodox or complementary practitioners at all. Thus, a community-based screening survey was carried out followed by a case-comparison study, as set out in Figure 13.4. The sample for the screening survey was drawn from a population of patients registered with five general practices in the local area. A postal questionnaire, which included screening questions on upper-limb pain taken from a previously validated instrument, was sent to a random sample of the working population aged 25 to 64.

Figure 13.5 thereafter shows the overall response rate (56 per cent) and illustrates the response to the two reminders, both of which elicited around a 10 per cent response rate. The first reminder was a postcard aimed at prompting those who were intending to take part. The second reminder was a letter, questionnaire and pre-paid envelope (identical to the first mailing) aimed at persuading the 'hard core' of non-responders to participate.

For this study, one of the major aims of the initial screening survey was to identify 'cases' for follow-up. These cases were selected according to predefined inclusion criteria to encompass those who had experienced arm pain during the previous 12 months; those who had had arm pain for longer than a month or not (a measure of duration); those with different levels of difficulty with undertaking activities (a measure of severity); those who had consulted a doctor and those who had not; and those who were in paid employment or not. For each group, informants were randomly selected from the survey sample. In all, 50 informants were contacted according to these criteria. It was only possible to interview 47 of the informants. Each had agreed to allow their medical records to be accessed and were invited for an examination by a nurse. In addition, participants were asked to nominate a health care worker they had seen for their upper-limb pain. This health worker was then approached for an interview. The interview focused initially on the participant's 'case' and then expanded to general policies and practices. This example illustrates how postal surveys can be used as precursors to qualitative methods by identifying groups for follow-up. Figure 13.4 and Figure 13.5 now follow.

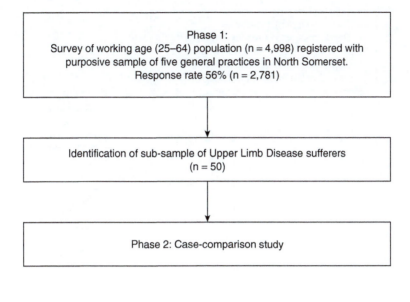

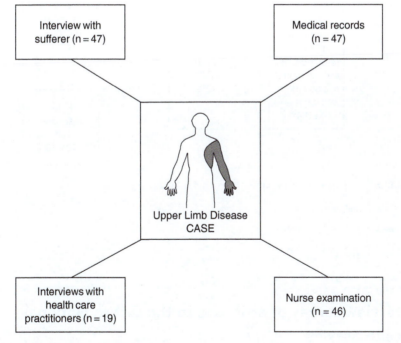

FIGURE 13.4 Study design for upper-limb pain sufferers

Source: Calnan et al. (2005)

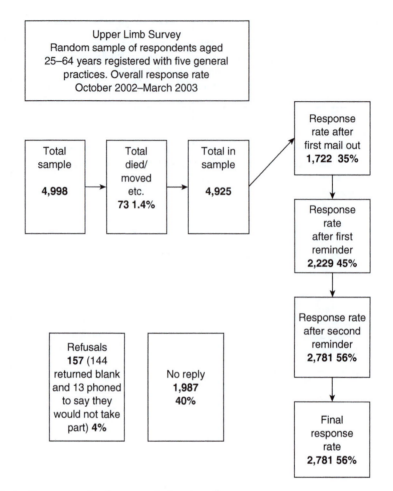

FIGURE 13.5   Response rates for upper-limb pain sufferers

Source: Calnan et al. (2005)

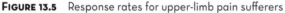

Interview survey of attitudes to the British National Health Service

Interview surveys take at least two forms, namely face-to-face interviews and telephone interviews. A typical example of an interview survey is the British Social Attitudes Survey, referred to earlier. This survey (Clery, Curtice and Harding 2016;

Park et al. 2003) began in 1983 and has been conducted annually to date except for 1988 and 1992. The survey is designed to produce annual measures of attitudinal shifts. One of its main objectives is to monitor patterns of continuity and change, and the relative rates at which attitudes, in respect of a range of social issues, change over time. It is a regular survey but samples from a new population each year. The interview questionnaire contains a number of core questions covering major topic areas, such as defence, the economy and the use of public services. The remainder of the questionnaire is devoted to a series of questions about social, economic, political and moral issues. The questions are predominantly structured and closed. Each year, the survey samples adults aged 18 and over, living in private households in Britain. It is based on a multi-stage stratified random sample. From 1993, the sample was drawn from the Postcode Address File, and for all years of the survey a weighting procedure is available to adjust for unequal selection probabilities. Sample sizes vary each year, and between 1983, 2002 and 2017 they ranged between 1,355, 3,469 and 3,998.

One strength of the British Social Attitudes Survey is that it can be used to monitor changes in attitude over time. This is clearly illustrated by respondents' attitudes to the National Health Service (NHS). A set of core questions have been included in the survey nearly every year since 1983. This is the general question: '*All in all, how satisfied or dissatisfied would you say you are with the way in which the NHS runs nowadays?*' It is followed by questions about specific services and more specific questions: '*From your own experience, or from what you have heard, please say how satisfied or dissatisfied you are with the way in which each of these parts of the National Health Service runs nowadays: local doctors or GPs, being in hospital as an inpatient, attending hospital as an outpatient, and NHS dentists*'.

Therefore, it is possible from the survey to monitor changes in attitude to the NHS as well as specific sectors of health care over time. For example, recent evidence shows that public satisfaction with the NHS overall was 57 per cent in 2017 – a 6 percentage point drop from the previous year. At the same time, dissatisfaction with the NHS overall increased by 7 percentage points to 29 per cent – its highest level since 2007. Older people were more satisfied than younger people: 64 per cent of those aged 65 and over were satisfied with the NHS in 2017 compared to 55 per cent of those aged 18 to 64. Between 2016 and 2017 satisfaction fell among all age groups (Robertson, Appleby and Evans 2018).

The British Social Attitudes Survey data have been shown to report higher levels of dissatisfaction than other surveys, which in general record a high degree of satisfaction with health care (see Judge and Solomon 1993). This is believed to be due to the context in which the questions are asked. In the interview, the questions on satisfaction were next to questions about government priorities and public expenditure. The British Social Attitudes Survey questions may elicit a more political response, whereas other satisfaction surveys may be more firmly grounded in local knowledge. It has been suggested that general attitudes to the NHS tell us as much about government popularity as they do about the NHS *per se* (Appleby and Rossete 2003).

An increasingly popular method of collecting interview data is via the telephone. The high level of access to a telephone, particularly a mobile phone, in the

(Continued)

(Continued)

United Kingdom coupled with concerns about security make the telephone an increasingly acceptable medium for interview. Baeza and Calnan (1998) used telephone interviews in a national study to evaluate the new health promotion arrangements introduced into general practice in England and Wales in 1996. Once again, a mixed-method design was employed, beginning with a national survey followed by a series of in-depth case studies using qualitative methods. The objective of the survey was to explore the extent and nature of health promotion activity being undertaken through a survey of all health authorities in England. A postal survey was not appropriate because many of the questions were semi-structured and the interviewee was the person responsible for the health promotion scheme in the health authority and could vary depending on the health authority. In the event, the response rate to the telephone interview was high with 89 per cent (n = 85) of the 96 health authorities in England taking part.

Reading health research based on quantitative survey methods

In the appraisal of published survey research, particularly if a hypothesis is being tested, the research questions should be both specific and precise and assessed in these terms. Other key issues are:

- What types of research questions are being addressed? Are they descriptive questions: what, who, when? Or are they explanatory questions: why?
- Is the survey structured in a way that is suitable for addressing these types of research question?
- Are there causal influences imputed in the question? If so, is there a temporal aspect to the survey?
- How are concepts operationalized and how are measures or indicators selected and why?
- How reliable and valid are the indicators used in the study?
- Is there any bias in the selection of respondents?
- Are details of the response rate described and the characteristics of the non-respondents presented?
- Is there any bias perceivable in the selection of questions?
- How are the methods for data collection specified and are they appropriate?
- How are the data analysed and was the statistical analysis appropriate and sufficient?
- Are the conclusions derived from the evidence?
- Are the limitations in the survey methodology taken into account in the interpretation of the findings?

Conclusion

The survey is probably the most widely used and well-tested method for obtaining data from a selected population. If correct sampling techniques are used, then findings can be generalized to very large populations. As has been argued, the survey can be particularly effective when used to compare changes over time. However, surveys can also be carried out on a modest scale and telephone surveys, in particular, can be a useful technique for students and other researchers. Questionnaire design with critical reflection on what a question is aiming to find out and pilot testing of questions are crucial aspects of conducting a survey. All surveys require careful planning and management and need to be underpinned by good administrative systems. If interviewers are being used, they should be properly trained and briefed prior to, and during, the course of a project. The unexpected often occurs during the course of the fieldwork or data collection phase and interviewers may require access to ongoing support and discussion with researcher leaders. The examples set out in this chapter highlight how different survey methods have been used in practice in health research. The reader also has the opportunity to complete an exercise on translating concepts into indicators in the health field.

Exercise 13.1   Translating concepts of health into indicators

The final section of this chapter provides a problem-solving exercise that readers are invited to complete. It follows the discussion presented in an earlier section about how concepts can be operationalized into indicators by using a descending ladder of abstraction. The focus of the exercise is on translating concepts of health into indicators or questions for a survey that aims to assess the health status of the adult population. Figure 13.6 provides a schema to encourage readers to break down the general abstract concept of health into various component parts. Reference back to Figure 13.1 may be helpful as a guide.

Fill in the empty boxes in Figure 13.6 which provide a ladder of abstraction by:

- Providing a number of different definitions of health
- Choosing one definition on which to focus
- Identifying the dimensions and sub-dimensions which emerge from the chosen definition
- Developing questions that would act as indicators of these dimensions and sub-dimensions in the sample survey of the adult population.

Once the exercise is completed, readers might like to evaluate their indicators against a standardized instrument for measuring physical and mental health status – such as the SF-36 or the Nottingham Health Profile (Jenkinson 1994).

(Continued)

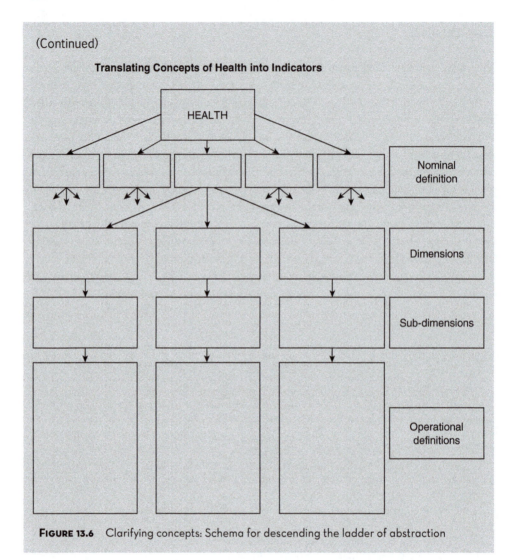

(Continued)

Translating Concepts of Health into Indicators

FIGURE 13.6   Clarifying concepts: Schema for descending the ladder of abstraction

Recommended further reading

This is a very accessible introductory textbook, setting survey methods within a general context of other research methods:

Babbie, E. (2016) *The Basics of Social Research*, International edition. London: Thomson/Wadsworth.

This book provides useful complementary reading to this chapter and is strongly recommended:
Bryman, A. (2016) *Social Research Methods*, 5th edition.Oxford: Oxford University Press.

This is a detailed guide specific to designing surveys:
Czaja, R. and Blair, J. (2005) *Designing Surveys: A Guide to Decisions and Procedures*. Thousand Oaks, CA: Pine Forge Press.

This text covers all the main issues discussed in this chapter in more detail and is strongly recommended:
De Vaus, D. (2014) *Surveys in Social Research*, 6th edition. London: Routledge.

References

Appleby, J. and Rosete, A. (2003) 'The NHS: Keeping up with public expectations', in A. Park, J. Curtice, K. Thomson, L. Jarvis and C. Bromley (eds), *British Social Attitudes: The 20th Report. Continuity and Change over Two Decades*. London: Sage.

Babbie, E. (2008) *The Basics of Social Research*, International edition. London: Thomson/Wadsworth.

Baeza, J. and Calnan, M. (1998) 'Beating the bands?', *Health Services Journal*, *108*(5623): 26–7.

Bourque, L. and Fielder, E. (2003) *How to Conduct Telephone Surveys*. London: Sage.

Bryman, A. (2016) *Social Research Methods*, 5th edition. Oxford: Oxford University Press.

Calnan, M., Cant, S. and Gabe, J. (1993) *Going Private*. Buckingham: Open University Press.

Calnan, M. and Rowe, R. (2008) *Trust Matters in Health Care*. Buckingham: Open University Press.

Calnan, M. and Sanford, E. (2004) 'Public trust in health care: The system or the doctor?', *Quality and Safety in Health Care*, *13*: 92–7.

Calnan, M., Wainwright, D., O'Neill, C., Winterbottom, A. and Watkins, A. (2005) 'Lay evaluation of health care: The case of upper limb pain', *Health Expectations*, *8*(2): 149–60.

Clery, E., Curtice, J. and Harding, R. (2016) *British Social Attitudes: The 34th Report*. London: NatCen Social Research. Available at: www.bsa.natcen.ac.u

Couper, M. P. (2008) *Designing Effective Web Surveys*. Cambridge: Cambridge University Press.

Czaja, R. and Blair, J. (2005) *Designing Surveys: A Guide to Decisions and Procedures*. Thousand Oaks, CA: Pine Forge Press.

De Vaus, D. (2014) *Surveys in Social Research*, 6th edition. London: Routledge.

Dragano, N., Siegrist, J. and Wahrendorf, M. (2011) 'Welfare regimes, labour policies and unhealthy psychosocial working conditions: A comparative study with 9917 older employees from 12 European countries', *Journal of Epidemiology and Community Health*, *65*(9): 793–9.

Edwards, P. J., Roberts, I., Clarke, M. J., DiGuiseppi, C., Wentz, R., Kwan, I., Cooper, R., Felix, L. M. and Pratap, S. (2009) 'Methods to increase response to postal and electronic questionnaires', *Cochrane Database of Systematic Reviews*, Issue 3: Art. No. MR000008.

Fink, A. (2003) *The Survey Handbook*, 2nd edition. London: Sage.

Jenkinson, C. (ed.) (1994) *Measuring Health and Medical Outcomes*. London: UCL Press.

Judge, K. and Solomon, M. (1993) 'Public opinion and the National Health Service: Patterns and perspectives in consumer satisfaction', *Journal of Social and Political Studies*, *22*(3): 299–322.

Litwin, M. S. (1995) *How to Measure Survey Reliability and Validity*. London: Sage.

Lozar Manfreda, K., Bosnjak, M., Berzelak, J., Haas, I., Vehovar, V. and Berzelak, N. (2007) 'Web surveys versus other survey modes: A meta-analysis comparing response rates', *International Journal of Market Research*, *50*: 79–104.

Mindell, J., Biddulph, J. P., Hirani, V., Stamatakis, E., Craig, R., Ninn, S. and Shelton, N. (2012) 'Cohort profile: The Health Survey for England', *International Journal of Epidemiology*, *41*(6): 1585–93.

Murnane, R. and Willett, J. (2010) *Methods Matter: Improving Causal Inference in Educational and Social Research*. Oxford: Oxford University Press.

Park, A., Curtice, J., Thomson, K., Jarvis, L. and Bromley, C. (eds) (2003) *British Social Attitudes: The 20th Report. Continuity and Change over Two Decades*. London: Sage.

Robertson, R., Appleby, J. and Evans, H. (2018) *Public Satisfaction with the NHS and Social Care in 2017: Results and Trends from the British Social Attitudes Survey*. London: King's Fund.

Shih, T. H. and Fan, X. (2008) 'Comparing response rates from web and mail surveys: A meta-analysis', *Field Methods*, *20*: 249–71.

Stait, E. and Calnan, M. (2016) 'Are differential consumption patterns in health-related behaviours an explanation for persistent and widening social inequalities in health in England?', *International Journal for Equity in Health*, *15*: 171. Available at: doi: 10.1186/s12939-016-0461-2

van der Schee, E., Braun, B., Calnan, M., Schnee, M. and Groenewegen, D. (2007) 'Public trust in health care: A comparison of Germany, The Netherlands, and England and Wales', *Health Policy*, *81*: 56–67.

Wilson, P., Petticrew, M., Calnan, M. and Nazareth, I. (2010) 'Effects of a financial incentive on health. Researchers' response to an online survey: A randomized controlled trial', *Medical Internet Research*, *12*(2): e13.

14

Randomized Controlled Trials

GEORGE LEWITH AND PAUL LITTLE

Chapter objectives

- To discuss the underlying principles and concepts governing randomized controlled trials (RCTs) and their place in clinical research
- To outline the different types of RCT
- To explore the process of protocol development
- To examine the practical problems of setting up a trial in a clinical setting
- To give a critical evaluation of the RCT.

Introduction

This chapter will focus on the underlying principles of randomized controlled trials (RCTs), some different types of RCT and the practical issues that arise in a clinical setting. In the main, examples will be drawn from complementary and alternative medicine (CAM), not only because this is the first author's area of expertise, but also because some philosophical and ethical issues occur in this setting in particularly stark form.

RCTs can be used in a number of different contexts, although they are used mostly in laboratory or clinical settings. For instance, the performance of two pieces of machinery or two devices that claim to perform the same function can be compared in a highly controlled environment to assess energy consumption and cost-effectiveness. Although it is more difficult to control the experimental environment, trials can be effective in health, social care or educational settings. For example, the impact of regular 'good-neighbour visits' to elderly people in improving their wellbeing could be assessed or the outcome of a new reading scheme could be compared with an existing scheme among 6-year-olds. The fundamental principles of the RCT remain the same in whichever context they are applied. This chapter aims to outline the steps that are fundamental to setting up an RCT.

How to approach setting up a randomized controlled trial

The historical and philosophical origin of the RCT centres on the desire to find an answer to a very specific question. It sets out to evaluate the effects of a particular treatment or management strategy in a population where an intervention is introduced, by comparing the outcome with a control group where no intervention has been made. The population must be clearly defined and the sample selection justified. A number of implicit assumptions underpin the RCT, as set out in Box 14.1.

Box 14.1   Assumptions underpinning randomized controlled trials

- We have an incomplete understanding of the world and knowledge evolves and develops. It is contingent and never definitive.
- Logically, cause precedes effect, or, put another way, A leads to B.
- Beliefs cannot influence random events, and in a well-designed study, the researcher's beliefs must not influence the outcome.
- A randomized trial aims to minimize the effects of confounding, particularly so-called 'confounding by indication' (confounding due to the fact that clinicians choose to give – or not give – treatments based on the particular characteristics of patients).
- Understanding treatment and developing model validity around its delivery is important so that the best intervention available can be evaluated.

Source: Adapted from Vickers et al. (1997)

These tenets lead to the claim that the RCT provides the 'gold standard' for research – and that it is the best means of attributing real clinical cause and effect, although not all researchers necessarily agree with all these assumptions (see, for example, Frank and Frank 1991; Ronsenzweig 1936).

Refining the research question

Setting up an RCT is a challenging task and researchers contemplating a trial must ask themselves:

- What is a good question?
- How can questions be matched to the research design?
- How can an appropriate interpretation of the results be made and an inappropriate interpretation avoided?

The first prerequisite for refining a research question is a thorough literature search (see Chapter 4). It will help to identify whether the question one wants to ask has already been answered, and also point out the strengths and weakness of previous research in addressing and answering the question. Regular attendance at academic meetings, reading journals and reviewing internet sources regularly will help to keep the researcher abreast of developments in the field too.

A question is likely to be answerable if it is explicit, focused and feasible, and where it is possible to link the effect of an intervention explicitly to a specific outcome. There should be a very clear, simple primary question and a research method that will provide an answer. If there are multiple questions, then the primary research question must be given priority. The primary research question must be framed so that it is both possible and practical to answer the question – as the examples given in Table 14.1 highlight – and is achievable within a reasonable period of time and within the bounds of the resources available.

TABLE 14.1 Different types of research question and their suitability for a randomized controlled trial

Category of question	Examples	Suitable for RCT
Attributing cause and clinical effect	Does homeopathically prepared grass pollen reduce symptoms of hay fever more than a non-active (placebo) treatment?	Y
What happens in clinical practice?	What is the cost-effectiveness of adding homoeopathic treatment to a standard care package in hay fever?	Y
	How common are serious neurological complications following chiropractic cervical manipulation?	N

(Continued)

TABLE 14.1   (Continued)

Category of question	Examples	Suitable for RCT
What do people do?	How many people visit practitioners of CAM each year?	N
	What do patients tell their primary care physician about usage of CAM?	N
What do people believe and how do they explain it?	What do nurses believe about therapeutic touch? What is the patient's experience of the acupuncture consultation?	N
By what mechanisms does a therapy work?	What are the effects of needling the Hoku point on the production of endogenous opiates?	Y
Does something proposed in a therapy actually exist?	Does peppermint oil reduce histamine-induced contractions of tracheal smooth muscle?	Y
	Can an acupuncture point be distinguished from non-acupuncture points by measuring the electrical resistance of the skin?	N
Is a diagnostic or prognostic test accurate?	How sensitive and specific is detection of gall bladder disease by examining photos of the iris?	N

Source: Adapted from Brien, Lewith and Bryant (2003) and Vickers et al. (1997)

Ways to develop a viable randomized controlled trial

The planning stages of any clinical trial are vital – not least in terms of establishing the suitability of the research question for an RCT. Some tips for a successful project are discussed here.

First, for all but the most simple, small and straightforward study, clinical research is usually best conducted in teams. This is not just because the best science is facilitated when several people contribute, but because the complexity of clinical governance, ethics, trial protocols, trial management, data handling and statistical analysis make it too much for a lone researcher (Mathews 2011). Even for well-established teams, advice may be needed from collaborators who are experts in particular areas. Working in a group with colleagues who meet on a regular basis provides an opportunity for supportive yet critical, ongoing review of projects, and helps to avoid making definitive decisions and mistakes too rapidly!

Second, unless the intervention is very straightforward and logistic issues well understood, carrying out an initial pilot, or feasibility trial, is often useful, and well within the remit of undergraduate and postgraduate students. This can help to refine the research question; develop hypotheses to be tested (for instance, including proposed mediators of effect); check whether an intervention is likely to be implemented with fidelity; check whether the intervention is acceptable to participants; and provide estimates of recruitment rates, follow-up rates, and the variance of the key outcome (this is used to inform the sample size calculation). Where the outcomes or intervention are likely to change, the pilot will be an 'external' pilot (and the results are not included in the analysis of the main trial). However, if the outcomes and intervention do not change, the pilot results can be used in the analysis of the main trial (termed an 'internal' pilot). Small-scale pilots or feasibility studies are unlikely to be generalizable as they are likely to be underpowered and should not be used to estimate effect sizes (see Chapter 12).

Third, it is essential to make sure that outcome measures can be completed by participants (termed the response burden): that the information sheet given to them to consent is written in clear and non-technical language and makes them fully aware of any risks and costs and state the time involved to complete the trial. Participants will need to sign a consent form and keep a copy of the information sheet, both of which will need to be approved by the appropriate ethics committee.

Fourth, researchers should make sure that the process of randomization, blinding and follow-up is feasible. It is particularly important to ensure that if a placebo – as a non-active treatment – is being used, it is appropriate for the control group concerned (Vincent and Lewith 1995; White et al. 2003). A feasibility study may be an RCT, but it can be uncontrolled. The advantage of randomizing at the feasibility stage is to determine the likely acceptability of randomization, and the likely impact of randomization on recruitment.

Common methodological issues

Key issues in starting to plan the trial need to be considered early in the process: a trial may not be ethical (for instance, an RCT of the benefit or not of using antibiotics to treat meningitis); or may not be practical (for example, the sample size may be unfeasible, or there is insufficient equipoise among clinicians); or is unlikely to provide clear answers (such as insufficient power to document key outcomes). Bias can occur in many stages of a trial and, unless anticipated and countered at the planning stage, will lead to false estimates of the effect of an intervention. There may be, as set out in Box 14.2, some forms of bias.

Box 14.2 Forms of bias in randomized controlled trials

- *Recruitment bias*: A population may be selected for recruitment that does not represent the key population of interest – in consequence, the results of the

(Continued)

(Continued)

study will only apply to the specific population recruited. The variable performance of individuals who put the inclusion criteria into operation (for example, an experienced highly trained researcher versus an untrained health worker) may also result in recruitment bias.

- *Selection bias*: This occurs where the intervention and control patient groups are not comparable.
- *Performance bias*: This occurs when groups within the intervention arm, for example in a multi-centre study, may receive a different quality or intensity of intervention – perhaps due to the expertise of the clinician or the time they allocate to providing the intervention.
- *Detection bias*: This refers to systematic differences in the outcome assessment between groups.
- *Attrition bias*: This occurs when withdrawals from a study distort the symmetry of the initial selection process and therefore the results. There must be proper reporting of those who withdraw from a trial in order to document possible bias (Feinstein 1985).
- *Researcher/participant bias*: This occurs when the behaviour or response of those involved in a trial is affected positively or negatively by the knowledge that they are in the intervention or control group. This is sometimes referred to as the Hawthorne effect. In order to offset this, a trial may be 'blinded'. Here, the researcher and/or the participant do not know which group the research participant is in, and in the case of medicinal products, whether they have been given the trial treatment or a placebo. However, for many non-medicinal trials, especially with complex health interventions, blinding of participants is not possible, so the trial is in effect 'open' – that is, not blinded (see below).

Assessing confounding factors

Confounding occurs when there is an association between an exposure to an intervention and the outcome as a consequence of an intervening variable, or third factor. An example is that more males over 60 years of age die of lung cancer than males under 40 years, but unless the important intervening variable of smoking is controlled for, the impact of age cannot be assessed. The control of confounding is why the RCT is advocated as the best evidence for therapeutic benefit, and potential confounders should be equally distributed between groups. By definition, unknown confounders cannot be measured. An RCT is a good way to attribute cause because it can allow for both known and unknown confounding variables. Randomization is discussed further below.

Phases within a classic randomized controlled trial

In the past, the classic clinical trial process was designed to test the efficacy of drugs, rather than surgical or manual interventions such as physiotherapy or osteopathy. It is essentially a prospective study. It looks forward in time. More recently, clinical trials have been divided into four main phases which represent vital progressive steps in testing the efficacy of modern pharmaceutical agents. These are pre-clinical trials and Phase I, II and III trials.

In pharmaceutical development, before a pre-clinical trial is launched, there will have been many years of very careful testing carried out both in vivo and in vitro to minimize the risk to humans of taking a particular drug and to maximize the potential therapeutic benefit. The primary aim of these studies is to assess the absorption (A) of a drug; its distribution (D) through the body; the effect on metabolism (M); and the extent of excretion (E) – collectively known as the ADME of a drug.

In *Phase I* clinical trials, the population is not randomized into two groups and the trials are usually carried out in individuals who have a pre-existing pathology. The aim of these studies is two-fold:

- First, to establish the maximum tolerated dose by very cautiously increasing the dose of the medication for patients with real pathology and to look for side-effects.
- Second, to assess whether the medication is effective.

The criteria used to define the 'maximum tolerated dose' and 'treatment efficacy' vary significantly depending on the illness. For instance, patients with terminal cancer may give consent to a trial even if there are uncomfortable side-effects because they wish to help future patients or because they believe the drug will be effective. This is less likely in the case of patients with an intermittent benign illness such as migraine.

Phase II studies are carried out with patients with a known illness and commonly involve four treatment groups recruited to a prospective RCT. While a Phase I study may estimate the likely doses of a potential therapeutic agent, a Phase II study carries this work further, usually looking at three different therapeutic doses in three different arms of the trial with a placebo in the fourth arm. With most conventional pharmaceutical agents, therapeutic benefit increases with the size of the dose, but so does the potential risk of adverse reactions. The aim is to find a dose that provides the best clinical effect with the lowest level of any common adverse reaction. Typically, in one arm of the trial patients will receive what is thought to be the therapeutic dose, a second arm will be given half that dose and a third arm double the optimal dose, while the fourth arm receives a placebo. The specific treatment efficacy will be evaluated by comparing the balance of therapeutic benefit and adverse reaction with the active agent versus a placebo.

A *Phase III* clinical trial mirrors most closely the classic RCT. It is commonly a study that involves two groups (arms) and compares the optimal dose of active treatment with a placebo (in the case of medicinal products) over a period of time. It uses outcome measures that will allow researchers to conclude that any effects observed will be the specific effects of the drug or intervention being evaluated.

The most common trial designs used within a Phase III RCT are two-armed comparative trials designed to evaluate the difference between a specific intervention and a comparative placebo or control intervention, with clearly defined primary and secondary outcomes. In some instances, particularly for chronic conditions, various adaptations on this central scheme may be applied. For instance, a run-in period may be used to establish baseline symptoms prior to trial entry. This allows for the general improvement that may occur as a 'trial effect' and will become apparent as patients record their symptoms over a period of a week or month (Lewith et al. 2002; White et al. 2004). It may also protect against a ceiling or floor effect as some level of symptoms is necessary to demonstrate that a clinical improvement has occurred as a consequence of the intervention.

The process of protocol development

The process of protocol development forms the foundation of any RCT. It provides a road map or process for a trial setting. It sets out the aims and rationale and includes: a detailed methods section covering recruitment; the process of the research over time; the end points for measurement, such as any risks to patients; and incorporates statistical advice. As suggested above, protocol development is generally a group activity with input required from clinicians, research methodologists, statisticians, Patient and Public Involvement (PPI) collaborators and commonly health economists and social scientists. PPI collaborators provide a crucial and different perspective from professional researchers and not only provide invaluable input into the framing of the problem, but also enhance the likely acceptability of the intervention and outcome measures. PPI collaborators are also invaluable in drafting the patient consent form to explain the research project in lay language. This must be signed by the patient and retained by them.

Protocols are designed to clarify the researcher's thoughts but also, more importantly, to convey the scientific essence of the research proposal to others as part of a peer-review process. A protocol must have clarity and focus with a logical flow that justifies the researcher's plan of investigation. It will form the basis for all relevant research applications going to ethics and governance committees, and is used to seek external or internal funding. The protocol will also be the basis for subsequent publications. Research protocol forms are usually obtained from the institution sponsoring the research. Forms may differ in detail, but generally cover broadly similar areas, as described below.

The background section

The aim of the background section is to show that the researcher has a complete understanding of the problem they wish to investigate. It provides the argument for why a particular research question is both important and relevant within the specific field. It should be clearly and concisely written, concluding with a focused research question in the context of existing knowledge. The researcher should demonstrate an understanding of the disease process in question, its natural history, its impact on both the patient and society, and give a clear description of issues that might impact on the disease outcome. For example, a study of one of the authors on stroke and the use of acupuncture required an understanding of stroke and its physiological and emotional impact on functioning, which might affect the outcome of the evaluation of acupuncture (Hopwood et al. 2008). A thorough review of the research literature is required so that the research question is appropriate and logical and fills a gap in knowledge. The quantity of previous studies does not rule out the need for another study. For example, many studies have evaluated the use of acupuncture for back pain (Manheimer et al. 2005; White et al. 2002; White et al. 2004). However, in some of these studies, the methodology was flawed and, arguably, there is still a need for a large, rigorous trial.

Developing a hypothesis

The design of a research project will be influenced by the primary hypothesis, or the proposition to be tested. This can be briefly stated but must be firmly based on the research question. Commonly, investigators wish to know if an intervention works or is 'superior' (a 'superiority' trial) to the control and formulate a 'null hypothesis' which assumes that unless it can be shown statistically that an intervention works (the 'alternative hypothesis'), the null hypotheses (that there is no effect) should be accepted. A Phase III 'superiority' clinical trial will inevitably have one main hypothesis, although there will almost certainly be a number of secondary research questions. However, sometimes, instead of wanting to show whether an intervention is superior to the control group, investigators wish to know that a new intervention is for all intents and purposes clinically equivalent to the normal or control condition (a so-called 'equivalence' trial). In this case, the margins below which clinical equivalence can be agreed are determined in advance. If the analysis shows that both the estimate of effectiveness and its 95 per cent confidence interval do not reach those margins, then the intervention is determined to be clinically equivalent to the control.

Outcomes expected and their measurement:
Validity and reliability

The research protocol will require a statement of how the effect of an intervention will be measured. This may be done by stating clinical measures of the results, such as blood pressure levels, air flow or exercise tests, or by using quality of life measures or patient questionnaires. You would not dream of measuring a patient's blood pressure with an uncalibrated sphygmomanometer; similarly, all health outcomes following a trial must measure what they are intending to measure (they must be valid) to be able to say anything meaningful for patients. There are major advantages in using existing well-validated and reliable primary outcome measures. The concept of validity has a number of dimensions, as outlined in Box 14.3.

Box 14.3 Dimensions of the concept of validity

- *Face validity*: On the 'face' of it, the outcome measure is relevant to the study questions.
- *Content validity*: The outcome measure includes the range of issues considered important by patients and experts in the field.
- *Construct validity*: The outcome measure used in previous studies behaves in an appropriate manner which is relevant to the factors that it is measuring based on previous literature or theories – for example, a knowledge outcome should relate to training.
- *Criterion validity*: The outcome measure is congruent with an acknowledged 'gold standard' measure.

It is also important that the outcome being measured gives reliable results. The means of showing this are set out in Box 14.4.

Box 14.4 Demonstrations of reliability

- *Test–retest reliability*: Measures show the same result when repeated after a short interval, such as two weeks after in a stable condition.
- *Internal reliability*: This refers to the degree of rigour or consistency in a measure. For example, where questionnaire items are combined in a scale or sub-scale, individual questionnaire items should relate well to each other and to the scale total (Streiner and Norman 2014).
- *Outcome sensitivity*: An outcome should be sensitive to changes.

New outcome measures may be developed in the context of a clinical trial, providing they are, or can be, compared and validated with a standard measure in the same group of patients. For example, in a study where acupuncture was used to treat neck pain, the primary outcomes used were well-validated scales measuring the quality of life perceptions of pain in a group of patients suffering from chronic, mechanical neck pain (White et al. 2004). A further process of 'scale validation' was developed. Therefore, this was a secondary outcome of the study. It is usual, particularly in large clinical trials, to have both primary and secondary outcomes. For instance, a study on acupuncture and pain may have a visual analogue of pain as its primary outcome, with secondary outcomes relating to quality of life and range of measures to assess the extent of movement.

It is important to specify a primary outcome in a research study so that so-called Type I 'errors' can be limited – that is a statistically significant outcome that has arisen due to chance alone. For example, if 20 outcome measures were used in one clinical trial, it is likely that one of these would show a significant difference between an active and a placebo treatment at the 5 per cent level (that is, 1:20 times). Consequently, this might be considered a significant outcome. It is, in fact, likely to be simply a random event if all the other 19 outcomes show no difference between the active and the placebo treatment. Similarly, if 20 clinical subgroups within the trial population are investigated a Type I error is also likely: that is, one out of 20 subgroups is likely to be statistically significant by chance alone (known as 'torturing the data until it confesses'), hence the importance of specifying key subgroups in advance.

The choice of primary outcome will be determined by the type of trial: thus, in a pragmatic trial where the beliefs and behaviour of the participants are as natural as possible, with minimal interference, then patient-based outcomes may be developed for use rather than through the objective measurement of outcomes by independent observers. It is also important to consider, measure and control if necessary by stratification (see below) what may predict or confound an outcome, particularly in small-scale trials. For example, if patients are receiving either acupuncture or physiotherapy for their neck pain, then outcomes may be predicted by the attitudes and beliefs that trial participants hold prior to a particular intervention. If possible, these attitudes should be established in the initial part of the study (White 2003).

Ideally, outcomes should be measured independently of the investigator and, if possible, blind to the group to minimize outcome assessment bias (see 'blinding' above). Outcomes should also be measured in the same way in each group to avoid bias, as the manner and timing of a measurement may affect that measurement. For example, in the British Family Heart Study, blood pressure was measured in the intervention group at the beginning and at the end, but only at the end in the control group. One finding was that a fall in blood pressure was observed in the intervention group. However, it was not possible to say whether this was due to the intervention alone, or also due to the effect of a measurement that had been repeated (Family Heart Study Group 1994). The design had been sub-optimal and led to measurement bias. In sum, both the measurement and placebo/control arms of a trial should be subject to the same set of measures.

The selection of research participants: Inclusion and exclusion criteria

The decision about who to include in and who to exclude from a trial is of key importance. An effect of an intervention is most likely to be found with a homogeneous group of patients and should include those who are most likely to benefit, if this can be predicted from previous research. If too varied a group is included, then the higher variance in the primary outcome measure will limit the ability of the treatment to show an effect, and may obscure real and important benefit. The disadvantage of using a highly selected group is that treatment effects observed in such groups may not apply to a broader group, as seen in the community. The results may be less generalizable. If, for instance, a study is conducted involving a new intervention for chronic obstructive pulmonary disease (COPD), but excludes all patients taking oral steroids, then how relevant is such a conclusion to general practice where many patients with COPD are likely to be using oral steroids? Thus, there is a continuing tension within any clinical trial between reducing variability by selecting patients with clearly defined clinical and social characteristics and providing evidence that is generalizable to the population managed in everyday practice. Inclusion and exclusion criteria require careful thought with respect to this balance.

The recruitment process

The recruitment process used in a clinical trial will affect the generalizability of findings. For instance, a group of volunteers selected via the web may be an entirely different population from those invited to participate in a clinical trial via a general practice. As a consequence, it is vital to keep a check on the information on patients during on the flow of recruitment (Brien, Lewith and Bryant 2003; Moher et al. 2012). A good clinical trial will have a pre-specified mechanism for recording and handling the data, and it is important to track missing data on the patients who drop out. The most important guiding principle is that once a patient has been entered into a clinical trial and randomized, then they must be followed up throughout the study. It is crucial to try very hard to achieve a follow-up of at least 80 per cent, otherwise attrition bias may seriously compromise the validity of the results. If patients are rejected during a baseline recording period, either because they do not ultimately fulfil the entry criteria for a study (Lewith et al. 2002), or have not otherwise entered the trial process, they do not need to be followed up throughout the study. Those who are eligible but decline to take part should be documented and reported as part of a CONSORT trial flow diagram, which is the standard mechanism for reporting the flow of patient recruitment for clinical trials.

During the development of a protocol, the calculation of sample size forms the basis of the numbers that will need to be recruited to a trial in order to answer the trial's primary and secondary hypotheses. This will provide the foundation for costing and development within the context of a clinical trial. The effect that the trial is powered to detect will need to be carefully justified (preferably the minimum clinically important difference (MCID) in the primary outcome will be known).

Figure 14.1 overleaf illustrates patient recruitment in a study involving homeopathic proving, the method used for determining which remedies are suitable for particular conditions. It records the number of people who were contacted about the study, those included in the initial baseline screening and those subsequently randomized within the study, and those who dropped out. This helps to highlight the generalizability of findings and sources of bias.

Randomization and related issues

Randomization is the key method to minimize confounding within an RCT. The initial aim is to select a homogeneous group of patients, while identifying within the introductory or background section to a protocol the important factors (potential confounders) that may independently predict outcome. The method of randomization, if at all possible, should separate whoever generates the randomization codes from the person carrying out the randomization to minimize any possibility that the clinician managing the patient could have any influence on the choice of group. In a placebo-controlled trial, this is accomplished by an independent pharmacy making-up randomization packs containing an active drug or placebo. In an open trial, this is best accomplished using an external telephone randomization line.

Stratification and minimization

For very large trials, such confounders will be equally distributed between groups. In small single-centre clinical trials, great attention must be paid to understanding both the illness and the effect of interventions, along with potential predictive factors that may independently influence treatment outcome. For these smaller trials, particularly where some variables strongly predict outcome, it is important to make sure that such variables are balanced between groups, either by 'stratification' or 'minimization'. Stratification in effect creates separate randomization strata for key subgroups, whereas minimization controls the allocation to each group as randomization proceeds. For instance, in our asthma study, we were aware that initial asthma severity and the presence of smokers would need to be balanced between the two treatment groups, as both these factors might significantly influence outcome. As a consequence, we randomized the first ten patients using sealed opaque envelopes to receive either real homeopathy or a placebo and then subsequently used a minimization programme. This allocated patients so that with each participant randomized, any difference between groups for the potential confounding variables was minimized. The two treatment groups were therefore balanced for all major known potential predictors of outcome (Lewith et al. 2002).

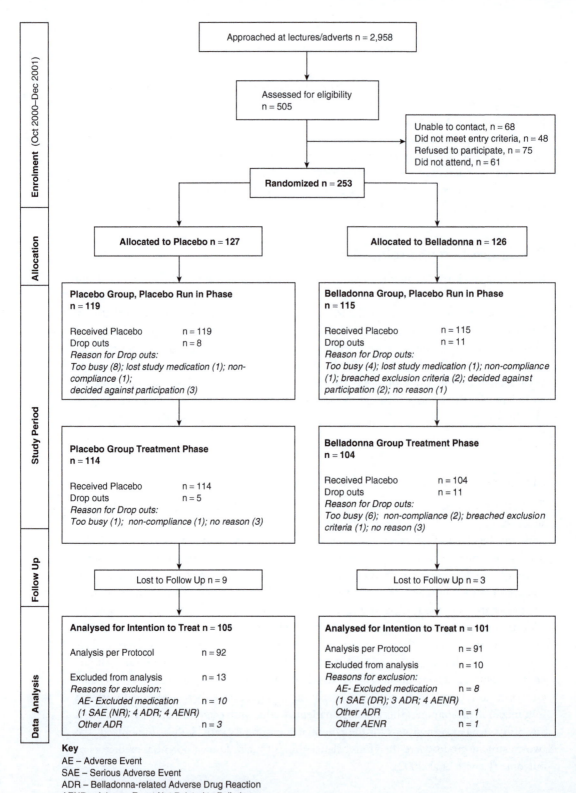

Enrolment (Oct 2000–Dec 2001)

Approached at lectures/adverts n = 2,958

Assessed for eligibility
n = 505

Unable to contact, n = 68
Did not meet entry criteria, n = 48
Refused to participate, n = 75
Did not attend, n = 61

Randomized n = 253

Allocation

Allocated to Placebo n = 127

Allocated to Belladonna n = 126

Study Period

Placebo Group, Placebo Run in Phase
n = 119

Received Placebo   n = 119
Drop outs   n = 8
Reason for Drop outs:
Too busy (8); lost study medication (1); non-compliance (1);
decided against participation (3)

Belladonna Group, Placebo Run in Phase
n = 115

Received Placebo   n = 115
Drop outs   n = 11
Reason for Drop outs:
Too busy (4); lost study medication (1); non-compliance (1); breached exclusion criteria (2); decided against participation (2); no reason (1)

Placebo Group Treatment Phase
n = 114

Received Placebo   n = 114
Drop outs   n = 5
Reason for Drop outs:
Too busy (1); non-compliance (1); no reason (3)

Belladonna Group Treatment Phase
n = 104

Received Placebo   n = 104
Drop outs   n = 11
Reason for Drop outs:
Too busy (6); non-compliance (2); breached exclusion criteria (1); no reason (3)

Follow Up

Lost to Follow Up n = 9

Lost to Follow Up n = 3

Data Analysis

Analysed for Intention to Treat n = 105

Analysis per Protocol   n = 92

Excluded from analysis   n = 13
Reasons for exclusion:
  AE- Excluded medication   n = 10
  (1 SAE (NR); 4 ADR; 4 AENR)
  Other ADR   n = 3

Analysed for Intention to Treat n = 101

Analysis per Protocol   n = 91

Excluded from analysis   n = 10
Reasons for exclusion:
  AE- Excluded medication   n = 8
  (1 SAE (DR); 3 ADR; 4 AENR)
  Other ADR   n = 1
  Other AENR   n = 1

Key
AE – Adverse Event
SAE – Serious Adverse Event
ADR – Belladonna-related Adverse Drug Reaction
AENR – Adverse Event Not Related to Belladonna

FIGURE 14.1   Patient recruitment in a study of homeopathic proving

In other studies, for instance with stroke, it was known that stroke severity would predict outcome irrespective of treatment. We therefore stratified patients so that the treatment groups were clearly balanced with similar numbers of patients with relatively severe, and relatively mild, stroke (Hopwood et al. 2008).

Clustering

Randomization in multi-centre trials can present a variety of different problems. The same treatments may not be delivered in the same way at every centre, or treatments may be delivered at some centres and not others, so the outcomes found might be centre-dependent with treatment effects 'clustered' in consequence. Thus, even an individually randomized trial can benefit from analysis taking account of clustering. Sometimes the intervention needs to operate at the level of a cluster (for example, changing the behaviour of several members within a general practice to optimize cardiovascular prevention); in these cases, unless the cluster is randomized, contamination between groups is likely to occur.

The disadvantage of cluster trials is that differential selection bias between intervention and control groups may occur. For instance, in the above example, intervention practices may be more engaged with the research and recruit a different spectrum of patients, resulting in selection bias. Equally, patients in control practices may be less engaged and less likely to complete follow-up outcome measures. This would result in an attrition bias. If possible, it is best to randomize by individual rather than by cluster and even accept the possibility of some contamination bias (this can be measured). However, individual randomization may simply not be sensible: if a cluster trial is necessary, then measures must be put in place to minimize selection bias, for example, by identifying participants prior to randomizing the cluster, or by having automated/standardized invitation procedures. Attrition bias can be minimized by paying particular attention to engaging participants at the consent stage about their willingness to complete any follow-up measures. Every effort should be made to standardize recruitment and both the sample size and analysis should allow for clustering (cluster trials need larger numbers). Those interested in multi-centre trials should refer to Campbell and Machin (1999).

The statistical analysis plan

Whatever the protocol and however the study is designed, a clear plan for data analysis must be presented at the protocol stage and a fuller analysis plan constructed later prior to any analysis being performed (see Chapter 17 on the statistics involved). An important principle is that the primary analysis should generally be an 'intention to treat' (ITT) analysis – that is, where all patients, whether they complied with the intervention or not, are included in the analysis according to their original study group. This is important because, to estimate the average effect patients can expect to receive from a treatment, the results should include both patients where it has worked and those where it has not worked or who have had to stop the treatment for whatever reason. This mirrors what is likely to happen in the real world: that is, the analysis reflects the point at which clinicians and patients are deciding to agree or intend to agree, following a course of treatment. Most studies usually also perform a so-called 'per protocol' analysis, where only those patients who have complied with the intervention are assessed. This will give an estimate of the effect of the intervention in ideal circumstances, but it has the disadvantage that by selecting a subgroup who comply in the intervention group, there may be no equivalent subset in the control group. In effect, you may not be comparing like with like since randomization has been undermined. This can be the case, particularly if the trial is not of a drug but concerns a complex pragmatic intervention.

Ethics and governance

The process of ethics and governance has changed radically with the introduction of the European Union clinical trial directive in April 2004 (see Chapter 19). Ethical issues must be addressed in any research protocol, particularly with respect to data protection, obtaining fully informed consent and by following the principles of good clinical practice. Great care should be taken in drafting the patient consent form with PPI collaborators so that the research is comprehensible in lay terms. Research ethics committees are often most critical of this aspect of a research protocol.

Methodological issues

The replicability of research

The essence of any scientific experiment is to describe, within the methods section, an experimental procedure that can be completely replicated by any other interested and properly trained researcher so that any other researcher would be able to carry out the same study using the same interventions and, hopefully, come to the same conclusions. This requires that the intervention is described specifically and exactly. In the case of a drug trial, the exact medication used must be defined, along with its specific manufacture, dosage and delivery method. In studies involving surgical or manual intervention, such as physiotherapy, a methodological prerequisite is to describe all the interventions in all arms to a high level of specificity. Where a complex intervention is being developed, it is vital that care is taken in describing the development, content and evaluation of the intervention, including process evaluations (Craig et al. 2008; Moore et al. 2015), and that the intervention development employs relevant theoretical understanding, prior evidence and extensive iteration with users in robust co-production methods using a person-centred approach (Geraghty et al. 2016).

Blinding and its problems

The process of blinding is designed to remove bias and retain patient equipoise. It is used to detect the specific effects of an intervention by removing any prior 'expectation' that the researcher or participant may have of the trial results from the active or placebo treatment. It is usually possible to blind a medicinal intervention. A placebo can usually be made to look, taste, feel and present as indistinguishable from the active treatment, although for some medication it can be difficult to generate the same taste. However, blinding with respect to a surgical intervention or pragmatic intervention such as physiotherapy, exercise prescription or reflexology is much more difficult. While it may have been ethical to blind patients about whether they had or had not received a real surgical intervention in the mid-1950s (Beecher 1955), it is no longer thought reasonable or ethical to do so. Within the context of a clinical trial, patients must consent to receive, or not to receive, medication, surgery or spinal manipulation.

A very pragmatic definition of a double-blind trial is where neither the investigating researchers nor the trial participants (volunteers/patients) are aware of who is receiving the active or placebo treatment. Both parties are blind to the nature of the intervention, hence expectation is removed and an equivalence created in terms of expectations about the treatment outcome.

A single-blind trial is where the therapist delivering the intervention knows which is the placebo and which is the active treatment, but the patient or volunteer thinks that both interventions are equally likely to be therapeutically effective. This has been achieved with some acupuncture studies (Wood and Lewith 1998). It is also the case where the primary outcome measure is achieved through, for example, a patient self-assessment questionnaire, a visual analogue scale or Short Form 36 (SF-36), or a generic quality of life measure. In this case, a patient can remain in equipoise, with an equal belief in the active and placebo treatment, although the groups receive two distinctly different treatments. Outcomes can be assessed either by themselves, or by an entirely objective or independent source (such as a blood test or a blinded third party). This may mean that a study can be legitimately described as a single-blind trial. However, where the key outcomes rely on a report from a patient (such as symptom severity for back pain), blinding an independent observer does not make a meaningful difference to the documentation of outcomes.

It has been estimated that approximately 70 per cent of clinical trials fail to report the details of blinding. As Schulz and Grimes (2002) argue, the removal of bias is the foundation upon which causal associations can be derived within clinical research. They point out that many conventional clinical trials fail to report the blinding and randomization process adequately, and indeed a proportion of researchers may have deliberately subverted the process (Grimes and Schulz 2002). However, it is possible to minimize the effect of open (unblinded) interventions by generating a placebo effect in each group, using the therapist/physician as a placebo. For example, in an open pragmatic trial of prescribing strategies for a sore throat, the placebo effect of prescribing antibiotics was empirically abolished by using structured advice sheets to support management in each group (Little et al. 1997) with similar findings for chest infections (Little et al. 2005; Little et al. 2013).

When carrying out a trial, researchers should aim to be sufficiently detached from preconceptions about the efficacy of a therapy, which is particularly important during data interpretation, and can be facilitated by the analysts remaining blind to the group during the analysis. The Jadad score (Jadad et al. 1996) and other such scores are widely used among systematic reviewers as the basis for summarizing major sources of bias in relation to blinding, randomization and the reporting of results. However, such quality scores rarely assess generalizability to the community of individuals suffering from the illness. The CONSORT group have provided essential checklists for reporting the details of trials (Moher et al. 2012).

Common variations of the randomized controlled trial

It has been argued above that the classic RCT is demanding on staff and resources and is often beyond the scope of the lone researcher. There are some variations, including cluster and equivalence trials as discussed above, as well as cross-over and step-wedge designs.

Cross-over studies

A cross-over study involves one treatment in a first phase, a washout period with no treatment and then a second randomized treatment with a control group in a further phase. Every individual takes part in both phases, but the order of treatments is randomized. The advantage is that it minimizes variation since each individual becomes their own control, and smaller numbers are needed. Cross-over designs are only appropriate for a stable disease and a therapy that has short-term effects (as exemplified by H2 blockers for gastro-oesophageal reflux). They would not be suitable in the case of antidepressants for mild depression because antidepressants' effects take time to work and to wear off, and with no treatment patients may no longer be depressed anyway. Similarly, acupuncture may have unpredictable long-term effects so a cross-over study is not appropriate (Lewith et al. 2002).

Step-wedge cluster trials

Where the target users are unlikely to accept not getting the intervention or where it will be rolled out anyway, as is the case with the implementation of a policy, a step-wedge design may still be possible. This would be the case with a cluster trial where intervention clusters all get the intervention but the timing of starting the intervention is randomized. Where there is leeway to consider a more traditional parallel cluster trial, caution should be used in opting for a step-wedge design in the case of: small clusters (where a step-wedge is inefficient compared with a simple 'parallel' cluster design); where there is consent to individual-level data collection without blinding (which may result in selection bias); or where clusters are unlikely to follow the randomization schedule.

Variations in control mechanisms and pragmatic studies

Some studies may attempt to control for an intervention by having an 'attention' control. This is where some patients simply spend time with a therapist, without the therapist providing a specific therapy. The methods section of the protocol may give information about the intervention, as was the case in a trial to assess the effect of exercise classes on the relief of fibromyalgia. The disadvantage of such studies is that the total effects of an intervention may involve both specific and non-specific effects, and it is the combined effect of these that the patient will experience in real life. These are also the most useful for clinicians in their decision to treat a patient. Cost-effectiveness cannot be reliably estimated in studies that use an attention control as this would not occur in actual practice: the increments compared to the control group of both effectiveness resource use (including, for instance, time to implement attention and thresholds for re-consultation) are likely to be different from a usual care control.

An efficacy study will concentrate on trying to show if the intervention is effective in the most controlled context. Conversely, a pragmatic effectiveness study is designed to more closely mimic what happens in real-world practice. The pragmatic context for patients with chronic lower-back pain is that they go to their conventional doctor to receive an analgesic or an anti-inflammatory and may also simultaneously visit an acupuncturist. As a consequence, a pragmatic trial of acupuncture would involve the randomization of patients to receive acupuncture plus conventional care as compared with those simply receiving the latter. Such a trial suffers from the disadvantage of being unable to define the specific effects of acupuncture, but it has the great advantage of being generalizable in a real-world context (Thomas et al. 1999; Thomas et al. 2005).

Factorial design in the evaluation of the Alexander Technique

It is generally the case that it is preferable to answer one question at a time. However, sometimes it will be important to ask more than one question. Factorial designs provide an excellent and efficient framework for asking several questions simultaneously and, to illustrate this, a case study is provided. For instance, in a study we conducted which evaluates the use of the Alexander Technique in chronic back pain, we had

(Continued)

CASE STUDY 14.1

(Continued)

eight groups within our clinical trial (Little et al. 2008). The Alexander Technique is a hands-on approach where the teacher, through both 'gentle' touch and explanation, helps pupils to release harmful muscle tensions, and improve muscle use and coordination. The questions asked in this trial were as follows:

- Primary research question: What is the effectiveness of introductory or longer courses of the Alexander Technique and of massage therapy in restoring normal activities which have been restricted by back pain?
- Then: What is the effectiveness of a general practitioner exercise prescription with a nurse follow-up appointment in restoring normal activities which have been restricted by back pain?
- What is the cost-effectiveness of these treatments compared with normal care?

We wanted to evaluate whether it was necessary to give a prolonged course (24 teaching sessions) of the Alexander Technique or whether six sessions could achieve the same clinical outcome. We did this as we believed that six sessions might be acceptable for NHS funding if the Alexander Technique proved to be cost-effective, while 24 sessions might not. However, we wished to retain the clinical assumptions prevalent among Alexander Technique teachers and evaluate the best possible intervention, and therefore considered that our trial would be completely inadequate if one group did not receive the complete set of Alexander Technique lessons (24 sessions).

Second, we wished to assess whether the educational element of the Alexander Technique was the key factor in improvement or whether this was simply due to a hands-on approach. For this we had one group of patients receive a massage, where there was a hands-on treatment but no education, as usually given in the Alexander Technique. The massage group was also useful to assess whether massage *per se* is helpful. A normal care group was required as the basic comparator for all groups. Without a normal care group, it would have been difficult to estimate differences in resource use between the groups and therefore difficult to estimate cost-effectiveness.

Thus, for one 'factor' we had four groups: longer Alexander Technique (24 lessons), shorter Alexander Technique (6 lessons), massage (6 sessions) and normal care. Each of these groups was split with random assignment of subjects into two sub-groups. One of these had additional exercise and the other did not. Designing the trial with the presence or absence of exercise in all four groups allowed us to compare the Alexander Technique with standard conventional treatment plus exercise. This is supported by prior studies which suggest that this is an effective and indeed cost-effective approach to the management of chronic lower-back pain (Frost et al. 2004).

The advantage of this factorial design is that several questions may be asked simultaneously. The statistical calculations associated with this design meant that a number of questions could be asked with slightly fewer trial participants. Inevitably, multifactorial studies are complex, difficult to execute and require considerable research expertise.

Reading health research based on randomized controlled trials

In appraising published research on RCTs in the health field – and recognizing that there are a variety of forms of RCT – the following points arising from this chapter should be considered, among others:

- Is there a clear and important primary question in the research?
- Has the study been sufficiently well justified based on the prior literature?

External validity and applicability

- Have participants been appropriately selected for the RCT?

  o Are the results relevant for your context – for instance, the patients seen?
  o What is the impact of the inclusion and exclusion criteria on the generalizability of the sample?
  o Have the key ethical bases been covered, including patient consent?

- Is the choice of intervention and control meaningful for your setting?

  o Can you do it – not least in terms of the resources required (including such aspects as the training of staff and time required by staff)? Is the study described with high-level specificity and capable of replication?
  o What are the implications of the type of control group for the results? This can be illustrated by attention control to assess the specific effect of the intervention as compared to usual care to assess the total effects.

Internal validity

- Did randomization work? (The baseline table should show trial groups are similar.)

  o If trial groups have different characteristics (that is, the potential for confounding) what did the authors do to deal with the issue? The simplest way to assess the issue is to control for the potential confounding variable in the statistical analysis model to see if the estimates of the study are altered when the potential confounder is included (if the estimates do not change the variable is not a confounder).

- Were all important outcomes included, and was evidence presented of their validity and reliability?

  o Are the various arms of the trial subject to the same set of measurements?

- How appropriate was the process of blinding and was there evidence that it worked?
- Was follow-up adequate (particularly for the primary outcome)?

- o 60 per cent is poor, 70 per cent moderate, 80 per cent good, and 90 per cent very good. Was there evidence of attrition bias? For example, were the characteristics of the people followed-up different from those lost to follow-up? If so, how did the authors control for it (for instance, by imputing missing values)?

- Do lower power (Type II error) or chance (Type I error) explain the results?
  - o If the trial is negative, with no evidence of statistical significance for the primary outcome, then was the study adequately powered (for example, to detect the MCID)?
  - o If the trial is positive, with evidence of a statistically significant change in the primary outcome, then could this be due to chance? (here the primary outcome needs to have been selected in advance; lower levels of significant p<0.01 or p<0.001 make chance much less likely; and if many secondary outcomes are either significant or at least going in a similar direction, then chance is also less likely).

- Are the estimates precise and do they come from an intention to treat (ITT) analysis?
  - o Large studies will usually have tighter 95 per cent confidence intervals for the estimates (which provide the 95 per cent probability bounds for where the 'true' estimate lies); for smaller studies with wider confidence intervals if the lower margins of the confidence interval reflect changes that might not be clinically important, then you will be much less secure about recommending the intervention.
  - o The ITT analysis best reflects the estimate to inform decision-making at the point that the intervention is being considered.

Are the results important?

- What does the change in outcome actually mean for a patient?

While the RCT is often projected as a 'gold standard', it is very important to remember that research using this method can be variable in quality.

Conclusion

This chapter describes an iterative process to enable and understand the development of RCTs. It centres on the importance of the protocol and how best to consider study development with respect to the essential issues that emerge during clinical trial development. The advent of the RCT is both a blessing and a curse. Undoubtedly, it has improved the evidence base to inform the delivery of clinical care, but inevitably any RCT is, by its nature, limited in scope. Furthermore, good science and clinical relevance do not always go hand in hand, and attempting to achieve both simultaneously requires clear thinking and the ability to work within a team. To underline the themes of this chapter, a short exercise has been included on evaluating the use of lavender essence as an alternative therapy.

Exercise 14.1   The evaluation of lavender essence using a randomized controlled trial

It has been suggested that *lavandula augustifolia* (lavender essence) may be of assistance in treating insomnia. Quite a number of people just put a few drops of lavender on their pillow when they are having difficulty sleeping and say that it 'works a treat'. Insomnia affects 20 per cent of the British population, but many conventional drugs used to treat it have the potential to become addictive.

Consider the issues that you would need to take into account if you wanted to evaluate the use of *lavandula augustifolia* using an RCT. Some of the questions you might wish to consider include:

- How would you search the literature to find out what has already been published?
- How would you construct a study to evaluate this?
- If you were going to use a placebo, how might you provide a convincing one?

Note

This chapter is written in memory of the late Professor George Lewith who was the co-writer of this chapter in previous editions of the book.

Recommended further reading

These articles in the epidemiology series give a concise introduction to research design:
Grimes, D. and Schulz, K. (2002) A series of articles in the *Lancet* on research design (359: 57–61; 145–9; 248–52; 341–5; 515–19; 614–18; 781–5; 881–4; and 966–70).

This book draws on the best of conventional research methods, including randomized controlled trials, and adapts them to complementary and alternative medicine:
Lewith, G. T., Jonas, W. and Walach, H. (2011) *Clinical Research in Complementary Therapies*, 2nd edition. Edinburgh: Churchill Livingstone.

This text provides clear coverage of statistical concepts and medical examples for those interested in clinical trials:
Mathews, J. N. S. (2011) *Introduction to Randomized Controlled Clinical Trials*, 2nd edition. London: Chapman & Hall/CRC.

References

Beecher, H. (1955) 'The powerful placebo', *Journal of the American Medical Association*, *159*: 1602–6.

Brien, S., Lewith, G. T. and Bryant, T. (2003) 'Ultramolecular homoeopathy has no observable clinical effects: A randomized, double-blind, placebo-controlled proving trial of Belladonna C30', *British Journal of Clinical Pharmacology*, *56*: 562–8.

Campbell, M. and Machin, D. (1999) *Medical Statistics: A Commonsense Approach*. Chichester: Wiley.

Craig, P., Dieppe, P., Macintyre, S., Michie, S., Nazareth, I. and Petticrew, M. (2008) 'Developing and evaluating complex interventions: New guidance', *British Medical Journal*, *337*: a1655.

Family Heart Study Group (1994) 'Randomised controlled trial evaluating cardiovascular screening and intervention in general practice: Principal results of British Family Heart Study', *British Medical Journal*, *308*: 313–20.

Feinstein, A. R. (1985) *Clinical Epidemiology: The Architecture of Clinical Research*. Philadelphia, PA: Saunders.

Frank, J. D. and Frank, J. B. (1991) *Persuasion and Healing: A Comparative Study of Psychotherapy*. Baltimore, MD: Johns Hopkins University Press.

Frost, H., Lamb, S. E., Doll, H. A., Taffe Carver, P. and Stewart-Brown, S. (2004) 'Randomised controlled trial of physiotherapy compared with advice for low back pain', *British Medical Journal*, *329*: 708–14.

Geraghty, A. W., Munoz, R. F., Yardley, L., McSharry, J., Little, P. and Moore, M. (2016) 'Developing an unguided Internet-delivered intervention for emotional distress in primary care patients: Applying common factor and person-based approaches', *JMIR Mental Health*, *63*(4): e53.

Grimes, D. A. and Schulz, K. F. (2002) 'Bias and causal associations in observational research', *Lancet*, *359*: 248–52.

Hopwood, V., Lewith, G., Prescott, P. and Campbell, M. J. (2008) 'Evaluating the efficacy of acupuncture in defined aspects of stroke recovery: A randomised, placebo controlled single blind study', *Journal of Neurology*, *255*(6): 858–66.

Jadad, A. R., Moore, R. A., Carroll, D., Jenkinson, C., Reynolds, D. J. and Gavaghan, D. J. (1996) 'Assessing the quality of reports of randomized clinical trials: Is blinding necessary?', *Control Clinical Trials*, *17*: 1–14.

Lewith, G., Watkins, A., Hyland, M. E., Shaw, S., Broomfield, J. and Dolan, G. (2002) 'A double-blind, randomised, controlled clinical trial of ultramolecular potencies of house dust mite in asthmatic patients', *British Medical Journal*, *324*: 520–3.

Little, P., Lewith, G., Webley, F., Evans, M., Beattie, A., Barnett, J., Ballard, K., Oxford, F., Smith, P., Yardley, L., Hollinghurst, S. and Sharp, D. (2008) 'Randomised controlled trial of Alexander technique lessons, exercise, and massage (ATEAM) for chronic and recurrent back pain', *British Medical Journal, 337*: a884.

Little, P., Moore, M., Kelly, J., Williamson, I., Leydon, G., McDermott, L., Mullee, M. and Stuart, B. (2013) 'Ibuprofen, paracetamol, and steam for patients with respiratory tract infections in primary care: Pragmatic randomised factorial trial', *British Medical Journal, 347*: f6041.

Little, P., Rumsby, K., Kelly, J., Watson, L., Moore, M., Warner, G., Fahey, T. and Williamson, I. (2005) 'Information leaflet and antibiotic prescribing strategies for acute lower respiratory tract infection: A randomised controlled trial', *Journal of American Medical Association, 293*: 3029–35.

Little, P., Williamson, I., Warner, G., Gould, C., Gantley, M. and Kinmonth, A. L. (1997) 'An open randomised trial of prescribing strategies for sore throat', *British Medical Journal, 314*: 722–7.

Manheimer, M. S., White, A., Berman, B., Forys, K. and Ernst, E. (2005) 'Meta-analysis: Acupuncture for low back pain', *Annals of Internal Medicine, 142*(8): 651–63.

Mathews, J. N. S. (2011) *Introduction to Randomized Controlled Clinical Trials*, 2nd edition. London: Chapman & Hall/CRC.

Moher, D., Hopewell, S., Schulz, K. F., Montori, V., Gotzsche, P. C., Devereaux, P. J., Elbourne, D., Egger, M. and Altman, D. G. (2012) 'CONSORT 2010 explanation and elaboration: Updated guidelines for reporting parallel group randomised trials', *International Journal of Surgery, 10*(1): 28–55.

Moore, G. F., Audrey, S., Barker, M., Bond, L., Bonell, C., Hardeman, W. et al. (2015) 'Process evaluation of complex interventions: Medical Research Council guidance', *British Medical Journal, 350*: h1258.

Ronsenzweig, S. (1936) 'Some implicit common factors in diverse methods of psychotherapy', *American Journal of Orthopsychiatry, 6*: 414–15.

Schulz, K. F. and Grimes, D. A. (2002) 'Blinding in randomised trials: Hiding who got what', *Lancet, 359*: 696–700.

Streiner, D.L. and Norman, G.R. (2014) *Health Measurement Scales: A Practical Guide to their Development and Use*, 5th edition. Oxford: Oxford Medical Publications.

Thomas, K. J., Fitter, M., Brazier, J., MacPherson, H., Campbell, M. and Nicholl, P. (1999) 'Longer term clinical and economic benefits of offering acupuncture to patients with chronic low back pain assessed as suitable for primary care management', *Complementary Therapies in Medicine, 7*: 91–100.

Thomas, K. J., MacPherson, H., Thorpe, L., Brazier, J., Fitter, M., Campbell, M., Roman, M., Walters, S. and Nicholl, J. (2005) *Longer Term Clinical and Economic Benefits of Offering Acupuncture to Patients with Chronic Low Back Pain. Final Report to NHS Health Technology Assessment Programme.* London: NHS Research and Develoment HTA (Health Technology Assessment).

Vickers, A., Cassileth, B., Ernst, E., Fisher, P., Goldman, P., Jonas, W., Kang, S., Lewith, G., Schulz, K. and Silagy, C. (1997) 'How should we research unconventional therapies?', *International Journal of Technology Assessment in Health Care*, *13*(1): 111–21.

Vincent, C. and Lewith, G. (1995) 'Placebo controls for acupuncture studies', *Journal of the Royal Society of Medicine*, *88*: 199–202.

White, P. (2003) 'Attitude and outcome: Is there a link in complementary medicine?', *American Journal of Public Health*, *93*: 1038.

White, P., Lewith, G., Berman, B. and Birch, S. (2002) 'Reviews of acupuncture for chronic neck pain: Pitfalls in conducting systematic reviews', *Rheumatology*, *41*: 1424–31.

White, P., Lewith, G., Hopwood, V. and Prescott, P. (2003) 'The placebo needle: Is it a valid and convincing placebo for use in acupuncture trials? A randomised, single blind, cross-over trial', *Pain*, *106*: 401–9.

White, P., Lewith, G. and Prescott, P. (2004) 'The core outcomes for neck pain: Validation of a new outcome measure', *Spine*, *29*: 1923–30.

White, P., Lewith, G., Prescott, P. and Conway, J. (2004) 'Acupuncture versus placebo for the treatment of chronic mechanical neck pain: A randomised, controlled trial', *Annals of Internal Medicine*, *141*: 911–20.

Wood, R. and Lewith, G. (1998) 'The credibility of placebo controls in acupuncture studies', *Complementary Therapies in Medicine*, *6*: 79–82.

15

Experimental Methods in Health Research

A. NIROSHAN SIRIWARDENA

Chapter objectives

- To consider the benefits of randomized controlled trials (RCTs) as an experimental method, alongside their shortcomings in health research
- To particularly highlight situations where it is not appropriate to use RCTs for methodological, practical or ethical reasons
- To outline a range of the techniques labelled as non-randomized experimental methods that provide a scientific alternative to RCTs
- To consider the strengths and weaknesses of such experimental methods in researching health.

Introduction

This chapter provides an overview of non-randomized experimental and quasi-experimental methods, particularly focusing on experimental techniques that provide alternatives to the randomized controlled trial (RCT). The RCT is a particular form of experimental method, and in the double-blind controlled trial ranks high in the hierarchy of evidence. Randomization can control for confounding variables and double-blinding can reduce certain types of bias. However, the chapter describes how RCTs suffer from their own potential biases and it is not always possible to conduct an RCT for methodological, practical or ethical reasons. 'Experimental methods' are defined as an umbrella term that includes a variety of techniques that aim to maintain scientific rigour in situations where it is not possible to introduce randomization, blinding or sometimes even a control group. The chapter will explain the language of experimentation and discuss the advantages and disadvantages, as well as how such methods should be applied. A range of experimental research designs based on published studies is described to illustrate the use of these methods in practice.

Non-randomized experimental designs and their rationale

Non-randomized experimental designs

The key feature of an experiment is that it assesses the effect of introducing a change, where the relationship between two or more measurements is investigated by deliberately prompting a change in one of them and observing the change in the other (Robson 1994). A change based on a hypothesis of cause is introduced in one variable (the independent variable), which may lead to a corresponding change, or effect, in another (the dependent) variable. The prediction of cause and effect (A leads to B) is termed the hypothesis. Experiments test hypotheses whereas other types of quantitative study using observational methods test the strength of associations between measurements (A is associated with B). Experiments are based on the scientific method of testing changes to establish a relationship between cause and effect, and they have advantages over other methods in their ability to test hypotheses, reduce bias and limit confounding. Arguably, they are also more robust in determining the true size of the effect of an intervention, the 'effect size' being the estimate of the magnitude of a change in a measure that may be calculated statistically.

Experimental methods should be distinguished from observational methods such as cross-sectional, case-control, cohort or related designs. Case-control studies aim to compare the characteristics of a particular phenomenon in the group of interest to a control or reference group. Thus, the health of one group of people exposed to risks, such as cigarette smoking or asbestos exposure, or a protective factor, such as an influenza vaccination, may be compared with another group that has not been exposed in order to assess for a specific outcome. Classic examples include the early studies linking lung cancer with smoking (Doll and Hill 1950; Wynder and Graham, 1950) or more recent studies confirming an association with asbestos (Villeneuve et al. 2012). More recent case-control studies have also shown that the influenza vaccine is associated with a reduced risk of heart attack or stroke (Siriwardena, Asghar and Coupland 2014; Siriwardena, Gwini and Coupland 2010).

Cohort studies involve a selected population studied over time to investigate the effect of a particular factor, which subgroups have different exposures to, on health outcomes. The landmark 'doctors' smoking study' established the relationship between smoking and lung cancer (Doll and Hill 1964; Doll and Peto 1978). Self-controlled case series studies, which are a more recently introduced form of study design, aim to determine the risk of a particular outcome over time by comparing periods of exposure with non-exposure in a single population rather than comparing groups with different exposures over the same period, for example in relation to an association between flu vaccination and reduced risk of heart attack (Gwini, Coupland and Siriwardena 2011) or stroke (Asghar, Coupland and Siriwardena 2015). Observational methods of this type should not be confused with the participant observer or ethnographic methods used in qualitative research, as described in Chapter 8

Non-randomized experimental methods include a range of study types including those where there is an intervention group only and others where an intervention group is compared to a non-randomized control group. The important characteristic is that the experimenter has some control over, or can deliberately manipulate, the introduction of the intervention (Deeks et al. 2003). These methods are summarized in Figure 15.1 that follows. They may also be classified into pre-experimental and quasi-experimental designs on the basis that the former are unlikely to provide valid evidence for effectiveness of an intervention, whereas the latter may do so in certain circumstances (Shadish, Cook and Campbell 2001).

Rationale for non-randomized experimental designs

RCTs are the gold standard for assessing whether health care interventions are effective because they address important sources of bias, particularly known or unknown baseline imbalance in (prognostic) factors associated with the outcome of interest, also called confounding. However, there may be practical or moral barriers to using randomized designs when health care practitioners or organizations have already, sometimes purposefully and sometimes inadvertently, introduced new health technologies or services without an established evidence base. Once these are applied, they are difficult to reverse from both ethical and practical perspectives. Once a new service is introduced or an intervention is established, there are limited possibilities for more structured experimental designs to determine the effectiveness or cost-effectiveness of the changes. In this situation, non-randomized experimental designs may provide the only possibility for evaluation. For example, randomization may not be possible due to factors that are either intrinsic to the study or external to it, such as some area-wide or organization-based interventions where randomization is not feasible, or where a higher-level (such as governmental) policy decision has been made to introduce a new service everywhere. In addition, RCTs are not immune to biases, which are discussed in more detail below.

Resources required for non-randomized experimental designs

Experimental designs in health care usually require formal independent ethical review. Sometimes, if a study is clearly shown to be an audit or an evaluation of existing services with no intervention other than a recommended quality improvement, this may not be required.

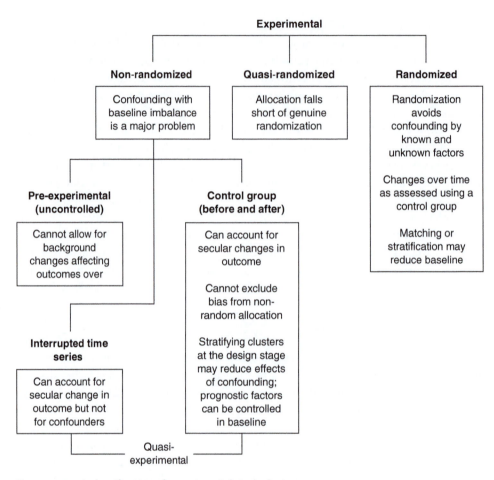

FIGURE 15.1 A classification of experimental study designs

Source: Adapted from Ukoumunne et al. (1999) and Deeks et al. (2003)

However, it is usually best to seek advice from the organization where the study is to take place and the local ethics committee. Experimental studies require good access to health care settings, close working relationships with health service partners and a skilled research team, including methodologists, statisticians and often health economists for larger-scale studies.

Pre-experimental study designs

Pre-experimental designs are non-randomized experiments where a particular outcome of interest is measured in the intervention group, either before-and-after or only post-test, that is, after the intervention. Occasionally this includes post-test measures in an intervention and a non-equivalent (non-randomized) comparison group. Such designs are often used to evaluate the feasibility or effect of certain types of intervention: an example would be an educational programme to improve the recognition of psychological illness in general practice (Hannaford, Thompson and Simpson 1996) or a complex intervention in which health visitors assess the risk of childhood obesity and promote preventive parental behaviours to reduce this risk in their infants (Redsell et al. 2017). Pre-experimental designs are also used by researchers wishing to evaluate the impact of large-scale changes. One such study examined the effect on general practitioner (GP) workload (in terms of hours spent on general practice work per week and time spent per patient in consultations) of the national introduction of a new contract for GPs in 1990 (Hannay, Usherwood and Platts 1992).

Quasi-experimental designs

These designs include two main types of study. These are:

- The non-randomized control group, before-and-after study
- The interrupted time series design.

The non-randomized control group before-and-after design involves one or more intervention groups with one or more non-equivalent comparator groups acting as controls with measurements of outcomes taken before and after the intervention. An example of a before-and-after study in relation to evaluating policy innovation is a study of the impact of legislation to ban smoking in public places in the Republic of Ireland. A before-and-after non-randomized control group study showed a reduction in passive smoking and respiratory illness in bar workers following the introduction of the ban (Allwright et al. 2005). Another study, this time based in the United Kingdom, found that the introduction of legislation restricting pack sizes of analgesics led to reductions in pack sizes on pharmacy shelves and that this was associated with a reduction in analgesic overdoses, the severity of the overdoses that occurred and other sequelae, such as the level of suicide deaths and of liver transplantation (Hawton et al. 2004).

   In the second type of study, using time series or interrupted time series designs, repeated measurements of the outcome of interest are taken over time from the population, beginning before the intervention and continuing afterwards. The time periods used can be continuous or discontinuous (that is interrupted). Measurements are taken to assess whether there is any change over and above that which would have been expected from the secular trend prior to the intervention. Measurements for time series studies may be taken from a whole population or by sampling from a cohort of the population. Alternatively, repeated cross-sectional samples can be taken from the whole population. This method need not necessarily involve a control group, but it can benefit from one in accounting for confounding external influences on the outcome to be assessed.

The strengths and weaknesses of non-randomized experimental designs

It is important to appreciate the advantages and disadvantages of the different types of experimental design. These are discussed, first, in relation to RCTs, then in non-randomized designs in general and, finally, for specific types of non-randomized design.

Strengths and weaknesses of randomized controlled trials

Large, well-designed and well-conducted RCTs ensure that intervention and control groups have a baseline of comparability. Differences in outcome can then be attributed to the intervention alone. Explanations for differences other than the intervention, or confounding factors, should be balanced equally between the intervention and control groups through randomization. The use of RCTs, despite their 'gold standard' epithet, can be hampered by a number of problems, which are illustrated in Box 15.1.

Box 15.1   Problems with the use of randomized controlled trials

- There may be such strong evidence for an intervention that a placebo group may be unethical.
- Randomization may be impossible because clinicians or organizations may advocate strongly one particular approach over another. In this situation, there is a lack of clinical equipoise, without true clinical equivalence between the intervention and control. A strong preference for either effectively prevents random allocation.
- Educational or other interventions when the active participation of subjects is required for the intervention to be effective may render randomization inappropriate or impossible.
- Randomized controlled studies may be ruled out on cost terms. They are more complex and more costly than non-randomized designs (Black 1996).

RCTs are also subject to a number of possible design flaws and are therefore not immune from bias. Bias may arise because:

- Those included are more or less likely to benefit from the intervention or may be unrepresentative of the population in which the intervention would usually be used.

- Participants have a preference for or against a particular treatment in unblinded RCTs.
- There are random allocation errors (due to a faulty allocation sequence or a failure to conceal allocation to intervention or control groups) (Dechartres et al. 2017).
- There are failures in blinding (of subjects or observers).
- There are problems with data collection (for instance, missing data) or data analysis (for example, not taking clustering into account).
- There are concerns about sponsorship (for example, trials sponsored by pharmaceutical companies are more likely to be positive) (Ahn et al. 2017).
- There are concerns about publication (positive trials are more likely to be published), all of which can increase effect size (Britton et al. 1998).

Taking participant selection as an example, those taking part in RCTs are often atypical. Only a small proportion of patients with a given condition can be included in a trial, either directly through selection and exclusion criteria or indirectly through having a greater likelihood of inclusion of certain types of patient, such as those attending academic centres. Women, elderly people, children and those with other illnesses or very severe illness are also less likely to be included in trials. This tends to augment treatment effects and to reduce the generalizability of a study. In treatment trials, there is a bias towards the inclusion of people who are less well-off and less well educated, whereas in preventive interventions, participants tend to be healthier, wealthier and better educated. The so-called 'healthy user' bias tends to increase effect size on proxy outcomes because of better compliance but, conversely, the 'healthy user' tends to reduce effect sizes on true outcomes because of a ceiling effect. Better baseline measures have less capacity to improve.

Non-randomized experimental designs can suffer from similar problems, but as they usually tend to be less restrictive in terms of inclusion and exclusion criteria, they exhibit better external validity and generalizability. Furthermore, there is no evidence that non-randomized studies have greater effect sizes than RCTs. Potentially, trial subjects, whether individuals or organizations, tend to benefit from an intervention. For this reason, it is more critical to the internal and external validity of an experimental study to ensure that the trial group is representative of the population from which it is drawn (Britton et al. 1998). Laboratory methods often involve experimental methods too. However, these cover a variety of methods of investigation and analysis that are outside the scope of this chapter.

Strengths and weaknesses of non-randomized designs

The key advantage of a non-randomized design is that randomization need not be undertaken in situations where it would not be ethical or acceptable for clients or other stakeholders to do so. Non-randomized studies may also be the only ethical option in some circumstances – for example, in situations where it can be argued that an educational intervention or treatment is likely to lead to a positive change, and therefore access should not be denied to a control group. In one non-randomized educational intervention study to investigate the effect of introducing decision rules for referral for x-ray in suspected ankle and foot fractures, under the so-called Ottawa ankle rules, it was decided that it was inappropriate to have a control group (Stiell et al. 1995). The results, following the educational programme, showed a reduction in requests for x-ray – and, while a decrease in waiting times and costs occurred, there was no increase in the number of missed fractures. It can be assumed that, pending further research, this was due to the education effect.

Although it is widely accepted that randomization in trials reduces some types of systematic error that may interfere with the results, it has also been argued that in certain circumstances there may be an advantage in allowing patients' preferences to play a part in determining which arm of a trial they enter, even if this leads to some loss in assessing the therapeutic treatment effect. One reason for allowing patient preferences to be taken into account is that some patients may have such strong preferences that they may refuse randomization, thus leading to selection bias. In studies where there are difficulties in recruiting patients, there may be advantages in following preferences even if this motivation may skew the results.

It could equally be argued that, where it is not possible to disguise which treatment arm patients are in, the results may also be skewed by low motivation. Furthermore, certain interventions require the active engagement of participants. This is the case where self-monitoring or self-medication is required; where rehabilitation or programmes for de-institutionalization are being assessed; where behavioural or cognitive treatments for anxiety and depression are being compared with each other; and where treatments involve drug medication. In these situations, comparisons may only work if participants have no preference, which may be an unlikely scenario. One solution to this problem has been to distinguish between patients who have no preference and to apply a randomization method in their case. Thus, a trial with two interventions will have four groups: randomized to A; prefer A; randomized to B; and prefer B. An example of this type of study was conducted by Chilvers and colleagues (2001) on the use of antidepressant drugs and generic counselling for the treatment of major depression in primary care.

Non-randomized methods are often most useful where an innovative practice is being introduced in a single or limited number of sites for an evaluation period or to assess the effect of legislative or policy changes. An example of this type of study was where non-randomized experimental methods were used to evaluate the impact of introducing an open-access walk-in centre for people needing first-line primary care. The Department of Health favoured the introduction of open-access walk-in clinics to reduce the pressure on Accident and Emergency departments, and general practices introduced this facility in certain localities in England. In order to estimate the effect of this intervention in one locality, a study using a controlled before-and-after design was used to evaluate the effect of introducing an open-access clinic on the use of Accident and Emergency departments and general practices (Hsu et al. 2003). In another study, this time with a control group, a mental health facilitator was employed in six general practices to train GPs to recognize and treat postnatal depression (Holden, Sagovsky and Cox 1989). The results were compared with six control practices where there was no facilitator. In this study, there were demonstrable improvements in terms of the identification of mental illness by GPs, but not in the management or outcomes of the illness.

Strengths and weaknesses of specific types of non-randomized design

Pre-experimental designs suffer from a serious and often fatal flaw. It is virtually impossible to determine whether the outcomes of such studies are due to the intervention or to some other confounding factor. Such factors can include: an unpredicted external influence or the effect of changes that occur naturally over time in the process of health care, such as increased awareness of new technologies, demographic changes, or local and national influences. These changes over time are often referred to as 'secular' trends. There may also be changes in the behaviour of study participants directly as a result of being observed, termed the Hawthorne effect, or the tendency called regression to the mean. This is for outlying measures to return to a central value. Studies may also be severely compromised by selection bias as there is a tendency for researchers to select participants who are likely to benefit from the intervention.

However, non-randomized designs do have a place, particularly in feasibility studies, for example where investigators are trying to determine whether an intervention is acceptable. Blenkiron (2001) used a pre-experimental design to investigate the efficacy of a self-help audio-cassette in helping patients to understand cognitive behavioural therapy (CBT) for depression (Blenkiron 2001). The study compared the extent of patient agreement with key messages on the audiotape, before and after use, and found an improvement in attitudes and knowledge about CBT following its use.

There are also a number of methodological problems with quasi-experimental studies. For instance, innovations are sometimes taken up inconsistently and comparisons can only be made between those that implement change and those that maintain the status quo. An example of this was a non-randomized control group study comparing the effect on financial control of prescribing in fundholding practices holding their own budget, with non-fundholding general practices (Bradlow and Coulter 1993). In this case, it was only possible to compare practices that took up the initiative with those that did not. It was found that fundholding practices were more likely to remain within their 'indicative' budget, but there may have been other intervening or confounding variables to explain the behaviour, such as differences in the level of organization or in the numbers of staff in fundholding, compared with non-fundholding, practices.

Other sources of bias in these types of study include external effects on outcome and secular (time-related) changes unrelated to the intervention. Although this source of bias can be minimized by having a control group, this may not be possible due to limited funding or because a new policy is introduced. In these circumstances, time series designs have been used to show, for instance, that media coverage can produce unwanted effects. For example, *Casualty*, a BBC television drama, once featured a drug overdose that led to an increase in real overdoses presenting to casualty departments (Hawton et al. 1999).

Time series studies using a particular cohort, although a useful quasi-experimental design, are more likely over longer periods of time to lead to bias due to non-response related to the Hawthorne effect, or to maturation where individual ageing is a factor, or to contamination. A study can be 'contaminated' when the change that is intended for the intervention group is inadvertently introduced to the control group. This could occur, for example, due to staff moving between health facilities, an unexpected movement of patients, or the introduction of a parallel intervention, which could skew the outcomes being measured. Although a control group in a time series design may not be possible, research using this method can strengthen the findings. This is exemplified by a recent interrupted time series study of the effect on specialist visits and hospitalizations of the introduction of primary care commissioning in England, where data from Scotland were used as a comparator (Lopez Bernal et al. 2017).

Pre-experimental studies may also be useful as a precursor to an RCT study to evaluate a complex intervention. This is where two or more interventions are combined in a single study. Many health care interventions are of this type and there is increasing evidence that multiple interventions may be more effective than a single intervention (Grimshaw et al. 2001; van der Wensing, van der Weijden and Grol 1998). The longstanding Medical Research Council framework for the design and evaluation of complex interventions is often used as the basis for the development of designs that may eventually lead to the classic RCT (Campbell et al. 2007). In this framework, a phased approach involving pre-clinical, theoretical modelling in Phase I and an exploratory study or studies in Phase II is the suggested approach before undertaking a definitive trial in Phase III. These initial phases could involve a qualitative study, such as a case study or interviews, a before-and-after experimental study (with or without controls), a time series study or a combination of these. An example is provided in one of the case studies given at the end of the chapter.

Analysis of data, writing up and presenting the findings

Data analysis in these study designs often requires considerable statistical expertise in deciding on the appropriate methods to correct for baseline imbalance, secular trends and changes over time as a result of the intervention in question. Although out of the scope for this chapter, where regression models are being used, decisions need to be made about whether to analyse for variables predicting the outcome of interest in the study as fixed or random effects.

Non-randomized designs in practice

Three examples of pre-experimental, non-randomized control, before-and-after studies and time series designs are presented here as case studies.

Feasibility of health visitors and parents using digital technology for proactive assessment of obesity risk during infancy: A before-and-after study

An example of a pre-experimental single group, before-and-after, design was this feasibility study of a complex intervention in which health visitors were trained to assess obesity risk in infants and prevent the development of obesity by working with parents (Redsell et al. 2017). The study took place in two settings, both with high rates of deprivation: one in a rural and one in an urban area of the East Midlands region of the United Kingdom. Health visitors were trained to recruit infants aged 6–8 weeks using a risk calculator to estimate the risk of obesity based on the infant's birth weight and length and the current weight measured at around 3–4 months, maternal and paternal height and weight, maternal smoking status during pregnancy and the breast-feeding status. Health visitors then used Proactive Assessment of Obesity Risk during Infancy (ProAsk), a therapeutic wheel located on a tablet computer, to agree evidence-based strategies with parents such as feeding practices and activities designed to prevent childhood obesity. The outcomes to be assessed included recruitment, response and attrition rates together with the proposed primary outcome measure, weight-for-age z-score, and secondary outcomes including parenting self-efficacy, maternal feeding style, infant diet and exposure to physical activity and sedentary behaviour.

In all, 28 health visitors were trained in the two sites and 22 participated in the study. They screened 324 infants and 66 of 226 eligible infants (29 per cent) were recruited. Assessment of overweight risk was completed on 53 infants: 40 per cent were identified as above population risk. Weight-for-age z-score (SD) between the infants at population risk and those above population risk differed significantly at baseline (−0.67 SD versus 0.32 SD). Health visitors were able to collect data and calculate the overweight risk for the infants. Health visitors and parents said in their feedback that the information provided in the therapeutic wheel was appropriate and acceptable. However, health visitors said they found it challenging to adhere to the protocol and apply the intervention in the way that it was intended.

An evaluation of an educational intervention to reduce inappropriate cannulation and improve cannulation techniques by paramedics

This study is an example of a non-randomized control group before-and-after design. It aimed to examine the effect of an educational intervention designed to improve both the appropriateness of the use of cannulation by paramedics and their expertise in the technique (Siriwardena et al. 2009). Intravenous cannulation involves the insertion of a synthetic tube into a vein using a needle that enables paramedics to administer fluids or drugs at home or in the ambulance, if patients are being transferred to hospital. When *cannulae* are used without good reason or inserted with inadequate infection control, there are potential risks for patients, including unnecessary pain or infection.

The hypothesis of the study was that following an education session for paramedics aimed at improving their understanding of when to use cannulation and to improve their technique, there would be a decrease in the use of (inappropriate) cannulation and an improvement in their cannulation technique. The primary outcome measure was the rate of appropriate cannulation, which for the purposes of the study was defined as cannulation where drugs or intravenous fluids were recorded as having been given. The secondary outcomes included the rate of cannulation overall and the correct use of the cannulation technique assessed by a trained observer. The outcomes were measured two months before and two months after the educational session took place to allow time for the intervention and for a change in practice to occur.

The comparative data were analysed using logistic regression to test for both the main and interaction effects between predictor variables. The first regression model included: data from the various sites (intervention versus control); the timing of testing (pre-intervention versus post-intervention); and the interaction between sites using the timing of testing as predictor variables. The overall cannulation rates were used as the outcome variable. The second regression model included: data from the sites (intervention versus control); the timing of testing (pre-intervention versus post-intervention); interaction between sites; and the timing of testing as predictor variables. In this case, inappropriate cannulation rates were the outcome variable.

There was a non-significant reduction in inappropriate cannulation rates – that is, in the intervention area (1.0 per cent decreasing to 0 per cent) compared to the control area (2.5 per cent increasing to 2.6 per cent). There was also a significant reduction in cannulation rates in the intervention area (9.1 per cent to 6.5 per cent) compared with an increase in the control area (13.8 per cent to 15.1 per cent) ($p<0.001$). Finally, paramedics in the intervention area were significantly more likely to use correct hand-washing techniques post-intervention compared with paramedics in the control area (74.5 per cent versus 14.9 per cent, $p<0.001$).

There were potential biases due to the non-equivalent group design. These included selection bias from non-random selection of intervention and control groups and confounding from possible other external influences on outcomes occurring between pre- and post-intervention phases. There were also possible existing differences between areas in cannulation technique. Biases, such as regression to the mean, would have been less likely, given that the baseline rate of cannulation was greater in the control than in the intervention area. Baseline differences in cannulation rates were adjusted for in the analysis. The study did not account for differences in secular trends in the intervention or control areas in the analysis. As the post-intervention assessment was not blinded, this was another potential source of bias. The measurement of outcomes was unchanged and consistent before, and after, the intervention.

CASE STUDY 15.3

Investigation of the effect of a countywide protected learning time scheme on prescribing rates of Ramipril: An interrupted time series study

The final example is of a time series study that aimed to investigate whether an area-wide educational intervention for general practice and primary health care workers increased prescribing of the drug Ramipril. This was advocated for reducing cardiovascular risk and preventing heart attacks (Siriwardena et al. 2007).

As a result of the benefits of specific drugs called angiotensin converting enzyme (ACE) inhibitors in improving clinical outcomes for patients at risk of heart disease, including those with diabetes, we used prescribing rates for Ramipril, an ACE inhibitor widely used for prevention at the time, as an outcome measure. This was based on the Heart Outcomes Prevention Evaluation (HOPE) trial, which provided evidence that patients with coexisting diabetes and hypertension or other cardiovascular risk factors, if treated with Ramipril, had lower rates of cardiovascular disease and death.

A time series design was used to analyse prescribing data in 101 practices in one county in England. Data were collected in one year, before and after the educational session, to assess changes in the rate of prescribing Ramipril. The time study showed a significant change in the rate of Ramipril prescribing at a therapeutic dosage following the educational intervention (OR: 1.50, 95 per cent; CI: 1.07 to 1.93), despite a background of secular change. Within this overall change, there were a number of patterns of change in prescribing. For instance, there were practices in which prescribing rates rose either a little or a lot after the intervention. There were practices that delayed prescribing the drug, in contrast to those where the rate of prescribing continued to rise.

The time series design was chosen for the study because it would have been inappropriate to randomize practices as all were invited to the educational session. It was difficult to provide an unbiased control group because of potential 'contamination'. The study took into account secular trends and assessed whether the intervention had a significantly greater effect than the underlying secular trend.

(Continued)

(Continued)

A change occurred, but this was partly related to increased Ramipril prescribing for diabetes and probably also for heart failure and hypertension. The data collection was retrospective to reduce the likelihood of a Hawthorne effect biasing the results. The design did not preclude effects other than the chosen intervention affecting the particular outcome.

Reading health research based on experimental methods

Despite their value, the reader needs to be able to critically appraise published health research based on experimental methods that are not RCTs, including non-randomized experimental and quasi-experimental methods. Key questions to ask include the following:

- Are the experimental methods used most suited to the research question and why?
- Are there good reasons for not conducting an RCT?
- Are the limitations of non-randomized experimental methods stated?
- How are these limitations addressed in the research design?
- What approach is taken to account for any potential confounding variables?
- How are internal and external validity improved?
- Are there plans for an RCT to follow in a phased approach?
- Has the study been ethically reviewed and approved?

The reader should also see the comments on health research based on RCTs in Chapter 14, given that the RCT is a specific form of experimental method.

Conclusion

In this chapter, it has been shown why and how experimental designs in health research extend beyond the traditional RCT. A number of pre-experimental, quasi-experimental and experimental designs have important potential applications for assessing and evaluating health technologies, interventions and services, and for modelling (that is, developing or refining) interventions prior to RCTs, particularly in the case of complex interventions. Finally, an exercise has been set out for the reader to complete. It asks which experimental methods can be applied to the ambulance service, and in what way.

Exercise 15.1　Non-randomized experimental designs

In 2004 in the United Kingdom the Healthcare Commission report on ambulance services noted that most patients (four out of five) said they had suffered pain from their presenting condition while in the ambulance. Although 81 per cent felt that the ambulance crew did everything they could to control pain, one in five wanted more pain relief; 14 per cent said the crew did this to some extent; and 5 per cent said that the crew did not do everything they could to control their pain.

As a result of this report, you are asked to design and implement a quality improvement protocol for improving the assessment and control of pain in an ambulance service in which you are working. Pain control is assessed in adults (aged 16 and over) using a verbal pain rating scale from 0 (no pain) to 10 (the most severe pain) and should be recorded for all patients. The NHS Trust board is keen to see improvements across the service and both you and they consider an RCT study to be neither ethical nor feasible.

In your report, address the following questions:

- Which patients or patient groups would you study in relation to pain? Who would you exclude, and why?
- What outcomes measures could you use for your evaluation?
- What methods could you use to improve pain control, and why?
- Consider what other experimental methods could be used in this situation.
- Which of these would you prefer to use, and why?
- Where would you find a control group for your study?
- Describe any sources of bias and confounding factors in your preferred study design. How might you address these?

Recommended further reading

This is an updated version of a classic text, in which experts in the field of quasi-experimentation discuss comprehensively key issues relating to the theory and practice of experimental and quasi-experimental designs:

Shadish, W. R., Cook, T. D. and Campbell, D. T. (2002) *Experimental and Quasi-experimental Designs for Generalized Causal Inference*. Boston, MA: Houghton-Mifflin.

This is a more recent, clearly written chapter focusing on social work research, which is relevant to a range of health and other disciplines:

Thyer, B. A. (2012) 'Quasi-experimental research designs', in T. Tripodi (ed.), *Pocket Guides to Social Work Research Methods*. New York: Oxford University Press.

For a very readable and accessible account of quasi-experimental methods, this is an excellent site written by an expert in quasi-experimental research methods:

Trochim, W. M. (2006) *Research Methods Knowledge Base*, 2nd edition. Available at: www. socialresearchmethods.net/kb/

This is a systematic review comparing randomized and non-randomized designs and supporting the use of well-designed quasi-experimental designs to answer particular types of research question:

Ukoumunne, O. C., Gulliford, M. C., Chinn, S., Sterne, J. A. C. and Burney, P. G. J. (1999) 'Methods for evaluating area-wide and organisation-based interventions in health and healthcare: A systematic review', *Health Technology Assessment*, 3(5): 9.

References

Ahn, R., Woodbridge, A., Abraham, A., Saba, S., Korenstein, D., Madden, E., Boscardin, W. J. and Keyhani, S. (2017) 'Financial ties of principal investigators and randomized controlled trial outcomes: Cross sectional study', *British Medical Journal*, 356: i6770.

Allwright, S., Paul, G., Greiner, B., Mullally, B. J., Pursell, L., Kelly, A., Bonner, B., D'Eath, M., McConnell, B., McLaughlin, J. P., O'Donovan, D., O'Kane, E. and Perry, I. J. (2005) 'Legislation for smoke-free workplaces and health of bar workers in Ireland: Before and after study', *British Medical Journal*, 331: 1117.

Asghar, Z., Coupland, C. and Siriwardena, A. N. (2015) 'Influenza vaccination and risk of stroke: Self-controlled case-series study', *Vaccine*, 33(41): 5458–63.

Black, N. (1996) 'Why we need observational studies to evaluate the effectiveness of health care', *British Medical Journal*, 312: 1215–18.

Blenkiron, P. (2001) 'Coping with depression: A pilot study to assess the efficacy of a self-help audio cassette', *British Journal of General Practice*, 51: 366–70.

Bradlow, J. and Coulter, A. (1993) 'Effect of fundholding and indicative prescribing schemes on general practitioners' prescribing costs', *British Medical Journal*, 307: 1186–9.

Britton, A., McKee, M., Black, N., McPherson, K., Sanderson, C. and Bain, C. (1998) 'Choosing between randomised and non-randomised studies: A systematic review', *Health Technology Assessment*, 2(13): 3.

Campbell, N. C., Murray, E., Darbyshire, J., Emery, J., Farmer, A., Griffiths, F., Guthrie, B., Lester, H., Wilson, P. and Kinmonth, A. L. (2007) 'Designing and evaluating complex interventions to improve health care', *British Medical Journal*, 334: 455–9.

Chilvers, C., Dewey, M., Fielding, K., Gretton, V., Miller, P., Palmer, B., Weller, D., Churchill, R., Williams, I., Bedi, N., Duggan, C., Lee, A. and Harrison, G. (2001) 'Antidepressant drugs and generic counselling for treatment of major depression in primary care: Randomized trial with patient preference arms', *British Medical Journal*, 322: 772–5.

Dechartres, A., Trinquart, L., Atal, I., Moher, D., Dickersin, K., Boutron, I., Perrodeau, E., Altman, D. G. and Ravaud, P. (2017) 'Evolution of poor reporting and inadequate methods over time in 20,920 randomised controlled trials included in Cochrane reviews: Research on research study', *British Medical Journal*, *357*: j2490.

Deeks, J. J., Dinnes, J., D'Amico, R., Sowden, A. J., Sakarovitch, C., Song, F., Petticrew M. and Altman D. G. (2003) 'Evaluating non-randomised intervention studies', *Health Technology Assessment*, *7*(27): iii–x, 1–173.

Doll, R. and Hill, A. B. (1950) 'Smoking and carcinoma of the lung; preliminary report', *British Medical Journal*, *2*(4682): 739–48.

Doll, R. and Hill, A. B. (1964) 'Mortality in relation to smoking: Ten years' observations of British doctors', *British Medical Journal*, *1*(5395): 1399–1410.

Doll, R. and Peto, R. (1978) 'Cigarette smoking and bronchial carcinoma: Dose and time relationships among regular smokers and lifelong non-smokers', *Journal of Epidemiology and Community Health*, *32*(4): 303–13.

Grimshaw, J. M., Shirran, L., Thomas, R., Mowatt, G., Fraser, C., Bero, L., et al. (2001) 'Changing provider behavior: An overview of systematic reviews of interventions', *Medical Care*, *39*(8, Suppl 2): 2–45.

Gwini, S. M., Coupland, C. A. and Siriwardena, A. N. (2011) 'The effect of influenza vaccination on risk of acute myocardial infarction: self-controlled case-series study', *Vaccine*, *29*(6): 1145–49.

Hannaford, P. C., Thompson, C. and Simpson, M. (1996) 'Evaluation of an educational programme to improve the recognition of psychological illness by general practitioners', *British Journal of General Practice*, *46*(407): 333–7.

Hannay, D., Usherwood, T. and Platts, M. (1992) 'Workload of general practitioners before and after the new contract', *British Medical Journal*, *304*(6827): 615–18.

Hawton, K., Simkin, S., Deeks, J., Cooper, J., Johnston, A., Waters, K., Arundel, M., Bernal, W., Gunson, B., Hudson, M., Suri, D. and Simpson, K. (2004) 'UK legislation on analgesic packs: Before and after study of long-term effect on poisonings', *British Medical Journal*, *329*: 1076.

Hawton, K., Simkin, S., Deeks, J. J., O'Connor, S., Keen, A., Altman, D. G., et al. (1999) 'Effects of a drug overdose in a television drama on presentations to hospital for self poisoning: Time series and questionnaire study', *British Medical Journal*, *318*(7189): 972–7.

Holden, J. M., Sagovsky, R. and Cox, J. L. (1989) 'Counselling in a general practice setting: Controlled study of health visitor intervention in treatment of postnatal depression', *British Medical Journal*, *298*: 223–6.

Hsu, R. T., Lambert, P. C., Woods, M. and Kurinczuk, J. J. (2003) 'Effect of NHS walk-in centre on local primary healthcare services: Before and after observational study', *British Medical Journal*, *326*: 530.

Lopez Bernal, J. A., Lu, C. Y., Gasparrini, A., Cummins, S., Wharham, J. F. and Soumerai, S. B. (2017) 'Association between the 2012 Health and Social Care Act and specialist visits and hospitalisations in England: A controlled interrupted time series analysis', *PLoS Medicine, 14*(11): e1002427.

Redsell, S. A., Rose, J., Weng, S., Ablewhite, J., Swift, J. A., Siriwardena, A. N., Nathan, D., Wharrad, H. J., Atkinson, P., Watson, V., McMaster, F., Lakshman, R. and Glazebrook, C. (2017) 'Digital technology to facilitate proactive assessment of obesity risk during infancy (ProAsk): A feasibility study', *BMJ Open, 7*(9): e017694.

Robson, C. (1994) *Design and Statistics in Psychology*, 3rd edition. Harmondsworth: Penguin.

Shadish, W. R., Cook, T. D. and Campbell, D. T. (2001) *Experimental and Quasi-experimental Designs for Generalized Causal Inference*. Boston, MA: Houghton Mifflin.

Siriwardena, A. N., Asghar, Z. and Coupland, C. C. (2014) 'Influenza and pneumococcal vaccination and risk of stroke or transient ischaemic attack-matched case control study', *Vaccine, 32*(12): 1354–61.

Siriwardena, A. N., Fairchild, P., Gibson, S., Sach, T. and Dewey, M. (2007) 'Investigation of the effect of a countywide protected learning time scheme on prescribing rates of ramipril: Interrupted time series study', *Family Practice, 24*(1): 26–33.

Siriwardena, A. N., Gwini, S. M. and Coupland, C. A. (2010) 'Influenza vaccination, pneumococcal vaccination and risk of acute myocardial infarction: Matched case-control study', *Canadian Medical Association Journal, 182*(15): 1617–23.

Siriwardena, A. N., Iqbal, M., Banerjee, S., Spaight, A. and Stephenson, J. (2009) 'An evaluation of an educational intervention to reduce inappropriate cannulation technique by paramedics', *Emergency Medical Journal, 26*(11): 831–6.

Stiell, I., Wells, G., Laupacis, A., Brison, R., Verbeek, R., Vandemheen, K. and Naylor, C. D. (1995) 'Multicentre trial to introduce the Ottawa ankle rules for use of radiography in acute ankle injuries: Multicentre Ankle Rule Study Group', *British Medical Journal, 311*: 594–7.

Ukoumunne, O. C., Gulliford, M. C., Chinn, S., Sterne, J. A. C. and Burney, P. G. J. (1999) 'Methods for evaluating area-wide and organisation-based interventions in health and healthcare: A systematic review', *Health Technology Assessment, 3*(5): 9.

van der Wensing, M., van der Weijden, T. and Grol, R. (1998) 'Implementing guidelines and innovations in general practice: Which interventions are effective?', *British Journal of General Practice, 48*: 991–7.

Villeneuve, P. J., Parent, M. E., Harris, S. A., Johnson, K. C. and Canadian Cancer Registries Epidemiology Research (2012) 'Occupational exposure to asbestos and lung cancer in men: Evidence from a population-based case-control study in eight Canadian provinces', *BMC Cancer, 12*: 595.

Wynder, E. L. and Graham, E. A. (1950) 'Tobacco smoking as a possible etiologic factor in bronchiogenic carcinoma: A study of 684 proved cases', *Journal of the American Medical Association, 143*(4): 329–36.

16

The Use of Economics in Health Research

STEVE PARROTT AND ALAN MAYNARD

Chapter objectives

- To understand resource limitations in health care and strategies for rationing
- To identify the main forms of economic evaluation including cost-effectiveness, cost–utility and cost–benefit analysis
- To outline the issues to be considered when designing an economic evaluation
- To describe the concept of Quality Adjusted Life Years (QALYs) and alternative methods of valuing health outcomes
- To consider economic evaluation and cost-effectiveness in assessing value for money in health care and informing resource allocation decisions.

Introduction

The scarcity of resources and the inevitability of illness and death are problems that face every society, both past and present. They impose difficult choices for decision-makers, from politicians to consumers. Either explicitly or implicitly anyone who has to make a choice between options is governed by the basic tenets of economics. Every choice we make has an opportunity cost: a value forgone. If a commissioner chooses to fund a drug to tackle a particular disease, given scarce resources, these funds will not be available to treat another health problem. For every treatment funded, another treatment must be withheld, and as a consequence some patients will not receive care. Therefore, health care must be rationed in some way.

Market forces, the invisible hand of demand and supply, have been shown to be inefficient, and can be deemed unethical, as access to health care is of such fundamental importance to individuals and societies. A completely free market in health care would mean that those without the ability to pay would not receive care. Individuals unable to work due to disability would be left to fend for themselves without the provision of any form of care whatsoever. The consequences are unthinkable, and therefore other means for allocating scarce resources, without total reliance upon the ability to pay, must be utilized. The methods that should determine who will receive care, who will be deprived of care and be left in avoidable pain and discomfort, and perhaps to die, have become central to the debate on how to ration health care and allocate resources.

A number of economic techniques have been used to develop principles and to evaluate the costs and benefits of different treatments. In this chapter, the rationale for economic evaluation is considered; the techniques for economic evaluation to prioritize treatments are described and their limitations discussed; different types of economic evaluation are outlined and a case study is provided to illustrate the process in practice.

What is health economics?

The discipline of economics examines the relationship between scarce resources and infinite wants. Demand and supply interact through the market to determine prices and levels of output, and the invisible hand solves the problem of what to produce, how to produce it and for whom to produce. However, a number of conditions are required for the invisible hand to drive the market to an efficient outcome. These conditions include many consumers and producers competing in a market with full information and certainty. They must also include trade in a homogeneous product where the costs and benefits of consumption fall wholly upon the consumer and producer who are party to the transaction. The analysis of economics and health is complicated because there is no market in health; health cannot be bought and sold. The relevant market in economic terms is the market for *health care*, health care being an intermediate good the demand for which is derived from the demand for health. Health care in itself does not generate utility or wellbeing as would, say, a chocolate bar or a holiday. It is the combination of both health care and time that enable the individual production of health, health being the outcome that yields utility – that is, benefit. The individual's consumption of health care was first put into a formal context in a seminal paper on the demand for health by Grossman (1972).

In health care the conditions for a free market are almost completely violated. In addition, modern societies believe that allocating health care entirely on the basis of the ability to pay is unethical, and to deny the sick any form of health care whatsoever does not sit well with their moral compass. Therefore, alternative means for allocating health care are required as the market is dismissed as undesirable. Policies to achieve these means have given rise to a whole new branch of economics – known as health economics. The main objective is to guide the allocation of scarce health care resources when the traditional forces of demand and supply are deemed to generate an inefficient and/or inequitable outcome.

The rationale for economic evaluation

In the National Health Service (NHS) in the United Kingdom (UK) and other publicly funded health care systems around the world, societies have rejected the use of the price mechanism and the willingness and ability of people to pay to determine access to health care. The free market outcome that would result from the interaction of demand and supply is deemed to be inefficient and inequitable. In these systems, it has been decided that 'need' and not ability to pay should be the dominant criterion for access, but this concept has to be carefully defined.

Rationing access to health care in the face of scarcity involves depriving some patients of care. Given that the demand for care usually exceeds supply, some argue that we should deliver those interventions that 'work', but this raises another definitional problem. How should this 'clinical effectiveness' be defined? For instance, with a hip replacement, the major benefits are the removal of pain and improved mobility. With some cancer care, the focus of doctors is on survival rates of perhaps months or years, often with little attention being paid to the quality of life during this period. Identifying and agreeing the 'end point' – that is, what outcomes should be evaluated and over what period of time would an outcome represent a gain for patients and society – are critical questions. How should outcomes be measured in clinical trials? It is never easy to answer these questions. This makes economic evaluation challenging, as we will discuss below.

Health economics provides an important contribution to health technology assessment (HTA), the systematic evaluation of properties, effects and impacts of health technology from a social, organizational and ethical perspective (Philips et al. 2004). The main purpose of HTA is to provide evidence to inform clinical decision-making. Commissioning cost-effective health care is a vital consideration in the face of limited resources and the health economist provides evidence of the potential value for money when choices must be made between different alternative courses of action.

Dilemmas of economic assessment

Clinical effectiveness is a critical criterion in determining access to care. The economic argument is that clinical effectiveness is a *necessary* characteristic for rationing access to care, but it is not *sufficient* – just because something works it is not an adequate argument that it should be funded. As argued by Maynard (1997), what is clinically effective may not be cost-effective, but what is cost-effective is always clinically effective. Economists have developed a measure for clinical effectiveness in terms of the number of Quality Adjusted Life Years (QALYs) that can be expected as an outcome from a particular treatment. All these words require definition but, put briefly, a QALY is one added year of perfect health. This measure must be set against the costs of treatment to assess clinical cost-effectiveness. QALYs provide the basis for comparing one treatment with another, as described in the example in Box 16.1.

Box 16.1   Purchasing cost-effective health care

Assume that there is a limited budget of £700,000. The costs of the alternative procedures X and Y for a particular disease are known. The benefits of each procedure are also known and measured in QALYs, where one QALY is one year of perfect health.

If therapy X produces five QALYs and therapy Y produces ten QALYs, on the basis of clinical effectiveness, Y is superior and will be preferred by the patient and their physician who, motivated by the individualistic Hippocratic Oath, wishes to do the best for the patient.

However, now consider the costs. What if therapy X costs £15,000 and therapy Y costs £70,000? The decision now should take into account costs as well as clinical effectiveness – we are now interested in cost-effectiveness. Therapy X produces a QALY at an average cost of £3,000, while therapy Y produces a QALY for £7,000. Therapy Y produces an additional five QALYs for an additional cost of £55,000 (£70,000 minus £15,000). The marginal cost of producing a QALY using Y is £11,000 (£55,000 divided by 5).

Therapy X is superior in terms of cost-effectiveness as it produces health QALYs at least cost, while therapy Y is clinically superior as it produces more QALYs. From the individualistic perspective of the patient and their agent, the doctor, therapy Y is preferred. However, from the social perspective of the economist and public health physician, therapy X is preferred as it produces the greatest health gain from a fixed budget. Thus, if a clinic had a fixed budget of £700,000, using therapy Y would produce 100 QALYs of health gain, but if it uses therapy X it will produce more than twice as many QALYs.

This example demonstrates how cost-effectiveness data can be used to achieve society's goal of maximum health gain from its finite health care budget. Indeed, the necessary and sufficient condition for resource allocation and determining access to health care is the relative cost-effectiveness of competing interventions. Those interventions that are cost-effective give the 'biggest health care bang for the NHS buck'. Decision-makers at the National Institute for Health and Care Excellence (NICE) use this criterion to determine access to the new technologies they evaluate (www.nice.org.uk). Cost-effectiveness data can be assessed against a benchmark or threshold; for example, in the UK a benchmark of £20,000 per QALY is often cited. Interventions generating a gain of one QALY for less than this benchmark are deemed to represent good value for money. Internationally, this approach is gradually challenging and eroding the narrow clinical perspective and the individualistic ethic reflected in the Hippocratic Oath, in which the medical practitioner swears to uphold specific ethical standards. However, the focus on the individual would be over-ridden for the greater good if treatment requires an intervention that is not cost-effective. Therefore, instead of being individually focused, treatment may be denied because resources could be utilized to create greater benefits for others – effectively a utilitarian approach.

While techniques of economic evaluation are increasingly used to prioritize interventions competing for funding in health systems, it is important that the evidence used to make decisions is of high quality. Checklists of good practice provide a useful way of elaborating the component parts of an economic evaluation and these guidelines have been refined and differentiated by a range of authors. Some examples are the checklists devised by Drummond and colleagues (2015) and the Consolidated Health Economic Evaluation Reporting Standards (CHEERS) (Husereau et al. 2013). The latter has become a frequently used checklist. A decision is only as good as the information on which it is based, and therefore ensuring that cost-effectiveness evidence is of the highest possible quality is a vital first step in any health economics research.

Specifying the evaluation methodology

When specifying a cost-effectiveness analysis, the first consideration is the selection of study data: whether we should use primary data, for example the data from a randomized controlled trial (RCT), or secondary data, such as data synthesized from previous trials in the relevant clinical area through a systematic review. These can be used to construct a model that will estimate cost-effectiveness. The factors that must be taken into account when deciding the type of analysis are, most obviously, the availability of data. The size of the budget available for the study and an assessment of various timescales are also important. When will the results of the study be required? What is the time-horizon in the study being evaluated? This could be 'a within trial one year' analysis or a projection of an assumed patient lifetime. In many clinical fields there are sources of data that can be used as a basis for model-based simulations. The Cochrane Collaboration is an international collaboration established to organize medical research findings to facilitate evidence-based decision-making by health professionals, patients and policy makers. Cochrane includes review groups and approximately 30,000 volunteer experts from around the world. The Collaboration has established good practice in the evaluation of 'what works' in clinical practice (see also Chapter 21).

The RCT is regarded as the 'gold standard' of measuring clinical effectiveness. However, clinical trials can be expensive to run, budgets are limited (scarce resources come into play again) so it is not always possible to determine effectiveness and cost-effectiveness. Decision-makers may not have the time required to design a trial, recruit patients, follow them up, and then evaluate data prior to a budget allocation in, for example, the service commissioning process in the UK. In addition, time horizons of 12 months are common-place for the final follow-up in many trials. A further problem is that a consideration of longer-term cost-effectiveness requires data on costs and consequences over a time period beyond the final measurements in some trials. In such cases the health economist must rely on models to investigate longer-term value for money.

The demand for longer-term cost-effectiveness data has given rise to the development of methods to extrapolate costs and utilities over a longer period in health economics research (Bojke et al. 2017). The ever-increasing capacity of new technology has made it possible to construct models based on data synthesized from trials and published research to project the future costs and consequences beyond the trial's time horizon, with inbuilt allowances for uncertainty in parameters. Uncertainty in such models can be accommodated by the use of probabilistic sensitivity analysis. Distributions are fitted to the parameters and values drawn in order to represent this uncertainty. A detailed explanation of decision-modelling and the extrapolation of longer-term cost and outcomes is beyond the scope of the current chapter. An excellent introduction to the background and methods of decision-analysis is provided by Briggs, Claxton and Sculpher (2006). The synthesis of evidence for cost-effectiveness analysis is explained in the classic paper by Ades and associates (2006). Bojke and colleagues (2017) provide an introduction to the methods of data extrapolation.

Cost-effectiveness studies evaluate interventions against a comparator. Any new service has to be compared with an alternative. The study description should not only define the alternatives being compared but also explain the choice of alternatives. Sometimes in drug evaluations a placebo or dummy drug is used. This is usually insufficient as we need to know not just whether the new treatment has an effect compared with using a placebo, but whether it is better than the accepted 'best available' treatment being used now. Whatever the alternative, its selection should be explicit and explained.

Study perspective: Which costs and benefits do we include?

The study perspective will determine the range of costs and outcomes that are to be eval-uated and should be clearly stated and justified. In England and Wales, guidance from the National Institute for Health and Care Excellence (NICE) (2017) states that all inter-ventions within an NHS setting should use both an NHS and Personal Social Services perspective to cost the health effects for patients and carers or family members, if these are relevant as outcome measures. NHS costs should include operating costs, capital costs and wider health care costs. Interventions with health and non-health outcomes such as those with a social care focus, should include costs to the public sector or employers and include the health effects on individuals.

Measuring outcomes

There are a number of important issues to be considered when specifying the benefits or outcomes of a health care intervention, in particular:

- The nature of the clinical trial method
- The measurement of the 'end point' or benefit
- The valuation of the benefit or end point
- How long these end points will persist.

Any review of a clinical area will immediately highlight the issue of selection of the end point, or benefit, from trial interventions. The health economist prefers to use direct evidence of improvement in the length and quality of life. However, trials often use intermediate or incomplete 'end points'. For instance, in cancer the principal focus is often on survival or additional months or years of life, with the quality of survival being ignored. For an outcome such as treatment to avoid myocardial infarction (heart attack), we would want to know the life years gained and the quality of life of those years. Economic evaluations build on the clinical evidence base. It is vital that clinical trials and medical research are conducted in a rigorous and scientific manner to ensure that findings can be used to improve current practice.

A complex issue in any economic evaluation is outcome measurement and the assignment of preferences and the valuation given to them. Ideally, we would like a benefit indicator that incorporates increased length and quality of life in a composite measure. However, patients themselves experience many health attributes, including dimensions such as physical and mental functioning and pain. If a single measure of health outcome can be measured, then it would enable comparisons to be made between health care interventions that would otherwise be denominated in different clinical outcomes. We will discuss a solution to this obstacle in the section on cost–utility analysis below.

The timings of costs and benefits

In terms of health benefits, an investment now may produce health benefits over decades. Preventive health care provides a good example. An individual who stops smoking will add years to his or her life and also improve the quality of those future years gained. For an individual, a diagnosis of hypertension involves costs for the rest of that person's life.

The question to be asked is: what is the opportunity cost of a pound spent now compared with a pound spent in ten years' time on this treatment? In these cases, it is expected that an individual would naturally prefer a gain now and a cost in the future. To cope with the time preferences of individuals and of a society, streams of benefits and costs are adjusted in a process called discounting. Economic evaluations that include costs or outcomes beyond the scope of a one-year time horizon should discount these. In the UK, guidance on the use of discounting in economic evaluation is provided by the National Institute for Health and Care Excellence (2017), employing the rate of 3.5 per cent per annum for costs and health outcomes.

Types of economic evaluation

The terms 'economic evaluation' and 'cost–benefit analysis' can be confusing if they are used loosely and without precision. In effect, there are several types of economic evaluation. The following four types of economic evaluation can be found in the literature and are explored further below:

- Cost minimization analysis
- Cost-effectiveness analysis
- Cost–utility analysis
- Cost–benefit analysis.

Before examining the main types of economic evaluation, we should note that studies in health economics that do not fulfil the criteria of a full economic evaluation because both costs and outcomes are not considered, are called 'partial' evaluations. These include 'cost of illness' studies. For example, such studies may estimate the cost to the health service of treating smoking-related disease, or the cost to society that arises from diabetes, but they cannot provide guidance on how to invest resources. They do not show how a disease can be treated efficiently to minimize costs and maximize benefits because they provide no information on the effectiveness of existing treatments. They are not a form of economic evaluation as there is no comparison with alternative interventions.

Cost-minimization analysis

Cost-minimization analysis (CMA) involves the identification, measurement and valuation of the costs of competing therapies. In such a study, it is assumed that the outcome of the alternatives is identical. Thus, the focus of the analysis is partial. It seeks to identify which of two alternatives is cheapest.

One of the early examples of the CMA approach was an analysis of alternative methods for treating varicose veins. Piachaud and Weddell (1972) identified two interventions:

surgery and injection-compression therapy in an outpatient clinic. They measured the cost of health service resource use and the individual cost to patients in terms of the time and cost of entering treatment. The authors also examined the wage cost losses of those treated but made no attempt to value unpaid activity such as the services provided by carers. The study was based on an RCT. After three years of follow-up, the results for patients under 60 showed that both interventions were equally effective. The authors concluded that as the cost of injections was less than a third of the cost of surgery, and the loss of earnings was much less than in the non-surgical arm of the trial. Injection therapy was therefore preferred as it was less costly and just as effective. However, a subsequent follow-up of the patients in the trial showed that at five years the equivalence of outcome was valid only for patients aged less than 35. In this group there were no signs of venous insufficiency. For the majority of patients, the longer-term outcomes of surgery were superior. Thus decision-makers faced the choice of whether to fund an intervention that was more expensive but gave better results in the longer term.

Cost-effectiveness analysis

Cost-effectiveness analysis (CEA) is an approach that has roots that are at odds with the goals of modern economic evaluations in health care. CEA was devised by the United States military during the Korean War to identify the cheapest way to kill enemy soldiers. For instance, what were the relative costs of bombing the enemy, using napalm gas, using tanks and using infantry, and how successful were these methods measured by 'body count'? Thankfully, more recent applications have measured lives saved or life years gained rather than lives lost. CEA involves the costing of alternatives and the use of an intervention-specific measure of success. In health care where our interest is in improving the length and quality of patients' lives, the CEA approach involves costing alternatives and using outcome measures such as reductions in blood pressure or lives saved.

CEA has a significant drawback that has led to a curtailment of its use in recent years. CEA does not enable us to make evaluative comparisons across specialities. For example, we may measure the outcome of a hip-replacement programme to improve a patient's mobility, but how would we assess the relative value for money compared to a programme that aimed to help individuals to stop smoking, measured by the quit rate? We cannot compare the two because we do not know the relative worth of an improvement in mobility and a reduction in the rate of smoking. Only when we measure the two competing alternatives using a common unit can we make decisions about their relative cost-effectiveness.

Cost-utility analysis

The absence of a generic benefit measure that informs choices between interventions in therapeutic areas in CEA has led to the development of cost–utility analysis (CUA) which is now a core element in the appraisal process for new technologies used by NICE (2017).

The construct that has been adopted to overcome this hurdle is the Quality Adjusted Life Year, or the QALY. The first stage of measuring QALYs is to measure patient outcomes, using a preference-based, multi-attribute, health status measurement. The most common instrument used is the EQ-5D (EuroQol Group 1990). EQ-5D has five dimensions (mobility, self-care, usual activities, pain/discomfort and anxiety/depression – see www. euroqol.org). The scores from EQ-5D can be used as a 'weighted health index' that gives a numerical value for quality of life in a given health state. Such scores can be used in the calculation of QALYs (for further explanation, see Drummond et al. 2015). A five-level version of EQ-5D, the EQ-5D-5L, is also available (van Hout et al. 2012). Besides EQ-5D there are other available methods of generating QALYs, with the SF-6D (Brazier and Roberts 2004) offering an alternative means of constructing utility-based health outcomes.

A QALY combines the estimated increases in survival with health status valuations using quality of life measures such as EQ-5D. One QALY stands for one year of perfect health and it is measured on an interval scale. Figure 16.1 shows the two dimensions incorporated into the QALY, the quantity of life measured in natural years of life (x-axis) and the quality of life, measured as an index between 0 and 1.0 on the y-axis. Plotting life years and quality of life enables us to calculate QALYs. In the figure, all three profiles show one QALY despite the patient living for different numbers of life years in each profile. For example, patient A survives for one year at quality of life index 1.0, hence has 1 × 1.0 = 1 QALY. Patient B survives for two years with a quality of life index of 0.5, so has 2 × 0.5 = 1 QALY

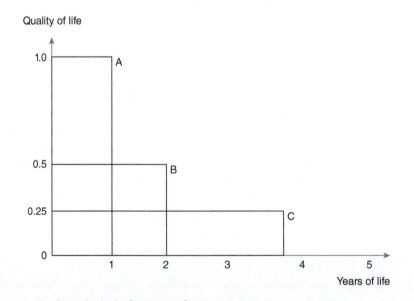

FIGURE 16.1   Quality Adjusted Life Year profiles

while patient C survives for four years at quality of life index of 0.25 and has 4 × 0.25 = 1 QALY. Hence, despite the three individuals having different numbers of natural life years, when adjusted for quality in terms of QALYs, they are all the same.

In using QALYs, a major issue is whose valuation of quality of life should be employed. Doctors and nurses are better informed about health states and interventions than patients. However, patients are informed about the health states they experience, but not about those that they have not experienced. Typically, patients rate health states higher than health care professionals. An alternative source of evaluation is the wider society, where a mix of informed and uninformed views can be obtained. The current EQ-5D values are based on those generated from a sample of the general public. Studies show that typically this gives values lower than those of patients.

There continues to be considerable argument about the validity of QALY estimates. Typical challenges include: Do they really measure what they claim to measure? Are they reliable (that is, reproducible and consistent)? Are they sensitive to small health state changes? Are they stable over time and independent of the duration of time in a health state? One pragmatic response of QALY adherents is that they may be imperfect, but they are the best approach available.

Cost-benefit analysis

Cost–benefit analysis (CBA) involves the identification, measurement and valuation of both the monetary costs of each alternative treatment considered in an evaluation, together with the monetary value of the benefits.

Translating the stream of benefits from any intervention into monetary equivalents can be done by contingent valuation (CV) or willingness to pay (WTP) studies, whose purpose is to apply a monetary valuation for common or societal goods, such as pollution and services, or, for example, the value patients place on being able to control their symptoms. These goods are not traded in markets. CV seeks measures to value all health factors, such as the length and quality of life outcomes, and non-health factors, such as privacy and politeness in the treatment process.

A CBA involves investigating how much individuals are willing to pay to avoid ill health or to improve their health. For instance, let us assume that you are in pain. There are two treatments: drug X and drug Y. You are informed that drugs X and Y are equally effective in controlling your pain. However, drug X gives 1 patient in 100 stomach bleeds, while drug Y gives bleeds to 3 in 100 patients. How much would you be willing to pay, to get drug X? How much will you pay to reduce the risk of a stomach bleed from 3 to 1 per cent?

The findings of a CBA are presented in terms of a net monetary cost or net monetary benefit. Expressing the overall result in monetary units gives rise to a key advantage of CBA, namely that programmes can be compared across different areas of spending.

For example, we can assess the net economic impact of a health care intervention compared with an educational programme, a road-building scheme or an environmental protection policy, provided that CBA is undertaken using the same guidelines across the different sectors.

The CBA approach poses many difficulties, most notably the valuation of health outcomes, translating physical and mental health into monetary units, with the associated ethical as well as methodological considerations. In terms of methods, there is evidence that the method used to elicit valuations affects the values given. There is also a risk that respondents may state high values for their preferred alternative as in the NHS they do not actually have to pay. Furthermore, given the societal perspective that requires all costs and outcomes to be measured and valued, difficulties arise in attributing impacts further afield from the intervention, given the multiplicity of causal links. For example, what is the value of lost output as a consequence of a patient's family taking time off work to take him or her to a hospital appointment? CBA requires vast quantities of data, and the execution of a CBA itself has an opportunity cost in terms of resources. Such methodological difficulties may give rise to the use of proxies for costs, such as using national average wage rates to value time or productivity costs and outcomes. CBA is rarely used in practice in health technology assessment.

Comparing value

Health utility, measured by instruments such as QALYs, is now required in technology appraisals by regulatory agencies such as NICE (2017). Studies denominated in a common unit can be used to compare value for money across clinical areas, areas which would be almost impossible to assess in a comparative way when measured in different clinical outcomes. Tables of health care interventions listed in terms of the cost per QALY are known as 'QALY league tables'.

The use of cost per QALY data, ranked in these league tables, has been criticized because, *inter alia*, such tables have previously been compiled from studies using differing methods. For example, there may be differences in the valuations made in QALYs, or in the estimation of costs. Different costing techniques or different categories of cost and study perspectives may be applied. The QALY league table approach illustrates how the relative ranking of technologies can determine a regulatory sanction or rejection, based on a benchmark cost per QALY. Some argue that the value of a QALY for different groups might be weighted to reflect equity concerns – for example, whether an additional QALY for a poor recipient as opposed to a rich one is of greater value to a society interested in decreasing health inequalities. Following this direction, research has focused on how equity can be built explicitly into economic evaluation (Cookson, Drummond and Weatherley 2009). Early literature in this area included conjecture of a 'fair innings' by Alan Williams (1997), whereby elderly citizens could give up the use of efficient interventions to fund the inefficient treatment of young people who would otherwise die prematurely after a short life span. Technology assessments typically do not use weights based on social class or age, but there continues to be a vigorous academic debate about whether they should take these factors into account.

Drummond and colleagues (2015) and Husereau and colleagues (2013) argue that studies should be subjected to a rigorous checklist before a QALY league table is compiled. This is because a range of methodologies can be used to undertake an economic evaluation and to make comparisons on value for money between different and competing interventions. Such checks are required to enable interventions to compete on a 'level playing field' and identify any inherent biases that may give rise to a misleading conclusion or comparisons made between the value for money afforded by different and competing interventions.

Efficiency, ethics and equity

Is economic evaluation ethical? From the economic perspective, waste or the inefficient use of society's scarce resources is unethical as it deprives potential patients of care. The application of techniques of economic evaluation assumes that the policy maker's objective is efficiency – namely, maximizing health gains (QALYs) from a finite budget. Nonetheless, society often chooses to act inefficiently, for example by intervening to save the lives of very low birthweight babies. This is inefficient because the incidence of disability is high, but it is funded as society values young lives highly.

Other social values may override the pursuit of efficiency. For instance, QALYs are weighted equally in routine economic evaluations but if your objective is to reduce health inequality, should QALYs accruing to the poor be weighted more highly than QALYs accruing to the rich? As noted earlier, Williams (1997), when considering the health care costs of elderly people, advocated the 'fair innings' argument. He claimed that life beyond the allocated 'three score and ten' was a bonus that should be discriminated against, such that the efficient treatment of elderly people should be forgone and resources shifted to the inefficient treatment of the young who might not have a fair innings due to, for example, to disability. Equity arguments such as these are generally ignored by health technology agencies such as NICE in the UK and parallel bodies in Europe, Canada and Australasia. Their concern, perhaps contentiously, remains the maximization of society's overall health status.

Reading health research based on economics

In this chapter advice has already been given on how to critically assess the role of economics in health research, especially in the evaluation of service or treatment interventions.

In this respect, the following questions are worth reiterating as key points to note when reading an economic evaluation and assessing the evaluation in terms of its usefulness in guiding decision-making:

- Are the research question and associated objectives clearly identified?
- What is the role of the particular service or treatment intervention?
- What would be the consequence of doing nothing?
- What is the comparator service or treatment intervention?
- Are all the costs of the new service or treatment identified?
- Have these costs been measured and valued against comparators?
- Are all the benefits identified, measured and valued?
- What are the political/ethical implications of the analysis?

Of course, health economists are not only concerned with the cost-effectiveness and cost–benefits associated with service or treatment interventions, but this is a very important part of their work. As demands on health care increase, due to advances in technology and the effects of increasing and ageing populations, the need to ensure that resources are not used wastefully becomes ever more important. It is not sufficient just to demonstrate that something works; it is also necessary to show that it is cost-effective and offers value for money. The latter is the domain of the health economist, providing cost-effectiveness data to guide decision making, adding another dimension to ensure that societies make the most of the limited resources at their disposal.

Conclusion

Limited resources and the seemingly endless demands placed upon them indicate that societies will always have to make choices. The development of the discipline of health economics and economic evaluation techniques offer an explicit framework into which evidence of cost and effect can be inserted, often as probabilistic statements. Decisions should be based on cost-effectiveness as opposed to solely effectiveness – just because something *can* be done effectively it does *not* mean that it *should* be done. The deployment of resources to satisfy one goal inevitably means that another goal is forgone, and the use of economic evaluation enables the commissioners (those who 'commission' health services in a quasi-market for their populations) to identify the opportunity cost – what is the value of the alternative that is foregone. As computing technology has advanced since the first economic evaluations were published, the longer-term projection of costs and consequences, based on combinations of trial data and published data, are put together to provide a synthesis of evidence.

Economic evaluations inform those charged with making the difficult rationing choices facing society. However, the health economist does not claim to have all the answers or to provide prescriptive guidance for the allocation of resources. Instead, the role is to provide unbiased cost-effectiveness evidence on which commissioners can make better informed decisions, incorporating value for money data with other criteria to guide resource allocation. The chapter has made a distinction between different types of economic evaluation and what they aim to do. It has also drawn attention to the weaknesses of many studies. The reader should look for rigour and objectivity in the research that underpins economic assessments. An exercise has been included in which the reader can apply some of the basic principles covered in this chapter.

Exercise 16.1 Which treatment should be funded?

A health care commissioner has a budget of £5,000,000. Table 16.1 shows three interventions that could be purchased with the budget, together with the cost per person and the QALYs gained per patient.

TABLE 16.1 The costs and benefits of health interventions

Intervention	Cost/patient	QALYs gained /patient	Patients treated	Cost/ QALY
Hospital haemodialysis for chronic renal failure	£20,000	1		
Smoking cessation advice and nicotine replacement therapy	£1,000	5.4		
Heart transplantation	£50,000	5		

Applying health economics to the problem:

- With each intervention, how many patients can be treated and what is the cost per QALY?
- What information would you seek as the commissioner to provide a case for increasing the budget allocation for these interventions?
- What are the costs and benefits of adopting interventions?
- Explain how equity and efficiency may conflict in the choices made by the decision-maker. Should the decision-maker aim for a 'fair' allocation of care or the maximum health gain?

Note

This chapter is written in memory of the late Professor Alan Maynard, who was the sole writer of this chapter in previous editions of the book.

Recommended further reading

This text provides an introduction to health economics for the beginner, including the rationale for evaluation, the types of evaluation, and measuring costs and benefits:

Drummond, M. F., Sculpher, M. J., Claxton, K., Stoddart, G. L. and Torrance, G. W. (2015) *Methods for the Economic Evaluation of Health Care Programmes*, 4th edition. Oxford: Oxford University Press.

This text reports standards for economic evaluations aiming at quality, consistency and comparability:

Husereau, D., Drummond, M., Petrou, S., Carswell, C., Moher, D., Greenberg, D., Augustovski, F., Briggs, A. H., Mauskopf, J. and Loder, E. (2013) 'Consolidated Health Economic Evaluation Reporting Standards (CHEERS) – explanation and elaboration: A report of the ISPOR Health Economic Evaluation Publication Guidelines Good Reporting Practices Task Force', *Value in Health*, 16(2): 231–50.

This book provides an introduction to decision-modelling for economic evaluation with examples. It demonstrates how to structure a decision model and the use of different types of models:

Briggs, A., Claxton, K. and Sculpher, M. (2006) *Decision Modelling for Health Economic Evaluation*. Oxford: Oxford University Press.

References

Ades, A. E., Sculpher, M., Sutton, A., Abrams, K., Cooper, N., Welton, N. and Lu, G. B. (2006) 'Bayesian methods for evidence synthesis in cost-effectiveness analysis', *Pharmacoeconomics*, 24(1): 1–19.

Bojke, L., Manca, A., Asaria, M., Mahon, R., Ren, S. and Palmer, S. (2017) 'How to appropriately extrapolate costs and utilities in cost-effectiveness analysis', *PharmacoEconomics*, 35(8): 767–76.

Brazier, J. E. and Roberts, J. R. (2004) 'The estimation of a preference-based index from the SF-12', *Medical Care*, 42(9): 851–9.

Briggs, A., Claxton, K. and Sculpher, M. (2006) *Decision Modelling for Health Economic Evaluation*. Oxford: Oxford University Press.

Cookson, R., Drummond, M. and Weatherly, H. (2009) 'Explicit incorporation of equity considerations into economic evaluation of public health interventions', *Health Economics, Policy and Law, 4*(2): 231–45.

Drummond, M. F., Sculpher, M. J., Claxton, K., Stoddart, G. L. and Torrance, G. W. (2015) *Methods for the Economic Evaluation of Health Care Programmes*, 4th edition. Oxford: Oxford University Press.

EuroQol Group (1990) 'EuroQol: A new facility for the measurement of health related quality of life', *Health Policy, 16*: 199–208.

Grossman, M. (1972) 'On the concept of health capital and the demand for health', *Journal of Political Economy, 80*(2): 223–55.

Husereau, D., Drummond, M., Petrou, S., Carswell, C., Moher, D., Greenberg, D., Augustovski, F., Briggs, A. H., Mauskopf, J. and Loder, E. (2013) 'Consolidated Health Economic Evaluation Reporting Standards (CHEERS) – explanation and elaboration: A report of the ISPOR Health Economic Evaluation Publication Guidelines Good Reporting Practices Task Force', *Value in Health, 16*(2): 231–50.

Maynard, A. (1997) 'Evidence based medicine: An incomplete method for informing treatment choices', *Lancet, 349*: 126–8.

National Institute for Health and Care Excellence (2017) *Developing NICE Guidelines: The Manual*. London: NICE. Available at: www.nice.org.uk/process/pmg20/chapter/about-this-manual

Philips, Z., Ginnelly, L., Sculpher, M., Claxton, K., Golder, S., Riemsma, R., Woolacott, N. and Glanville, J. (2004) 'A review of guidelines for good practice in decision analytic modelling in health technology assessment', *Health Technology Assessment, 8*(36): 1–158.

Piachaud, D. and Weddell, J. M. (1972) 'The economics of treating varicose veins', *International Journal of Epidemiology, 1*: 287–94.

van Hout, B., Janssen, M. F., Feng, Y. S., Kohlmann, T., Busschbach, J., Golicki, D., Lloyd, A., Scalone, L., Kind, P. and Pickard, A. S. (2012) 'Interim scoring for the EQ-5D-5L: Mapping the EQ-5D-5L to EQ-5D-3L value sets', *Value in Health, 15*(5): 708–15.

Williams, A. (1997) 'The rationing debate: Rationing health care by age – the case for', *British Medical Journal, 314*: 820–5.

17

Quantitative Data Analysis

GEORGE ARGYROUS

Chapter objectives

- To give a basic introduction to the statistical methods for analysing health data, including the factors that govern the choice of appropriate methods
- To provide an understanding of basic statistical analysis and presentation of descriptive statistics, including graphs, tables, and numerical measures of central tendency and dispersion
- To describe measures of association and correlation and the logic of inferential statistics through hypothesis testing and the use of confidence intervals
- To illustrate the application of this knowledge to a given data set.

Introduction

This chapter provides a basic introduction to statistics for analysing health data. Although there are a number of texts that detail the use of statistics in the health field, the distinguishing feature of this chapter is its accessibility in introducing the subject of data analysis – what we do with quantitative research information once we have gathered it. More specifically, this chapter helps us to describe data more effectively. As such, it focuses on the first step in statistical analysis – straightforward statistical description – pointing the way to more advanced methods for those who wish to undertake further reading on the subject. For example, if we have collected measurements for the sex, age, amount of weekly exercise, smoking history and health status of patients visiting a clinic on a certain day, this chapter should help us to communicate this information more effectively, beyond simply listing the individual measurements that give the distribution for each of these variables.

Data analysis and research questions

We do not gather quantitative data for their own sake. We do so to help us answer research questions, to inform our understanding of the world so as to improve health outcomes. For example, we might be interested in the following four research questions that have prompted us to gather data through a survey:

- What is the health status of respondents in the survey?
- Is there a relationship between the health status of respondents and their smoking level?
- Is any relationship between health status and smoking level affected by other factors, such as amount of regular exercise?
- Can we generalize the results from our sample survey to the whole population?

These four questions follow a pattern: they begin with the simple and become more complex. The first question is only interested in a single variable, which is the survey respondents' health status. We call this a *univariate question*, since it is interested in the distribution of a single variable (i.e. health status). We then ask whether this overall health status is somehow related to respondents' smoking levels; a question that addresses the possible *relationship* between two variables requires *bivariate statistical analysis*. At a higher level of complexity *multivariate analysis* takes into account many other factors, such as age and exercise. And lastly, if the data come from a sample survey, we ask whether the answers to the earlier questions tell us something about the whole population.

This general sequence of research questions corresponds to the way in which data analysis should progress, that is from simple to complex analysis (Pryjmachuk and Richards 2007). This chapter is organized this way. As a general point, it is usually best not too 'dive into the deep end' and do complex quantitative analysis without having done some simple analysis first. There are aspects to the data that we may miss if we do the complex analysis first. The sequence of questions listed above allows us to 'build a story' about what the data tell us to inform our understanding of the world.

Descriptive statistics

You will notice that the first three questions listed above involve analysis of the data we have collected for survey respondents. There is a whole class of statistics – descriptive statistics – that help us answer such questions by summarizing the data in particular ways.

Descriptive statistics are the numerical, graphical and tabular techniques for organizing, analysing and presenting data. The major types of descriptive statistics are listed in Table 17.1, broken down by the question types we listed above. The great advantage of descriptive statistics is that they make a mass of research material easier to 'read' by reducing a large set of data into a few statistics, or into a graph or table.

TABLE 17.1   Types of descriptive statistics

Type	Function	Examples
Graphs	Provide a visual representation of the distribution of a variable or variables	Pie, bar, histogram, polygon (univariate)
		Clustered pie, clustered/stacked bar (bivariate, nominal/ordinal scales)
		Scatterplot (bivariate, interval/ratio scales)
Tables	Provide a frequency distribution for a variable or variables	Frequency table (univariate)
		Cross-tabulations (bivariate/multivariate)
Numerical measures	Mathematical operations used to quantify, in a single number, particular features of a distribution	Measures of central tendency (univariate)
		Measures of dispersion (univariate)
		Measures of association and correlation (bivariate/multivariate)

Levels of measurement

As well as the complexity of the research question, the main factor that determines the type of quantitative analysis undertaken is the level at which each variable is measured (Stevens 1946). To illustrate what is meant by *levels of measurement*, assume that the health status of the patients in our study is measured in three different ways, based on the simplified measures used in the Australian Bureau of Statistics (2014–2015):

*   By classifying patients according to the organ of the body affected by their disease (for example, blood and blood-forming organs, the nervous system, the respiratory system)
*   By classifying patients according to whether they rate themselves as Very Unhealthy, Unhealthy, Healthy or Very Healthy
*   By counting the number of times in the previous year a patient has consulted a doctor or other health professional.

Each of these scales provides a different amount of information about the variation in health status among patients. The first scale of measurement classifies patients according to the organ system where the disease is located. This scale only allows us to say that patients are qualitatively different according to the location of the disease and, as such, is an example of a *nominal* scale: it classifies cases into categories that have no quantitative ordering.

Compare this to the second scale for measuring health status. The four categories that make up the scale have a logical order, starting with the lowest point, Very Unhealthy, and moving up to the highest point, Very Healthy. This scale allows us not only to talk about patients being different in terms of their health status, but also to say that the health status of individual patients is better or worse than others. This ability to *rank-order* cases according to the quantity or intensity of the variable expressed by each case makes this an *ordinal* scale. We cannot, however, measure how much healthier one person is relative to another.

The third scale for measuring health status does allow us to measure such differences. As with nominal and ordinal scales, measuring the number of times in the past year someone has consulted a health professional allows us to classify patients into different groups. As with ordinal (but not nominal) scales, we can rank patients according to their respective scores from lowest to highest. But unlike both nominal and ordinal scales, we can measure the differences – the intervals – between them. We now have a unit of measurement, the number of consultations, which allows us to quantify the difference in health status. This is therefore an example of an *interval/ratio* scale (sometimes called a *metric* scale).

This example of measuring health status illustrates that any given variable can be measured at different levels, depending on the particular scale that is used. This is important. We must be clear about the level at which a variable has been measured. The descriptive statistics we calculate to express any variation across cases may be limited by this fact.

We will begin our discussion by focusing on those descriptive statistics that help us answer the *first* of the four questions listed above. This asks about the distribution of a single variable, in this case health status.

Graphs

Graphs or *charts* are the simplest, and often the most striking, method for describing data, and there are some general rules that apply to their construction. Most importantly, a graph should be a self-contained bundle of information. This can be achieved in various ways. We need to:

- Give the graph a clear title indicating the variable displayed and the cases that make up the study
- Clearly identify the categories or values of the variable
- Indicate, for interval/ratio data, the units of measurement
- Indicate the total number of cases

- Explain any difference between the total in the graph and the total number of cases in the study
- Indicate the source of the data.

There are different ways of presenting data, such as pie charts and bar graphs.

Pie charts

The pie graph drawn for the patient survey in Figure 17.1 illustrates these rules of presentation. A *pie graph* presents the distribution of cases in the form of a circle. The relative size of each slice of the pie is equal to the proportion of cases within the category represented by the slice. Pie charts can be constructed for all levels of measurement and their main function is to emphasize the relative importance of a particular category to the total. They are therefore mainly used to highlight distributions where cases are concentrated in only one or two categories. For example, the pie chart in Figure 17.1 highlights the heavy concentration of patients who have a disease of the respiratory system.

Pie graphs begin to look a bit clumsy when there are too many categories for the variable. As a rule of thumb, there should be no more than five slices to the pie. Thus, the pie chart in Figure 17.1 has grouped together a number of categories with low frequencies into an 'Other' category.

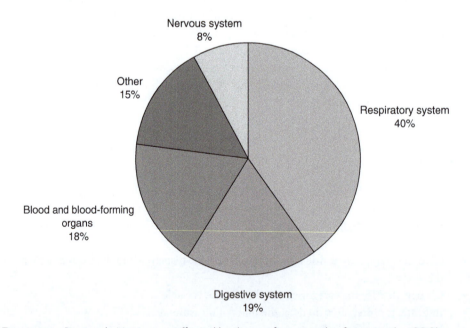

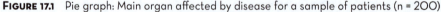

FIGURE 17.1   Pie graph: Main organ affected by disease for a sample of patients (n = 200)

Bar graphs and histograms

Bar graphs and *histograms* emphasize the frequency of cases in each category relative to each other. Along one axis of these graphs are the categories or values of the scale. This axis is called the *abscissa* and is usually the horizontal base of the graph. Along the other axis are the *frequencies*, expressed either as the raw count or as percentages of the total number of cases. This axis is known as the *ordinate*. This is usually the left, vertical axis. A rectangle is erected over each point on the abscissa, with the area of each rectangle being proportional to the frequency of the value in the overall distribution.

The difference between bar graphs and histograms is that bar graphs are constructed for discrete variables, such as the sex of patients, which are usually measured on a nominal or ordinal scale, as illustrated by Figure 17.2.

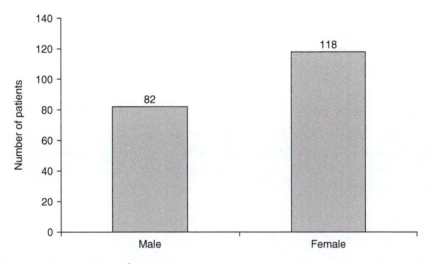

FIGURE 17.2   Bar graph: Sex of patients

With bar graphs, there are always gaps between each of the bars: there is no gradation between male and female, for example. A person's age, on the other hand, is a continuous variable: it increases progressively. As a result, the bars on the histogram for age in Figure 17.3 are 'pushed together'.

As an alternative to a histogram, Figure 17.3 also presents the distribution for age of patients in the form of a *frequency polygon*. This is a continuous line formed by plotting the values in a distribution against the frequency for each value.

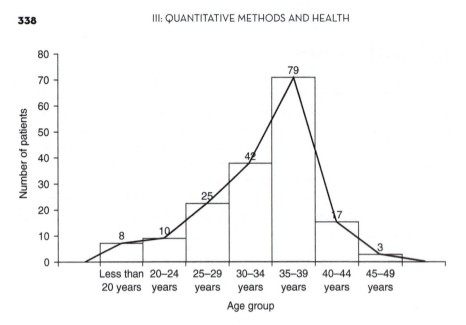

FIGURE 17.3   Histogram: Age of patients

Interpreting graphs

Once we have constructed the relevant graph, we then need to interpret it in a way that helps us answer the first type of research question we listed above. When we look at a graph, we generally try to identify one or more of the following four aspects of the univariate distribution it represents:

- The shape
- The centre
- The spread
- The existence of outliers.

There are certain common *shapes* that appear in research. For example, the histogram for age in Figure 17.3 is 'bell shaped' or 'mound shaped'. For a distribution that has this 'bell shape', we also describe its *skewness*. If the curve has a long tail to the right, it is *positively skewed*, or, as is the case with the age distribution of patients, a long tail to the left indicates a *negatively skewed* distribution. If the tails on either side look reasonably similar, we describe the shape as *symmetrical*.

To gauge the *centre* of a distribution, imagine that the bars of the histogram are lead weights sitting on a balance beam. Where would we have to locate a balance point along the bottom edge of the graph to prevent it from tipping either to the left or right? This, in a loose fashion, identifies the average or typical score. In the example in Figure 17.3, we might say that the average age of patients is around 35–39 years of age.

We can also observe how tightly clustered our measurements are around the central point. Do the scores *spread* very widely across the range of possible values (that is, the distribution is *heterogeneous*) or are most of them similar to each other (that is, the distribution is *homogeneous*)?

Lastly, we can also note the existence of any *outliers* that are not just at the upper or lower end of the tails but are disconnected from the rest of the group. Figure 17.4, for example, presents the annual frequency of visiting a health professional. We can immediately see an outlier with 12 visits to a health professional in the previous year. Where we identify such an outlier, we can isolate the reason why it appears (data entry error or real case) and exclude it from further analysis so that it does not distort other statistics. But when we exclude an outlier from further analysis, in any account we need to always make it clear that we have done so.

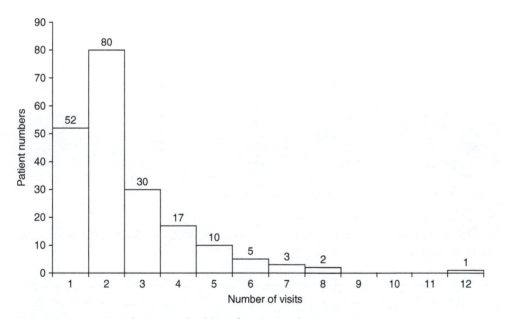

FIGURE 17.4 Number of visits to a health professional in the past year

Frequency tables

The power of graphs is their simplicity; the visual impact of a graph can convey a message better than the most advanced statistics. The simplicity of graphs can also be their weakness.

We often do want to 'dig deeper' to extract more precise understandings of the data than can be gleaned from a chart. Obtaining a more detailed breakdown of a distribution usually begins with the construction of *frequency tables*. At the very least, a frequency table tallies up the number of times (*f*) each value of the variables appears in a distribution. Such a table has in the first column the name of the variable displayed in the title row, followed by the categories or values of the variable down the subsequent rows. Then, the second column presents the frequencies for each category or value. Table 17.2 presents the same distribution as Figure 17.4 but provides much more detail about the frequency of cases across the range of scores for the number of visits to the doctor.

TABLE 17.2   Number of visits to doctor or other health professional in the previous year

Number of visits	Frequency	Per cent*	Cumulative frequency	Cumulative per cent
1	52	26	52	26
2	80	40	132	66
3	30	15	162	81
4	17	9	172	86
5	10	5	182	95
6	5	3	187	97
7	3	2	197	99
8	2	1	199	99
More than 8	1	<1	200	100
Total	200	100		

Note: * Does not add up to 100 per cent due to rounding error.

Frequency tables follow the same rules of presentation that we listed above for graphs, with the addition of the following points:

- Arrange the values of ordinal and interval/ratio scales so that the lowest score in the distribution appears in the first row and the scale then increases down the page. Thus, in Table 17.2, which presents the distribution of an interval/ratio scale, we have as the first row those who visited a health professional only once.
- Arrange the categories of nominal scales so that the category with the highest frequency (referred to below as the mode) is the first row. The category with the second highest frequency is the second row, and so on. The modal category is often of specific interest when analysing the distribution of a nominal variable, and therefore it is convenient to present it first.

Table 17.2 also provides the *relative frequencies*. These express the number of cases within each value of a variable as a percentage or proportion of the total number of cases. *Percentages* are statistics that standardize the total number of cases to a base value of 100, whereas *proportions* standardize the total to a base of 1. The formulae for calculating a percentage (%) or proportion (p) respectively are:

$$\% = \frac{f}{n} \times 100$$

$$p = \frac{f}{n}$$

where *f* is the frequency of cases in a particular category and *n* is the total number of cases.

An alternative to percentages and proportions for expressing relative frequencies is to use *rates*. Rates express the frequency of something in terms of a number larger than 100, such as 1,000 or 100,000 or 1,000,000. Rates are often used in health data analysis to express the incidence of diseases. The number of women experiencing breast cancer, for example, relative to the total population in any given country, is small. When expressed as a percentage we would have a very small fractional number, such as 0.021 per cent. A better way to express this is to say 21 per 100,000 females. It is easier to think in terms of whole-number comparisons than fractions to many decimal places, and the use of rates allows us to do this. The base upon which the rate is expressed, such as per 100,000, is determined by whatever multiple of 10 will give the incidence as a whole number.

Notice that the column of percentages in Table 17.2 should add up to 100 per cent, since all cases must fall into one classification or another. The actual percentages listed in the table, however, sum to 101 per cent, as the numbers have been 'rounded off'. Where this occurs, a footnote should be added to the table that states 'Does not sum to 100 due to rounding error', or words to that effect, as is done in Table 17.2.

With ordinal and interval/ratio data, one further extension to the simple frequency table can be made, which is also illustrated in Table 17.2. This is the addition of columns providing *cumulative frequencies* and *cumulative relative frequencies*. Since ordinal and interval/ratio scales allow us to rank-order cases from lowest to highest. It is sometimes interesting to know the number, and/or percentage, of cases that fall above or below a certain point on the scale. For example, in Table 17.2 we can see that 162 patients (81 per cent) visited a health professional three times or less. This is the sum of the frequencies in the first three rows of the table. By implication, this means that 19 per cent of patients visited a health professional more than three times in the last year. Cumulative frequencies are not appropriate where we have a nominal scale, as the ordering of the categories is not fixed, or where there are only two categories, as the simple frequencies and cumulative frequencies will be the same.

One additional point needs to be made about tabulating interval/ratio data: we often use *class intervals* rather than individual values to construct a frequency distribution. A class interval groups together a range of values for presentation and analysis. We use class intervals if the range of values that appears in the distribution is so large that it makes presentation and analysis difficult. For example, if we have many individual ages for the patients in our study, we may first group them into five-year intervals, such as 1–5 years, 6–10 years, and so on, before constructing the table or graph. Generally, class intervals should have the same width, although at the lower and upper end of the data range we often have open-ended intervals, such as '60 years or over'. The exception is the value of 0, which is usually listed separately. It is common for readers of tables to be specifically interested in the number of cases that have a zero value for a particular variable. The actual width of class intervals depends on the particular situation, especially the amount of information required. The wider the class intervals, the easier it is to 'read' the table, since this will reduce the number of rows. However, this increase in 'readability' comes at the cost of information, and therefore should not be undertaken if the data collected are already in a few, easily presented, values.

Measures of central tendency

We mentioned above that graphs and tables give us a quick visual sense of key features of a distribution. But we sometimes want to be more precise about the centre of a distribution. For instance, rather than stating that 'the scores tend to centre around an average of 35–39 years', we may need to be more precise about the average score. *Measures of central tendency* indicate the typical or average value for a distribution.

There are three common measures of central tendency: mode, median and mean. Each measure embodies a different notion of the 'average'. Choosing the measure to calculate on a given set of data is restricted by the level at which a variable is measured.

The mode

The *mode* (M_o) is the simplest measure of central tendency and can be calculated for all levels of measurement. The mode is the value in a distribution that has the highest frequency. The great advantage of the mode over other measures of centre is that it is very easy to calculate. A simple inspection of a frequency table is enough to determine the mode. In Table 17.2, for example, we can see that the most frequent number of times a patient visited a health professional is 2, which accounts for 80 patients. However, the mode has one major limitation that arises, especially when it is used to describe interval/ratio data that have many values. Take, for example, the following scores that represent the time in seconds for a drug to take effect on a sample of patients, arranged in rank order:

$$36, 36, 81, 82, 84, 85, 86, 89, 91, 95, 97, 98$$

It is clear to the naked eye that the data are 'centred' somewhere in the range of 85–90 seconds. Yet the mode is 36 seconds since this appears twice in the distribution, whereas every other score appears only once. The mode is not really reflecting the central tendency of this distribution. We should either use another measure of central tendency, such as those we are about to discuss, or else organize the data into suitable class intervals, and report the modal class interval, rather than the individual modal score.

The mean and median

With interval/ratio data, the *mean* and *median* can be calculated as measures of central tendency rather than the mode. The mean is the sum of all scores in a distribution divided by the total number of cases. The actual formula we use to calculate the mean depends on whether we have the data in listed form or tallied in a frequency table. If we have the raw data with each individual score listed separately, the equations for the mean of the population and the mean of a sample respectively are:

$$\mu = \frac{\sum X_i}{N}, \bar{X} = \frac{\sum X_i}{n}$$

where μ (pronounced 'mu') is the mean for an entire population, N is the size of the population, X (pronounced 'X-bar') is the mean for a sample, n is the size of the sample, and X_i is each score in a distribution. The Greek alphabet symbol Σ (pronounced 'sigma') means 'the sum of' (or 'the total from the addition of'), so we read these equations in the following way: 'the mean equals the sum of all scores divided by the number of cases'.

Alternatively, where the scores are already grouped into a frequency table, such as in Table 17.2, the relevant formula for a sample is:

$$\bar{X} = \frac{\sum fX_i}{n}$$

This formula instructs us to multiply each score by the frequency with which it appears in the table and to sum these products before dividing by the number of cases. For Table 17.2, the calculations will be:

$$\bar{X} = \frac{\sum fX_i}{n}$$

$$= \frac{(1 \times 52) + (2 \times 80) + (3 \times 30) + (4 \times 17) + (5 \times 10) + (6 \times 5) + (3 \times 7) + (2 \times 8)}{199}$$

$$= \frac{487}{199}$$

$$= 2.4 \text{ visits}$$

The mean has two major limitations because it is calculated using *every* score in the distribution. The first limitation is that it is affected by the presence of outliers, and therefore we generally exclude outliers from the calculation of the mean. Thus, when calculating the mean number of visits to a health professional, we exclude the one 'outlier' who visited a health professional more than eight times. When presenting a 'trimmed' mean as the centre of distribution, this should be noted in the text.

The other limitation to the use of the mean as a measure of central tendency, even where outliers are excluded, is that its value is pulled away from the centre of a distribution when it is skewed. For example, in Figure 17.4 we can see that the spread of scores for number of health visits is skewed to the right and this has produced a value for the mean that is higher than that we might expect from a quick visual inspection.

An alternative measure of central tendency to the mean is the *median* (M_d). This is especially useful where a distribution is heavily skewed. If all the cases in a distribution are ranked from lowest to highest, the median is the score in the middle of the sequence. The actual calculation of the median will differ according to whether we have an odd or even number of scores. For an odd number of rank-ordered cases, the median is the middle score. For an even number of rank-ordered cases, the median is the mean of the two middle scores. Thus, if I lined up the 200 patients in my study according to the frequency with which they visited a doctor in the previous year, starting with patients that attended a health professional only once, the middle scores in this line-up are those for the 100th and 101st patients, both of which have a value of 2 visits. We have an even number of cases, so the median is the mean of these two middle scores, which is 2.

If a cumulative relative frequency table such as Table 17.2 has been generated, an easier way to calculate the median is to identify the value at which the cumulative per cent first passes 50 (i.e. 2 visits). We can see that the median depends solely on the value of these scores in the middle and is not 'pulled' in one direction or another by the long tail of a skewed distribution or the presence of any outliers, factors which we have seen affect the value of the mean.

Measures of dispersion

Measures of dispersion are descriptive statistics that indicate the spread or variety of scores in a distribution. Most of these require interval/ratio-level measurement (a measure for nominal scales). The Index of Qualitative Variation is not covered here, but further details can be found in Argyrous (2011). The simplest measure of dispersion is the *range*, which is the difference between the lowest score and highest score. This is an easily calculated measure of dispersion because it involves a straightforward subtraction of one score from another. This advantage of the range is also its major limitation: it only uses the extreme scores, and therefore changes with the values of the two extreme scores.

The *inter-quartile range* (IQR) overcomes this problem with the simple range by ignoring the extreme scores of a distribution. The IQR is the range for the middle 50 per cent of cases in a rank-ordered series: the difference between the lower limit of the first quartile and the upper limit of the third quartile. Unlike the simple range, the IQR will not change dramatically if we add one or two cases to either end of the distribution.

The *standard deviation* is a more complex measure of spread, the value of which captures the average distance each score is away from the mean. It is calculated for a sample and population respectively by the following equations:

$$s = \sqrt{\frac{\Sigma\left(X_i - \bar{X}\right)^2}{n-1}}, \; \sigma = \sqrt{\frac{\Sigma\left(X_i - \mu\right)^2}{N}}$$

where *s* represents the standard deviation for a sample, and σ (pronounced 'sigma') represents the standard deviation for a population.

A close look at these equations indicates how they capture the notion that the standard deviation is the average distance of each score from the mean. The numerator is the difference between each score and the mean, and the denominator adjusts those differences by the number of cases. Unfortunately, we cannot simply add all the *positive deviations* (scores above the mean) to all the *negative deviations* (scores below the mean) since, by definition, these will sum to zero. This is why the equation for the standard deviation squares the differences: it turns all the deviations into positive numbers, so that the larger the differences, the greater the value of the standard deviation. But the general idea is clear. Distributions that are more spread out will have many scores that are different from the mean, producing numerous large deviations and thereby a high value for the standard deviation. Another set of scores may have the same mean, but with the scores more tightly clustered around it. In this case, the deviations between each score and the mean will thereby generally be small, producing a lower value for the standard deviation.

Bivariate descriptive statistics: Simple comparisons

The previous section looked at methods for describing the distribution of a single variable. *Univariate analysis* can help address simple questions such as 'What is the age distribution of patients?' or 'What is the health status of patients visiting a clinic?' As we discussed above, this simple analysis is usually a precursor to a more complex analysis that asks whether the health status of patients is related to another variable, such as their smoking history.

Probably everyone has a common-sense notion of what it means for two variables to be 'related to' each other. We know that older children also tend to be taller: age and height are related. This example expresses a general concept for which we have an intuitive feel: as the value of one variable changes, the value of the other variable also changes. If we believe two variables such as health status and smoking are related, we need to express this relationship in the form of a *theoretical model* before we undertake bivariate analysis to measure the relationship. A theoretical model is an abstract depiction of the possible relationships among variables. For this example, the model is easy to depict. If there is a relationship, it is because a patient's smoking history affects their health level. It is not possible for the relationship to 'run in the other direction' – a patient's smoking history will not change as a result of a change in their health level. In this instance, we say that smoking history is the *independent variable* and health status is the *dependent variable*.

Once we have specified the model that we believe underpins any relationship between two variables, we can then generate appropriate statistics to see if such a relationship does in fact appear in the data we have collected. There are two ways we can assess whether a relationship exists between two variables:

- For each of the groups defined by the independent variable, calculate univariate descriptive statistics to summarize the dependent variable and compare the differences
- Calculate the measures of association and correlation.

The first method is the simpler since we generate the univariate statistics we have already discussed, but rather than doing so for the whole data set, we generate these statistics for each of the groups defined by the independent variable. For example, if I wished to see whether health status is affected by smoking history, I would calculate summary statistics for health status, but I would do so separately for smokers and for non-smokers. This is illustrated by the *stacked bar chart* in Figure 17.5. The same comparison between smokers and non-smokers can be made using the *bivariate table* in Table 17.3, also known as a *contingency table* or *cross-tabulation*, or 'cross-tab' for short (see Reynolds 1977 for a more detailed discussion).

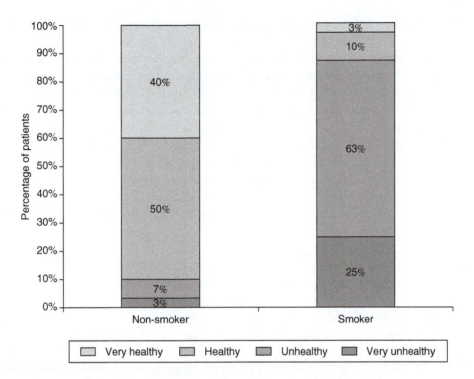

FIGURE 17.5 Stacked bar chart: Health rating by smoking history of clinic patients

TABLE 17.3 Health rating by smoking history of clinic patients

Health rating	Smoking history		
	Non-smoker	**Smoker**	**Total**
Very Unhealthy	3%	25%	12%
Unhealthy	7%	63%	29%
Healthy	50%	10%	34%
Very Healthy	40%	3%	25%
Total	100%	100%	100%
	(120)	(80)	(200)

NB Percentage figures are rounded up and may come to more than 100%

It should be noted that with cross-tabs we follow these two rules for arranging the information:

- Place the appropriate variables in the rows and columns. If there is reason to believe that one of the variables is dependent on the other, the categories of the independent variable should be arranged across the columns and the categories of the dependent variable down the rows. In this example, we have specified that smoking history is the independent (column) variable and health status is the dependent (row) variable.
- For scales that can be ranked, ensure the scale increases down the rows/across the columns. Notice that one of the variables, 'Health rating', is ordinal. Thus, the categories that make up this scale can be ordered from lowest to highest. We therefore place the lowest point on the scale, the 'Very Unhealthy' category, on the first row, so that the scale increases down the page until we reach the highest point on the scale, which is the 'Very Healthy' category.

To help us compare the difference in the health levels between smokers and non-smokers, the cross-tab presents the *column percentages*. For example, we can see that of all 120 non-smokers in the study, 3 per cent were Very Unhealthy. This compares with the 25 per cent of all 80 smokers who were Very Unhealthy. Figure 17.5 similarly presents the breakdown of each group's health status as a percentage of the total number of cases in that group, rather than the actual number of people that are Very Unhealthy, Unhealthy, Healthy or Very Healthy. In both the cross-tab and the bar chart, these percentages adjust for the different total number of smokers and non-smokers in the data, and thereby allow for a more valid comparison than just using the raw counts.

Where the dependent variable is measured on an interval/ratio scale, we can also compare the groups defined by the categories of the independent variable in terms of summary statistics such as the mean and median, as illustrated in Table 17.4.

Table 17.4 Average annual number of visits to health professional by smoking history of clinic patients

Measure of average	Non-smoker	Smoker
Mean number of visits to health professional	1.2	3.1
Median number of visits to health professional	1	3

Once we have generated graphs, tables or summary statistics such as a mean to compare the relevant groups, the task is then to interpret the differences. We must assess whether they reveal a relationship between the two variables. When comparing differences between the relevant groups, we look at the *pattern* and *strength* of any relationship that such differences reveal. For example, the cross-tab in Table 17.3 shows that the health status of smokers is lower than for non-smokers and smokers are more heavily concentrated in the Unhealthy category than non-smokers. We can thus say that there is a relationship between these variables and that the relationship is negative: a higher level of smoking is associated with lower health status.

Bivariate descriptive statistics: Measures of association and correlation

In the previous section, we detected a relationship between smoking and health status by observing a difference in the set of percentages in each column of a cross-tab. The next step is to ask: what is the *strength* of this relationship? We can make an arbitrary assessment of a relationship's strength by arguing that the two sets of column percentages are very different from each other and therefore suggest a moderate-to-strong relationship. Alternatively, we can arrive at a more precise and objective measure of the strength of a relationship by calculating numerical *measures of association and correlation*. These measures are descriptive statistics that quantify a relationship between two variables. Table 17.5 lists the most common measures.

TABLE 17.5 Measures of association and correlation

Measure	Data consideration
Lambda	At least one variable nominal
Goodman and Kruskal tau	At least one variable nominal
Eta	Independent variable is nominal and dependent variable is interval/ratio
Somer's d	Both variables at least ordinal
Gamma	Both variables at least ordinal
Kendall's tau-b	Both variables at least ordinal
Kendall's tau-c	Both variables at least ordinal
Spearman's rho	Both variables at least ordinal with many points on the scale
Pearson's r	Both variables interval/ratio with many points on the scale
Kappa	Both variables at least ordinal and measured on the same scale

Detailing the logic of each of these measures and the methods for calculating them is beyond the scope of this chapter, but for a comprehensive guide see Liebetrau (1983). However, we should note here that, as with most other statistics, the appropriate choice is affected by the level at which the variables under analysis have been measured, as indicated in Table 17.5.

The general point to note about these measures is that they give a precise value on a scale from 0 to 1, indicating the *strength* of any relationship observed between two variables. Rather than just relying on a visual impression of a cross-tab or graph, measures of association provide a single figure to show the strength of association. In addition, where both variables are measured at least at the ordinal level, a + or a – sign also indicates the *direction* of association – that is, whether an increase in the quantity of one variable is associated with an increase (positive association) or decrease (negative association) in the quantity of the other variable. For instance, in the previous part of the chapter we observed that the health level decreases as the smoking level increases, and therefore we observe a negative relationship between them.

It is important to remember that the measures only detect a *statistical association*. They do not necessarily show whether one variable causes a change in another. We may suspect theoretically that one variable causes a change in the other, but the measures listed in Table 17.5 cannot prove causation. They only provide supporting evidence for a theoretical model. For example, a relationship between the number of storks in an area and the birth rate in that area has been observed, and we may calculate a measure that quantifies this statistical relationship. However, we cannot go from this statistical regularity to a conclusion that the presence of storks determines the birth rate!

Descriptive statistics: Advanced methods for analysing many variables

The simple statistical techniques we have discussed above can take us a long way into data analysis and help answer many of the research questions we wish to answer. However, there are many more methods of analysis that are available to the researcher willing to learn and use them. One such technique readers may frequently encounter is *regression analysis*, which seeks to depict the relationship between an independent variable and one or more dependent variables in the form of a *regression equation*. For example, we may have data for the number of minutes of weekly exercise undertaken by a sample of people, along with their respective rested pulse rates. To see whether these two variables are related, we use regression analysis to yield the following equation:

Rested pulse rate = 89 – 0.3 (minutes of weekly exercise)

This equation allows us to estimate the rested pulse rate for an individual given their respective exercise level. For example, where the amount of weekly exercise is 0, we expect the rested pulse rate to be 89 beats per minute (bpm). For every minute of weekly exercise above

0, we expect the rested pulse rate to decrease by 0.3. Thus, for someone who exercises for 30 minutes per week, we predict their pulse rate to be:

$$\text{Rested pulse rate} = 89 - 0.3(30) = 89 - 9 = 80 \text{ bpm}$$

Regression analysis can be extended to take into account even more complex relationships involving three or more variables. For example, the relationship between regular exercise and pulse rate may be affected by a person's sex and also their age in years, and *multiple regression analysis* produces a single equation that will measure the extent to which each of these variables affects rested pulse rate.

Table 17.6 lists the main techniques for such *multivariate analysis*. To detail these choices for is beyond the limits of this chapter, but see Argyrous (2011) for a more detailed introduction.

TABLE 17.6 Types of multivariate analysis

Multivariate technique	Data considerations
Multiple regression	Interval/ratio independent and dependent variables Categorical independent variables can be included as dummy variables
Logistic regression	Dependent variable is categorical and independent variables are interval/ratio
Loglinear analysis	All variables are categorical

Inferential statistics

We have discussed at some length various ways of describing our data. These data often come from a sample rather than from the whole population, so that we are faced with a problem, namely: are the sample statistics 'representative' of the population from which the sample is drawn? The operation of *sampling error* may cause the sample to be 'off'. Sampling error occurs when random factors cause us to include in our random sample members of the population that have relatively low or high scores for the variable we are investigating. This sampling error then causes the overall sample statistics to be different from those we would have obtained if we had studied the whole population. Given that sampling error is always a possibility, on what basis can we make a valid generalization from the sample to the population?

We address this problem with *inferential statistics*. Inferential statistics are the numerical techniques for making conclusions about a population based on the information obtained from a random sample drawn from that population. The nature of inferential statistics can be illustrated by an example. Assume that we have randomly selected 200 people who perform regular weekly exercise and we find that this sample has a mean resting pulse rate of 60 bpm, and standard deviation of 10 bpm. What can we infer about the population of all people who exercise regularly?

We may have information that the general population has a mean rested pulse rate of 72 bpm. On the basis of the sample result, can we say that the *population* of all people who exercise regularly is lower than that for the general population? Maybe it is not, and our sample of 200 has produced a relatively low mean rested pulse rate as a result of sampling error. Alternatively, maybe the population of regular exercisers does have a lower mean rested pulse rate and the sample of 200 reflects this. The process of *hypothesis testing* helps us decide between these inferences by calculating the *statistical significance* of the sample result (also called the *p*-value). Statistical significance is the probability that the sample did indeed come from a population of regular exercisers whose mean rested pulse rate is the same as that for the general population, and that the low sample mean is due to sampling error alone.

Another way of making an inference from a sample result to the whole population is to ask: from what kind of population it is reasonable to assume the sample was derived? If the sample mean is within the 'normal' bounds of sampling error, what range of values can we confidently believe includes the population mean? Answering this type of question involves the calculation of *confidence intervals*. In our example, we may calculate the confidence interval to be 60 ± 1.4 bpm. In other words, if we assume that the sample is not greatly affected by sampling error, the population from which it is drawn has a mean rested pulse rate between 58.6 and 61.4 bpm. Underlying the calculation of such a confidence interval is the simple logic that random samples will only rarely produce a result that is very different from the value for the population from which it is drawn.

This section gives some general idea about the role of inferential statistics in quantitative analysis, but the issues and calculations involved in the application of inferential statistics are far more complex than we can discuss here (see Hauer 2003; Sterne and Smith 2001).

Reading health research based on statistics

The following is a useful checklist of questions to ask when reading statistics in the literature. When reading simple summary statistics, you should ask:

- Which average is calculated: mean or median? (ideally both!)
- If the mean, then is this with or without outliers/extreme scores? If yes, note the bias this produces in the calculation of the mean.
- If the mean, is this for a skewed distribution? If yes, note the bias this produces in the calculation of the mean.

- Are measures of spread provided along with measures of the average? If not, question the usefulness of averages if the data are very dispersed.
- Have the authors used averages or percentages? Averages should always be calculated using the raw data, rather than taken from summary statistics that have already been calculated from their data.

When reading inferential statistics, you should ask:

- What is the practical significance of any *statistically significant* difference? A result may be statistically significant, especially when it comes from very large samples, but the measured effect in practical terms may be too small to worry about.
- What is the confidence (alpha) level at which statistical significance is decided? Is it sufficient relative to the importance of the results or consequences of being wrong? Ideally, results should present the exact *p*-value for any significance test so that readers can judge for themselves whether this is statistically significant, by selecting an alpha level that is appropriate to their needs.
- What is the confidence interval around the sample result?
- Was the sample randomly selected?
- What is the population to which a generalization is being made?

Conclusion

The chapter has covered a wide range of tools for quantitative data analysis in health research. A key element in determining which of these tools is appropriate is the question we want to answer: univariate, bivariate, multivariate, or inferential. In addition, we also need to identify the way in which our variables of interest have been measured. In particular, we first need to determine whether our variables have been measured at the nominal, ordinal or interval/ratio levels.

We introduced three broad classes of statistical techniques that can help us describe the data that we collect, namely graphs, tables and numerical calculations, and within each of these broad groups we have further choices. For example, we saw that there are different classes of numerical calculations depending on whether we are trying to identify the central tendency of a distribution or the amount of dispersion it contains. Choices also depend on how complicated the analysis is that we wish to undertake – whether we are interested in describing the distribution of a single variable, or the relationship between two variables, or indeed the relationship among many variables. The chapter concludes with an exercise in which the reader is invited to apply some of the statistical methods outlined to the health data set out in Table 17.7.

TABLE 17.7 Health data set

ID	Height	Weight	Age	Sex	Smokes	Exercise	Pulse
1	180	77	18	F	No	15	47
2	186	87	23	M	No	12	49
3	188	87	20	M	No	14	50
4	171	71	41	M	No	15	52
5	173	64	20	F	No	12	55
6	182	63	20	M	No	8	56
7	169	68	19	M	No	12	58
8	175	75	20	M	No	10	59
9	175	65	19	M	No	11	60
10	182	85	20	M	No	14	60
11	170	54	20	F	No	8	60
12	175	54	18	F	No	10	61
13	170	60	18	M	No	11	62
14	183	73	20	M	No	5	63
15	164	78	28	F	No	5	64
16	173	70	20	M	No	9	64
17	170	56	19	M	No	9	64
18	170	62	20	F	No	4	64
19	165	58	23	F	No	8	64
20	180	75	20	M	No	4	65
21	184	65	21	M	No	8	65
22	167	75	20	F	No	10	65
23	174	60	19	F	No	8	66
24	162	60	19	F	No	8	66
25	175	66	20	M	No	11	66
26	158	51	18	F	No	8	68
27	180	85	19	M	Yes	10	68
28	191	78	19	M	No	8	68
29	164	56	19	F	No	5	68
30	176	59	19	M	No	6	68
31	162	57	20	F	No	7	68
32	170	65	18	M	No	10	69
33	180	72	18	M	No	4	69

ID	Height	Weight	Age	Sex	Smokes	Exercise	Pulse
34	157	41	20	F	No	11	70
35	177	74	18	F	No	5	70
36	140	50	34	F	No	6	70
37	163	55	20	F	No	7	70
38	163	51	18	F	No	10	70
39	182	85	20	M	Yes	2	70
40	170	68	22	M	No	5	70
41	178	62	21	M	No	1	70
42	163	47	23	F	No	4	71
43	195	84	18	M	No	4	71
44	169	55	18	F	No	1	71
45	175	57	20	F	No	2	72
46	172	53	20	M	No	5	72
47	167	63	28	M	No	2	72
48	164	66	23	F	No	1	74
49	168	55	24	F	No	3	74
50	180	76	21	M	No	2	74
51	189	88	45	M	No	5	74
52	178	58	19	M	No	6	74
53	160	57	19	F	No	4	75
54	185	85	19	M	No	2	75
55	194	110	25	M	No	1	75
56	170	75	20	M	No	5	76
57	166	50	19	F	Yes	2	76
58	182	98	19	M	No	3	76
59	179	80	20	M	No	2	76
60	180	102	20	M	No	1	76
61	190	82	19	M	Yes	0	76
62	171	67	18	F	No	1	76
63	171	70	26	F	No	1	76
64	178	86	21	M	Yes	4	76
65	185	110	22	M	No	0	77
66	172	59	18	F	No	5	78

(Continued)

TABLE 17.7   (Continued)

ID	Height	Weight	Age	Sex	Smokes	Exercise	Pulse
67	186	96	19	M	No	6	78
68	184	74	22	M	No	2	78
69	189	60	19	M	No	1	78
70	163	55	20	F	Yes	0	78
71	155	50	19	F	No	3	78
72	187	59	18	M	No	4	78
73	185	90	18	M	No	1	80
74	180	70	18	M	No	0	80
75	160	49	19	F	No	0	80
76	192	105	21	M	No	1	80
77	182	75	26	M	Yes	1	80
78	164	54	18	F	No	0	80
79	170	60	19	F	No	2	80
80	180	80	21	M	No	2	80
81	170	59	20	M	No	2	80
82	172	60	21	F	Yes	3	81
83	179	58	19	F	No	1	82
84	155	55	20	F	No	0	82
85	166	56	21	F	Yes	0	83
86	165	48	19	F	No	2	83
87	194	95	18	M	No	1	84
88	165	63	18	F	No	1	84
89	178	63	23	M	No	3	84
90	151	42	22	F	No	4	85
91	175	79	19	M	No	0	85
92	178	56	21	F	No	1	86
93	182	60	22	M	Yes	0	86
94	173	57	18	F	No	2	86
95	165	60	19	F	Yes	3	88
96	68	63	19	M	No	4	88
97	180	65	20	M	No	0	88
98	168	60	23	M	No	1	88
99	175	60	19	M	No	2	88

ID	Height	Weight	Age	Sex	Smokes	Exercise	Pulse
100	162	50	19	F	Yes	1	90
101	170	58	21	M	Yes	1	90
102	173	64	18	F	Yes	1	90
103	161	43	19	F	No	1	90
104	170	63	20	F	No	0	92
105	167	70	22	M	Yes	0	92
106	167	62	18	F	Yes	2	96
107	155	49	18	F	No	1	104
108	164	46	18	F	Yes	0	104
109	155	65	19	F	Yes	0	119
110	179	80	20	M	Yes	2	145

Exercise 17.1   Statistical tests on a health data set

The data in Table 17.7 are the results from a random sample of 110 people. The rested pulse rate of each person is measured and also their height in centimetres, weight in kilograms, age in years, sex, whether each considers themselves a regular smoker and the amount of regular weekly exercise each undertakes in hours. Either consider the data directly or enter them into a computer program of your choice. (The data are available from the companion website.) Then complete the following questions:

- What is the level of measurement for each variable?
- Produce appropriate descriptive statistics to assess the distribution of rested pulse rate. Your statistics should allow you to analyse the shape, centre and spread of the distribution, as well as the existence of any outliers. How might you explain any outliers, and how should they be handled in further analysis?
- Compare the mean pulse rate for smokers and non-smokers. In this analysis, which variable is the independent variable and which is the dependent variable? What is the appropriate measure of association?

Recommended further reading

This book provides reasonably comprehensive coverage of the descriptive statistics introduced in this chapter, as well as an entry point for the more advanced measures of association and inferential statistics that have only briefly been outlined here:

Argyrous, G. (2011) *Statistics for Research*. London: Sage.

This text gives a clear and simple introduction to more advanced topics for those wanting to undertake regression analysis:
Kahane, L. H. (2008) *Regression Basics*. London: Sage.

This book provides a more detailed discussion of statistics for health professionals:
Scott, I. and Mazhindu, D. (2009) *Statistics for Health Care Professionals: An Introduction*. London: Sage.

References

Argyrous, G. (2011) *Statistics for Research*. London: Sage.

Australian Bureau of Statistics (2014–2015) *National Health Survey*. Cat. No. 4364.0. Canberra: ABS.

Hauer, E. (2003) 'The harm done by tests of significance', *Accident Analysis and Prevention*, *36*: 495–500.

Kahane, L. H. (2008) *Regression Basics*. London: Sage.

Liebetrau, A. M. (1983) *Measures of Association*. Beverly Hills, CA: Sage.

Pryjmachuk, S. and Richards, D. A. (2007) 'Look before you leap and don't put all your eggs in one basket: The need for caution and prudence in quantitative data analysis', *Journal of Research in Nursing*, *12*: 43–54.

Reynolds, H. T. (1977) *The Analysis of Cross-Classifications*. New York: Free Press.

Scott, I. and Mazhindu, D. (2009) *Statistics for Health Care Professionals: An Introduction*. London: Sage.

Sterne, J. A. C. and Smith, G. D. (2001) 'Sifting the evidence – what's wrong with significance tests?', *British Medical Journal*, *322*: 226–31.

Stevens, S. S. (1946) 'On the theory of scales of measurement', *Science*, *103*: 677–80.

18

Researching Health Care Management Using Secondary Data

IAN KIRKPATRICK AND GIANLUCA VERONESI

Chapter objectives

- To highlight gaps in research on the characteristics and impact of managers in health care
- To define and provide a taxonomy of administrative data sources relevant to researching health care management
- To review the range of statistical techniques used to analyse administrative data
- To illustrate how the analysis of administrative data sources can advance knowledge about the characteristics of managers in health care and their impact
- To discuss the limitations of administrative data and avenues for future research.

Introduction

This chapter focuses on how emerging new 'administrative' data sources might enhance research into the changing management of health services. Since the early 1980s, most developed countries have given priority to reforming management (Mintzberg 2017). Costs have risen due to ageing populations and the technologies developed to meet their changing (and rising) expectations, concerns and needs (Kuhlmann et al. 2015). These demands have been especially acute in tax-funded health care systems. For instance, in the United Kingdom National Health Service (NHS), the government has most recently set targets for a 2 per cent annual efficiency gain (£9 billion in total) from providers in the five years up to 2021 (NHS England 2016). Concerns have also been raised about high levels of 'unwarranted variation' in the productivity and efficiency in non-specialist acute services, according to one review (Carter 2016), costing £5 billion per annum.

Despite these mounting policy concerns, attempts to reform management have been highly controversial and, in most health care systems, they continue to be questioned and criticized. The introduction of managers in executive roles in hospitals, with a mandate to control resources, has often been resented by the medical profession, which views this as a challenge to its dominance and autonomy (Kirkpatrick, Ackroyd and Walker 2005). For example, in the NHS, even after three decades of reforms, there still remains a pressing need for 'dialogue and conflict resolution' to improve 'doctor–manager relationships' (Powell and Davies 2016). The level of cynicism about managers in the NHS has spilled over into public debate. In the United Kingdom media, headlines such as 'death by bureaucracy', 'greed of NHS fat cats' or 'cure the NHS with fewer managers' are increasingly commonplace (Kirkpatrick, Veronesi and Altanlar 2017). Most recently, Max Pemberton (himself a doctor), writing in the *Daily Mail*, has criticized the recruitment of managers at the expense of frontline clinical staff such as nurses and doctors. Managers, he suggests, have proliferated in the NHS and add little or no value: 'Put a manager in a room with a clipboard and they will find work' (Pemberton 2017).

While these assumptions are widely held, what do we really know about the nature and impact of managers and management in health systems? Who are these managers and what roles do they perform? More importantly, what impact have managers had on the performance of health services? Are they a largely unproductive overhead, as many recent accounts would have us believe, or do managers add value as 'the people who keep the show on the road, day-in day-out' (see www.miphealth.org.uk/home-/Home.aspx)?

In this chapter, we explore some of the challenges these questions pose in terms of what research methods are appropriate. In recent years there has been a proliferation of studies focusing on the dynamics of leadership and management in the NHS – some of it funded through the National Institute for Health Research (NIHR) – and much of this work has been predominantly qualitative (see NIHR 2013 for a summary). This research has deepened our understanding of how management and leadership roles have developed in specific cases, although, with some exceptions (Bloom and van Reenan 2010), we still know little about the wider characteristics of management (for example, in terms of size and different functions) and even less about its impact.

To address these concerns, we highlight the usefulness of alternative 'administrative data' sources that are increasingly available for conducting research on the nature and impact of health care management (Smith et al. 2004). While such data are not designed exclusively for research purposes, they have been used extensively within public management research. Examples of this include studies focusing on the size and characteristics of administrative functions in public organizations ('administrative intensity') (Andrews and Boyne 2014) and on the impact of management policies and practices (Walker 2013). By contrast, in health care, despite a growing interest in the use of human resource data such as payroll information to assess the nature and outcome of nurse staffing levels (Griffiths et al. 2015), and issues associated with organizational climate and culture (West et al. 2015), less attention has been paid explicitly to management.

In this chapter, we illustrate the potential of an alternative research agenda that focuses on managers in the English NHS using the growing availability of 'administrative data sources' (Smith et al. 2004). In what follows we first set the scene by identifying certain gaps in the current research on managers and management in health care, focusing specifically on the case of the English NHS. We then turn to a discussion of administrative data in the NHS, the methods used for analysis, and provide examples from our own research on the nature and impact of managers.

Managers and management in the NHS: Key questions for research

In this section we outline some of the key questions relating to the development of managers and management in health care systems and the challenges this poses for data and research methods. As we noted earlier, health care systems around the world have been subject to demands to improve efficiency and develop enhanced management capabilities. These reforms are frequently described in terms of the New Public Management (NPM), as set out in Box 18.1. While the NPM implies multiple changes, a key development has been the greater emphasis on management in hospitals and other health care organizations. This topic has been widely researched in the literature, but certain questions have still not been addressed as fully as they might. The characteristics of management within health care organizations and the variations that occur have been largely ignored so we know little about the impact of these variations on outcomes in terms of efficiency and service quality.

Box 18.1   The New Public Management

In response to challenges associated with multi-morbidity, rising costs and population ageing, there has been a common emphasis on reforming the management of

(Continued)

(Continued)

health services to increase control over input mix and level, outputs and scope of activities (McKee and Healy 2002). These reforms fall under the rubric of the New Public Management (NPM). This refers to a cluster of doctrines and practices that are held to constitute a paradigm of management distinct from 'traditional modes of public administration' (Verbeeten and Speklé 2015). According to Hood (1995), an NPM agenda means empowering managers and stressing their 'right to manage' with fewer constraints such as those imposed by rules and bureaucracy. These reforms have been associated with a transformation in the organizational landscape of health systems, moving away from vertically integrated hierarchies to a situation where hospitals and other agencies have their own governing boards and increased formal autonomy, similar to private firms (Lindlbauer, Winter and Schreyögg 2015; Saltman, Durán and Dubois 2011). There have also been changes in the funding of health care organizations (linked to variable budgets associated with activity or performance) and attempts to increase 'competition' between providers (so-called quasi markets). Reforms have sought to strengthen the internal management capabilities of health care organizations such as public hospitals (Ackroyd, Kirkpatrick and Walker 2007). The latter bore many of the hallmarks of a 'professional bureaucracy', with management formally separated from the 'worlds' of care and cure (Glouberman and Mintzberg 2001). More recently, the trend has been to make management more integral, developing specialist (non-clinical) management functions and also co-opting doctors and other professionals into management and leadership work (for instance, through clinical directorates) (Kirkpatrick et al. 2013).

Nature and antecedents of management

In the recent literature, terms such as 'management' and 'managerialism' are sometimes used loosely. Often it is assumed that NPM reforms have led to the employment of more managers and managers themselves are a unified group with a well-defined agenda for controlling costs and regulating professional practice. However, there are obvious difficulties with these assumptions. The important questions that they raise are now considered.

What exactly do we mean by managers and management?

In wider public administration the need to differentiate between these terms is noted (Diefenbach 2009). While 'management' is a general process that might conceivably be performed by anyone, 'manager' denotes a 'distinctive occupation' (Grey 1999). In the NHS, management as a process that implies performance management, focusing on greater accountability for achieving results and targets at levels (Verbeeten and Speklé 2015). From this perspective, a large proportion of staff including clinical professionals are involved in 'management', a tendency exaggerated by the growing emphasis on 'leadership' from ward to board (Spurgeon and Clark 2017). A recent study by Buchanan and colleagues (2013) found that around one in three clinical staff had some kind of 'managerial' role associated with administration or staff supervision, even if they did not hold formal 'management' job titles.

By contrast, 'managers' is a narrower category, referring to people who occupy job roles with the title of 'manager'. Historically, this has been less apparent in health care organizations, which have tended to be 'bureaucracy-lite' (Hales 2002), with parallel hierarchies for administrators and clinical professionals and decisions made through consensus (Ackroyd, Kirkpatrick and Walker 2007). In the NHS, the appearance of general (or 'pure play') managers dates mainly back to 1983 when the then Prime Minister, Margaret Thatcher, commissioned Sir Roy Griffiths, the Director of the supermarket chain Sainsbury's, to conduct a review. His solution was to recruit dedicated managers with the executive authority to run hospitals, holding them accountable for budgets and, later, performance (Ham 2009).

What is the background of these general or 'pure play' managers?

In some accounts, managers are often treated as a unified block of outsiders, recruited into the NHS to challenge the (legitimate) decisions of clinical professionals. However, this image of managers is clearly problematic given the emergence of hybrid professional-manager roles within health care systems (see Kirkpatrick 2016). An important development was the creation of clinical directorates at the middle level of hospitals, delegating some budgetary responsibilities to professionals, usually doctors. At the strategic level, doctors and nurses were also recruited onto the boards of hospitals in roles such as medical and nursing director (Kirkpatrick et al. 2013). While there is a mounting body of research on these hybrid roles, much of it focuses on issues of identity (see, for example, Croft, Currie and Lockett 2015; Spyridonidis, Hendy and Barlow 2015) and surprisingly little is known about the backgrounds of these 'managers' or about how significant these 'hybrids' are as a proportion of all managers.

What is the overall size and composition of the 'management' function and what conditions that have influenced its development?

As we noted in the Introduction, there is an assumption in the media and some political circles that expenditure on management in the NHS has grown exponentially in recent years. It is also widely believed that this growth has been most pronounced in organizations such as Foundation trusts or Clinical Commissioning Groups, which have been given greater formal autonomy (Kirkpatrick, Veronesi and Altanlar 2017). Yet, while general estimates of the number of managers in the NHS are available, our understanding of these issues remains limited.

All three questions pose challenges in terms of available research methods and data. An obvious limitation of the qualitative research on this topic – that is largely based on case studies – is a lack of any accurate measure of the size and characteristics of management functions across the NHS. To some extent, the latter information can be obtained from official sources. In 1995, using official figures, a Kings Fund report (2011) found that there were 20,842 'managers and senior managers' in the NHS, accounting for 1.9 per cent of the workforce. Since then, in a context of growing financial constraints and a major re-organization of primary care management, numbers have fluctuated. By 2017, there were approximately 31,113 managers employed, accounting for 2.97 per cent of the workforce (NHS Confederation 2017). Walshe and Smith (2011) also found that, in 2010, in England, the largest proportion of managers (53.6 per cent) were located in 'provider' organizations, with less than 6 per cent in central functions (including regional authorities) and 40.8 per cent in primary care (commissioning roles). However, while these figures are a useful starting point, they are based on very crude definitions of 'management' and administration' and do not provide a clear breakdown of different roles *within* management, including hybrids.

Impact on performance

A further deficiency of the existing research is that few studies to date have focused on the impact of managers on the performance of health care organizations. As noted earlier, the assumed costs of management in the NHS have become an issue of growing media and political concern. A recent poll published by Lord Ashcroft KCMG (2015) asked respondents what they believed the biggest problems facing the NHS are today. Appearing first on the list of public concerns was 'too much being spent on management and bureaucracy'. This ranked higher than issues such as 'hospital closures and other cuts', 'staff shortages' and 'patients being denied drugs or treatment because of cost'. Many politicians have also jumped onto the anti-management bandwagon. Most recently, in a speech to the NHS Annual Conference in 2017, the Minister for Health, Jeremy Hunt, declared: 'we should today ask whether the NHS made a historic mistake in the 1980s by deliberately creating a manager class who were not clinicians' (*Guardian* 2016).

The view that managers are largely ineffective (or even irrelevant) is also widespread in some academic literature (Greener et al. 2013). However, not all studies are equally disparaging about the motivations and contributions of managers. While some have emphasized quite stark differences in values between managers and doctors (Degeling et al. 2006), others point to many areas of shared commitment, and a strong public service orientation of middle managers (Crilly and LeGrand 2004). This research also highlights the possibilities for more productive relationships between medicine and management that can be negotiated locally, and it supports service improvement (Kirkpatrick et al. 2008).

There has been debate on the motivations and experiences of managers in the NHS and research focusing on the impact of management practices, such as human resource management, as well as on the effect of leadership styles on performance and staff satisfaction (Bloom and van Reenen 2010; Bloom et al. 2015; see West et al. 2015 for a summary). In collaboration with the global management consulting firm McKinsey & Co., Bloom and van Reenen (2010) developed a 20-point scale of management practices. Although designed initially for manufacturing, this survey has been applied to over 2,000 public and private hospitals in nine countries, including the United Kingdom. The results show that high management scores correlate strongly with better clinical outcomes and a range of financial outcomes, including profitability, especially in private hospitals (Bloom et al. 2015). However, while useful, this research is cross-sectional, making it hard to impute the direction of causality – that is, whether management practices generate improved hospital performance or are a result of it. It also relies on subjective self-assessments of practices by managers themselves.

Administrative data sources and methods for researching health care management

In this section we now turn to the matter of how knowledge in this field might be advanced though the use of an alternative research designs that draw on and combine a range of 'administrative' data sources. We describe these data sources and their advantages and explore a range of analytical techniques that may be used to exploit them.

What are administrative data?

'Administrative data' refer broadly to information collected primarily for administrative (not research) purposes (Smith et al. 2004). According to Connelly and colleagues (2016: 2), it relates to 'data which are derived from the operation of administrative systems (for instance, data collected by government agencies for the purposes of registration, transaction and record keeping)', so essentially this is a form of 'Big Data' (Mayer-Schonberger and Cukier 2013). In the United Kingdom, government departments are the main controllers of large administrative databases, including welfare, tax, educational record systems and, crucially, health. Although these data sets are used primarily to inform policy making, their potential for research has also been realized.

Administrative data have many strengths (Connelly et al. 2016). They have already been collected and there are few additional costs associated with collection. The coverage of such data across populations (say, organizations in a sector) is often complete, sometimes including 100 per cent of the records in question, with information regularly updated in a standardized and consistent format to ensure comparability. More often than not, administrative data are longitudinal, making it possible to address research questions about change over time. Data are usually also subject to rigorous quality checks and are generally not that intrusive for the target population. Lastly, there are potential advantages in matching administrative data sets to conduct analysis. This avoids many of the pitfalls of using a single source, with its attendant possibility of bias.

Administrative data have certain weaknesses. Most importantly, the information collected is limited to whatever data are required for administrative purposes and is therefore beyond the control of the researchers. There are also risks of frequent changes in the administrative procedures used to collect such data – for example, in how they are classified and coded. This may make some data sets hard to use over a longer time period. As we have seen, not all administrative data are free for public use, with some important sources held by commercial organizations (see Angrave et al. 2016).

Administrative data relating to health care management

In the English NHS context, there are different strands of administrative data. Some are easy to access. Data have already been collected, collated and made available for download to any potentially interested researcher (for example, from NHS Digital, the main NHS data repository). An advantage of existing data sets is that all the information included - from number of patient admissions to percentage of bed occupancy, and so on - can be traced at the organization level, and each organization has a unique identifier that is constant across databases.

By contrast, other data are still publicly available, but need to be extracted and re-organized before they can be used for analytical purposes. An example here are the official communications of NHS organizations, such as annual reports and related financial statements, board meeting minutes and any other formal document available on the organization website. This would, for instance, include information on educational background and the professional expertise of members (directors) of hospital trust governing boards.

Other data sources are privately owned and are subject to fee payments or special access arrangements. A prime example of the latter is the Binley's database of NHS managers (owned by Wilmington Healthcare Ltd). This is a directory containing information on the personal details of individual managers (such as salutation, gender and professional belonging), as well as their formal managerial role (for instance, financial director, estates manager and clinical director). Published since 1991, the database is periodically compiled every four months and updated through a survey of employees of NHS organizations, containing more than 30,000 individuals and over 100 job functions - including clinically qualified managers.

An outline of the different sources of publicly available administrative data relating to management in the English NHS is provided in Table 18.1, which includes data relating to the nature and antecedents of management. The latter includes sources that provide estimates of management numbers (for example, NHS Workforce statistics and the Binley's database) and those providing information on potentially relevant organizational conditions (such as financial information and hospital episode statistics).

TABLE 18.1 Administrative data sources relevant to the nature and antecedents of management in the NHS

Database name	Source	Content
Estates and Returns Information Collection	NHS Digital	Trust type and location, number of sites used, and contracted-out (non-clinical) services
NHS Bed Availability and Occupancy Data	NHS England	Average daily numbers of available and occupied beds (day and overnight) by sector
Hospital Episode Statistics	NHS Digital	Number of consultant episodes, number of admissions, aggregated patient-level data (including time waited and length of stay), day cases, and bed days
NHS Workforce Statistics (staff management and numbers)	NHS Digital	Staff divided into professional groups and contractual arrangements, sickness and absence rates, joining and leaving rates, and stability index
NHS Workforce Statistics (staff earnings)	NHS Digital	Mean annual earnings divided by staff groups
NHS Trusts Accounts Data	GOV.UK	Statements of comprehensive income, financial position, and cash flows
Binley's database of NHS managers	Wilmington Healthcare Ltd	Database of NHS managers, including 30,000 individuals and over 100 job functions

Table 18.2 describes sources that can be used primarily as outcome or performance measures, including efficiency data and patient experience scores. Of course, these distinctions are not hard and fast. NHS Staff Survey data provide information on the nature of management practices, including Heath Resource Management policies and assessments of leadership styles. NHS Trust Accounts Data might also be used to assess levels of investment in management, or associated activities, such as the use of management consultants (see Kirkpatrick et al. 2019).

TABLE 18.2   Administrative data sources relevant to the performance of NHS organizations

Database name	Source	Content
Clinical Indicators	NHS Digital	Hospital care, NHS Outcomes Framework, and Summary Hospital-level Mortality Indicator
NHS Patient Experience Survey	Care Quality Commission	Annual survey of inpatients, outpatients, accident & emergency patients on the quality of services provided
NHS Staff Survey	NHS England	Annual survey of staff divided by professional groups
National Patient Safety Incident Reports	NHS Improvement	Patient safety incidents

Analytical methods

There are a wide range of analytical methods to exploit these 'administrative' data sources to investigate the nature and impact of management on performance outcomes. In what follows, rather than review all these possibilities, we summarize instead some of the more obvious methodological approaches, including those that feature in our own research – see Table 18.3 for a summary.

TABLE 18.3   Example of analytic techniques for interrogating administrative data in NHS management research

Technique	Description	Examples
Descriptive statistics	Summary of the data sample, including central tendency, spread and shape	General characteristics of NHS managers (Walshe and Smith 2011)
Cross-sectional regression analysis	Regression analysis using information about different observations at the same point in time or during the same time period (for example, ordinary least squares and logistic regressions)	Relationship between human capital of hospital board members and performance (Veronesi, Kirkpatrick and Vallascas 2013) The impact of business experts on performance (Kirkpatrick, Veronesi and Vallascas 2017)

Technique	Description	Examples
Time series cross-sectional analysis	Method to investigate the nature of a sequential set of data points, measured typically over successive times (for instance, panel corrected standard errors)	The impact of different hospital types (Foundation and non-Foundation trusts) on the nature and size of management functions (Kirkpatrick, Veronesi and Altanlar 2017) The effect of clinical leadership and organizational status on patient experience (Veronesi, Kirkpatrick and Altanlar 2015)
Times series longitudinal analysis	Method to examine changes in variables over time and differences in variables between observations, either through static or dynamic panel data estimations	The impact of managers, pay and employment tenure on hospital performance (Veronesi, Altanlar and Kirkpatrick 2018)
Structural equation modelling (including Partial Least Squares)	Multivariate statistical analysis technique that is used to analyse (sometimes inductively) structural relationships	The consequences of 'board heterogenity' for performance (Blanco-Oliver, Veronesi and Kirkpatrick 2016)
Fuzzy set/Qualitative Comparative Analysis (fsQCA)	Configurational comparative method based on the analysis of membership of cases in a population with given characteristics	The importance of elite status for advancement to senior medical manager roles (Kirkpatrick, Veronesi and Zardini 2016)

A first possibility is to simply look at descriptive statistics such as measures of central tendency (for instance, mean, median and mode) and indicators of variability or dispersion (including standard deviation/variance, minimum and maximum values, and kurtosis and skewness). These are most revealing when a whole population is considered but are also useful even for smaller representative samples. For example, in their report on the NHS management workforce for the King's Fund, Walshe and Smith (2011) use the Binley's NHS Directory to present trends on the composition and characteristics of senior and middle management, over a period of 14 years (1997–2010).

Beyond descriptive analysis, a more revealing approach is to investigate the existence and magnitude of the effect of one or more explanatory variables upon a dependent variable at a given point in time. This analytical approach usually requires the formulation of hypotheses, grounded in theory and looking for statistically significant associations between variables. Goodall (2011), for example, employs a linear regression model to focus on the relationship between the background of hospital Chief Executive Officers (CEOs), medical or otherwise, and the effect on the quality ranking of the top 100 United States hospitals in 2009. Also using data related to the United States health care system, Bai (2013) utilizes ordinary least squares (OLS) to analyse the relationship between governing board size and the presence of doctors measured as a binary variable with the social performance (community benefits) of 703 hospitals, accounting for confounding factors such as patient mix, location, workforce and the range of services offered.

Our own research has also used cross-sectional analysis, based on data collected by observing many organizations at the same point in time, to focus on the impact of clinical representation on the governing boards of English NHS acute care trusts (Veronesi, Kirkpatrick and Vallascas 2013). Following a similar research design with matching databases, we looked at the effect of clinical directors on the board of 102 hospital trusts over the period 2006–2009 on two outcome measures: the Healthcare Commission (now Care Quality Commission) rating for the quality of care provided and Dr Foster's (a commercial provider of health care benchmarking data) hospital-related mortality rates. In the first instance, due to the characteristics of the dependent variables, the analysis employed pooled regression (that is, observed cross-sectional data of the same organization at different points in time) via an ordered logit model (that is, a regression model for ordinal independent variables), whereas for the morbidity rates (a continuous variable), an OLS regression (that is, a method for estimating the unknown parameters in a linear regression model) was used.

An approach that is arguably more sophisticated is to exploit the longitudinal nature of data sets using a technique called panel corrected standard errors (that is, a class of estimators for the variance-covariance matrix – a square matrix containing the variances and covariances associated with the variables – of the OLS when there are many observations per year in a relatively short time period). In our own research, this was used to analyse the effects of clinical leadership in governing boards on the experience of patients in acute care hospital trusts (Veronesi, Kirkpatrick and Altanlar 2015). This methodology has the advantage of controlling for prior levels of the dependent variable (essentially, the existence of path dependency) as well as accounting for potential correlation of the errors across trusts within the same time period (autocorrelation), and unequal variances across different subsets of hospitals (heteroskedasticity). To confirm the main results, separate robustness tests can be run that apply panel data with fixed effects and random effects estimations. The former is useful to address the possibility of an omitted variable bias (that is, unobserved heterogeneity or not including alternative explanatory factors), whereas the latter controls for the likelihood that variation across trusts is random and not correlated to the explanatory variable. To address the concern of reverse causality (essentially a two-way causal relationship), one can also treat the main independent variable – the presence of clinicians on the board – as endogenous (that is, its values are affected by other functional factors) – by applying the Arellano–Bover/Blundell–Bond dynamic panel data estimations.

An extension of this approach is the system Generalized Methods of Moments (a type of dynamic panel data model), where the dependent variable is dynamic, meaning that its lagged values are entered in the estimation regressions, and the predictors are treated as not strictly exogenous (that is, potentially correlated with past and possible current realizations of the error). This methodology becomes particularly useful when the association between certain factors (for example, management size and board composition) and organizational performance is explored, as it allows the researcher to account for the possible feedback loop between variables (management can influence performance, but this in turn can also influence management).

A different method employed in our body of research on NHS management consists of structural equation modelling. This is a statistical technique used mainly for confirmatory testing of hypotheses based on a general linear model. Related to this is partial least squares path modelling (based on predicted and observable variables), which operates similarly to multiple regression analysis. As a soft modelling technique, this method is particularly suited for exploratory research purposes as well as dealing with formative indicators (that is, the indicators causing the construct). In our case, we use this methodology as it allows modelling the relationship between 'board heterogeneity' (the mix of skills and backgrounds of members) and hospital trust performance while exploring the mediating and mutually reinforcing role of line managers' styles and practices and levels of staff satisfaction (see Blanco-Oliver, Veronesi and Kirpatrick 2016).

Lastly, we have also employed a data analysis technique applying the rules of logical inference to examine the characteristics of those members of governing boards of NHS acute trusts with a medical background. Specifically, we use fuzzy-set/qualitative comparative analysis (fsQCA), which combines case-oriented and variable-oriented quantitative analysis. Based on the analysis of set relations, this technique allows a greater degree of freedom to examine causal complexities and focuses on a joint causal system that accommodates interaction effects among characteristics in a case.

Managers and performance: Emerging research

In this section we turn to some of the applications of this research using administrative data and the range of analytical methods described above, conducted by ourselves and others. This provides an insight into the challenges posed by this kind of research and how the substantive findings are useful for advancing knowledge about management in the NHS. To achieve this, we focus on studies relating to the two central questions described earlier – the characteristics of management and antecedents and the impact of managers on performance.

Managers in the NHS: Characteristics and antecedents

As we noted earlier, while data relating to the overall size and composition of management in the NHS are available, little attention has been given to exploring these in more detail. Our own research draws on the administrative data sources shown Tables 18.1 and 18.2 and has helped to advance the debate on the effect of general management as a whole and, more specifically, the composition (or human capital) of boards on outcomes.

Managers in the acute hospital trust sector

Building on the debates mentioned earlier, research by Kirkpatrick, Veronesi and Altanlar (2017) sought to explore the characteristics and antecedents of (or factors explaining) the development of management in the NHS, drawing on the Binley's database and other sources. This study focused on English acute trusts over a five-year period (2007–2012), with a panel of 158 hospital trusts in 2012. It made use of a variety of administrative data sources, especially those described in Table 18.1, and of different analytical methods, including descriptive statistics and Panel corrected standard errors (see Table 18.3). Using categories adopted from Mintzberg (1993), the study found that 'strategic apex' managers accounted for around 27 per cent of the total, with middle-tier managers (mainly in clinical director-ates) another 33 per cent. In 2012 clinical managers, or 'hybrids' (including roles such as Clinical and Medical Director and senior nurse managers), accounted for 30 per cent of all managers. Further analysis revealed some interesting variations in the development of these management functions within trusts. For example, both specialist trusts and teaching trusts tended to have higher proportions of managers to staff.

However, most interesting and surprising was the divergence in practice between Foundation trusts, with greater formal autonomy, and non-Foundation trusts. Contrary to what one might expect, Kirkpatrick, Veronesi and Altanlar (2017) found that the shift to Foundation trust status had a statistically significant *negative* impact on the size of management functions, despite challenges associated with increased delegation and account-ability. At the same time, it showed that Foundation trusts tended to deploy more managers involved in strategic roles. The latter underscores the trend towards developing board-level governance arrangements and the additional work associated with satisfying the demands of regulators and other external stakeholders, such as commissioners (Klenk and Pavolini 2015). More generally, the results question the idea that NPM-style reforms aimed at 'cor-poratizing' public organizations are necessarily leading to an expansion in the number of managers. While these organizations are more 'managed' in terms of processes and account-ability regimes, it is possible that they are also *under-managed*.

To explore some of the reasons for this outcome, additional tests were conducted focusing on the possible mediating impact of media scrutiny. This was motivated by the idea that growing public and political concern about the value and impact of managers might have a negative impact on the willingness of decision-makers in Foundation trusts, which might be concerned about bad press, to recruit managers. In the event, we found some evidence to support this proposition.

Using the LexisNexis database which covers all published media, we noted that Foundation trusts were significantly more likely to attract media scrutiny calculated as the number of times mentioned in the LexisNexis database. This in turn was found to be a powerful mediating factor explaining the relatively lower proportion of managers-to-staff. Such findings highlight the political sensitivities associated with moves towards Foundation trust status and how this may be impacting on decisions concerning the relative size and resourcing of management functions. They also highlight another key advantage of administrative data, namely the ability to combine multiple and diverse data sources.

Board-level management

A second strand of research has focused on the characteristics of managers who sit on the boards of NHS acute trusts, in particular, with regard to their human capital – such as whether their background is clinical or non-clinical (see, for example, Veronesi, Kirkpatrick and Vallascas 2013, 2014). In this area, publicly available administrative data were less useful, making it necessary to extract this information manually from hospital trust websites and annual reports covering the four years from 2005/06 to 2008/09. A limitation of this approach is that in earlier years many hospital trusts provided less detailed information on their governance structures, making it hard to develop a complete data set for the entire population.

Using mainly descriptive statistics in the first instance, this research yielded some interesting results. In 2008/09, the average board size stood at 12.45, with the ratio of non-executive directors on the board being just over 50 per cent. Women made up a minority of board members (33.8 per cent in 2008/09). Although representing only a slight increase since the later 1990s (Walshe and Smith 2011), the gender mix of NHS boards compares favourably with those of leading commercial organizations. Even more revealing was the proportion of hospital board members with non-public sector or business and commercial backgrounds. The drive to recruit business specialists is a hallmark of NPM reforms (Petrovsky, James and Boyne 2015), notably so in the NHS following the Griffiths report (Department of Health and Social Security, 1983). Our own analysis revealed that, on average, 52.12 per cent of board members came from outside the NHS, ranging from 20 per cent in some trusts and 80 per cent in others. Interestingly, however, business experts made up only 3 per cent of CEOs (Kirkpatrick, Veronesi and Vallascas 2017).

Given the above, it is perhaps not surprising that our analysis indicated that clinicians made up a minority of board members. Overall, clinicians accounted for 26.4 per cent of membership in English Trusts in 2008/09, roughly evenly split between doctors and those with other clinical backgrounds including nursing. In most cases, board participation was limited to the statutory roles of nursing and medical director, although in roughly a quarter of cases they made up more than 30 per cent of board members. Interestingly, over the four years, only around a fifth of the CEOs had a clinical background (Veronesi, Kirkpatrick and Vallascas 2013). Such figures highlight the dominance of non-clinical management in the highest echelons of the NHS, although the involvement of clinicians (general practitioners) is higher in primary care organizations such as clinical commissioning groups.

However, even more intriguing were the findings of a study (Kirkpatrick, Veronesi and Zardini 2016) that focused on the backgrounds of medical board members in one year. This study employed a more sophisticated method of fsQCA described earlier. Matching information from the Binley's database and the General Medical Council (GMC) register, the study was able to categorize medical directors according to their medical specialization and educational background. Using national and international rankings of universities and specialisms, this information was then used to assess the status backgrounds of medical directors. Initial analysis found that in 2012, from a population of approximately 150 medical directors, 85 per cent came from either a top-three ranked specialism (surgery, general medicine and anaesthesiology) or the top-three medical schools (Oxford, Cambridge and London). In addition, 34.6 per cent of medical directors combined *both* of these status credentials, compared with only 4.2 per cent of the GMC population of doctors in England as a whole. Hence, while medical leaders represent only a minority of hospital trust governing boards, those that occupy these roles hail from the upper echelons of the profession. Such findings again highlight the ways in which multiple administrative data sources (Binley's and the GMC register) can be combined in innovative ways to advance knowledge about health care management.

Managers and performance

In this section we turn to research focusing on the second question of what impact, if any, managers in the NHS might have on performance. To do so, we built on the earlier distinction between the management function overall and the specific context of board-level managers. For both themes, this research drew on data relating to the characteristics of managers (as above) and a range of organizational outcome or performance statistics summarized in Table 18.2.

Board human capital and performance

For some time, the broader literature on boards and governance has sought to explore the impact of different mixes of human capital – for example, generic versus sector-specific expertise – on corporate performance (Sundaramurthy, Pukthuanthong and Kor 2014). This theme has also been picked up in research focusing on CEO appointments in public organizations such as local authorities and the relative importance of 'publicness fit' (Petrovksy,

James and Boyne 2015). In the NHS context, while there has been growing interest in board governance (Chambers et al. 2013), with the exception of studies focusing on board culture (Dixon-Woods et al. 2013; Jacobs et al. 2013), less attention has been paid to performance outcomes. Our research has sought to fill this gap, focusing on two key themes: the impact of business experts (Kirkpatrick, Veronesi and Vallascas 2017) and clinicians (Blanco-Oliver, Veronesi and Kirkpatrick 2016; Veronesi, Kirkpatrick and Altanlar 2015; Veronesi, Kirkpatrick and Vallascas 2013, 2014) on NHS boards. These studies employed a range of different methods including cross-sectional regression and structural equation modelling (see Table 18.3).

Starting with business experts, our analysis of four years of data found that the presence of these board members had no negative (or positive) impact on service quality and patient wellbeing. On the other hand, business expertise did appear to have a positive impact on a more specific range of financial management and efficiency outcomes. Our findings therefore suggest a need for caution when assuming that the influx of managers with non-public backgrounds will necessarily have damaging consequences. On the contrary, this expertise may be useful in terms of helping to respond to demands for improved efficiency, at least on those trust boards that are less experienced (Kirkpatrick, Veronesi and Vallascas 2017).

Turning to the question of clinical involvement on boards, more research has been conducted in health care settings, notably in the United States (see Sarto and Veronesi 2016 for a review). For example, Jiang and colleagues (2009) show how greater medical participation in hospital committees improves performance in terms of the care process (measured as quality of care of heart attack, heart failure, pneumonia and surgical infection prevention) and mortality rates. Goodall (2011) also found that having a CEO with a medical background generates greater quality improvements and results in higher hospital rankings.

Our own work, focusing on the NHS, largely confirms and extends these findings. An initial study by Veronesi, Kirkpatrick and Vallascas (2013), using cross-sectional data and pooled regression, found a very strong relationship between the now redundant Healthcare Commission's quality ratings and clinical involvement on trust boards. Similar results were obtained using an alternative indicator of quality – the hospital standardized mortality ratio published by Dr Foster. An additional test (marginal effects) was conducted to quantify the benefits of having a higher share of doctors on boards. This showed that if the proportion of doctors increases by roughly 10 per cent, the probability that a hospital trust will achieve the maximum score of four is increased by 7.34 per cent.

Surprisingly, despite the critical importance of nursing for the delivery of high-quality care, the research found that the influence of nurse directors on performance was negligible. The results also suggest that the qualifications of the CEO may be less significant than previously assumed. Contrary to the findings of Goodall (2011), for example, there was no significant relationship between CEOs who are doctors and performance. Instead, what appears to count for more is having a larger group of clinicians on boards collectively contributing to decision making.

Other papers, extending this work, looked at the impact of clinical involvement on a range of other performance outcomes, including efficiency and patient experience (Veronesi, Kirkpatrick and Altanlar 2015; Veronesi, Kirkpatrick and Vallascas 2014). Against expectations, we found that the higher participation of doctors on boards had a positive, albeit weak, impact on Healthcare Commission financial ratings. Medical participation was also strongly related to improved patient experience, in terms of care: access, coordination, information, relationships with clinical staff and comfort (Veronesi, Kirkpatrick and Altanlar 2015). However, further tests revealed that these positive relationships were limited only to the boards of Foundation trusts. Implied here is that the voice and influence of doctors in strategic decision making may be greatly enhanced in organizational contexts where hospital trusts also exercise greater formal autonomy.

General managers and performance

As noted earlier, with the possible exception of Bloom and van Reenen (2010), far less has been written about the impact of managers. To address this, we built on an earlier study of the management function in acute trusts (Kirkpatrick, Veronesi and Altanlar 2017) to also look at whether the proportion of managers to staff, their pay and job tenure had an impact on performance (Veronesi, Altanlar and Kirkpatrick 2018). The study used a longitudinal database, drawn from Binley's, for all English acute trusts spanning six years (2007–2012), combining this with data from NHS Digital on annual manager salaries (mean of £52,000) and average annual turnover for managers (a mean of roughly one in ten). This research used the generalized method of movements described in Table 18.3 and also multiple organizational performance data (see Table 18.2).

To explore the impact of managers on performance two main tests were conducted: one looked at our key explanatory variables (management size, pay and job tenure) in isolation and a second looked at them in combination. The results of this analysis question the popular assumption that managers represent an essentially unproductive overhead in the NHS. Specifically, we found that a higher manager-to-staff ratio in hospital trusts led to a reduction in infection rates and greater efficiency, and these results were not affected by issues of reverse causality due to endogeneity concerns.

Patient experience also seemed to be positively affected by having more managers in relation to staff, although the statistical confidence in this finding was less robust. Management pay and job tenure did not have any significant association with performance outcomes. Further analysis revealed that even a small increase in the proportion of managers (1 per cent above the average) could lead to significant improvements, placing an average performing hospital trust in the top third in terms of efficiency and infection rates. For an average size hospital trust (employing 3,900 staff), a 1 per cent growth in this ratio would mean employing approximately 39 more managers at a basic gross salary cost of £2.03 million.

Reading health research about managers based on secondary data

Various administrative data sources now make it possible to research a range of aspects of health care management from its core characteristics to its impact on performance. In such studies, it is vital at a generic level, among other things, that:

- The interpretation of secondary data is made with appropriate circumspection
- Researchers have not been lured into 'gaming' in the system through their data usage
- Care is taken in using associations between data to infer causal relationships
- There is an adequate theoretical and methodological framework
- Multi-method approaches are used where appropriate to forge connections
- In an associated way, there is not an excessive reliance simply on one data set.

These points are variously amplified further in relation to health care managers in the extended Conclusion that follows and complement those on quantitative statistical techniques in the previous chapter.

Conclusion

Our point of departure in this chapter is debates concerning health care management and its contribution, if any, to performance. We noted that, while NPM reforms have been ongoing for some time, relationships between managers and clinical professionals continue to be fraught with difficulty. These concerns have also spilled over into policy debates, with politicians and media critiquing managers as rent-seeking bureaucrats or unproductive overheads (Kettl 2017). However, while these claims are often made, the research evidence both on the nature and characteristics of managers and their impact is limited.

In this chapter, we have illustrated the potential of an alternative research agenda, one which also draws on a growing availability of 'administrative data sources' (Smith et al. 2004). These data have numerous advantages. As we saw, it is possible to combine data sources to understand the characteristics, antecedents and performance consequences of management. Often, administrative data allow for large, almost complete, coverage of relevant populations (such as NHS hospital trusts) and are relatively standardized and consistent over time. The latter also means it is possible to perform longitudinal analysis, making it easier to determine the broad direction of association (or causality) over time.

As we saw from the examples of our own and other research focusing on the English NHS, using administrative data can help to advance knowledge of management in a number of key respects. First, this can be taken with regard to the growth of both clinical and non-clinical managers. According to Nigel Edwards (2016), previously head of the NHS Confederation, the view that there are 'too many chiefs' is one of the five myths of the NHS that we need to dispel. Our analysis confirms this assumption, showing how organizations such as Foundation trusts are often under-managed – despite having greater responsibilities delegated to them – and how this is accentuated by (mainly negative) media scrutiny (Kirkpatrick, Veronesi and Altanlar 2017).

Second, an even more significant contribution is to our understanding of the impact that managers have on performance. Research using administrative data adds to existing research on board governance, noting the positive impact of hybrid professional managers on boards - notably doctors (Goodall 2011; Jiang et al. 2009). However, it also qualifies this work, noting how these benefits may be restricted to certain organizational contexts, such as foundation trusts (Veronesi, Kirkpatrick and Altanlar 2015). In addition, new data sources have made it possible to explore the impact of management functions more generally on performance. This calls into question the assumption that managers are an unproductive overhead and points instead to their importance for the coordination of complex services. While the practice of managers is certainly not beyond criticism, as Hyde and colleagues (2016: xiv) suggest, they play 'vital roles in the daily functioning of healthcare organizations'.

When noting these advances, it is of course important to also acknowledge certain risks associated with the greater use of administrative data sources. Often these data only offer very crude proxies for actual management practice and could also be more fine-grained. For example, a particular criticism of Health Commission ratings is that they failed to adequately capture the quality of the health care provided (Bevan and Hood 2006), focusing too much on subjective assessments of process. More worryingly, it is suggested that these reviews generated perverse incentives for hospitals to 'game' the system by inflating their scores and that consequently more qualitative aspects of performance were ignored or given only secondary importance. Criticisms have also been lodged against measures such as the hospital mortality ratio collected by Dr Foster Intelligence (www.drfoster.com), which fails to differentiate between preventable and non-preventable deaths (Lilford and Pronovost 2010), and the Reference Cost Index as an accurate measure of efficiency (Deloitte 2014).

A more significant challenge in terms of the explanatory power of the kind of analysis we have reviewed here is that, while we can establish strong associations (even causal) between variables (for instance, management and performance), this does not explain *why* these relationships exist. This limitation underscores the need for research using this type of data to be guided by theory. It also highlights the usefulness of multi-method research strategies, perhaps combining the interrogation of administrative data to identify patterns and associations followed by more targeted qualitative research using ethnographic or comparative case study designs.

There is obvious potential for further research adopting the approach we have outlined here. This may probe deeper into questions relating to the antecedents and impact of management, perhaps drawing on yet untapped administrative data sources. It would be useful to focus on the experience of primary care organizations, such as Clinical Commissioning Groups, where there has been an explicit policy drive to recruit clinicians (general practitioners) on to boards. Future research might also look at the issue of chief executive turnover and succession events in NHS organizations, or the role played by external management consultants. Some initial work on the latter theme has already been conducted, drawing on the financial accounts of hospital trusts to quantify annual expenditure on consultants and the negative relationship between this spending and efficiency (Kirkpatrick et al. 2019). There is scope to explore this topic further, to understand the factors which mediate the use of consultants by NHS organizations.

Lastly, it would be beneficial to replicate this approach in other national health systems. Studies conducted by ourselves and other colleagues (Sarto, Kirkpatrick and Veronesi 2018), focusing on management in Italian public hospitals, demonstrate similar dynamics to the English NHS. Further work of this kind will depend on the availability of relevant administrative data. The potential for more national case studies of health care management and, in the longer term, even comparative research based on multi-country studies is clearly evident, helping to inform both theory and policy.

Exercise 18.1 Analysing health data

The following activities are intended to offer you a practical example of searching data related to researching health care management that can be used for analytical purposes and to undertake some descriptive and preliminary analysis of the collected data.

Search for data

Access the NHS Digital website at https://digital.nhs.uk/. Click on the View data and publications link. Click on the All our publications hyperlink on the next page. In the Search option field, type Hospital Episode Statistics and in the following page click on Hospital Episode Statistics (HES). Scroll down the next page until you find HES publications and then click on Admitted Patient Care. Subsequently, click the hyperlink under the heading Latest Version which, at the time of writing this chapter, is Hospital Admitted Patient Care Activity, 2016–17. Once reaching the next page, in Resources, click on Hospital Admitted Patient Care Activity, 2016–17: Hospital Providers. An Excel spreadsheet will open containing episode groups related to activity in English NHS Hospitals and English NHS commissioned activity in the independent sector. This data will be used for the exercises that follow as part of the preliminary descriptive analysis, which can be cross-referenced to Chapter 17.

Preliminary and descriptive analysis

Measures of central tendency

The raw data set includes information on providers' activity, including Finished consultant episode, Admissions, Patient characteristics, and so forth. To better

(Continued)

(Continued)

understand the data in hand, it is useful to summarize the information, particularly in relation to the centre of that set of data. Central tendency describes the tendency of the observations to bunch around a particular value or category. The three common ways of describing the central tendency of a data set is to calculate the mean (the average value of a group of numbers), median (the middle number in a group) and mode (the most commonly occurring number in a group).

Compute these three measures for any of the activity information provided in the data set (for example, for Finished consultant episodes) using the relevant function in Excel, which can be found in the Formulas tab.

Measures of dispersion

The mean is the value generally used to indicate the centre of a distribution. However, when dealing with quantity variables, a description of the data set would not be complete without a measure of the extent to which the observed values are spread out from the average.

The three most common measures of dispersion are range, the variance and the standard deviation. The range of a set of data represents the size of the smallest interval which contains all the data - in between the lowest and highest value. The variance measures how far a set of (random) numbers are spread out from their average value. Lastly, the standard deviation is a measure employed to quantify the amount of variation or dispersion of a set of data values. It entails the average of each observed values deviation from the mean.

Compute these three measures for any of the activity information provided in the data set (for instance, for Finished consultant episodes) using the relevant function in Excel, which can be found in the Formulas tab.

Measures of correlation

A correlation coefficient is a numerical value that indicates how strongly related two variables are. A common form is represented by the Pearson Correlation Coefficient (usually defined by 'r'). It can vary between −1 and +1 and the sign before the number indicates the direction of the relationship: a positive (negative) value means that as one variable increases, the other variable increases (decreases). The closer the value is to 1, the stronger the linear relationship and the closer it is to 0, the weaker the linear relationship. The Pearson Correlation Coefficient assumes that the relationship between two variables is linear.

Compute the Pearson Correlation Coefficient r for any of the activity information provided in the data set: as an example, you could look at the relationship between mean age of patients and mean length of stay. Use the relevant function in Excel, which can be found in the Formulas tab.

Further recommended reading

This book provides a preliminary introduction to econometrics in data analysis without resorting to matrix algebra, calculus or statistics beyond elementary level:
Gujarati, D. N. and Porter, D. C. (2009) *Basic Econometrics*, 5th edition. Columbus, OH: McGraw-Hill Education.

This article assesses the contribution of business experts in board-level activities in the public sector, including in the health care environment:
Kirkpatrick, I., Veronesi, G. and Vallascas, F. (2017) 'Business experts on public sector boards: What do they contribute?', *Public Administration Review*, 77: 754–65.

This article provides key research-based insights into the importance of clinical leadership for patients in the health sector:
Veronesi, G., Kirkpatrick, I. and Altanlar, A. (2015) 'Clinical leadership and the changing governance of public hospitals: Implications for patient experience', *Public Administration*, *93*(4): 1031–48.

References

Ackroyd, S., Kirkpatrick, I. and Walker, R. (2007) 'Public management reform and its consequences for professional organisation: A comparative analysis', *Public Administration*, *85*(1): 9–26.

Andrews, R. and Boyne, G. A. (2014) 'Task complexity, organization size, and administrative intensity: The case of UK universities', *Public Administration*, *92*(3): 656–72.

Angrave, D., Charlwood, A., Kirkpatrick, I., Lawrence, M. and Stuart, M. (2016) 'HR analytics: Why HR is set to fail the big data challenge', *Human Resource Management Journal*, *26*(1): 1–11.

Bai, G. (2013) 'How do board size and occupational background of directors influence social performance in for-profit and non-profit organizations? Evidence from California hospitals', *Journal of Business Ethics*, *118*: 171–87.

Bevan, G. and Hood, C. (2006) 'What's measured is what matters: Targets and gaming in the English public health care system', *Public Administration*, *84*(3): 517–38.

Blanco-Oliver, A., Veronesi, G. and Kirkpatrick, I. (2016) 'Board heterogeneity and organisational performance', *Journal of Business Ethics*. Available at: http://dx.doi.org/10.1007/s10551-016-3290-8

Bloom, N., Propper, C., Seiler, S. and van Reenen, J. (2015) 'The impact of competition on management practices: Evidence from public hospitals', *Review of Economic Studies*, *82*(2): 457–89.

Bloom, N. and van Reenen, J. (2010) 'Measuring and explaining management practices across firms and countries', *Quarterly Journal of Economics*, *122*(4): 1351–408.

Buchanan, D. A., Denyer, D., Jaina, J., Kelliher, C., Moore, C., Parry, E. and Pilbeam, C. (2013) *How Do They Manage? The Realities of Middle and Front Line Management Work in Healthcare*. Health Services and Delivery Research (Project Ref: 08/1808/238). Southampton: National Institute for Health Research.

Carter, P. (2016) *Operational Productivity and Performance in English NHS Acute Hospitals: Unwarranted Variations*. Available at: https://www.gov.uk/government/uploads/system/-uploads/attachment_data/file/499229/Operational_productivity_A.pdf

Chambers, N., Harvey, G., Mannion, R., Bond, J. and Marshall, J. (2013) *Towards a Framework for Enhancing the Performance of NHS Boards: A Synthesis of the Evidence about Board Governance, Board Effectiveness and Board Development*. Health Services and Delivery Research, *6*(1). Southampton: National Institute for Health Research. Available at: doi: 10.3310/hsdr01060

Connelly, R., Playford, C., Gayle, V. and Dibben, C. (2016) 'The role of administrative data in the big data revolution in social science research', *Social Science Research*, *59*: 1–2.

Crilly, T. and Le Grand, J. (2004) 'The motivation and behaviour of hospital trusts', *Social Science and Medicine*, *58*(10): 1809–23.

Croft, C., Currie, G. and Lockett, A. (2015) 'Broken "two-way windows"? An exploration of professional hybrids', *Public Administration*, *93*(2): 380–94.

Degeling, P., Zhang, K., Coyle, B., Xu, L. Z., Meng, Q. Y., Qu, J. B. and Hill, M. (2006) 'Clinicians and the governance of hospitals: A cross-cultural perspective on relations between profession and management', *Social Science and Medicine*, *63*(3): 757–75.

Deloitte (2014) *Reference Cost Data Quality: A Final Report for Monitor*. London: Deloitte.

Department of Health and Social Security (1983) *NHS Management Inquiry*. London: HMSO.

Diefenbach, T. (2009) 'New public management in public sector organizations: The dark sides of managerialistic enlightenment', *Public Administration*, *87*(4): 892–909.

Dixon-Woods, M., Baker, R., Charles, K., Dawson, J., Jerzembek, G., Martin, G., McCarthy, I., McKee, L., Minion, J., Ozieranski, P., Willars, J., Wilkie, P. and West, M. (2013) 'Culture and behaviour in the English National Health Service: Overview of lessons from a large multimethod study', *BMJ Quality and Safety*, *23*: 2.

Edwards, N. (2016) 'Wasteful, too many chiefs: Five myths about the NHS we need to dispel', *Guardian*, 26 January. Available at: www.theguardian.com/society/commentisfree/2016/jan/26/-five-myths-nhs-health-service

Glouberman, S. and Mintzberg, H. (2001) 'Managing the care of health and the cure of disease – Part I: Differentiation', *Health Care Management Review*, *26*(1): 56–69.

Goodall, A. (2011) 'Physician-leaders and hospital performance: Is there an association?', *Social Science and Medicine*, *73*: 535–9.

Greener, I., Harrington, B., Hunter, D., Mannion, R. and Powell, M. (2013) *A Realistic Review of Clinic–Managerial Relationships in the NHS: 1991–2010*. Health Services and Delivery Research (Project 08/1808/245). Southampton: National Institute for Health Research.

Grey, C. (1999) '"We are all managers now", "we always were": On the development and demise of management', *Journal of Management Studies*, *36*(5): 561–85.

Griffiths, P., Ball, J., Bloor, K., Briggs, J., Pryterch, D., Smith, G., Meredith, P., Sinden, N., Böhning, D., Maruotti, D., de Longh, A. and Schmidt, P. (2015) *Nurse Staffing Levels, Missed Vital Signs Observations and Mortality in Hospital Wards: Modelling the Consequences and Costs of Variations in Nurse Staffing and Skill Mix. Retrospective Observational Study Using Routinely Collected Data.* Health Services and Delivery Research (Protocol 13/114/17). Southampton: National Institute for Health Research.

Guardian (2016) 'Why would doctors and nurses put themselves through the ordeal of NHS management? ', 2 December. Available at: www.theguardian.com/healthcare-network/2016/dec/02/-doctors-nurses-ordeal-nhs-management

Hales, C. (2002) '"Bureaucracy-lite" and continuities in managerial work', *British Journal of Management*, *13*(1): 51–66.

Ham, C. (2009) *Health Policy in Britain*, 6th edition. Basingstoke: Palgrave Macmillan.

Hood, C. (1995) 'The "New Public Management" in the 1980s: Variations on a theme', *Accounting, Organizations and Society*, *20*(2–3): 93–109.

Hyde, P., Granter, E., Hassard, J. and McCann, L. (2016) *Deconstructing the Welfare State.* Abingdon: Routledge.

Jacobs, R., Mannion, R., Huw, T., Davies, O., Harrison, S., Konteh, F. and Walshe, K. (2013) 'The relationship between organizational culture and performance in acute hospitals', *Social Science and Medicine*, *76*: 115–25.

Jiang, H. J., Lockee, C., Bass, K. and Fraser, I. (2009) 'Board oversight of quality: Any differences in process of care and mortality?', *Journal of Healthcare Management*, *54*: 15–29.

Kettl, D. F. (2017) 'The clumsy war against the "administrative state"', *Public Administration Review*, *77*(5): 639–40.

King's Fund (2011) *The Future of Leadership and Management in the NHS: No more Heroes.* London: The King's Fund.

Kirkpatrick, I. (2016) 'Hybrid managers and professional leadership', in M. Dent, I. L. Bourgeault, J.-L. Denis and E. Kuhlmann (eds), *The Routledge Companion to the Professions and Professionalism.* Abingdon: Routledge.

Kirkpatrick, I., Ackroyd, S. and Walker, R. (2005) *The New Managerialism and Public Service Professions.* Basingstoke: Palgrave Macmillan.

Kirkpatrick, I., Bullinger, B., Lega, F. and Dent, M. (2013) 'The translation of hospital management reforms in European health systems: A framework for comparison', *British Journal of Management*, *24*: S48–61.

Kirkpatrick, I., Shelly, M. S., Dent, M. and Neogy, I. (2008) 'Towards a "productive" relationship between medicine and management: Reporting from a national inquiry', *International Journal of Clinical Leadership*, *16*(1): 27–35.

Kirkpatrick, I., Sturdy, A., Reguera, N., Blanco-Oliver, A. and Veronesi, G. (2019) 'The impact of management consultants on public service efficiency', *Policy and Politics* , *47*(1): 77–96.

Kirkpatrick, I., Veronesi, G. and Altanlar, A. (2017) 'Corporatisation and the emergence of (under managed) managed organizations: The case of English public hospitals', *Organization Studies, 38*: 12.

Kirkpatrick, I., Veronesi, G. and Vallascas, F. (2017) 'Business experts on public sector boards: What do they contribute?', *Public Administration Review, 77*: 754–65.

Kirkpatrick, I., Veronesi, G. and Zardini, A. (2016) 'The emergence of professional-management hierarchies in public hospitals: Reinforcing and changing the professional status order', paper presented at 31st European Group for Organizational Studies Colloquium, July.

Klenk, T. and Pavolini, E. (2015) *Restructuring Welfare Governance: Marketisation, Managerialism and Welfare State Professionalism.* Cheltenham: Edward Elgar.

Kuhlmann, E., Blank, R., Bourgeault, I. and Wendt, C. (eds) (2015) *The Palgrave International Handbook of Healthcare Policy and Governance.* Basingstoke: Palgrave Macmillan.

Lilford, R. and Pronovost, P. (2010) 'Using hospital mortality rates to judge hospital performance: A bad idea that just won't go away', *British Medical Journal, 340*: c2016.

Lindlbauer, I., Winter, V. and Schreyögg, J. (2015) 'Antecedents and consequences of corporatization: An empirical analysis of German public hospitals', *Journal of Public Administration Research and Theory, 26*(2): 309–26.

Lord Ashcroft KCMG (2015) *The People, the Parties and the NHS.* London: Lord Ashcroft KCMG PC.

Mayer-Schonberger, V. and Cukier, K. (2013) *Big Data.* London: John Murray.

McKee, M. and Healy, J. (2002) *Hospitals in a Changing Europe.* Buckingham: Open University Press.

Mintzberg, H. (1993) *Structure in Fives: Designing Effective Organizations.* Englewood Cliffs, NJ: Prentice-Hall.

Mintzberg, H. (2017) *Managing the Myths of Health Care.* Oakland, CA: Brent-Koehler.

National Institute for Health Research (2013) *New Evidence on Management and Leadership.* Health Services and Delivery Research. London: NIHR. Available at: www. journalslibrary.nihr.ac.uk/downloads/research-programmes/HSDR/New-Evidence-on-Management-and-Leadership.pdf

NHS Confederation (2017) *NHS Statistics, Facts and Figures.* Available at: www.nhsconfed. org/resources/key-statistics-on-the-nhs

NHS England (2016) *NHS Five Year Forward Review.* London: NHS England.

Pemberton, M. (2017) 'Dr Max the mind doctor: It is nurses working at the coalface of the NHS that we need, not more bosses', *Daily Mail*, 3 March. Available at: www.dailymail. co.uk/health/article-5456701/It-nurses-need-not-bosses-says-Dr-Max-Pemberton. html#ixzz59uBcnSLl

Petrovsky, N., James, O. and Boyne, G. A. (2015) 'New leaders' managerial background and the performance of public organizations: The theory of publicness fit', *Journal of Public Administration Research and Theory, 25*(1): 217–36.

Powell, A. and Davies, H. (2016) *Managing Doctors, Doctors Managing.* London: Nuffield Trust.

Saltman, R. B., Durán, A. and Dubois, H. F. W. (2011) *Governing Public Hospitals: Reform Strategies and the Movement Towards Institutional Autonomy.* Copenhagen: European Observatory on Health Systems and Policies.

Sarto, F. and Veronesi, G. (2016) 'Clinical leadership and hospital performance: Assessing the evidence base', *BMC Health Services Research,* 16. Available at: https://doi.org/10.1186/s12913-016-1395-5

Sarto, F., Kirkpatrick, I. and Veronesi, G. (2018) 'Organising professionals and their impact on performance: The case of public health doctors in the Italian SSN', *Public Management Review.* Available at: doi:10.1080/14719037.2018.1544270.

Smith, G., Noble, M., Anttilla, C., Gill, L., Zaidi, A., Wright, G., Dibben, C. and Barnes, H. (2004) *The Value of Linked Administrative Records for Longitudinal Analysis.* Report to the ESRC National Longitudinal Strategy Committee.

Spurgeon, P. and Clark, J. (2017) *Medical Leadership: The Key to Medical Engagement and Effective Organisations.* Abingdon: CRC Press.

Spyridonidis, D., Hendy, J. and Barlow, J. (2015) 'Understanding hybrid roles: The role of identity processes amongst physicians', *Public Administration, 93*(2): 395–411.

Sundaramurthy, C., Pukthuanthong, K. and Kor, Y. (2014) 'Positive and negative synergies between the CEO's and the corporate board's human and social capital: A study of biotechnology firms', *Strategic Management Journal, 35*(6): 845–68.

Verbeeten, F. H. and Speklé, R. F. (2015) 'Management control, results-oriented culture and public sector performance: Empirical evidence on New Public Management', *Organization Studies, 36*(7): 953–78.

Veronesi, G., Altanlar, A. and Kirkpatrick, I. (2018) 'Managers in the public sector: A bureaucratic burden? The case of English public hospitals', paper presented at the Organisational Behaviour in Healthcare Conference, Montreal, May.

Veronesi, G., Kirkpatrick, I. and Altanlar, A. (2015) 'Clinical leadership and the changing governance of public hospitals: Implications for patient experience', *Public Administration, 93*(4): 1031–48.

Veronesi, G., Kirkpatrick, I. and Vallascas, F. (2013) 'Clinicians on the board: What difference does it make?', *Social Science and Medicine,* 77: 147–55.

Veronesi, G., Kirkpatrick, I. and Vallascas, F. (2014) 'Does clinical management improve efficiency? Evidence from the English NHS', *Public Money and Management, January*: 1–8.

Walker, R. M. (2013) 'Strategic management and performance in public organizations: Findings from the Miles and Snow framework', *Public Administration Review, 73*(5): 675–85.

Walshe, K. and Smith, L. (2011) *The NHS Management Workforce.* London: King's Fund.

West, M. A., Armit, K., Loewenthal, L., Eckert, R., West, T. and Lee, A. (2015) *Leadership and Leadership Development in Health Care: The Evidence Base.* London: Faculty of Medical Leadership and Management.

PART IV
Issues in Health Research

19

Ethics in Health Research

PRISCILLA ALDERSON

Chapter objectives

- To provide a brief history of health research ethics
- To summarize the main concerns of formal ethics reviews and the meaning of voluntary and informed consent
- To consider professional ethics guidelines and their purpose
- To discuss the relevance of health research ethics and potential conflicts of interest
- To conclude with a critique of current research ethics and their fitness for purpose.

Introduction

This chapter aims to review the history and development of health research ethics. It considers the role and purpose of formal ethics review in health research and discusses what is meant by voluntary and informed consent. In the chapter, procedural and substantive health research ethics are compared, and it is argued that a consideration of ethics is both a method and a topic for research, and social research can contribute to health research ethics. Ethics has relevance to a range of health-related activities, such as regulatory governance and policy making. Particular attention is paid to the ethics of research with disadvantaged groups and how formal health research ethics systems can support researchers. The conclusion raises doubts about whether, without reform, present health research ethics systems can cope adequately with current developments in health research.

In the chapter, terms are used that require definition. The term 'participant/subject' is used to acknowledge that not everyone taking part in research has been a fully informed and is a willing 'participant', despite this being the standard set. There are still research 'subjects' who have not given informed and willing consent. 'Medical' will refer to clinical scientific research on the body and body parts, its processes, tests and treatments, including preventative and public health research, while 'social' includes research about people's views and experiences of health and illness. 'Bioethics' refers to the more philosophical, abstract version of health ethics.

A brief history of health research ethics

Ethics is defined as the formal moral standards set by professional associations and other institutions to help to maintain and evaluate high standards in practice and research. 'Ethics' is also used interchangeably with the broader term 'morals', which are concerned with principles of right and wrong behaviour. One of the oldest binding ethics documents concerns relations between doctors and patients, the Hippocratic Oath (around 400 BCE), which is still taken in modern versions by doctors today (for example, General Medical Council 2014). Although it is mainly about medical etiquette and professional solidarity, the Oath respects the ethics of patients' confidentiality and aims to benefit the sick according to the doctor's ability and judgement and keep them from harm and injustice. These promises, based on 'do no harm', relate to research, although the Oath does not mention it.

Before 1950, there were few formal ethics guidelines or committees. During the 1930s and 1940s formal guidelines in Germany did little to prevent harmful research. This was also the case in the United States, Europe and the Far East (McNeill 1993). Eugenics (good birth) was widely practised, to protect the purity of the race by preventing the birth and survival of 'inferior' children. The Nazi Holocaust began with Hitler's personal physician organizing the euthanasia (good death or mercy killing) of disabled children in schools and hospitals, many run by churches (Proctor 1988). The most caring professionals can hold misleading dangerous ideals, so that formal and effective ethics guidance and systems are always vital. These are set out in the Nuremberg Code (1947) and the Declaration of Helsinki (World Medical Association [1964] 2013).

From the 1970s onwards, Institutional Review Boards (IRBs) and Research Ethics Committees (RECs) began to be introduced widely to review ethical standards in medical research, along with new university bioethics centres, courses, journals and conferences (Beauchamp and Childress 2013; National Commission for the Protection of Human

Subjects in Medical and Behavioral Research 1978). Ethics guidelines were issued and updated frequently. There was rapid change from largely unregulated research to far more careful and critical regulation. Health care professionals and hospitals led the way, driven by anxiety about the rising costs of litigation from patients who alleged they had been harmed by research or had not been fully informed about the risks before they consented. Radical change came when patient representatives were appointed as 'lay members' to IRBs/RECs and they promoted greater caution about risk-taking and higher standards of informed consent than doctors alone had previously accepted.

Today, the context for health research has changed in several ways. There is great pressure to guard against complaints and costly litigation from aggrieved participants/subjects. One approach is to subject all proposed research projects, including those by graduate students, to formal ethics review. Another is to try to ensure that the informed consent forms clearly transfer responsibility for any risks from the researchers on to informed research participants/subjects. IRBs/RECs may protect their institutions by rejecting medical research with 'vulnerable' groups, including children and women who might be pregnant. This increases the risk of excluding their experiences, and of limiting their access to medications of proven safety and efficacy. Academic and commercial research institutions now rely on vast research funding from governments, businesses and philanthropic trusts.

At first, IRBs/RECs were fairly independent, but they are now run by research administration departments. Compared with the 1980s, in large RECs, and reported on websites (see, for example, University College London 2018), there seems to be much greater use of chair's action that bypasses a whole committee discussion. There is less time given to training REC members, and more waiving of consent forms that need not be used with anonymized secondary data. This means that secondary research can be done on the data of hundreds of thousands of people without their knowledge, consent or approval. During public protests about Facebook's invasive and commercial exploitation of personal data, some academics have questioned the routine hiring out by universities of very detailed, though anonymized, personal data for secondary analysis, without the donors' specific knowledge or consent or the need for REC oversight (see, for instance, Holmwood 2018).

The main concerns in formal health research ethics

In the three frameworks shown in Box 19.1, principles (or deontology) and rights set clear general standards, although these can be flexible in how they are interpreted to fit different local needs and contexts. There is no right to health, since that cannot be willed or enforced, for example when someone is terminally ill. However, there are rights to the highest attainable standard of health and health care and to an adequate standard of living, such as to housing, nutritious food and clean water (United Nations 1948, 1989).

Box 19.1   Three frameworks in health research ethics

These three frameworks can be set out as follows:

- Principles of ethics centre on respect for autonomy, justice, doing no harm and beneficence.
- Rights provide for basic needs, including access to the best available health care and an adequate standard of living; they protect people from harm, abuse, neglect and discrimination; they respect privacy and freedom of information, expression, thought and conscience; and they promote social inclusion and self-determination.
- Outcomes aim to avoid or reduce harm and costs and to promote benefits.

Source: Beauchamp and Childress 2013; National Commission for the Protection of Human Subjects in Medical and Behavioral Research 1978; United Nations 1948, 1989 (see also Alderson and Morrow 2011; Biggs 2009; Cave and Brazier 2016; Cornstock 2013; Emanuel, Grady and Crouch 2011).

In contrast to principles and rights, outcomes (or utilitarianism) involve calculating the greatest benefit to the greatest number of people, or balancing the harms, risks, costs and inconvenience to participants/subjects against the hoped-for benefits from research. The balance between harms and benefits is further complicated in that participants/subjects bear the risks, but future patients will receive the benefits if the treatment or health promotion being tested proves to be effective, the research is published and implemented, and possibly also if official bodies approve and fund the new procedures. Patients might benefit from the treatment being tested on them, but that is not certain, otherwise the treatment would not be the object of research. A problem with these risk/benefit equations is the logical assumption that the higher the potential benefit, then the higher the permitted risks (see also Chapter 16). In practice, this can mean that if a new medication might cure end-stage cancer (very high potential benefit), then it can be trialled on extremely ill patients (very high risk that it could kill them or increase their suffering). This logic potentially exposes the most vulnerable.

Whereas health care practitioners provide direct benefits and services to their patients or clients, in research the process is reversed when participants/subjects confer benefits on researchers by giving them data. This reversed relationship requires that participants/subjects should have more rights than patients/clients. These rights centre on voluntary and informed consent, as outlined in Box 19.2 in the next section.

The ethical frameworks, including other approaches, such as virtue ethics, all have strengths but leave gaps. They are widely analysed and debated. Moral questions about power, honesty and respecting or abusing participants/subjects, arise throughout the research process. Formally or less consciously, researchers tend to resolve questions by thinking about principles. They are concerned with the right thing to do: with human rights, with respecting and protecting people, and with the outcomes of research. What might be the benefits to promote and the harms to avoid? Many researchers combine the three frameworks shown in Box 19.1 and, although they do not provide easy answers to ethical problems, they can help to identify and clarify problems and suggest ways to solve or reduce them.

Voluntary and informed consent

If consent is to be voluntary, researchers must avoid exerting any pressure or inducements that could affect a freely made decision. The Nuremberg Code (1947), written in reaction to Nazi medical experiments, was about 'healthy volunteers', not about those participants/subjects who are also patients receiving the treatment that is being tested. The Code also excluded people such as young children and others without 'legal capacity'. The Declaration of Helsinki (World Medical Association 2013) covered patients and children and mainly kept to the Nuremberg standards of informed consent.

Box 19.2   Voluntary and informed consent

Voluntary consent

The Nuremberg Code (1947) begins:

> The voluntary consent of the human subject is absolutely essential.
>
> This means that the person involved should have legal capacity to give consent; should be so situated as to be able to exercise free power of choice, without the intervention of any element of force, fraud, deceit, duress, over-reaching, or other ulterior form of constraint or coercion.

Informed consent

The Nuremberg Code (1947) also states that:

> the human subject should have sufficient knowledge and comprehension of the elements of the subject matter involved, as to enable him [sic] to make an understanding and enlightened decision. This latter element requires that ... there should be made known to him the nature, duration, and purpose of the experiment; the method and means by which it is to be conducted; all the inconveniences and hazards reasonably to be expected; and the effects upon his health or person, which may possibly come from his participation in the experiment.

Professional ethics guidelines

In recent decades, numerous research ethics guidelines have been agreed for a range of professions. These are mainly developed along the lines of Nuremberg and Helsinki, although they vary considerably.

The question arises: Who draws up and takes decisions on ethical guidelines? The general public might be wary of police ethics guidelines written entirely by the police and suspect them of being self-serving and a defence for the police rather than for the public. In a recent exercise in the United Kingdom, the police drew up their clear, rigorous guidance (College of Policing 2014) after a series of consultations with the public and academics. In an initial public survey with over 2,000 responses, they received hundreds of responses to their draft guidelines, which were openly published online and amended further. Similarly, strong ethical guidance for health research has been co-written by doctors, lawyers, philosophers and patients' representatives. Yet the ethics guidance by the British Sociological Association (2017a, 2017b) was written by sociologists, mainly ethnographers, social constructionists or ethnomethodologists, and favour relativist and 'situational ethics' over universal concepts of justice, autonomy and rights. Public consultation was not reported. The style and standards tend to be somewhat vague and evasive, emphasizing personal perceptions over realities, slippery 'personal worlds', 'wrongs' that are somehow not 'harms', and 'apparent' intrusions. For example:

> 23. Even if not harmed, those studied *may* feel wronged by aspects of the research process. This can be particularly so if they perceive apparent intrusions into their private and personal worlds, or where research gives rise to false hopes, uncalled for self-knowledge, or unnecessary anxiety. (British Sociological Association 2017a: 6, my emphasis)

There are numerous let-out clauses for sociologists to use their discretion, for example: '*Where appropriate and practicable*, methods for preserving anonymity should be used' (British Sociological Association 2017a: 31, my emphasis). Guidance on digital online research from the British Sociological Association (2017b) addresses the new complexities on how the 2018 European Union General Data Protection Regulation replaces the 1998 Data Protection Act, with a new stress on privacy rights. There are also valuable references to legislation and a range of other professions' guidelines. The British Psychological Society (2018) issues similar guidance.

When applying to an IRB or REC, researchers should start by checking the relevant website guidelines, such as those of the Medical Research Council (2017), and forms for making applications and then check their own profession's ethics guidance. A further step for novice applicants is to consult detailed guidance. Alderson and Morrow (2011) break research projects into ten stages and discuss the many ethical questions that can arise for researchers at each stage. Their book is relevant to research with all age groups and has extra questions relating to children. Among other useful sources, Bioedge (2017) sends out general weekly news on bioethics, and there are many specialist online sites, such as for genetics-related research (Center for Genetics and Society 2017; GeneWatch UK 2017). These provide forums to debate ethical problems about rights, privacy, data protection, consent, patenting and many other matters, which are pressing – as illustrated by the dialogue in Box 19.3.

Box 19.3   Giving informed consent in large surveys: An example of potential difficulties

Researcher:	Thank you for agreeing to meet me to discuss enrolling your baby in our research.
Annette:	I'm wondering what is involved.
Researcher:	Interviews with you every three years and then with your child when she is older.
Annette:	So what is the point of the research?
Researcher:	Well, it is always useful to know how children are growing up, their life course.
Annette:	Who will analyse the interviews?
Researcher:	We will do initial analysis, then other teams will be involved.
Annette:	Other teams?
Researcher:	Yes. It is good to make full use of the data and when other teams pay to use our data sets that helps to fund this large study. Don't worry, you and your child will be anonymous.
Annette:	What sort of questions will the other teams ask?
Researcher:	We do not know.
Annette:	I am an immigrant on benefits. How can I be sure they will not use my interviews negatively?
Researcher:	They will be objective.
Annette:	How can I give informed consent, if I do not know how our data will be used?

Ethics and research with disadvantaged groups

There is great concern in the poorer majority world about how researchers can request consent to carry out research among 'non-literate communities' (see Box 19.4). At all levels, from researchers to national ethics committees, there tends to be a lack of training and knowledge about basic and applied health care ethics (Social Science Academy of Nigeria 2008). Distributive injustice is another great concern, when pharmaceutical corporations conduct clinical trials in Africa and Asia, where recruitment to trials is easier, running costs are lower and there are lower risks of litigation if research subjects are harmed. As there is a lack of local resources, many African researchers search for funding from the United States and Europe. Yet the participants may be least able to enjoy any benefits from trials, as successful medicines are sold mainly in wealthier countries. Africans bear high risks and personal costs of research, shown for instance in Pfizer's trial of treatment for meningitis, when some Nigerian children died, others were severely disabled, and the families' efforts to gain compensation dragged on for years (Boseley 2010). Boseley (2017) has more recently reported how ethical standards are further compromised by corruption within pharmaceutical companies.

Extreme inequalities between researchers and researched occur when post-colonized indigenous groups are researched as there are differences of power and status that lead to a lack of trust. There have been instances of abuse both within and between countries (Faulkner 2016; Flicker and Worthington 2012).

Box 19.4   Consent to vaccine research in Kampala

Akello and Mirembe live in Kampala, Uganda. One of their children has died of diarrhoea, and their other five children are often infected. Their main work is picking recyclable materials from rubbish tips and they cannot afford health care. When they heard that free medicines were being offered 'to stop children ever having diarrhoea' they hurried to join the long queue of waiting families. Eventually they met a nurse who said that only children aged under-6 years could enter the trial. Uncertain of the exact ages of his small, malnourished children, Akello said that four were aged under 6. The nurse tried to explain to them about experimental vaccinations, double-blind randomized trials, placebos, risks, informed consent and other complexities. She showed them the consent form and asked Akello to sign it. 'You are a nurse,' Akello replied. 'I know you work to help children. I cannot read your form, Sister, so let me shake your hand. That will show you I agree to you giving my children this good medicine.'

Can formal health research ethics systems support researchers?

British ethics committees have been responsible for: setting standards; defining ways to deliver standards; monitoring and assessing the arrangements; improving research quality; safeguarding the public by promoting good practice; reducing and preventing poor practice and misconduct; and ensuring that lessons are learnt from adverse incidents (Department of Health 2004). However, today's IRB/RECs tend to be under-resourced, under-funded and many of the unpaid members lack training or much time to serve on these committees. Their work may be limited to correcting poorly written information sheets, seeing that interpreters will be used, or that researchers working with children have Disclosure and Barring Service (DBS) checks in the United Kingdom.

The views of health researchers about research ethics vary from active interest and support, through resignation and unwilling compliance with ethics committees' requirements, to direct criticism. Much depends on researchers' own commitment to ethics. On zero-sum assumptions, it has been argued that ethics committees undermine and can partly usurp researchers' own ethical responsibilities, although the committees are intended to support and extend researchers' ethical concerns. Uncertainty about interpreting ethical guidelines is an important reason for having formal reviews and discussion, which helps to clarify complex arguments instead of leaving decisions to individual researchers and research teams alone.

Learning from social research ethics

Insights from social research can inform medical bioethics when its rules and systems are too abstract and impersonal, as the next example shows. Seventeen clinical bioethicists devised a 'zone of parental discretion' (ZPD), a tool for dealing with disagreement between parents and doctors about medical treatment for a child (McDougall, Delany and Gillam 2016). They almost entirely ignored the views of children and young people aged up to 18 years. This is unethical. It contravenes the Convention on the Rights of the Child (United Nations 1989), which was ratified by every country except the United States and asserts the need to inform and involve children in all matters that affect them. English Common Law influences the 53 Commonwealth countries and includes the Gillick case ruling in 1985 that children's informed and 'wise' decisions must be respected. Yet the ZPD ignores these decades of law as well as the ethical guidelines that require American doctors to respect the informed refusal of even young children to take part in medical research (United States National Commission for the Protection of Human Subjects of Biomedical and Behavioral Research 1977).

Social science research has demonstrated the vital importance of keeping children informed and, to different degrees, involved in decisions about their health care (Alderson 1993). This is partly to avoid a child's fearful resistance, which may make adults feel they have to enforce treatments. ZPD assumes that clinical ethicists' analysis, their abstract harm–benefit calculations, and their advice to clinicians can replace meeting and listening to parents and children. Examples from social research show why meeting and listening are vital if clinicians and researchers are to understand each unique child's complex experiences, hopes and feelings, and what 'harm' and 'benefit' really mean to each child (Alderson 1993). Grounded in practical everyday experiences, social research ethics can introduce practical, realistic insights that are too often ignored in abstract ethics (Petersen 2011; Sayer 2011).

Researchers may also contribute to the development of practical research ethics by:

- Learning from feelings and emotions during the research process
- Acknowledging practical problems throughout the research
- Explicitly acknowledging ethics in the social, political and economic contexts of research.

Learning from 'moral' emotions

Researchers develop insights through learning from their own moral emotions. This can be achieved by looking inwards at their hopes and fears about their work, as well as acknowledging their anxiety about possible mistakes and the stress induced by a lack of time and resources. Researchers gain from sharing both their concern and their satisfaction about new data and theories and also by responding to the hopes and fears of participants/subjects. Although emotions can mislead and cloud judgement, there are grave dangers if researchers lose empathy and pity. MacIntyre (1966) analysed how overly rational Kantian ethics, which dismissed emotions, contingencies and empathy, ended by validating Nazism, which was notorious for its inhumane research. Researchers can become detached from their 'moral self constituted by responsibility' and become blindly obedient to rules, instead of carefully negotiating a way forward through unpredictable and ambiguous interactions (Bauman 1993). During stressful challenges, researchers can learn from supporting and debriefing one another through shared research analysis sessions.

Acknowledging practical problems

On the numerous practical and unpredictable problems that arise during research projects, solutions can be developed in several ways: through researchers respecting participants and colleagues, negotiating relationships, achieving a complicated balance between opposing ethical options, working together to interpret and apply ethical codes, and reflecting together on the research process in their efforts to reach high standards (Halliwell, Lawton and Gregory 2005).

Explicitly examining ethics in the social world

Social researchers crucially expand the economic and political dimensions of health care ethics. For example, they can take account of the different effects on families of receiving care in private health care systems or in publicly funded ones where they have greater freedom of choice (Alderson 2016). Conventional bioethics tends to take justice to mean enforcing present rules, whereas many social researchers question unjust rules and examine current economic, political and ecological systems that undermine health and wellbeing (Alderson 2016; Curry 2011; Dorling 2017; Evans et al. 2011; Faulkner 2016; Levy 2015). In an ethnography of antenatal clinics, Thomas (2017) shows how research about prenatal screening for Down's syndrome was not driven by public need or demand, but by researchers being able to devise screening methods and push for these to be widely funded. They took the view, 'we can do it, therefore we will'.

Bioethics tends to avoid examining power differences explicitly both between researchers and participants/subjects and within research teams. Power has greatest force when it is least obvious, visible or acknowledged, and when it is exerted through subtle persuasion, or when knowledge is withheld. Power is weaker when it is overt and can be countered by open resistance (Lukes 2005). It is therefore important to be aware of the exercise of power in research.

Conflicts of interest in health research

The interests of health care researchers and researched might seem to be mutual, with more data for more research providing more benefits for all. Yet central to ethics are attempts to address conflicts of interests between researchers, individual participant/subjects, and the countless potential future beneficiaries, as shown in the next example in Box 19.5.

The students who are recorded as excluded, referred to in Box. 19.5, are ten times more likely to suffer mental health problems than average students (Institute for Public Policy Research 2017). They face very high risks in future of being homeless or being in mental hospital or prison. Yet are mental health problems the main cause of exclusions? Alternatively, are schools that exclude students part of a pathologizing context that damages students' mental wellbeing?

Social health research can too easily confuse causes with interacting effects and symptoms. Medical science, however, aims primarily to identify and treat the causes of disease, such as cancer, beyond treating only the symptoms. Yet efforts to address the social cancers and social causes of ill health, such as poverty, inequality and discrimination, tend to be dismissed as 'political', and therefore outside the remit of reliable, 'objective' social and natural science. News of the school exclusion example attracted agencies that are anxious to treat students' mental illness but to overlook the political causes (Defend Digital Me 2017).

Box 19.5 Mental illness and school exclusions

The English government and researchers favour health care records being added to the education records of children and young people who are excluded from school. Surely it would help all the students if more is known about correlations between possible reasons for their exclusion and their health difficulties, in order to help them more effectively.

Yet an alliance of charities helping excluded young people protested that more detailed and shared records of mental illness or teenage pregnancy could increase life-long difficulties for the young people whenever they applied for work or education placements. Their data at present are stored forever and are never deleted. They are not anonymized but named individual records. Neither parents nor children aged from 2 to 18 years are asked for their consent or offered any choice before the data are handed out. With over 23 million entries, the National Pupil Database is one of the richest education data sets in the world, and is hired out hundreds of times each year to academic and commercial research agencies – although official records of exclusion rates may be one fifth of the actual total (Defend Digital Me 2017; Institute for Public Policy Research 2017).

Does health research ethics apply to other activities?

Some professional guidelines (such as American Psychological Association 2016; British Sociological Association 2017a) expand a concern with ethics into all professional activities in relations between colleagues and the public. For example, Faden and colleagues (2013) support the belief that American health care increasingly needs to be organized as a 'learning health care system' where knowledge generation is embedded into, and 'naturally' grows out of, practical medicine, leading to continual improvement in care. They propose a new ethics framework designed to increase this integration and to help to ensure high ethical standards across health care and research. In the report *Ethics in Epidemics, Emergencies and Disasters* by the World Health Organization (2015), it is noted that testing, surveillance, recording and learning from challenging procedures, such as triage, are expected to pervade all emergency clinical care. Other procedures, such as clinical audit and other routine evaluations where there is a degree of uncertainly, should also be subject to ethics review.

Clinical ethics committees (CECs), modelled on IRBs/RECs, now advise on dilemmas in the care of patients. Whereas IRBs/RECs may helpfully mediate between researchers and researched, there is a risk that CECs will undermine practitioner/patient relations when they can strongly influence what should be done for patients whom they may never have met or listened to (see McDougall, Delaney and Gillam 2016).

Formal ethics guidelines and advice may also be relevant to other staff in research departments. Large research departments employ administrators, finance staff and public relations officers, and hope to hit the headlines with attention-grabbing, sometimes exaggerated accounts of research findings in order to impress the public, rival research groups and potential future funders. All these staff deal with ethical questions of respect for the original participants/subjects, and with honesty, accuracy and protecting the integrity of research and other records.

Many researchers doing secondary analysis of anonymized data sets argue that they do not need to consider ethics, as these only apply to direct-contact research with participants. Yet their research raises many questions in common with primary research and, it could be argued, that they also should be reviewed by IRBs/RECs. Researchers who deny that this is necessary appear to be those most in need of reminders about ethics standards. Their work and reports could help or harm the original participants/subjects and possibly the whole (often disadvantaged) group to which they belong. Crucially, formal ethics review reminds professionals of basic ethical standards, of the potential conflicts between the common good and individual autonomy, and between participants' privacy and the need to publicize research findings. There is the difference between service users who receive benefits and participants/subjects who provide data. This highlights the importance of treating them all as dignified, and often vulnerable, persons and not mere objects.

Procedural or substantive health research ethics

Modern medical ethics began with the Nuremberg Code (1947), which was written by lawyers who aimed to prevent harmful and useless research. It was soon taken over by procedural ethics that concentrates on the rules of informed consent, harm–benefit equations, and IRB/REC review (Beauchamp and Childress 2013; National Commission for the Protection of Human Subjects in Medical and Behavioral Research 1978). Health care ethics is rarely substantive ethics, which would examine the kinds of research that participants consent to or that IRB/RECs review. Procedural ethics can be an excuse or mask for endemic problems in health research, indicated by the following five substantive (or real) examples.

First, IRBs/RECs support health services and associated research that spend billions more on treating diseases than on preventing them. Health research relatively rarely tackles the root causes of ill-health, such as the vast and growing inequalities between richer and poorer groups (Dorling 2017; Nuffield Trust 2017), austerity economics (Alderson 2016), pollution, the effects of climate change in floods, droughts and heat waves, and forced migration (Levy 2015). These are seldom seen as questions for health research ethics, and neither are the products of the food, drinks, drugs and petro-chemical global industries (Curry 2011). Alternative ethics systems are largely ignored by health researchers.

Second, IRBs/RECs help to sustain systems that ignore the primary causes of illness and concentrate on effects and symptoms. Each year they approve thousands of research projects to develop and redevelop medications, including many that have limited efficacy and dangerous 'side-effects'. Just one example is the rise in deaths from addictive medically prescribed opioids (Seelye 2017). Health research that aims to counteract dietary and lifestyle causes of illness is relatively rare. IRBs/RECs also support the research industry that spends fortunes on marketing medicines, which most people in the world, including millions of United States citizens, cannot afford to buy.

Third, when ethics concentrates on the personal rather than the political, as if the former is somehow more neutrally objective, ethics can favour research into individual treatments and screen out questions of the common good. Two examples are research into efforts to extend longevity and into IVF reproduction, in the highly populated world with millions of hungry and ill children in great need.

Fourth, ethics reviewers may approve substandard methodologies of social health research that tend:

- To underestimate either individuals' agency or their determining social contexts and structures, and the interactions between structure and agency
- To confuse correlations with causes
- To set aside values and truths that are integral to their research, either in 'objective' positivism or in relativist social constructionism
- To be over-confident about statistical variables and under-confident about the powerful explanations that well-conducted small studies can offer
- To take their theories and methods for granted instead of critically, explicitly examining them (Alderson 2016; Bhaskar 1998, 2008; Porpora 2015; Sayer 2011).

Fifth, with its philosophical origins, bioethics favours scientific curiosity, and supports countless experiments in, for instance, genetics and neuro-imaging, despite informed criticisms that many of the findings are unscientific and worthless. The sociologist and neuro-scientist Hilary and Steven Rose (2014, 2016) examine how the basic ethics for genetics and neuroscience review has not yet been worked out. Can often hasty ethics review, without adequate scientific scrutiny of proposals, be ethical? The Cochrane Collaboration (2017) regularly subjects quantitative health research reports to systematic reviews and finds a high proportion are inadequately designed and conducted. These produce flawed statistics and uncertain or negligible results (see, for instance, Glasziou and Chalmers 2009; Macleod et al. 2014).

To continue this line of argument, Goldacre (2018) lists many examples of 'bad' health research. High numbers of research reports simply echo earlier projects, and only small numbers of clinical research reports can be replicated and validated. Many medical and psychological treatments are therefore based on false research evidence. There is deep concern about this among distinguished doctors, for example Professors Paul Glasziou and Sir Iain Chalmers (2009), the latter a founder of the evidence-based Cochrane Collaboration. Medical research worldwide costs nearly $200 billion annually, and half the research remains unpublished. Weak design means that of the millions of published research papers, an estimated 85 per cent is worthless (Gasziou and Chalmers 2009; Macleod et al. 2014). Most reports are seen by Ionnidis (2016) as variously lacking context placement, information gain, pragmatism, patient centredness, value for money, feasibility and transparency. Farsides and Sparks (2016) conclude that many psychology findings are 'buried in bullshit' and that there are great pressures on psychologists to overstate statistical significance, publish unfinished work and avoid attempting to test and replicate colleagues' findings or publish critical reports. These problems apply to other health research disciplines too. Although not necessarily deliberate fraud, countless unethical and invalid research papers undermine those services that affect people's health, wellbeing and survival across the world.

There are risks in channelling research funds away from cost-effective public health research that benefits the majority into developing costly medical, surgical and genetic interventions for the relatively few who can afford them. This will increase inequalities and consign the majority into becoming second-class citizens with second-class health. There could be more questioning of scientists' collusion with the mass media and commercial interests that raise false hopes with news headlines about miracle cures (Evans et al. 2011; Rose and Rose 2014, 2016).

Conclusion

Unless they are reformed, research ethics systems will not cope adequately with current developments in health research, such as the exporting of much research activity to low-income countries, and the growing collections and use of vast data banks that can compromise participants' consent and privacy. Sayer (2011) argues that social scientists should recognize the value-laden nature of all social life, and work to understand and promote social health and flourishing. Just as clinical research is normative in aiming to promote health and reduce ill-health, Sayer contends that the illusion of 'value-free' social science, like politics without ethics, can 'embrace genocide as easily as democracy'. Greater understanding of social flourishing, especially listening to the views of groups targeted by research, is vital for effective health research.

Yet ethics and values have effectively been removed from being a central and substantive concern for much social health research into being a weak set of rules about research procedures. Abstract bioethics concepts of justice and informed consent can be defined flexibly to serve ulterior purposes. Research ethics may give health research a respectable veneer, but it excuses much poorly designed, useless or harmfully misleading research at great public cost, both financial and social. Better research might have helped to prevent much suffering.

The multibillion dollar health research industry tends to support, or at least does little to counter, the global problems of growing inequality and corporate promotion of for-profit services and unhealthy lifestyles. Yet more informed interdisciplinary work between expert statisticians, lawyers and philosophers, with health service users and carers and general public representatives, working with the range of clinical, scientific and social health researchers could help to bring reforms and raise standards of health research ethics – thereby improving the actual standards of research. Three different exercises have been included in this chapter to allow you to test out your understanding of the points raised about the role of ethics in health research.

Exercise 19.1   Exploring ethics in research

Different frameworks of ethical guidance

Compare the British Sociological Association (2017a) guidance with the guidelines of the Medical Research Council (2017).

- First, as a researcher and, second, as a research participant/subject, which guidelines would you prefer to have supporting you, and why?
- How do the guidelines differently address power and accountability, and the use of personal data?

Ethics and personal data

Discuss the ethics of the questions raised in Box 19.3 on the open-ended, secondary use of personal data.

- Each time a research team applies to hire participants'/subjects' data for secondary analysis, should the donors be informed and asked for their consent?
- Are there some kinds of secondary research for which donors' consent should always be requested and other kinds when the requests would be unnecessary? Do you have examples?
- What are the commercial and scientific reasons for and against always requesting consent for secondary analysis?

Obtaining consent from disadvantaged groups

List some of the ethical problems raised in Box 19.4 on obtaining consent from dis-advantaged groups.

- Discuss how the associated problems might be resolved.
- Is ethics mainly about interpersonal relations of respect and trust between researchers and researched or does it also involve larger concerns?
- If so, what are they, how can they affect health research ethics in this example, and how can they be addressed?

Recommended further reading

This text provides a practical guide to the ethics of research with children:

Alderson, P. and Morrow, V. (2011) *The Ethics of Research with Children and Young People: A Practical Handbook*, 3rd edition. London: Sage.

This book is a useful guide to the more general application of ethics to research:

Cornstock, G. (2013) *Research Ethics: A Philosophical Guide to the Responsible Conduct of Research*. Cambridge: Cambridge University Press.

This declaration makes a fundamental statement of ethical principles in health research on a longstanding and global scale:

World Health Association ([1964] 2013) *Declaration of Helsinki*. Fernay Voltaire: WMA. Available at: www.wma.net/policies-post/wma-declaration-of-helsinki-ethical-princi ples-for-medical-research-involving-human-subjects/

References

Alderson, P. (1993) *Children's Consent to Surgery*. Buckingham: Open University Press.

Alderson, P. (2016) *The Politics of Childhoods Real and Imagined*. Abingdon: Routledge.

Alderson, P. and Morrow, V. (2011) *The Ethics of Research with Children and Young People: A Practical Handbook*, 3rd edition. London: Sage.

American Psychological Association (2016) *Ethical Principles of Psychologists and Code of Conduct*. Washington, DC: APA. Available at: www.apa.org/ethics/code/

Bauman, Z. (1993) *Postmodern Ethics*. Oxford: Blackwell.

Beauchamp, T. and Childress, J. (2013) *Principles of Biomedical Ethics*. New York: Oxford University Press.

Bhaskar, R. (1998) *The Possibility of Naturalism*. London: Verso.

Bhaskar, R. (2008) *Dialectic: The Pulse of Freedom*. Abingdon: Routledge.

Biggs, H. (2009) *Healthcare Research Ethics and Law: Regulation, Review and Responsibility*. Abingdon: Routledge Cavendish.

BioEdge (2017) Available at: bioedge@bioedge.org

Boseley, S. (2010) 'Nigeria: drug trial tale of "dirty tricks"2', *Guardian Weekly*, 17 December. Available at: www.theguardian.com/business/2010/dec/09/wikileaks-cables-pfizer-nigeria

Boseley, S. (2017) 'Drugs firms are accused of putting patients at risk over price hikes', *Observer*, 28 January. Available at: www.theguardian.com/society/2017/jan/28/

British Psychological Society (2018) Available at: www.bps.org.uk/news-and-policy/general-data-protection-regulation-gdpr-%E2%80%93-faqs

British Sociological Association (2017a) *BSA Statement of Ethical Practice*. Durham: BSA.

British Sociological Association (2017b) *Ethics Guidelines and Collated Resources for Digital Research: Statement of Ethical Practice Annex*. Durham: BSA. Available at: www.britsoc.co.uk/media/24309/bsa_statement_of_ethical_practice_annexe.pdf

Cave, E. and Brazier, M. (2016) *Medicine, Patients and the Law*. Manchester: Manchester University Press.

Center for Genetics and Society (2017) Available at: cgs@geneticsandsociety.org

Cochrane Collaboration (2017) Available at: www.cochrane.org

College of Policing (2014) *Code of Policing*. Leamington: CoP. Available at: www.rcn.org.uk/professional-development/publications/pub-003138

Cornstock, G. (2013) *Research Ethics: A Philosophical Guide to the Responsible Conduct of Research*. Cambridge: Cambridge University Press.

Curry, P. (2011) *Ecological Ethics*. Cambridge: Polity Press.

Defend Digital Me (2017) Available at: http://defenddigitalme.com/

Department of Health (2004) *Research Governance Framework for Health and Social Care: Implementation Plan for Social Care*. London: HMSO.

Dorling, D. (2017) *The Equality Effect*. Oxford: New Internationalist.

Emanuel, E., Grady, C. and Crouch, R. (2011) *The Oxford Textbook of Clinical Research Ethics*. Oxford: Oxford University Press.

Evans, J., Meslin, E., Marteau, T. and Caulfield, T. (2011) 'Deflating the genomic bubble', *Science*, 331: 861–2.

Faden, R., Kass, N., Goodman, S., Pronovost, P., Tunis, S. and Beauchamp, T. (2013) *An Ethics Framework for a Learning Health Care System*. New York: Hastings Center Report, 43: S16–S27. Available at: doi:10.1002/hast.134

Farsides, T. and Sparks, P. (2016) 'Buried in bullshit', *The Psychologist*, 29: 368–71.

Faulkner, J. (2016) *Young and Free: [Post]colonial Ontologies of Childhood, Memory and History in Australia*. London: Rowman & Littlefield.

Flicker, S. and Worthington, C. (2012) 'Public health research involving aboriginal peoples', *Journal of Public Health*, 103: 19–22.

GeneWatch UK (2017) Available at: www.genewatch.org

General Medical Council (2014) *Good Medical Practice*. London: GMC. Available at: www.gmc-uk.org/guidance/good_medical_practice.asp

Glasziou, P. and Chalmers, I. (2009) 'Avoidable waste in the production and reporting of research evidence', *The Lancet 374*(9683): 86–9.

Goldacre, B. (2018) *I Think You'll Find it's a Bit More Complicated than That*. London: Fourth Estate.

Halliwell, N., Lawton, J. and Gregory, S. (2005) *Reflections on Research*. Buckingham: Open University Press.

Holmwood, J. (2018) 'Big data needs bigger oversight', *Times Higher*, 12 April.

Institute for Public Policy Research (2017) 'New programme to reduce exclusions in England and make the difference for vulnerable students'. Available at: www.ippr.org/news-and-media/press-releases/new-programme-to-reduce-exclusions-in-england-and-make-the-difference-for-vulnerable-students

Ioannidis, J. (2016) Why most clinical research is not useful, *PLoS Medicine, 13*(6): e1002049. Available at: doi: 10.1371/journal.pmed.1002049.

Levy, B. (ed.) (2015) *Climate Change and Public Health*. Oxford: Oxford University Press.

Lukes, S. (2005) *Power: A Radical View*, 2nd edition. Basingstoke: Palgrave Macmillan.

MacIntyre, A. (1996) *A Short History of Ethics: A History of Moral Philosophy from the Homeric Age to the Twentieth Century*. London: Macmillan.

Macleod, M., Michie, S., Roberts, I., Dirnagl, U., Chalmers, I., et al. (2014) 'Biomedical research: Increasing value, reducing waste', *The Lancet, 383*(9912): 101–4.

McDougall, R., Delany, C. and Gillam, L. (2016) *When Doctors and Parents Disagree: Ethics, Paediatrics and the Zone of Parental Discretion*. Sydney: Federation Press.

McNeill, P. (1993) *The Ethics and Politics of Human Experimentation*. Cambridge: Cambridge University Press.

Medical Research Council (2017) *Good Research Practice: Principles and Guidelines*. London: MRC. Available at: www.mrc.ac.uk/publications/browse/good-research-practice-principles-and-guidelines/

National Commission for the Protection of Human Subjects in Medical and Behavioral Research (1978) *The Belmont Report: Ethical Principles and Guidelines for the Protection of Human Subjects of Research*. Washington, DC: DHEW.

Nuffield Trust (2017) *Admissions of Inequality: Emergency Hospital Use for Children and Young People*. London: Nuffield Trust. Available at: www.nuffieldtrust.org.uk/research/admissions-of-inequality-emergency-hospital-use-for-children-and-young-people

Nuremberg Code (1947) Available at: ohsr.od.nih.gov/guidelines/nuremberg.html

Petersen, A. (2011) 'Can and should sociology save bioethics?', *Medical Sociology News, 6*(1): 2–14. Available at: www.medicalsociologyonline.org/resources/Vol6Iss1/MSo-Volume-6-Issue-1.pdf

Porpora, D. (2015) *Reconstructing Sociology*. Cambridge: Cambridge University Press.

Proctor, R. (1988) *Racial Hygiene: Medicine under the Nazis*. Cambridge, MA: Harvard University Press.

Rose, H. and Rose, S. (2014) *Genes, Cells and Brains*. London: Verso.

Rose, H. and Rose, S. (2016) *Can Neuroscience Change our Minds?* Cambridge: Polity Press.

Sayer, A. (2011) *Why Things Matter to People: Social Science, Values and Ethical Life*. Cambridge: Cambridge University Press.

Seelye, K. Q. (2017) 'As overdose deaths pile up, a medical examiner quits thee morgue', *New York Times*, 7 October. Available at: www.nytimes.com/2017/10/07/us/drug-over-dose-medical-examiner.html

Social Science Academy of Nigeria (2008) *Ethics for Public Health Research in Africa*. Abuja: SSAN. Available at: https://assets.publishing.service.gov.uk/media/57a08bad40f0b-64974000cdc/ethics-public-health.pdf

Thomas, G. (2017) *Down's Syndrome Screening and Reproductive Politics*. Abingdon: Routledge.

United Nations (1948) *Universal Declaration of Human Rights*. New York: UN.

United Nations (1989) *Convention on the Rights of the Child*. New York: UN. Available at: www.ohchr.org/EN/ProfessionalInterest/Pages/CRC.aspx

United States National Commission for the Protection of Human Subjects of Biomedical and Behavioral Research (1977) *Research Involving Children: Report and Recommendations*. Washington, DC: DHEW, 77-0004 and 5.

University College London (2018) *Research Ethics Committee*. Available at: https://ethics.grad.ucl.ac.uk/

World Health Organization (2015) *Ethics in Epidemics, Emergencies and Disasters: Research, Surveillance and Patient Care. WHO Training Manual*. Geneva: WHO. Available at: http://apps.who.int/iris/bitstream/10665/196326/1/9789241549349_eng.pdf?ua=1

World Medical Association (2013) *Declaration of Helsinki*. Fernay-Voltaire: WMA. Available at: www.wma.net/policies-post/wma-declaration-of-helsinki-ethical-princi ples-for-medical-research-involving-human-subjects/

20

Identity and Health Research

TERESA CARVALHO AND TIAGO CORREIA

Chapter objectives

- To discuss the concept of identity in health research
- To consider different dimensions of identity – from gender and ethnicity to age and social class
- To analyse the use of the concept at the macro, meso and micro levels
- To evaluate the balance of quantitative and qualitative approaches to this subject
- To draw on groups in health care, such as doctors and nurses, as exemplars.

Introduction

In this chapter, we analyse and discuss the concept of identity and its use in health research. Identity is a significant concept in the social sciences across various fields of study: in psychology, sociology and anthropology, among others. Identity is based on the idea that the 'self' is linked to identification with certain social groups. A sense of identity or of belonging may be associated with social class, ethnicity, age, gender or other communities. In health research, the concept of identity has been used to collect data and make comparisons. This raises an issue of how identity has been used by researchers.

We start by identifying the approaches taken in the literature on identity studies and their relationship to different research methods. These approaches are analysed on three distinct levels – namely, macro (including at a wider political level), meso (as exemplified by professional identity in the health arena) and micro (as constructed through interaction between health professionals and patients). The strengths and weaknesses of different theoretical perspectives and research methods are considered in researching identity in health care. Finally, an empirical study of the impact on nurses' sense of professional identity following the introduction of the New Public Management is presented as an illustrative case study, with a particular focus on the use of qualitative methods for data collection and analysis.

Identity as a concept and its use in health research

Identity has been studied from the ancient Greeks through to contemporary philosophy. One characteristic of human beings is their self-awareness and the fact that they live in groups. An understanding of how people see themselves is the key to understanding the way that individuals and groups both self-identify and identify with others. The notion of identification was developed in the psychoanalytic context in the classical studies of Sigmund Freud (1984). Later this was explored through the sociological theories of Robert Merton (1957) and the empirical studies of symbolic interactionists such as Anselm Strauss (1959) and Erving Goffman (1961).

In the 1960s, the term became widely diffused across other disciplinary areas and was associated with the rise of political movements. For example, in the United States the rise of the Black Power movement was explained in terms of self-awareness, consciousness of identity and group formation (Cross 1985). In the 1980s studies of race, class and gender adopted a similar terminology and, more recently, extended this concept to sexuality, religion, ethnicity, nationalism, immigration, new social movements, culture and identity politics (Brubaker and Cooper 2000).

In the 1970s in the field of social psychology, Henry Tajfel and colleagues made a significant contribution to the epistemological and ontological discussion on the phenomenon of identity (Tajfel 1970, 1978; Tajfel and Turner 1979). The authors related cognitive processes to behavioural motivation based on group studies. Participants in these studies were distributed into groups at random and were invited to assign points to other participants. The findings showed that participants systematically awarded more points to in-group members. This suggested that the act of placing people into groups made them think of themselves and others as group members instead of individuals. Group membership supported people in defining who they were and determined how they related to each other.

The process of social categorization tended to result in dichotomous classifications by identifying those who belong to the same in-group (us) as opposed to those who belong to an out-group (them). This in turn led to the stereotyping of people and groups as it exaggerated the differences between groups and the similarities in the same group, thus contributing to processes of social exclusion. Educational processes, both formal and informal, contribute through internalized psychological processes to the construction of the self. They are based on the identification of a similar characteristic within a specific group that can be assigned or acquired.

Social scientists also use social categories, such as status, sex, age and ethnic group, as a way to classify behaviour and organize opinions (Tajfel and Turner 1979). This provides a basis for selective data collection and comparison between groups in health research.

These initial approaches were sustained in a positivist or quantitative frame of reference with the assumption that identity was a rigid concept that could be adopted by an external researcher. More recent constructivist approaches note that identification is not simply related to a single list of socio-demographic characteristics (as, for instance, gender, ethnicity, religion, class or profession). It also includes the dynamic relationship between many aspects of identity. From this perspective, identity is relative to a specific social context and is always in flux. Therefore, what it means may change over context and time. In consequence, it has been argued that the specific content of the concept of identity depends on the context of how the term is used (Antaki and Widdicombe 1998; Benwell, and Stokoe 2006). In this regard, identity is typically seen as constructed in action and through talk, with the main interest being on how people find and construct meaning to make sense of who they are in everyday living. From this vantage point, qualitative rather than quantitative methods are usually considered the most suitable and are widely used in research on identity.

Nonetheless, the concept of identity remains controversial. As Brubaker and Cooper (2000: 1) state: '"Identity" tends to mean too much (when understood in a strong sense), too little (when understand in a weak sense), or nothing at all (because of its sheer ambiguity).'The relevance of studying identity in health is associated with the fact that 'the health of every person is intimately tied to the conditions of group life' (Jetten et al. 2017: 789). In addition, the responsibility for personal health is, ultimately, both a collective and individual responsibility.

The conviction that people's self-understanding and self-image are related to their social group and have important consequences for their health and wellbeing has led to a specific field of research known as 'social cure' (Jetten, Haslam and Haslam 2012). The main premise of social cure is as follows:

> ... because people's self-understanding and behaviour is fundamentally intertwined with the social groups to which they belong, those group memberships, and the social identities that people derive from them, have important consequences for their health and well-being. (Jetten et al. 2017: 789–90)

Here, the importance of the group in health has been acknowledged not only by sociology and social psychology, but also by other social scientific disciplines, such as economics and political science (Jetten, Haslam and Haslam 2012). In short, these studies reveal how social status, inequality, poverty and disadvantage can be powerful predictors of health and wellbeing – and call for governments and policy makers to responsibly attend to the social dimensions of health and wellbeing (Jetten et al. 2017; Marmot 2015). In recent years, research on social identity and health has become more popular, albeit still with considerable differences in the theoretical approaches and the form of empirical analysis.

Different approaches and different research methods

The various historical and theoretical perspectives on how the concept of identity is framed are embedded in different epistemological and methodological paradigms. Previously, most studies have been carried out from a macro social scientific perspective – mainly using quantitative methods to study group identity as an explanatory and predictive variable for class, gender, race and other social categories. As suggested above, though, there has been a more recent shift towards interpretivist social constructivist theoretical approaches and to qualitative methods in studies on identity in health.

Many contemporary empirical studies therefore rely on the premise of social constructivism. Different authors acknowledge that the terms and practices of describing or classifying someone are constructed through discourse (Alasuutari 2000; Antaki and Widdicombe 1998; Brubaker and Cooper 2000). This perspective presents 'identity as an "essential", cognitive, socialised, phenomenological or psychic phenomenon that governs human action' (Benwell and Stokoe 2006: 3). This radical shift is integrated in a 'postmodern' perspective in the social sciences and humanities.

From this perspective, identity is not an inner self acquisition based on cognition and experience, but, instead, a public phenomenon constructed within a process of interaction. Identity results from a performance or construction that is interpreted by other people and is embodied in human conduct. This is expressed in the way we move, what we wear, what we discuss and how we talk, and so on. Thus, there is seen to be continuous construction and reconstruction in the realms of discourse and other semiotic systems that make meaning. It is not simply reflected in discourse but is dynamically constituted *in* discourse (Alasuutari 2000; Antaki and Widdicombe 1998; Benwell and Stokoe 2006).

These studies use an ethnomethodological method (Antaki and Widdicombe 1998; Malone 2013), and mainly employ discourse analysis or conversation analysis to interpret data. Conversation analysis (CA) is a recent approach that examines the sequential accomplishments of interaction, analysing actions by noting preceding and following actions (Hutchby 2008). It is based on the analysis of interactional patterns and of their contribution to ongoing social actions. Harvey Sacks (1992), the pioneer researcher of CA, developed his work in the health field by scrutinizing 'talk' in calls made to suicide prevention centres. CA focuses on how identities are used in practice – including when and how talk is employed. It emphasizes how social life is achieved through talk and the human capacity to create reality, such as in the construction of sexuality (Jackson 2006; Weeks, Holland and Waites 2003).

Adding to CA, discourse analysis (DA) is also used in analysing qualitative data in studies about identity. DA is predicated on the view that any particular account or version of the world is intimately related to the circumstances of its production, and that the complexity of these circumstances should be included in any analysis (Gilbert and Mulkay 1984). Based on the classical studies of Althusser (1971) and Foucault (1982), DA relies on a more structural perspective in assuming that discourses have a concrete life which results from attempts to impose specific arguments on reality. Studies using DA focus on the analysis of one particular identity category, such as gender (Johnson and Meinhof 1996; Litosseliti 2014), sexuality (Cameron and Kulick 2003; Weeks, Holland and Waites 2003), age (Nikander 2002), and ethnic and national identities (De Fina 2003; Joseph 2004). In health studies, identity is identified as occurring in different contexts and at various levels.

Identity in health research: The three levels of analysis

Identity in health research can be analysed at three different levels, each with distinct approaches to conceptualization and methodology: the macro, meso and micro levels.

The macro level: Health and society

At the macro level, identity is helpful in indicating the extent to which health systems, including their structure and functioning, are linked to, and produce, social differentiation. The study of social categories based on identity highlight why some social groups suffer more illness than others; how the very organization of health services may promote social inequality; and how these inequalities are commonly perceived by populations.

Gender, age, race/ethnicity and professions are visible expressions of identity-related classifications and categories of socioeconomic position at the macro level, which in turn influence individual behaviours, and individuals' exposure to different material constraints and opportunities. It is relatively well accepted that such material constraints and opportunities have a multiplier effect on health outcomes, such as mortality and morbidity rates (Bury 1997).

One interpretation of the interplay between identity-related classification and categorization in health research requires making judgements on the criteria for inclusion and exclusion. Both in-depth qualitative and quantitative studies conducted in different countries tend to agree that citizenship status, country of origin and ethnicity (Quan et al. 2006; Tarraf, Jensen and González 2016), and age and gender (Rodin 2013) condition individuals' formal enrolment in health services and how they navigate a way through them. The interplay between identity-related classifications and categories in health systems can be seen in how people are grouped. For example, differential access to preventive screening services can be found by sex, age and class, as, for instance, in the case of mammography for women and prostate screening for men. Age categories are used in screening programmes for colon cancer and gender categories are employed in screening for sexually transmitted diseases and the risk of developing genetic diseases (Rose 2001; Schueler, Chu and Smith-Bindman 2008; Singer and Clair 2003).

As a social variable, gender can be shown to influence access to health professions. In the past, women had restricted access to the high-status professions. Nursing was seen as women's work and medicine was a predominantly male profession (Davies 1995). Nowadays, while this difference is less marked, research data indicate that a cleavage is found in most health professions in relation to women's access to leadership positions. Although there is growing feminization of the health professions in most countries, women's presence in senior positions in professional hierarchies continues to be uneven (Kuhlmann and Annandale 2010).

In fact, gender-sensitive health studies have moved to the mainstream of health research (Kuhlmann and Annandale 2010). They do not rely on a single method or research design and are undertaken using different epistemological assumptions. In the 1970s and 1980s, feminist researchers criticized positivism for claiming that science could be neutral and objective (Lagro-Janssen 2012) and drew attention to the importance of studies that were sensitive to differences in power relations (Haraway 1988; Harding 1986; Kuhlmann and Annandale 2010). In this context, interpretivist and constructivist approaches became more dominant with qualitative analysis based on interviews and direct observation being assumed to be more suitable to analyse the complexity of gender relations in society. Nevertheless, it is important to highlight the strong tradition in this field in conducting quantitative research, especially through large-scale surveys on health-related issues (Annandale 2010).

These methods are also used to research both sex and gender. While sex is a biological characteristic, frequently used as an independent variable, gender includes a social dimension integrating differing expected social roles. Gender studies are not based on a simple divide between male and female categories, but instead investigate the social construction of femininity and masculinity. For instance, it is known from quantitative studies that the dominant forms of masculinity can lead men not only to find it difficult to seek help, but also to have undiagnosed and untreated depressive symptoms, as demonstrated in quantitative studies (Kilmartin 2005). However, Emsliea and colleagues (2006) carried out a qualitative study with 16 in-depth interviews with men diagnosed with depression in the UK and found that the generalizations about depressed men being silent are misleading. Based on the content analysis of these interviews, they found that depressed men can also re-interpret their experiences as masculine. The possibility of expanding the scope of attention from sex as a variable to gender, including men's health care, has led to the emergence of gender mainstreaming approaches – that is, where gender as a concept is an integral part of the research objectives in studying how health institutions work and health policies are implemented (Annandale and Riska 2009).

Qualitative analyses that integrate gender into health care studies make use of not only conventional techniques like interviews, focus group and participant observation, but also more innovative approaches based on images, written material and participant-generated data (Bourgeault, Dingwall and de Vries 2010). Data analysis using these new approaches employs such techniques as CA and DA to analyse data (Wooffitt 2005). An example of these new approaches is the study developed by Johnson, Sharkey and Dean (2011) on diet-related chronic diseases in women of Mexican origin. The authors used a visual method, based on participant-driven photo-elicitation, to understand the food choices of mothers, since they were the people who determined food choices and health activities within their family.

Research on identity and gender in health may employ all the types of research and data collection techniques, depending on the way identity is interpreted, as an explanatory variable or as integrated in the discourses about the self. The choice of method will depend on the research questions since, as in other research fields, different questions call for different methodological approaches and there is an increasing awareness of the merits of using 'mixed methods' (Kuhlmann and Annandale 2010).

Gender is a relevant variable in identity studies, but it does not operate alone. We are far from the initial feminist approach based on the assumption that women are an oppressed and homogeneous group. New perspectives are framed on an intersectional approach based on the view that there is a mutual construction of relations in the formation of social identities (Shields 2008). Gender as a variable operates in combination with others, such as ethnicity, social class, sexuality and age, all of which are relevant when analysing vulnerability or resistance to ill health, as well as access to care and assessments of the quality of care.

Gender is used here as an example of the way a socially constructed concept to categorize people or groups in society can promote inequalities not only in access to health but also in health status and treatments. Identity can be identified as relevant at other levels too, particularly at the organizational or meso level – or even at the micro level, as we shall see in the following sub-sections.

The meso level: Professionals and managers

At the meso level the notion of professional identity is particularly relevant. In the last decades, changes in the political and social organization of health services, along with the increasing technical domain in society, can affect the status and power of professional groups as well as their sense of identity. At this level, identities are governed by the norms, rules and regulations that underlie socialization processes, underpin the standards set and tend to structure relationships (Allsop and Mulcahy 1998).

Professions build on shared learning processes and experiences that create similarities among its members and dissimilarities with the outsiders, be they the members of other professional groups or non-professionals. One of the key references in this respect is to professional socialization that reflects how individuals and groups self-define as professionals and act accordingly. In this way they construct a collective professional identity.

The concept of professionalism builds originally on the notion of professional autonomy – that is, a space for decision making free from bureaucratic and market forces where there is the opportunity to define, organize and perform the work to be done (Freidson 2001). Professionalism thus appears as a 'third' logic, different from managerialism and the market. However, a number of studies argue that this static understanding of relationships should be replaced by a more dynamic approach that is able to capture more nuanced boundaries and influences. In industrialized societies, organizations are the primary sites of work, and practitioners are necessarily subjected to many organizational rules with diverse rationales (Muzio and Kirkpatrick 2011). One aspect of organizational functioning that potentially affects health professionals, especially in relation to nurses' and physicians' professional identity, is the growing pressure from managerialism, which brings greater hierarchical control and standardization in work practices.

Empirical evidence, mostly driven by qualitative approaches involving close and ongoing contact with professionals in organizational settings, identifies complex patterns of articulation between medical-based communities and organizational-based hierarchies (Adler, Kwon and Hecksher 2008). Accordingly, physicians' identity is determined by the relationship in play between medical professionalism and managerialism (Correia 2013). Medical professional values include the defence of professional authority, legitimacy and prestige and the exercise of knowledge-based competence with discretion to deal with complex cases and maintain collegial relations. However, with the growth of managerialism, medical professional values must now include respect for external forms of regulation that allow for exposure to audit and measurement with performance-based targets; the acceptance of work standardization; and openness to inter-professional collaboration (Evetts 2009). This is more fully discussed in Chapter 18.

Other aspects of organizational functioning that can potentially affect physicians' identity in their day-to-day performance occur in their contacts with patients, managers and allied health professionals. For example, practitioners' real work experiences can be disruptive to the learning process (Cuff and Vanselow 2004), especially as medical school curricula and residency training often lack exposure to the behavioural and social sciences. There may be a mismatch between students' learning about their future practice and the experiences they actually face in the diagnosis and treatment of patients. Health care organizations are complex, with specific organizational cultures and subcultures, and medical practice involves interaction with a range of other professional groups (Correia 2017).

Using research methods that included video ethnography and individual interviews with staff, empirical evidence on inter-professional practices throws up apparently contradictory findings. Some studies show that inter-professional work can enhance savings, improve health care outcomes and increase staff satisfaction. However, it can also act as a trigger to conflict between groups and poorer performance among professionals.

According to McNeil, Mitchell and Parker (2013), these differences demonstrate that important variations take place in different organizational settings. The outcome depends on the workplace setting. Where intra- and inter-profession relationships are built on relatively stable institutions with harmonious relationships, inter-professional working can have positive outcomes, but this cannot be predicted or predetermined in advance (Long, Lee and Braithwaite 2008).

The evidence collected by Correia (2013) supports these findings on the effect of organizational dynamics on both professional and managerial relationships and inter-professional working. He used a qualitative approach composed of interviews and daily observations on two medical wards in a public hospital (one internal medicine and one surgery). He found significant differences in the way physicians from the two wards defined their work and dealt with pressures from management: some accepted and made use of managerial requirements, while others did not. These differences can be understood by examining characteristics of medical work on each ward. The variables were the patients' condition (chronic or acute), the degree of technological involvement in medical practice (low or high), patients' turnover (low or high) and selection (indiscriminate or selective). The study found that physicians tend to accept and integrate the managerial rationale and values when they dealt with acute conditions, had high dependence on technological procedures and experienced high patient turnover. On the other hand, physicians tended to oppose the managerial rationale and values when their patients had long-term conditions, with low technological involvement and low patient turnover.

Based on the same empirical study, Correia and Denis (2016) consider further the exposure of physicians' identity to managerial values and rationale, whose effects are visible in the way they think, perform and interact with peers and outsiders. According to their findings, physicians' identities do not necessarily either encompass or oppose the managerial rationale and the market. They may integrate aspects of managerialism into their thinking. Muzio and Kirkpatrick (2011) describe this as a process of 'hybridization'. It is clear that, in medicine, there are various subcultures where professionals express different aspects of their professional identity (Fitzgerald and Teal 2004), and therefore research studies must investigate interactions and aspects of identity within specific work contexts.

Inspired by perspectives on feminist post-structuralism and critical realism respectively, Correia (2017) argues that the theoretical framework to study physicians' professional identity needs to go beyond the assumption of professionals' passive reproduction of shared ideologies and experiences. He suggests that empirical research using qualitative methods should explore differences in how professionals see themselves; how they behave as professionals, and how they make use of their stock of knowledge. While all physicians have been socialized into some attitudes, practices and behaviours that are shared due to their medical education, there are nevertheless differences in their professional identity within specific work contexts. Using qualitative methods in his studies, Correia found that medical specialties had diverse ways of practising medicine according to the workplace setting, thus confirming earlier work by Freidson (1970). This had an effect on their professional identity as well as relations with their peers, patients and other professionals.

Correia (2017) suggests that the key message for the study of physicians' professional identity, and indeed the study of other health professional groups, is to find out how each professional rationalizes the practice of being a member of that profession. This follows the Weberian standpoint that individual action reflects specific influences. In conducting research on professionals, researchers must therefore investigate both the personal intentions and expectations of the individual professional and assess how their intentions and expectations are translated into practice in specific situations or contexts. This approach can help operationalize theoretical propositions about being a professional. As Correia (2017: 1064) comments, 'personal intentions and how these are played out in context, relate to cognitive processes that involve both personal projects and the general values and ideologies of the organizations within which physicians work'.

The micro level: Professional–patient interaction

The perspective on identity that we next develop relates to the micro-level interaction between professionals and patients. It is widely accepted that effective interaction in the clinical encounter is critical to health outcomes. However, several expressions of social discrimination, such as those based on sexual orientation, ethnicity and social class may affect the nature of that encounter. This is one factor that can contribute to the inequalities in health care outcomes, even in developed countries (Graham 2004). It is also important to acknowledge that forms of social discrimination in micro-level health interactions are a driver of social identity – that is, how individuals construct their view of themselves and others. Thus, professional–patient interaction not only reproduces, but also produces social identities.

Gengler and Jarrell (2015) provide an extensive review analysis of studies that address this issue. Both qualitative and quantitative studies conducted with patients and their relatives and with professionals show that ethnicity, gender, sexual orientation and class background affect how professionals communicate with patients. This affects the level of emotional engagement in encounters and may lead to verbal dominance, which in turn affects the time spent with a patient and the extent of information shared. Accordingly, professionals differ in their diagnostic approach and consequently there is variation in their patients' access to treatment. Patients, in their turn, differ in the way they express their symptoms and find possible explanations for their own condition. This may be shaped by gender, ethnicity and social class.

The micro level of analysis of identity has been the most extensively studied in empirical research, using a range of methodologies. Therefore, summarizing the main traits discovered is not straightforward. In contrast to the macro and meso levels, though, quantitative and qualitative studies tend to agree on the overall results, namely that social identities influence, as much as they are influenced by, encounters between professionals and their patients. Such identity-driven differences also necessarily reflect individuals' different material constraints and opportunities and health outcomes.

Regardless of conducting qualitative or quantitative studies, researching into micro-level interactions related to identity in health requires a clear identification of the rationale underpinning the choice of research methods:

- The first issue to take into account here is the research question.
- The second issue is to accept that the micro level of analysis is exposed to cultural and social biases.

Therefore, researchers need to acknowledge which strategies allow them to address the research question, while coping with sensitive issues.

The most important lesson from these empirical studies is that there is no predetermined formula for the best way forward. Researchers must reflect on their choice of method and their technique for data collection. The pros and cons of qualitative and quantitative methods are well known. Their own interpretation needs to avoid epistemological obstacles – namely, individualism, naturalism and ethnocentrism (Bachelard 1986):

- The obstacle of individualism is to assume that an individual's behaviour is detached from social, political and cultural influences.
- The pitfall of naturalism is to assume that an individual's behaviour is predetermined by 'natural' influences, such as age, sex or ethnicity.
- The shortcoming of ethnocentricism is where an assumption is made about an individual's overt behaviour or demeanour or how they present themselves. Researchers here should interpret without pre-judgement; think about the categories and classifications they are using and on what these are based; try to understand which past events may help to explain current behaviour and opinions; and be aware that similar behaviours can be perceived and labelled as a consequence of social and cultural factors.

Professional identity and nursing in a managerial context

The way professional identity has been influenced by managerialism and New Public Management narratives, and policies and practices in the health sector have been widely reported in qualitative and in quantitative studies. As different authors (Evetts 2003, 2006, 2009; Muzio and Kirkpatrick 2011; Noordegraaf 2007) acknowledge, there is an urgent need to reconsider the way professionalism and managerialism have been considered as dual and contradictory concepts.

In a study of professional values and norms in the nursing profession, Goodrick and Reay (2010) found that nurses do not reject or contradict older identities when new ones emerge.

Instead they tend to incorporate managerial values into their practice, while at the same time maintaining professional values absorbed at an earlier career stage. Both identities can coexist. The studies by Carvalho (2012, 2014) reached similar conclusions. The position is explored further in the following case study.

Professional identity and nursing in a managerial context

Using a qualitative approach, based on 103 interviews with nurses with management duties in district hospitals located in urban areas in Portugal, Carvalho (2012, 2014) provided a detailed account of the way both managerialism and professionalism influence professional identities. She showed that the construction of identity is highly complex and can integrate several components that are often presented as contradictory. For instance, the legitimation of the profession in scientific knowledge creates a professional identity more centred in objective and technical principles. These are assumed as being opposite to the humanistic and altruistic values of care, although both can exist alongside each other in nurses' discourses about their professional identity.

Carvalho (2012, 2014) suggests that a vocational ideology continues to exist in the profession, albeit in hybrid ways. Ethical or altruistic values are combined with both specific personality characteristics and attitudes derived from experiences in daily practice. Nurses do not interpret the profession as a gift to be bestowed on patients and some even distance themselves from having a special talent for the profession. Nevertheless, they still value the ideals of a vocation, but as based on accumulated knowledge and experience drawn from the daily practice of caring for patients. Ethical and altruistic values are present, but are based on practical learning.

Distinct conceptions of care were found, which could be relational and/or technical and scientific:

- Care as a relational concept is mainly associated with the interaction established with patients and results from an extension of female work, undertaken on a daily basis in the domestic domain.
- Care as a technical and scientific concept is more associated with the scientific knowledge and expertise obtained through education which embeds daily practices.
- This includes a holistic perspective – that is, a global perspective of the patient that does not rest only on disease, but includes their personal, social, economic and cultural context.

To integrate all these different dimensions of care as a core value in professional identity, nurses must have a professional project to change formal training to more closely relate theory to practice. This can also be seen as an attempt to integrate different values in professional identity. The same tendency to incorporate different values emerges with managerialism, since nurses are able to intertwine management values, such as efficiency, efficacy and value for money, with more traditional ones in the definition of their professional identity.

The way nurses used these values interchangeably within their narratives could only be captured through the content analysis of their discourse. When asked directly about what it meant for them to be a nurse, they gave accounts of their daily practice. This suggests that notions of professional identity are fluid and dynamic and change as a consequence of daily practice, thus confirming the theoretical position that identities are changeable and generated in the work process. In this way, values and norms that appear contradictory can be integrated. The core professional value of care as an altruistic and ethical value can therefore coexist with the managerial values of efficiency and efficacy.

Conclusion

The concept of identity has been widely used in the social sciences. This chapter has shown the usefulness of the concept in health research. Historically, different theoretical and epistemological perspectives have framed the dominant definition of identity. More recently, identity has been assumed from a social constructivist perspective to be a fluid concept, as the result of a performance or construction interpreted by other actors. This signals a general shift towards interpretivist and social constructivist theoretical approaches and qualitative methods in recent studies on identity in health.

In the health domain, identity is used at different levels with different theoretical and methodological approaches. At a macro level, there has been a tendency to use identity to identify differences between social groups, even without deeply questioning the classifications used. In this domain, the way gender has been included in health research is particularly illustrative of the shift from studies centred on quantitative approaches, based on simple interpretations of the divide between men and women, to more complex interpretative and qualitative approaches, which question gender categories, their construction and their relevance to health. At a meso level, qualitative and interpretative approaches have also been dominant in the contemporary context, especially in what concerns health organizations and professionals. At this level, the interactions between organizations and professionals in (re)defining professional identities are particularly relevant as objects of analysis. Finally, at the micro level, the social classification of people in different groups has been recognized as influencing the interaction between patients and professionals – and, in consequence, health outcomes. However, the method of research adopted will depend on the research questions. In planning studies on identity and health – even knowing that interpretative perspectives are rather more used at the present time – there needs to be reflection on the best way to collect and analyse data in terms of the research objective(s).

Exercise 20.1   The values and norms of managerialism in health care

Evaluate how the values and norms of managerialism are being incorporated in health professional identities. Develop a literature review on identity, professionalism and managerialism and explore whether the published studies point towards relevant changes in identity in your chosen health profession, and, if so, in which direction. Some main questions might be:

- What are the key references in discourses concerning professional identity?
- Are there relevant differences in health professional discourses related to the context within which they are produced?
- Do the professionals in question have the same discourses when they talk with other colleagues or when they address the public?
- How do they perceive the impact of potential changes in their identity in daily caring practices?
- How do changes in professional identity intersect with other dimensions, such as the age, gender, class and culture of patients?
- Do the selected health professional group act differently when they engage in inter-professional relations?
- Are there any differences when they interact with doctors or when the interaction is with managers?
- How do managerialist discourses affect nurses' subjectivity?

What are the explanations for your findings? Discuss different theoretical approaches, including macro-, meso- and micro-level influences and consider the merits of quantitative and qualitative studies. Reflect especially on identity as a dynamic concept. When does it appear to be in flux and in what context? How can this be shown through discourse analysis? On the basis of your findings, what are your policy recommendations for improving the work of health professionals and for enhancing care for citizens? What recommendations do you have for further research and methodological investigation?

Further recommended reading

This book contains a collection of studies reflecting on how professions and professionalism are transformed by managerialism. Both quantitative and qualitative approaches are used in the analyses, which include doctors and nurses:

Carvalho, T. and Santiago, R. (eds) (2015) *Professionalism, Managerialism and Reform in Higher Education and the Health Services: The European Welfare State and Rise of the Knowledge Society*. Basingstoke: Palgrave Macmillan.

Based on ethnography, this study sheds light on the way a doctor's identity builds on workplace-level contingencies and the extent to which professional identities have a performative scope, echoing reflexive deliberations and situated interests:

Correia, T. (2017) 'Doctors' reflexivity in hospital organisations: The nexus between institutional and behavioural dynamics in the sociology of professions', *Current Sociology*, 65(7): 1050–69.

This book reflects on the way group membership, and the social identities associated with it, can represent a relevant determinant of individual health and wellbeing. Reference is made to theoretical and empirical insights associated with identity and health:

Jetten, J., Haslam, C. and Haslam, S. A. (eds) (2012) *The Social Cure: Identity, Health and Well-being*. New York: Psychology Press.

References

Adler, P. S., Kwon, S. W. and Heckscher, C. (2008) 'Perspective – professional work: The emergence of collaborative community', *Organization Science*, 19(2): 359–76.

Alasuutari, P. (2000) *Researching Culture: Qualitative Method and Cultural Studies*. London: Sage.

Allsop, J. and Mulcahy, L. (1998) 'Maintaining professional identity: Doctors' responses to complaints', *Sociology of Health and Illness*, 20(6): 802–24.

Althusser, L. (1971) *Lenin and Philosophy and Other Essays*. London: Monthly Review Press.

Annandale, E. (2010) 'Health status and gender', in W. C. Cockerham (ed.), *The New Blackwell Companion to Medical Sociology*. Hoboken, NJ: John Wiley & Sons.

Annandale, E. and Riska, E. (2009) 'New connections: Towards a gender-inclusive approach to women's and men's health', *Current Sociology*, 57(2): 123–33.

Antaki, C. and Widdicombe S. (eds) (1998) *Identities in Talk*. London: Sage.

Bachelard, G. (1986) *The Formation of the Scientific Mind: A Contribution to a Psychoanalysis of Objective Knowledge*. Boston, MA: Beacon Press.

Benwell, B. and Stokoe, E. (2006) *Discourse and Identity*. Edinburgh: Edinburgh University Press.

Bourgeault, I., Dingwall, R. and de Vries, R. (eds) (2010) *The Sage Handbook of Qualitative Methods in Health Research*. London: Sage.

Brubaker, R. and Cooper, F. (2000) 'Beyond "identity"', *Theory and Society*, 29(1): 1–47.

Bury, M. (1997) *Health and Illness in a Changing Society*. London: Routledge.

Cameron, D. and Kulick, D. (2003) *Language and Sexuality*. Cambridge: Cambridge University Press.

Carvalho, T. (2012) 'Managerialism and professional strategies: A case from nurses in Portugal', *Journal of Health Organization and Management*, 26: 524–41.

Carvalho, T. (2014) 'Changing connections between professionalism and managerialism: A case study of nursing in Portugal', *Journal of Professions and Organization*, *1*(2): 176–90.

Correia, T. (2013) 'The interplay between managerialism and medical professionalism in hospital organizations from the doctors' perspective: A comparison of two distinctive medical units', *Health Sociology Review*, *22*(3): 255–67.

Correia, T. (2017) 'Doctors' reflexivity in hospital organisations: The nexus between institutional and behavioural dynamics in the sociology of professions', *Current Sociology*, *65*(7): 1050–69.

Correia, T. and Denis, J.-L. (2016) 'Hybrid management, organizational configuration, and medical professionalism: Evidence from the establishment of a clinical directorate in Portugal', *BMC Health Services Research*, *16*(Supp 2): 161.

Cross, W. E. (1985) 'Black identity: Rediscovering the distinction between personal identity and reference group orientation', in M. B. Spencer, G. K. Brookins and W. R. Allen (eds), *Beginnings: The Social and Affective Development of Black Children*. Hillsdale, NJ: Lawrence Erlbaum.

Cuff, P. and Vanselow, N. (eds) (2004) *Improving Medical Education: Enhancing the Behavioral and Social Science Content of Medical School Curricula*. Washington, DC: National Academy of Sciences.

Davies C. (1995) *Gender and the Professional Predicament in Nursing*. Buckingham: Open University Press.

De Fina, A. (2003) *Identity in Narrative: A Study of Immigrant Discourse*, Volume 3. Amsterdam: John Benjamins.

Emsliea, C., Ridge, D., Ziebland, S. and Hunt, K. (2006) 'Men's accounts of depression: Reconstructing or resisting hegemonic masculinity?', *Social Science and Medicine*, *62*(9): 2246–57.

Evetts, J. (2003) 'The sociological analysis of professionalism: Occupational change in the modern world', *International Sociology*, *18*(2): 395–415.

Evetts, J. (2006) 'Short note: The sociology of professional groups: New directions', *Current Sociology*, *54*(1): 133–43.

Evetts, J. (2009) 'New professionalism and new public management: Changes, continuities and consequences', *Comparative Sociology*, *8*(2): 247–66.

Fitzgerald, A. and Teal, G. (2004) 'Health reform, professional identity and occupational sub-cultures: The changing interprofessional relations between physicians and nurses', *Contemporary Nurse*, *16*(1–2): 71–79.

Foucault, M. (1982) 'The subject and power', in H. L. Dreyfus and P. Rabinow (eds), *Michel Foucault: Beyond Hermenutics and Structuralism*. Brighton: Harvester.

Freidson, E. (1970) *Profession of Medicine: A Study of the Sociology of Applied Knowledge*. New York: Harper & Row.

Freidson, E. (2001) *Professionalism. The Third Logic*. Chicago, IL: University of Chicago Press.

Freud, S. (1984) *On Metapsychology: The Theory of Psychoanalysis*. Harmondsworth: Pelican.

Gengler, A. M. and Jarrell, M. V. (2015) 'What difference does difference make? The persistence of inequalities in healthcare delivery', *Sociology Compass*, *9*(8): 718–30.

Gilbert, G. N. and Mulkay, M. (1984) *Opening Pandora's Box: A Sociological Analysis of Scientists' Discourse*. Cambridge: Cambridge University Press Archive.

Goffman, E. (1961) *Encounters: Two Studies in the Sociology of Interaction*. Indianapolis, IN: Bobbs Merrill.

Goodrick, E. and Reay, T. (2010) 'Florence Nightingale endures: Legitimizing a new professional role identity', *Journal of Management Studies*, *47*(1): 55–84.

Graham, H. (2004) 'Social determinants and their unequal distribution: Clarifying policy understandings', *The Milbank Quarterly*, *82*(1): 101–24.

Haraway, D. (1988) 'Situated knowledges: The science question in feminism and the privilege of partial perspective', *Feminist Studies*, *14*(3): 575–99.

Harding, S. (1986) *The Science Question in Feminism*. Ithaca, NY: Cornell Press.

Hutchby, I. (2008) *Conversation Analysis*. Hoboken, NJ: John Wiley & Sons.

Jackson, S. (2006) 'Interchanges: Gender, sexuality and heterosexuality: The complexity (and limits) of heteronormativity', *Feminist Theory*, *7*(1): 105–21.

Jetten, J., Haslam, S. A., Cruwys, T., Greenaway, K. H., Haslam, C. and Steffens, N. K. (2017) 'Advancing the social identity approach to health and well-being: Progressing the social cure research agenda', *European Journal of Social Psychology*, *47*(7): 789–802.

Jetten, J., Haslam, C. and Haslam, S. A. (eds) (2012) *The Social Cure: Identity, Health and Well-being*. New York: Psychology Press.

Johnson, C. M., Sharkey, J. R. and Dean, W. R. (2011) 'It's all about the children: A participant-driven photo-elicitation study of Mexican-origin mothers' food choices', *BMC Women's Health*, *11*(1): 41.

Johnson, S. and Meinhof, U. H. (eds) (1996) *Language and Masculinity*. Oxford: Wiley-Blackwell.

Joseph, J. (2004) *Language and Identity: National, Ethnic, Religious*. London: Springer.

Kilmartin, C. (2005) 'Depression in men: Communication, diagnosis and therapy', *Journal of Men's Health and Gender*, *2*(1): 95–99.

Kuhlmann, E. and Annandale, E. (eds) (2010) *The Palgrave Handbook of Gender and Healthcare*. Basingstoke: Palgrave Macmillan.

Lagro-Janssen, A. L. M. (2012) 'Sex, gender and health: Developments in medical research', in E. Kuhlmann and E. Annandale (eds), *The Palgrave Handbook of Gender and Healthcare*, 2nd edition. Basingstoke: Palgrave Macmillan.

Litosseliti, L. (2014) *Gender and Language Theory and Practice*. London: Routledge.

Long, D., Lee, B. B. and Braithwaite, J. (2008) 'Attempting clinical democracy: Enhancing multivocality in a multidisciplinary clinical team', in C. R. Caldas-Coulthard and R. Iedema (eds), *Identity Trouble: Critical Discourse and Contested Identities*. New York: Palgrave Macmillan.

Malone, M. (2013) *Worlds of Talk: The Presentation of Self in Everyday Conversation*. Hoboken, NJ: John Wiley & Sons.

Marmot, M. (2015) *The Health Gap: The Challenge of an Unequal World*. London: Bloomsbury.

McNeil, K., Mitchell, R. and Parker, V. (2013) 'Interprofessional practice and professional identity threat', *Health Sociology Review*, *22*(3): 291–307.

Merton, R. K. (1957) *Social Theory and Social Structure*, 2nd edition. Glencoe, IL: Free Press.

Muzio D. and Kirkpatick I. (2011) 'Introduction: Professions and organizations – a conceptual framework', *Current Sociology*, *59*(4): 389–405.

Nikander, P. (2002) *Age in Action: Membership Work and Stage of Life Categories in Talk*. Helsinki: Academia Scientiarum Fennica.

Noordegraaf, M. (2007) 'From "pure" to "hybrid" professionalism: Present-day professionalism in ambiguous public domains', *Administration and Society*, *39*(6): 761–85.

Quan, H., Fong, A., De Coster, C., Wang, J., Musto, R., Noseworthy, T. W. and Ghali, W. A. (2006) 'Variation in health services utilization among ethnic populations', *Canadian Medical Association Journal*, *174*(6): 787–91.

Rodin, J. (2013) 'Accelerating action towards universal health coverage by applying a gender lens', *Bulletin of the World Health Organization*, *91*: 710–11.

Rose, N. (2001) 'The politics of life itself', *Theory, Culture and Society*, *18*(6): 1–30.

Sacks, H. (1992) *Lectures on Conversation*, Volumes *I* and *II*. Oxford: Blackwell.

Schueler, K. M., Chu, P. W. and Smith-Bindman, R. (2008) 'Factors associated with mammography utilization: A systematic quantitative review of the literature', *Journal of Women's Health*, *17*(9): 1477–98.

Shields, S. A. (2008) 'Gender: An intersectionality perspective', *Sex Roles*, *59*(5–6): 301–11.

Singer, M. and Clair, S. (2003) 'Syndemics and public health: Reconceptualizing disease in a bio-social context', *Medical Anthropology Quarterly*, *17*: 423–41.

Strauss, A. L. (1959) *Mirrors and Masks: The Search for Identity*. Glencoe, IL: Free Press.

Tajfel, H. (1970) 'Experiments in intergroup discrimination', *Scientific American*, *223*: 96–102.

Tajfel, H. (ed.) (1978) *Differentiation between Social Groups: Studies in the Social Psychology of Intergroup Relations*. London: Academic Press.

Tajfel, H. and Turner, J. C. (1979) 'An integrative theory of intergroup conflict: The social psychology of intergroup relations', in W. G. Austin and S. Worchel (eds), *The Social Psychology of Intergroup Relations*. Monterey, CA: Brooks/Cole.

Tarraf, W., Jensen, G. A. and González, H. M. (2016) 'Impact of Medicare age eligibility on health spending among U.S. and foreign-born adults', *Health Services Research*, *51*(3): 846–71.

Weeks, J., Holland, J. and Waites, M. (2003) *Sexualities and Society: A Reader*. Cambridge: Polity Press.

Wooffitt, R. (2005) *Conversation Analysis and Discourse Analysis: A Comparative and Critical Introduction*. London: Sage.

21

Public Involvement in Health Research

ANNELIESE SYNNOT AND SOPHIE HILL

Chapter objectives

- To discuss what is meant by the term 'public' and 'involvement' in health research
- To outline the competing rationales for public involvement in health research and the main reasons why the public and researchers might want to work together on research
- To consider the challenges and barriers to public involvement, including current debates surrounding this
- To identify activities in which the public could be involved and the methods for such involvement
- To examine the practicalities of public involvement in health research and conditions for success.

Introduction

The idea that patients, families, carers, their representatives and the public more broadly can and should have a say in health research is one whose time has well and truly come. While individuals and organizations have long championed and practised public involvement in health research, it has only recently reached a tipping point. We are witnessing cultural and policy shifts among the health research community, whereby public involvement is increasingly expected, and sometimes mandated, by research institutions, funders and publishers. The literature is now filled with examples of public involvement, methodological discussions about research and practice, and, more recently, 'how to' guides for researchers. Yet public involvement in health research is still in its infancy and there are many conceptual, cultural and practical challenges. The shift to make public involvement a requirement in health research are likely to spur further activity, presenting both opportunities and risks.

In this chapter, we describe the genesis of public involvement in health research and explore the shifts in terminology and meaning of the terms such as 'public' and 'involvement' with increasing prominence given to the notion of 'co-production'. We explore the competing rationales for public involvement in health research and outline why both researchers and the public might want to work together. We then consider the 'how' of public involvement, introducing the research cycle or stages, and provide examples of the kind of activities the public can be involved in at each stage, and the possible methods for involvement. Practical considerations are part of public involvement and research has contributed to identifying the conditions for success, as well as common barriers and challenges. We conclude with a summary of the current debates and criticisms of public involvement. Throughout the chapter examples are given of public involvement drawn from the work of ourselves and others.

A history of public involvement in health research

Over the second half of the twentieth century, many of our social structures and institutions, including health care, have moved from paternalistic to more democratic and participative models. As patients and users of health care, many of us now take for granted that we have a right to participate in decisions about our health and that of our families with our doctors and other health providers. But this right did not come about easily. Some of these changes we owe to broader social movement like 'the push for women's rights', but equally important have been the sustained efforts of individuals and groups advocating for the human and health care rights of people with disability, people with mental illness or HIV, and indigenous people (Brown and Zavestoski 2004; Sepkowitz 2001). Activism within the health system has also drawn energy from the public's awakening to the extent of adverse events and substandard practice (Coulter 2002a; Kohn, Corrigan and Donaldson 1999; Ocloo and Matthews 2016). These movements have seen patients and families, and the organizations which represent them, demand a say not only in their individual care, but in how the health services and health programmes they use are governed and made accountable (Coulter 2002b). Policy responses from governments and agencies around the world (for example, World Health Organization 2013) have led to at least an expectation in many health systems that people who use health care services should be actively involved in all levels of governance, service planning and design, programme implementation and evaluation, in addition to participation in individual care (Coulter 2002b; Ocloo and Matthews 2016).

In parallel, we have seen increasing interest and activity in bringing together patients, families and the organizations who represent them along with researchers and research funders to work together on the planning, conduct and dissemination of health research. Indeed, there has been a veritable recent explosion of activity and literature about the need for, and value of, public involvement in health research – what it is and is not, and how to do it, report it and evaluate it (Shippee et al. 2015; Staniszewska et al. 2017).

Organizational support is now integrated into some health systems, such as the INVOLVE national advisory group, which is part of, and funded by, the National Institute for Health Research (NIHR) in the United Kingdom. In recent years, developments here have been so rapid that it has led to 'National Standards for Public Involvement in Research', published in 2018 (Public Health Agency, Chief Scientist Office, Health and Care Research Wales and National Institute for Health Research 2018).

The progress in the implementation of public involvement should not be exaggerated, despite so much activity. It is a public health irony that the social movements most connected with efforts to seek greater participation may not have led to the greater inclusion of diverse participants, as might be expected. For example, Ocloo and Matthews (2016) report that those who are most marginalized in society are still the least represented in public involvement activities. However, while still in its early stages and unevenly distributed in practice, the fact that we are seeing critiques of public involvement, new theories about how it works, and a proliferation of primary research into it, indicates that public involvement in health research is coming of age as a legitimate discipline in research in its own right. This is underlined by Box 21.1.

Box 21.1 Major research organizations that involve the public in their work

Around the world, many of the leading research organizations have established policies and extensive programmes to support the involvement of patient and carer representatives in health or medical research. Here is a brief overview of some innovative practices.

NICE, United Kingdom

In the United Kingdom, NICE (the National Institute for Health and Care Excellence) provides national guidance and advice to improve health and social care. NICE involves members of the public in all levels of its work and through various participatory and

(Continued)

(Continued)

consultative mechanisms. It supports involvement through training and offers pay-ment. Engagement and the two-way flow of information and advice is ensured through maintaining an extensive set of relationships with various types of community organi-zations. All its advisory committees and working groups have at least two lay members, defined as 'patients, service users, carers or members of the public' (see nice.org.uk and related pages).

INVOLVE, United Kingdom

INVOLVE is part of the National Institute for Health Research (NIHR), which supports public involvement in the NHS and in public health and social care research. It has a 15-member National Advisory Group that has a role to 'bring together expertise, insight and experience in the field of public involvement in research, with the aim of advancing it as an essential part of the process by which research is identified, prioritized, designed, conducted and disseminated'. Policy and resource documents on its site include explanatory documents for researchers and the public, evidence about public involvement, payment policies, and advice on training and support. As described earlier, in 2018, it published the results of its major project on defining the principles and key features of co-production to aid the work of the NIHR (see Hickey et al. 2018; and invo.org.uk).

PCORI, United States

In the United States, the Patient-Centered Outcomes Research Institute (PCORI) produces evidence for the American health system through comparative clinical effectiveness research. PCORI uses the term 'engagement in research' for strategies to involve patients, caregivers, clinicians and people representing health professional organizations in all stages of research. PCORI has Methodology Standards for patient-centredness that are applicable to all research applicants. Members of the public can be ambassadors for PCORI, advisory panel members, and peer reviewers, and training and other resources are provided to researchers and the public on their site (see pcori.org).

CADTH, Canada

The Canadian Agency for Drugs and Technologies in Health (CADTH) provides evi-dence, analysis, advice and recommendations to the Canadian health system to ensure informed decision making about the optimal use of drugs and medical devices. When projects commence, for example, a review of a new drug, CADTH seeks input from patient groups. Once recommendations are drafted, feedback is sought more widely from patient groups or from members of the public. Members of the public are represented on the Board and expert committees. There is a Patient Community Liaison Forum with rep-resentatives of patient umbrella groups to advise on engagement strategies. Research strategies are also used to inform decision-making with a synthesis of qualitative studies of views and experiences (see cadth.ca).

What do we mean by 'public' and 'involvement'?

From patient to health consumer to person and the public

In recent decades, many terms have been used to refer to the person at the receiving end of health care. This partly reflects the range of roles that a person can inhabit at any one time as patient, potential patient, advocate or representative, family member, carer, lay person, health service user, volunteer, citizen or member of the public (Hill 2011). People can contribute their own lived experience or personal views or can represent the collective voice of a group of individuals, or an organization to which they are accountable (National Health and Medical Research Council and Consumers Health Forum of Australia 2016). There is considerable variation in preferred terms between countries – for example, 'consumer and community member' is often used in Australia, whereas 'patients and the public' is more common in the United Kingdom. There is also variation according to the health care setting within groups and between individuals. For example, 'service user' is common in mental health, but not necessarily elsewhere.

In this chapter, we will use the terms 'people' and 'public', by which we mean: patients and potential patients; people who use health, social and community services; carers, parents and guardians; people with disabilities; members of the public targeted by health promotion programmes; organizations that represent the interests of the public; communities that are affected by health, public health or social care issues; and

---

Box 21.2   Individuals and groups who might be involved in research

Individuals may participate as:	Local groups may participate through:
• Service users and carers • Patient representatives • Patient advocates • Citizens • Members of the public who are potential users of health services	• Population groups • Support groups • Groups convened to discuss health matters such as citizens' juries • (Inter)national consumer organizations • Statutory bodies • Charities • (Inter)national support groups

Source: Boote, Telford and Cooper (2002)

groups asking for research because they believe they have been exposed to circumstances, products or services that are potentially harmful (INVOLVE 2012; National Health and Medical Research Council and Consumers Health Forum of Australia 2016). This range of involvement in research is reflected in Box 21.2 above.

Participation, involvement, engagement or co-production?

In the past, public involvement in health research occurred through participation by patients and members of the public as 'subjects' in research that was carried out by professional or clinical researchers. Typically, they gave their informed consent to being a subject in a research project, but had no part in setting up the research or contributing to the design process. Nor were they necessarily informed about the outcomes.

The emphasis has now shifted to a more 'active involvement' or 'partnership' in all stages of the research process, from setting priorities, to designing and conducting the research, to disseminating the findings (PCORI 2015). There has been a language shift from 'participation' to 'involvement', 'engagement' and 'partnership'. The meaning of these terms reflects subtle shifts in power with patients and members of the public undertaking a range of new activities in health care research. In the United Kingdom, INVOLVE defines public involvement in research as research being carried out 'with' or 'by' members of the public rather than 'to', 'about' or 'for' them (INVOLVE 2012). In Australia, it is described as 'consumers, community members, researchers and research organizations working in partnerships, to improve the health and wellbeing of all Australians through health and medical research' (National Health and Medical Research Council and Consumers Health Forum of Australia 2016: 2). These are the definitions and terminology we will use in this chapter.

More recently, the terminology of involvement has shifted again, and we increasingly see involvement referred to as 'co-production' and 'co-design'. Co-production is not usually described as an activity but rather as a set of principles that underpin the way the public and researchers can work together. In doing so, the focus is moving from the 'what' to the 'how' of involvement. In 2018, INVOLVE published guidance on the principles of co-production and proposed some of its key features (Hickey et al. 2018). Their principles of co-production include:

- *Power is shared*: The research is jointly owned and everyone works together to achieve a joint understanding
- *Diverse perspectives and skills are included*: The team includes people who bring different perspectives, skills, knowledge and experiences and is inclusive
- *Everyone's contribution is valued and respected*: Everyone is of equal importance
- *Reciprocity*: Contributions are recognized and everyone gets something out of working together

- *Emphasis on building and maintaining relationships*: Trust is built on a joint understanding and consensus and clarity over roles and responsibilities, where people feel valued.

Their key features of co-production include: 'establishing ground rules; ongoing dialogue; joint ownership of key decisions; a commitment to relationship building; opportunities for personal growth and development; flexibility; continuous reflection; and valuing and evaluating the impact of co-producing research' (Hickey et al. 2018: 4).

Readers taking even a brief glimpse at the public involvement literature will quickly see the plethora of different terms used to describe public involvement. However, when you look closely at how involvement is defined or described, and how it should optimally be done, we are usually all talking about the same thing. We see the following commonalities with all these terms:

- The emphasis has shifted from tokenistic to active, meaningful involvement
- Attention to relationships is paramount
- Involvement can be at all research stages
- Power and influence over decisions should be, and can be, shared.

Involvement as a spectrum

Involvement activities are often described as existing on a spectrum, from minimal involvement through to shared leadership. For example, Oliver and colleagues (2008) say the 'degree of public engagement' can vary from minimal consultation (asking people for their views, which the researchers use to inform their decisions), collaboration (an active, ongoing partnership with researchers) and lay control (where the public designs, conducts or disseminates the research, and researchers are involved by invitation only). Another model, by the International Association for Public Participation (IAP2) Federation, describes five different roles that the public can have in their 'Public Participation Spectrum' (International Association for Public Participation 2014). These include: inform (provided with information only), consult (provide feedback on aspects of the research), involve (work directly with researchers throughout the process to ensure public concerns are understood and considered), collaborate (partner with researchers in all aspects of decision-making) and empower (final decision-making is in the hands of the public).

While many such spectrums exist, at their core they are concerned with the level of influence (or power) over the decisions that the public has. Such involvement spectrums are helpful for researchers and the public alike to think critically about how they plan to involve the public in their work, and what methods are most appropriate to inform the kind of influence they as researchers, and the public, want to have.

What is the rationale for public involvement in health research?

Broadly speaking, there are two competing rationales for public involvement in research. Drawing on the literature about 'community engagement' to develop public health interventions, Brunton and colleagues (2017) describe these two perspectives as:

- 'Utilitarian', where public involvement is thought to lead to more acceptable and appropriate research, thereby improving health outcomes
- 'Social justice', where the emphasis is less instrumental and the focus is on empowerment and the development of the community itself.

With a utilitarian or instrumental rationale, involving the public in health research is thought to lead to improved relevance, quality and uptake of research. For example, involving patients to set priorities for research is thought to better align research with the needs of the lives of the people the research affects, thereby improving its relevance (Chalmers et al. 2014). Research quality may be improved by patients and the public contributing to more user-friendly patient information materials or by providing a deeper interpretation of what the study results mean (Brett et al. 2014b). Partnering with patient groups and their networks to champion the findings can also assist in dissemination and increase uptake of the research into policy and practice (Brett et al. 2014b). More recently, patient and public involvement in the agenda-setting stage of research has been proposed as a strategy to reduce avoidable waste in research (Chalmers et al. 2014). Through these mechanisms, the ultimate aim of public involvement from the utilitarian perspective is for the research to improve health outcomes.

Brunton and colleagues (2017) explain that the ultimate aim within a social justice rationale may include improvements in health but it is broader than this. It is also concerned with addressing inherent imbalances in power, democracy and accountability. The social justice rationale also has a considerable moral imperative. Miller and colleagues (2017) argue that given that patients and the public are ultimately most affected by health research, they must have a say in what research is funded, and how it is conducted. Further, patients and the public are also the ultimate payers of research through their taxes (given that so much research is government funded). According to the social justice rationale, the process of involving patients and the public in a democratic and empowering way can be the end and not just the means. We can see many of these ideas expressed in the spectrums of involvement, and the principles of co-production, described earlier.

In reality, researchers and research institutions often cite both arguments as reasons for involving the public, although they may have a stronger emphasis on one or the other (Brunton et al. 2017). While these two competing rationales can sit side-by-side, they have led to tensions in determining what success looks like, and what aspects of public involvement we should evaluate, and how (see Edelman and Barron 2016).

What is in it for researchers?

In a systematic review, Brett et al. (2014a) identified numerous self-reported benefits, or positive impacts, of public involvement for researchers. Researchers reported gaining new insights into issues they were exploring, for example gaining a greater understanding of the community's needs and better identifying barriers to their research. By spending time and building a good rapport with community members, they learnt more about how community members think and feel. They expanded their networks for future research studies and remained focused on the issues important to the community they were researching. Involving patients and the public provided greater diversity within the research team and, in the case of more collaborative public involvement approaches, often reduced the workload of researchers.

As it becomes increasingly expected that public involvement in research will be funded and published (Richards and Godlee 2014), it may become more instrumentally necessary for researchers and research institutions to be so engaged. It can be argued that the fact that researchers have involved the public, irrespective of whether this has had any impact on their research, enhances their standing as researchers. They are more credible and have a greater chance of being financially supported and having their work accepted and cited. It is therefore possible that public involvement may become a largely symbolic exercise for some researchers.

What is in it for patients and the public?

In their systematic review, Brett and colleagues (2014a) identified a range of benefits reported by the patients and the public who were directly involved in research. They referred to feeling valued, being listened to and empowered, and being able to give something back to the research community. After being involved in research, other benefits included greater confidence and self-worth, gaining a sense of mutual support from other people, feeling involved and being part of a team. People also reported gaining a better understanding of research (when they had received training as part of their role) and increasing their knowledge about their condition and current developments. Finally, being involved in research presented an opportunity to gain life skills in public speaking, interviewing and group facilitation that could be useful for gaining employment.

In our own experience, we found working in partnership with patient representatives on research projects to be incredibly rewarding. In the Integrating and Deriving Evidence Experiences and Preferences (IN-DEEP) study, we partnered with a three-member consumer advisory group to develop online summaries of evidence on treatments for multiple sclerosis (MS) for Australians affected by the condition. The group included two women with MS and a representative from the state-based MS organization. We subsequently published an article with advisory group members describing how we worked together and the impact on the research itself and on everyone involved (Synnot et al. 2018b).

In this article, we concluded that partnering with consumers improved the research in various important and unforeseen ways. First, we felt that the quality of the research was improved, in that we were more responsive to, and reflective of, the needs and experiences of Australians with MS. For example, on the advice of the advisory group, we held separate focus groups for people who were newly diagnosed with MS, and those who had lived with MS for longer, to access different views. Partnering with our advisory group expanded the project's depth and reach. We could utilize their networks to assist with focus group recruitment and identify potential themes for discussion. We also felt that the outputs of the research through online summaries of evidence of MS treatment were both appropriate and sensitive as a result of the cooperation. As researchers, we gained in confidence and capacity to manage study challenges, while the advisory group felt they could assist the MS community and that their contributions were valued and respected, rather than tokenistic. The research concluded with a celebratory dinner and advisory group members spoke at the project launch.

What are the challenges of, and barriers to, public involvement?

For both patients and the public, and researchers, there is overlap in what they consider to be the challenging aspects of public involvement. For example, two systematic reviews by Brett and colleagues (2014a) and Domecq and colleagues (2014) found that the public can experience considerable frustration with the lengthy processes and time commitment required to contribute to research as well as the additional resources and costs of involvement. Recruiting, training and providing ongoing support to patients and the public, running meetings and more formal involvement activities may require additional funding.

Both the public and researchers fear involvement being tokenistic (Domecq et al. 2014). Brett and colleagues (2014a) found that where involvement is not well done, the public can feel devalued, not listened to, or that their contributions are not taken seriously, while researchers described difficulties in relinquishing their decision-making power and managing conflicting views. They concluded that many of the challenging impacts are underpinned by misunderstandings, mismatched expectations or tensions between academic and patient perspectives.

How people are involved in research

The research cycle or stages

The various steps are common to health care research and are often described as the research cycle or research stages. For example, Shippee and colleagues (2015) use a linear model, describing three phases with eight stages of research. These include the preparatory phase (stage 1: agenda setting and funding), the execution phase (stages 2 to 5: study design and procedures; study recruitment; data collection; and data analysis) and the translational phase (stages 6 to 8: dissemination; implementation; and evaluation). Another commonly used example is provided by INVOLVE (2012), which describes a circular model with seven research stages: identifying and prioritizing; commissioning; designing and managing; undertaking; disseminating; implementing; and evaluating impact.

Examples of the kind of activities the public can be involved in at each stage are listed below:

- *Preparatory phase*: Suggesting or voting on priorities for future research, being on a steering committee or being co-investigators on research projects, being on grant review panels at research funders.
- *Execution phase*: Reviewing project materials and plans, being a lay member of an ethics committee, assisting with project recruitment, undertaking interviews, reviewing interpretation of focus group data.
- *Translational phase*: Patient reviewers of journals, co-authoring manuscripts, contributing to lay project summaries, being a patient panel member for clinical guidelines, and planning for future research.

Such frameworks help to understand and plan the different points in the research process in which the public might be involved. Public involvement is possible at every stage, although it can be selective. Reviews of the evidence suggest the public are more commonly involved in the earlier research stages, agenda setting, protocol development, participant recruitment and some translational stages, such as dissemination, rather than in the 'doing' stages (Domecq et al. 2014; Shippee et al. 2015).

A project that we conducted for the Cochrane Consumers and Communication Review Group (cccrg.cochrane.org) provides an example of involving people in the preparatory phase of research, namely setting priorities for future Cochrane Reviews published by the Cochrane Consumers and Communication Review Group (Synnot et al. 2018a). To do this, we invited patients, the public, health professionals, policy makers, and anyone who was interested, to tell us their ideas for future priority Cochrane Review topics. We conducted an international online survey, followed by an Australian workshop to identify and refine priority topics. However, this priority setting project was itself a research study, so we wanted to involve the public and other important stakeholder groups to help us undertake it. As such, we convened an 11-member steering group to oversee the project, which included people who represented the range of stakeholders who might use, or be affected by, the resulting Cochrane Reviews, including consumers, consumer groups, health policy makers, health professionals, health service representatives, and research funders.

With the exception of stage 1 (agenda setting and funding) and stage 8 (evaluation), the steering group was involved in all stages of the research. In the execution phase, steering group members played a role in: study design and procedures (defining project scope, approving proposed methods, and refining the sampling frame for participant selection); study recruitment (advising on networks for recruitment, and directly sharing recruitment materials); data collection (co-facilitating the workshop); and data analysis (offering their interpretations of study results). In the translational phase, steering group members were involved in dissemination (advising on dissemination formats, such as infographics, and reviewing the final report), as well as implementation. Some steering group members are now active as co-authors or advisory group members on the current Cochrane Reviews.

Involvement beyond individual research projects

There are increasingly roles for the public, together with research funders and research institutions, in research governance. Some international research funders ask patients and members of the public to assess grant applications and/or to suggest strategic priorities for funding (Nasser et al. 2017). Increasingly, research institutions, such as universities and research centres, appoint members of the public in advisory committees and some universities, particularly in the United Kingdom, employ 'patient and public involvement advisors' who support researchers and the public in working together. We are also seeing greater public involvement embedded in the research publishing community, with roles such as co-editor-in-chief, patient editors and lay reviewers. Journals also expect that patients will be included as authors, or that their contribution to the research will be clearly described. Examples include *Research Involvement and Engagement* (Stephens and Staniszewska 2015), the *British Medical Journal* (Richards and Godlee 2014), and the Cochrane Collaboration (Cochrane 2017).

Methods of involvement

Public involvement can take myriad different forms, and methods vary considerably. Formal research methods, such as interviews, focus groups and surveys can be used, or the increasingly popular consensus methods. Delphi studies may use iterative individual survey rounds that can be conducted online (see Vernon 2009). The nominal group technique based on facilitated group activity with idea generation, clarification and individual voting (see McMillan, King and Tully 2016) and citizens' juries comprising structured fora for citizens to discuss information provided by experts are further techniques (see Gooberman-Hill, Horwood and Calnan 2008). Predominantly, informal methods are used, such as advisory or steering group meetings, project team discussions, and written consultations or peer review. These may draw on selected individuals or a larger group. Such activities can also be undertaken using different modes, from online to face-to-face, one-off or a series of meetings activities.

In the IN-DEEP project, numerous methods of involvement were employed (Synnot et al. 2018b). Informal involvement methods in different modes were used. Across the two-and-a-half-year project, we met face-to-face with the consumer advisory group in a series of meetings and sought *ad hoc* input by email. We worked directly with our advisory group, which included people with MS, and we partnered with the group in some of the major decisions following guidance of the IAP2 Public Participation Spectrum (International Association for Public Participation 2014). We also sought input from a wider group of people affected by MS as part of the core stages of the project itself. To do this, we used formal research methods, including focus groups and an online forum conducted with 60 people affected by MS (see Synnot et al. 2016). These were one-off activities, conducted either face-to-face or online. Then, when the website content was being developed, we undertook structured face-to-face feedback sessions with 'review panels', with 16 people, most of whom were affected by MS. We then pilot tested the website via an online survey with follow-up phone interviews (Synnot et al. 2018c).

While there has been little research directly comparing methods of involvement to support one method over another (Domecq et al. 2014), the involvement method chosen should reflect the aims of engagement and the stage of the research (Oliver et al. 2008). Participants should be asked how they wish to be involved. Some people with illness, disability or caring responsibilities might prefer to take part from home, while others prefer group meetings.

Bringing it all together: A framework for undertaking public involvement in research

Oliver and colleagues (2004, 2008) developed a comprehensive framework for categorizing involvement in research. It has eight key features that explore a range of roles, functions and methods, and has wide applicability (see Nilsen et al. 2006; Paterson 2004). The framework can assist in analysing the dimensions of consumer involvement by using a checklist such as that shown in Box 21.3.

Box 21.3 Categorizing involvement in research

- *Who is involved?* Individuals or people representing a consumer organization?
- *Who initiated the involvement?* Consumers or researchers?
- *What was the degree of involvement?* Information giving and consultation or some form of power sharing through collaboration or consumer control?
- *What are the forums for exchanging ideas?* For example, citizens' juries, focus groups or consensus conferences?
- *What are the methods used for collective decision-making?* For instance, this can be through developing a method for ranking research priorities.
- *What are the practical arrangements for user involvement?* For instance, transport, financial resources, or opportunities for training and skill development?
- *What is the context for agenda setting?* Institutional type, geographical coverage or the background of participants in consumer activism?
- *What theory underpins the strategy for consumer involvement?* Is this researcher-led, consumer-led or even professionally led?

Source: Oliver et al. (2004, 2008)

The practicalities of public involvement and conditions for success

There are some practical details to be considered in health research. A common question is: who should I involve and how do I find them? Researchers should consider whether to offer training and support to participants or offer to meet costs and reimburse expenses. Researchers should also document, share and formally publish their public involvement activities and seek feedback from participants. Box 21.4 lists sources for advice.

Box 21.4 Practical guidance for public involvement: Guides and toolkits

Patient and Public Involvement in Health and Social Care Research: A Handbook for Researchers is a practical guide on planning and undertaking public involvement published by the NIHR Research Design Service (2014). It includes templates for advertisements and role descriptions, and advice on costs, payment and evaluation.

Imperial College London in the United Kingdom maintains a rich PPI Resource Hub (www.imperial.ac.uk/patient-experience-research-centre/ppi-resource-hub/). This includes introductory material on the stages of public involvement, supported by real-life examples of activities along with templates for forms from payment to setting ground rules for meetings.

The Change Foundation (2015a) report in Canada, *Rules of Engagement: Lessons from Panorama*, provides 15 experienced-based and practical tips. Examples include: 'Expect the unexpected' and 'Be prepared for lulls, and how to navigate them'. The report includes an infographic outlining 'Ten ground rules for dialogue'.

It also provides a decision tool 'to help organizations answer the payment/non-payment question' to include a range of factors: time, equity, vulnerable-group status, challenges, accountability, positive impact, access and other forms of recognition (The Change Foundation 2015b). It generates an overall score to determine whether payment is appropriate (changefoundation.ca/patient-compensation-report/).

The Public Involvement Impact Assessment Framework (PiiAF) (Popay and Collins 2014) focuses on impacts. It suggests first exploring shared values, outlining the approach and agreeing its intended impacts, and then devising an impact assessment plan,

The Guidance for Reporting Involvement of Patients and the Public (GRIPP2) checklist (Staniszewska et al. 2017) is the first consensus-based reporting guideline. It includes a five-item short form for use when reporting public involvement within a study, and a 34-item long form for studies that are mainly about public involvement in research.

The literature of 'how to' guides has proliferated and much of this practical guidance provides both positive and negative examples. The importance of building trusting and reciprocal relationships in which researchers and the public learn together has been highlighted as a key 'condition for success' (Brett et al. 2014a; Shippee et al. 2015). There is greater focus on nurturing good relationships in the shift towards co-production and in the UK Standards for Public Involvement in Research (Public Health Agency, Chief Scientist Office, Health and Care Research Wales and National Institute for Health Research 2018). Six national standards include:

- Inclusive opportunities (accessible opportunities that allow people from diverse backgrounds to participate)
- Working together (all contributions are valued and relationships are mutually respectful and productive)
- Support and learning (to build confidence and skills)
- Communications (timely, two-way and targeted communication using plain language)
- Impact (capture and share the difference that public involvement makes)
- Governance (the public is involved in governance and leadership).

Current debates and criticisms of public involvement in health research

The involvement of the public in health research represents the intersection of two phenomena: on the one hand, the emergence of health social movements (Brown and Zavestoski 2004) and, on the other hand, the development of theories, methods and knowledge in the clinical sciences. Activities are therefore contingent on researchers, but also politicized in the sense that the power to create new knowledge – formerly lying with researchers – is now expected to be shared (Locock et al. 2017). This is the expectation of funding bodies and consumer groups but may be less apparent among researchers.

The last few decades can be categorized by the developmental, voluntary and the increasingly political nature of public involvement, which in many instances is not well documented or researched. Recently, researchers with a commitment to public involvement have sought to conceptualize and theorize to build a coherent body of work and examine how and when public involvement can have an impact on a future research agenda, particularly for those most in need of access to effective health care. Ocloo and Matthews (2016) outline a framework for empowerment and to increase inclusiveness to reach a wider range of voices.

Efforts to conceptualize the field have linked with the need to demonstrate that public involvement has an impact and so increase its legitimacy. This has centred on the claim that public involvement can contribute to knowledge by articulating the 'lifeworld' of patients and the public alongside professional knowledge (Edelman and Barron 2016). We consider evaluating the quality of the involvement processes (how meaningful and satisfactory it was for all parties) to be just as important.

Earlier debates on terminology appear to have receded (see Boote, Telford and Cooper 2002; Henderson and Petersen 2002; Herxheimer and Goodare 1999), possibly because organizations have formalized agendas (moving the discourse away from advocacy to expected business) and newer, more 'generic' terms have come into use. Key among these are co-production or co-design (Hickey et al. 2018) and stakeholders (Concannon 2012). This language has the benefit of general applicability to various forms of partnership between a range of parties in health care.

The issue of whose interests are well served by public involvement may get muddied with the inclusion of consumer or illness groups who receive funding from a pharmaceutical company for projects and activities that provide access to information on recent research or products. Some groups where the management or cure is dependent on the company's products may have a shared interest with pharmaceutical companies. The dilemma is the potential for loss of integrity and independence in a relationship where there is inequality in terms of power and wealth and where profit is a primary goal for companies (Lipworth and Kerridge 2013). There have been concerns about the lack of transparency for several years, resulting in various codes of conduct (Baggott, Allsop and Jones 2005; Consumers Health Forum of Australia and Medicines Australia 2008; Herxheimer 2003).

Finally, an emergent issue is the blurring of roles associated with public involvement, particularly as co-design models take hold. In these cases, members of the public may be research advisers, research subjects and research analysers – all in one study (Liabo et al. 2018). This may lead to a need for different forms of research protocol, authorship and accountability structures.

We have now chosen to present two short case studies. One is of public involvement in a research organization, representing a more macro perspective. The second is public involvement in a single research project.

Public involvement in an institution: The consumer and community engagement framework of the South Australian Health and Medical Research Institute

The South Australian Health and Medical Research Institute (the 'Institute') in Australia is a major organization where a broad range of health issues are researched – from biomedicine through to public health. Information for this case study comes from Miller and collegues (2017). (Interested readers may also look up documents and examples on the Institute's website at sahmri.org, particularly at ww.sahmri.org/consumer-community-engagement/ and www.sahmri.org/research-theme/resource-13/).

In 2014 the Institute implemented a comprehensive new Consumer and Community Engagement Framework to support and increase 'consumer engagement' (their terminology) in its work at all levels, from governance to projects. In this case study, we describe the background, process and outcomes, and conclude with a brief commentary on how this example illustrates some of key lessons presented in the chapter.

Background

The Institute was established in 2009, and when new, the need was identified for integrating consumer engagement into its policies and operations. Despite research policies being supportive of consumer participation in Australian research, there are few structures or mechanisms to support it, and so the reality of participation is patchy and project- or researcher-dependent.

Process

A team at the Institute undertook a mixed-methods process with several iterative stages. A partnership was established between the Institute and the main body for

(Continued)

(Continued)

health consumers in South Australia, and, following this, a Steering Committee was formed with scientists, researchers and consumers. A literature review to establish 'What strategies have been effective for consumers and researchers?' commenced. The review's findings were complemented by intelligence gathered from interviews with consumers, carers and researchers with experience of consumer engagement. The findings from both stages were discussed by the Steering Committee and a full-day consensus conference was held to develop the Framework.

Outcomes

A comprehensive Framework was the result. It has four organizational dimensions:

- Governance (including partnership with consumers, partnership committee, policies and accountability)
- Infrastructure (including resources, engagement facilitators, tools, guidance and a consumer register)
- Capacity building (including information and community education, researcher and consumer training, evaluation and research)
- Leadership and culture (including leadership and advocacy, principles, organizational culture and translational strategy).

Commentary

In discussing the achievements and challenges of their Framework, Miller and her co-authors emphasize the need for attention to each of the organizational dimensions, in the context of having strong organizational 'will and commitment'. This experience and advice may resonate with early adopters of consumer engagement in research where opposition or apathy may be present in the organization (Greenhalgh et al. 2004). It may also signal the changes which are required in organizational cultures, to ensure indirect impacts over time, such as leading to a pool of more cognizant researchers for assessing innovative projects that seek to co-produce research.

Public involvement by co-production to update a systematic review on physiotherapy for stroke

A team led by Cochrane author, editor and researcher Dr Alex Pollock, at Glasgow Caledonian University, updated a Cochrane review with user involvement (their terminology) on the question of the effects of physiotherapy after stroke. Their

CASE STUDY 21.2

Cochrane review and the involvement approach and its impact are reported in Pollock et al. (2014, 2015).

Approach

Pre-planning contributed to a viable process, with three stroke survivors, one carer and nine physiotherapists recruited to join a Stakeholder Group, which reflected the broad range of users of the final review. Participants received a role description, with the skills, experience and knowledge they needed, the expected time commitment, and confirmation that travel expenses would be met. Four physiotherapists joined the Group as non-voting members as they were all authors. Meeting dates were set in advance and formal decision rules for consensus decision making (based on nominal group techniques) were established from the outset.

Three meetings were held. The first was used to explore and reach consensus on the scope and methods for the update – not least how physical rehabilitation approaches should be categorized and whether international approaches should be included. In the second meeting the Group explored and agreed on the specific strategies to 'operationalize' the decisions made in the first meeting. The review update was then conducted, and the third meeting was used to discuss the clinical implications of the findings and informed dissemination activities.

Impacts

A high degree of consensus was achieved, underscoring all key decisions. The Stakeholder Group influenced the scope, methods and analysis of the review update, and significant changes in direction were made from the first version. International trials were therefore added into the scope of the review and methods were identified for unpacking and designing the intervention components of what is a complex therapeutic intervention. This also influenced the comparisons made and the subgroup analyses performed. Key messages from the analyses were agreed. A post-review evaluation, albeit small in scale, identified positive views on the role and impact of the Stakeholder Group.

Dr Pollock commented on the experience and subsequent developments as follows:

This 12-month project demonstrated that involving people in a complex systematic review is feasible and valued; can significantly impact on review structure and methods; and is perceived to increase the clinical relevance of evidence synthesized within a review. Based on our experiences, we would definitely recommend similar models of involvement within other systematic reviews and evidence syntheses. Members of our stakeholder group would agree with this. One consumer said: 'I have taken part in quite

(Continued)

(Continued)

a number of things of this nature over the past 20 years and this is the first time that I have really felt that it has been successful and that I have been listened to'. One of the physiotherapists said that the approach 'links clinicians with researchers, allowing research to be more clinically relevant'. (Pollock et al. 2018)

Dr Pollock went on to add that 'as a review author, what was most challenging was the lack of information or resources relating to how to involve people in a meaningful way. It was this lack of resources that led us to carry out further work aiming to bring together information to help systematic review authors involve people in their reviews'.

In consequence, this work included the development of a free online learning resource ('Involving People'), which is designed to support authors in getting people engaged in the production of their reviews. It is available at: training.cochrane.org/involving-people.

Commentary

In discussing their achievements, Pollock and colleagues (2018) say that they sought to have a more equal number of health professionals and the consumer/carer members, but that time pressures and electronic distribution may have prevented them from reaching a wider number of the latter. However, the commitment by the author team to listen to, give equal value to and enact the decision of the whole group may have meant that there was a high level of satisfaction among the stakeholders.

Conclusion

As we have seen above, the public involvement landscape is moving very quickly. There are now a considerable number of frameworks and guidance documents designed to help researchers better understand the key concepts of public involvement, and how to do it, and do it well. As public involvement becomes a requirement, not just an 'optional extra' for research funding, new and established researchers will need to sharpen their skills in public involvement and follow good practice. The key organizations cited in this chapter provide a way of keeping abreast with the latest developments.

Public involvement in research can be incredibly powerful and beneficial to those concerned, but it usually requires considerable investment of time and resources. If not done well, it can have a negative impact for everyone concerned. Involving the public in your research does not have to be complicated, nor involve huge numbers of people. It is better to do something achievable, working in partnership with the public and do it well than be over-ambitious.

Exercise 21.1 Planning for public involvement in health research

Imagine you need to develop a plan for public involvement in a research study, or in a research institution, like a research centre or a funder. Using the frameworks described above, consider the following questions to help you develop your plan:

- Why do you want to involve people? What is your rationale?
- Describe your aims of involvement? What do you hope involvement will result in?
- Who will you involve? What are the characteristics of the people you would like to involve? And how will you find or recruit people?
- In what stages of the research will you involve people? What activities could you invite them to take part in?
- Describe the methods, mode and timing of your involvement. Think about the degree to which your methods will allow power to be shared between research-ers and the public. Consider the time it may take to ensure participation and discussion is meaningful.
- What sort of budget would you need for such an approach?
- Where does your approach lie on the involvement spectrum?
- What steps or activities could you undertake so your involvement activities meet the principles of co-production?
- Describe your plans for covering expenses and reimbursement for people's time and expertise.
- What training and support will you provide for the public or for your research colleagues?
- How can you evaluate the process or impact of the involvement?
- How will you share what you have done?

Note

We would like to thank Drs Caroline Miller and Alex Pollock for reviewing the case studies pertaining to their work.

Recommended further reading

This is good reading in acquiring a sociological understanding of health social movements: Brown, P. and Zavestoski, S. (2004) 'Social movements in health: an introduction', *Sociology of Health and Illness*, 26(6): 679–94.

This is a highly readable report that summarizes current thinking about the principles and features of co-production of research:

Hickey, G., Brearley, S., Coldham, T., Denegri, S., Green, G., Staniszewska, S., Tembo, D., Torok, K. and Turner, K. (2018) *Guidance on Co-producing a Research Project*. Southampton: INVOLVE.

This is a helpful paper in exploring the issue of power and how patients and the public attain status and respect:

Locock, L., Boylan, A., Snow, R. and Staniszewska, S. (2017) 'The power of symbolic capital in patient and public involvement in health research', *Health Expectations, 20*: 836–44.

The issue of representativeness in public involvement is contested. This is an enjoyable article that highlights the impossibility of true representativeness in public involvement:

Maguire, K. and Britten, N. (2017) '"How can anybody be representative for those kind of people?" Forms of patient representation in health research, and why it is always contestable', *Social Science and Medicine, 183*: 62–69.

References

Baggott, R., Allsop, J. and Jones, K. (2005) *Speaking for Patients and Carers: Health Consumer Groups and the Policy Process*. Basingstoke: Palgrave Macmillan.

Boote, J., Telford, R. and Cooper, C. (2002) 'Consumer involvement in health research: A review and research agenda', *Health Policy, 61*: 213–36.

Brett, J., Staniszewska, S., Mockford, C., Herron-Marx, S., Hughes, J., Tysall, C. and Suleman, R. (2014a) 'A systematic review of the impact of patient and public involvement on service users, researchers and communities', *Patient, 7*: 387–95.

Brett, J., Staniszewska, S., Mockford, C., Herron-Marx, S., Hughes, J., Tysall, C. and Suleman, R. (2014b) 'Mapping the impact of patient and public involvement on health and social care research: a systematic review', *Health Expectations, 17*: 637–50.

Brown, P. and Zavestoski, S. (2004) 'Social movements in health: An introduction', *Sociology of Health and Illness, 26*(6): 679–94.

Brunton, G., Thomas, J., O'Mara-Eves, A., Jamal, F., Oliver, S. and Kavanagh, J. (2017) 'Narratives of community engagement: A systematic review-derived conceptual framework for public health interventions', *BMC Public Health, 17*: 994.

Chalmers, I., Bracken, M. B., Djulbegovic, B., Garattini, S., Grant, J., Metin Gülmezoglu, A., Howells, D. W., Ioannidis, J. P. A. and Oliver, S. (2014) 'How to increase value and reduce waste when research priorities are set', *The Lancet, 383*: 156–65.

The Change Foundation (2015a) *Rules of Engagement: Lessons from Panorama*. Toronto: The Change Foundation. Available at: www.changefoundation.ca/rules-of-engagement/

The Change Foundation (2015b) *Should Money Come into It? A Tool for Deciding Whether to Pay Patient-Engagement Participants*. Toronto: The Change Foundation. Available at: www.changefoundation.ca/patient-compensation-report/

Cochrane (2017) *The Statement of Principles for Consumer Involvement in Cochrane*. Available at: http://consumers.cochrane.org/news/statement-principles-consumer-involvement-cochrane

Concannon, T. W. (2012) 'A new taxonomy for stakeholder engagement in patient-centred outcomes research', *Journal of General Internal Medicine*, *27*: 985–91.

Consumers Health Forum of Australia and Medicines Australia (2008) *Working Together: A Guide to Relationships between Health Consumer Organisations and Pharmaceutical Companies*. Revised edition. Available at: www.chf.org.au/497-working-together-guide-manual-2008.chf

Coulter, A. (2002a) 'After Bristol: Putting patients at the centre', *BMJ Quality and Safety*, *11*: 186–8.

Coulter, A. (2002b) *The Autonomous Patient*. Research report. London: Nuffield Trust.

Domecq, J. P., Prutsky, G., Elraiyah, T., Wang, Z. et al. (2014) 'Patient engagement in research: A systematic review', *BMC Health Services Research*, *14*: 89.

Edelman, N. and Barron, D. (2016) 'Evaluation of public involvement in research: Time for a major re-think?', *Journal of Health Services Research and Policy*, *21*: 209–11.

Gooberman-Hill, R., Horwood, J. and Calnan, M. (2008) 'Citizens' juries in planning research priorities: Process, engagement and outcome', *Health Expectations*, *11*: 272–81.

Greenhalgh, T., Robert, G., Macfarlane, F., Bate, P. and Kyriakidou, O. (2004) 'Diffusion of innovations in service organizations: Systematic review and recommendations', *Milbank Quarterly*, *82*(4): 581–629.

Henderson, S. and Petersen, A. (2002) 'Introduction: Consumerism in health care', in S. Henderson and A. Petersen (eds), *Consuming Health: The Commodification of Health Care*. London: Routledge.

Herxheimer, A. (2003) 'Relationships between the pharmaceutical industry and patients' organizations', *British Medical Journal*, *326*: 1208–10.

Herxheimer, A. and Goodare, H. (1999) 'Who are you and who are we? Looking through the eyes of some key words', *Health Expectations*, *2*: 3–6.

Hickey, G., Brearley, S., Coldham, T., Denegri, S., Green, G., Staniszewska, S., Tembo, D., Torok, K. and Turner, K. (2018) *Guidance on Co-producing a Research Project*. Southampton: INVOLVE.

Hill, S. (2011) 'Preface', in S. Hill (ed.), *The Knowledgeable Patient: Communication and Participation in Health*. Chichester: Wiley-Blackwell.

International Association for Public Participation (2014) *IAP2's Public Participation Spectrum*. Available at: www.iap2.org.au/Tenant/C0000004/00000001/files/IAP2_Public_Participation_Spectrum.pdf

INVOLVE (2012) *Briefing Notes for Researchers: Involving the Public in NHS, Public Health and Social Care Research*. Southampton: INVOLVE.

Kohn, L., Corrigan, J. and Donaldson, M. (eds) (1999) *To Err is Human: Building a Safer Health System*. Washington, DC: National Academy Press.

Liabo, K., Boddy, K., Burchmore, H., Cockcroft, E. and Britten, N. (2018) 'Clarifying the roles of patients in research', *British Medical Journal, 361*: k1463.

Lipworth, W. and Kerridge, I. (2013) 'Do consumer groups really advocate for the public interest?', *The Conversation*, 23 August 2013. Available at: https://theconversation.com/do-consumer-groups-really-advocate-for-the-public-interest-16423

Locock, L., Boylan, A., Snow, R. and Staniszewska, S. (2017) 'The power of symbolic capital in patient and public involvement in health research', *Health Expectations, 20*: 836–44.

McMillan, S. S., King, M. and Tully, M. P. (2016) 'How to use the nominal group and Delphi techniques', *International Journal of Clinical Pharmacy, 38*: 655–62.

Miller, C. L., Mott, K., Cousins, M., Miller, S., Johnson, A., Lawson, T. and Wesselingh, S. (2017) 'Integrating consumer engagement in health and medical research: An Australian framework', *Health Research Policy and Systems, 15*: 9.

Nasser, M., Clarke, M., Chalmers, I., Brurberg, K. G., Nykvist, H., Lund, H. and Glasziou, P. (2017) 'What are funders doing to minimise waste in research?', *The Lancet, 389*: 1006–7.

National Health and Medical Research Council, Consumers Health Forum of Australia (2016) *Statement on Consumer and Community Involvement in Health and Medical Research*. Canberra: NHMRC/CHFA.

NIHR Research Design Service (2014) *Patient and Public Involvement in Health and Social Care Research: A Handbook for Researchers*. Available at: www.rds-yh.nihr.ac.uk/wp-content/uploads/2015/01/RDS_PPI-Handbook_2014-v8-FINAL-11.pdf

Nilsen, E. S., Myrhaug, H. T., Johansen, M., Oliver, S. and Oxman, A. D. (2006) 'Methods of consumer involvement in developing healthcare policy and research, clinical practice guidelines and patient information material', *Cochrane Database of Systematic Reviews*, Issue 3. Art. No. CD004563.

Ocloo, J. and Matthews, R. (2016) 'From tokenism to empowerment: Progressing patient and public involvement in healthcare improvement', *BMJ Journal of Public Safety*. Avaliable at: http://dx.doi.org/10.1136/bmjqs-2015-004839.

Oliver, S., Clarke-Jones, L., Rees, R., Milne, R., Buchanan, P., Gabbay, J., Gyte, G., Oakley, A. and Stein, K. (2004) 'Involving consumers in research and development agenda setting for the NHS: An evidence-based approach', *Health Technology Assessment, 8*(15): 1–148. Available at: www.ncchta.org/fullmono/mon815.pdf

Oliver, S. R., Rees, R. W., Clarke-Jones, L., Milne, R., Oakley, A. R., Gabbay, J., Stein, K., Buchanan, P. and Gyte, G. (2008) 'A multidimensional conceptual framework for analysing public involvement in health services research', *Health Expectations, 11*: 72–84.

Paterson, C. (2004) '"Take small steps to go a long way": Consumer involvement in research into complementary and alternative therapies', *Complementary Therapies in Nursing and Midwifery, 10*: 150–61.

PCORI (2015) 'What we mean by engagement'. Available at: www.pcori.org/engagement/what-we-mean-engagement

Pollock, A., Baer, G., Campbell, P., Choo, P. L., Forster, A., Morris, J., Pomeroy, V. M. and Langhorne, P. (2014) 'Physical rehabilitation approaches for the recovery of function and mobility following stroke', *Cochrane Database of Systematic Reviews*, Issue 4. Art. No. CD001920.

Pollock, A., Campbell, P., Baer, G., Choo, P. L., Morris, J. and Forster, A. (2015) 'User involvement in a Cochrane systematic review: Using structured methods to enhance the clinical relevance, usefulness and usability of a systematic review update', *Systematic Reviews, 4*(55). Available at: https://dx.doi.org/10.1186%2Fs13643-015-0023-5

Pollock, A., Campbell, P., Struthers, C., Synnot, A., Nunn, J., Hill, S., Goodare, H., Morris, J., Watts, C. and Morley, R. (2018) 'Development of the ACTIVE framework to describe stakeholder involvement in systematic reviews', *Journal of Health Services Research and Policy, 7:* 208.

Popay, J. and Collins, M. (eds) (2014) *PiiAF: The Public Involvement Impact Assessment Framework Guidance*. Available at: www.rds-yh.nihr.ac.uk/wp-content/uploads/2015/01/RDS_PPI-Handbook_2014-v8-FINAL-11.pdf

Public Health Agency, Chief Scientist Office, Health and Care Research Wales and National Institute for Health Research (2018) *National Standards for Public Involvement in Research V1*. Available at: www.invo.org.uk/wp-content/uploads/2018/03/71110_A4_Public_Involvement_Standards_v4_WEB.pdf

Richards, T. and Godlee, F. (2014) 'The BMJ's own patient journey', *British Medical Journal, 348*: g3726.

Sepkowitz, K. A. (2001) 'AIDS: The first 20 years', *New England Journal of Medicine, 344*(23): 1764–72.

Shippee, N. D., Domecq Garces, J. P., Prutsky Lopez, G. J. et al. (2015) 'Patient and service user engagement in research: A systematic review and synthesized framework', *Health Expectations, 18*: 1151–66.

Staniszewska, S., Brett, J., Simera, I., Seers, K., Mockford., C. et al. (2017) 'GRIPP2 Reporting checklists tools to improve reporting of patient and public involvement in research', *Research and Public Engagement, 3*-13.

Stephens, R. and Staniszewska, S. (2015) 'One small step...', *Research Involvement and Engagement, 1*: 1.

Synnot, A., Hill, S., Garner, K. A., Summers, M. P., Filippini, G., Osborne, R. H., Shapland, S. D. P., Colombo, C. and Mosconi, P. (2016) 'Online health information-seeking: How people with multiple sclerosis find, assess and integrate treatment information to manage their health', *Health Expectations, 19*: 727–37.

Synnot, A., Bragge, P., Lowe, D., Nunn, J. S., O'Sullivan, M. et al. (2018a) 'Research priorities in health communication and participation: International survey of consumers and other stakeholders', *BMJ Open*. Available at: doi: 10.1136/bmjopen-2017-019481

Synnot, A., Cherry, C. L., Summers, M. P., Stuckey, R., Milne, C. A., Lowe, D. and Hill, S. J. (2018b) 'Consumer engagement critical to success in an Australian research project: Reflections from those involved', *Australian Journal of Primary Health*, *24*: 197–203.

Synnot, A. M., Hawkins, B. A., Merner, M. P., Summers, G. et al. (2018c) 'Producing an evidence-based treatment information website in partnership with people affected by multiple sclerosis', *Health Science Reports*, *1*(3): e24.

Vernon, W. (2009) 'The Delphi technique: A review', *International Journal of Therapy and Rehabilitation*, *16*: 69–76.

World Health Organization (2013) *Exploring Patient Participation in Reducing Health-care-related Safety Risks*. Available at: www.euro.who.int/__data/assets/pdf_file/0010/185779/e96814.pdf

22

Comparative Health Research

VIOLA BURAU

Chapter objectives

- To identify different approaches to comparative health research at the macro, meso and micro levels
- To consider the relative strengths of exploration, explanation and evaluation in comparative research
- To explore the politics of comparative health research in using evidence from different countries
- To assess strategies for sampling to ensure that the choice of country cases is fit for purpose
- To describe how to tackle challenges of equivalence so data from different countries are comparable
- To indicate how to manage complex comparative data based on typologies of health systems.

Introduction

Health, health care and policies have become more international over recent decades, reflecting a number of factors. The development of mass media and communication technologies means that information about health problems and health services in individual countries has become more readily available. This trend is supported by the work of international organizations such as the World Health Organization (WHO) and the Organization for Economic Cooperation and Development (OECD). These organizations not only gather but also disseminate information about health care across a wide range of countries. Increasingly, health policy is made at the international level. For example, the European Union (EU) is now involved in a wide range of areas from public health to pharmaceutical policies. Finally, many health problems are shared across countries, such as chronic diseases, and there is a shared a concern about how to control infectious diseases that cross country borders, such as H1N1 or swine flu. With the internationalization of health care, the cross-country, comparative perspective has become increasingly significant in understanding contemporary issues in health. Although there are methodological challenges, comparative health research allows the evidence from more than one country to be used in a systematic way. The notion of comparison may be incorporated into a flexible research design that draws on a range of different methods.

Approaches to comparative health research

Comparative health research can deal with a wide range of substantive areas in health and take a range of perspectives. Researchers should be aware of different approaches prior to embarking on a study and Clasen (2014), Øvretveit (1998) and Vassy and Keller (2011) provide useful overviews. An important substantive area of study in comparative health research is the needs of patients. For example, the needs of stroke patients can be analysed from three perspectives. First, the study can examine the organization of hospital-based care and the increasing introduction of early discharge teams working in the homes of patients (for example, Douw, Nielson and Pedersen 2015). Second, the study can analyse the day-to-day professional practice of patient-centred stroke care and how the professional groups involved in the teams strengthen inter-professional working (for example, Burau et al. 2017). Finally, the study can assess how patients experience the stroke care delivered in their homes and the role played by families (for example, Lou et al. 2017).

Studies can be undertaken at three different organizational levels:

- Macro-level studies may test a hypothesis and use statistical analysis, drawing on Big Data
- Meso-level studies tend to focus on the organization of health services
- Micro-level studies are concerned with specific aspects of health care behaviour and practice with a focus on users and providers.

This is illustrated by Box 22.1.

Box 22.1   Examples of comparative health research

- *Macro-level studies*: Wendt (2015) looks at the financial resources that OECD countries allocate to health care to examine whether there are any distinct trends in health care expenditure. The analysis finds considerable differences in health care spending and suggests, among other findings, that the share of public financing influences the level of total health care costs.
- *Meso-level studies*: There is a large literature on health policy and reform. Blank, Burau and Kuhlmann (2017) and Scott (2011), for example, use the categories of funding, provision and regulation of health care to understand why policy responses to health problems vary across countries. They, as well as other authors, suggest that public control over provision and funding offers states better leverage in containing costs and pursuing organizational reform.
- *Micro-level studies*: In their study of hospital governance in seven European countries, Kuhlmann and colleagues (2013) analyse the relationships between medicine and management. They identify three types of patterns of control, which reflect differences within the specific organizational settings of hospitals as well as in the overall health systems. These are: 'integrated' control with strong coordination and coherent cost and quality controls (Denmark and the Netherlands); 'partly integrated' control with many different types of coordination (Germany and Spain); and 'fragmented' control with limited coordination and frictions between cost and quality controls (Greece, Poland and Portugal).

The purpose of comparison

Beyond the choice of substantive area and level of analysis, another important consideration is the purpose of comparison. Comparison may be about:

- Exploration
- Explanation
- Evaluation.

Each of these will now be discussed in turn.

Exploratory studies

Exploratory comparative health research aims to investigate the same 'phenomenon' in different countries. This can be anything from the organization of palliative care and public health policies to cancer survival rates and public expenditure on hospital care. Here, the aim is to broaden the 'basis of evidence' by considering cases from very different contexts and so capture the potential underlying variation in service delivery.

Exploratory studies help to avoid both false particularism ('everywhere is unique') and false universalism ('everywhere is the same') as they aim to identify what is different and what is similar (Saltman 2012). In this respect, studies may adopt a static perspective and focus on the differences and similarities as such. For example, a central aim of the Health System Reviews series published by the European Observatory on Health Systems and Policy is to analyse the differences and similarities in the organization of health services across countries in Europe. The profiles describe the individual health systems in terms on four key dimensions: organization and governance; financing; physical and human resources; and the provision of services (Rechel, Thomson and van Ginneken 2010).

A study may adopt a more dynamic perspective and analyse how countries are becoming more different, or similar. This approach is particularly dominant in studies that analyse processes of convergence, whereby health problems, policies or services tend to become more similar over time (Tuohy 2012). Schmid and colleagues (2010) analyse health reforms across OECD countries and suggest that there are increasing similarities across different types of health system, with individual health systems becoming more hybrid in form. Convergence has a range of causes, including increasing international interdependence between countries as a result of the diffusion of ideas about health policies across countries (Okma et al. 2010). This may be based on knowledge about mechanisms to encourage competition, coercion, emulation and learning (Dobbin, Simmons and Garrett 2007).

Explanatory studies

Explanatory studies investigate deeper questions, notably about why it is we find certain differences and similarities (Klein 2009). For example, a study by Kirkpatrick and colleagues (2009) of the relationship between medicine and management in Denmark as compared to England, observes that while doctors across countries increasingly take on managerial responsibilities, which they term 'hybrid management', there can be differences in the level of support for this from front-line doctors in hospitals. They suggest that the timing and the objectives of the reforms have been similar, but hybrid management roles are more advanced in Denmark than in England. The study examines various explanations for this difference. Although exploratory studies give an indication of findings, explanatory studies make better use of the analytical potential of comparative research designs. The particular explanations considered depend on the specific theories underlying the research questions. For example, path dependency theory is the basis for the central assumption of Kirkpatrick and colleagues (2009). This theory suggests that the national health institutions and the political system shape the professional development of doctors and determine the ways in which reforms have been implemented in each country.

Evaluation studies

Finally, some health studies use comparison as a method of evaluation. Here, the main aim is to assess the impact of health care and policies in different countries against the specific criteria of relative success, or failure. An example is the report by the World Health Organization (2013) on research on universal coverage; that is, the extent to which health systems guarantee health care to all people regardless of the way health services are financed. The report analyses the challenges facing the promotion of universal health coverage and identifies what steps countries, within existing resources, can undertake to increase coverage. This can include strengthening their research capacity to transform existing knowledge into practice.

Evaluative studies build on two more or less explicit assumptions. First, the evaluation of health involves making judgements, often by identifying exemplary cases or so-called 'best practice'. This suggests implicitly that there is a best way of doing things. Examples would be a policy to promote health workforce planning to tackle shortages of particular health personnel, such as nurses, or to address shortages in specific geographical areas, such as in rural areas where it is difficult to attract staff. The European Union Joint Action on Health Workforce Planning and Forecasting has published a handbook that reviews methodologies across EU countries (Malgieri, Michelutti and van Hoegaerden 2015). The handbook discusses country experiences, such as policy aims, forecasting models, data sources and the organization of health workforce planning, and completes each section with a review of 'good practices'. The underlying assumption of evaluative studies like this handbook is that best practice can be transferred across countries and that in this way countries can learn from each other in very practical ways. However, both assumptions are problematic, as the next section shows.

The politics of comparative health research

The interest of both governments and international organizations in comparative health research has led to an increasing politicization of comparative studies. This is reflected particularly in more applied studies where the aim is explicitly to evaluate evidence from different countries in order to identify what works best. In relation to medical technologies, a well-established methodology is 'health technology assessment', which combines an assessment of clinical, economic and organizational effects (for example, Goodman 2014). The underlying rationale is to use such assessments as an evidence-based management tool with the aim to reduce variations in care and improve outcomes. For example, as part of a cross-country collaboration called 'European Network for Health Technology Assessment', Jefferson, Cerbo and Vicari (2015) examined a tool to structure telephone support for adult patients with chronic heart failure. It had a focus on safety, clinical effectiveness, costs, ethics, and effective organization as well as addressing the social and legal implications of the technology. According to Marmor, Freeman and Okma (2005) and Rose (2000), governments commonly identify existing problems and seek 'solutions' by looking at other health systems. For instance, in the United Kingdom in the early 2000s, the National Health Service was seen as 'underfunded' when compared with other countries that spent higher levels of GDP on health care (Dunne 2002). For policy makers, the attraction of cross-country comparison lies in the fact that it resembles a kind of 'natural experiment' that allows for 'testing' individual reform instruments and assessing their relative suitability and success.

This is especially attractive in two respects. First, policy making informed by comparative research has the potential to allow learning from the mistakes of others, and thereby holds the implicit promise of avoiding policy failure altogether. This is an attractive promise in any policy area, not least health, which is high on the political agenda of many countries, reflecting the importance of health services to the general public. Second, policy making informed by comparative research enjoys greater credibility because it is informed by more than the personal judgement of policy makers (Klein 2009). Comparison can be part and parcel of a more 'evidence-based' style of policy making. The introduction of cancer pathways is an example (Probst, Butt and Andersen 2012). For example, Denmark has long had a higher incidence of cancer and poorer cancer survival rates than many other European countries. In 2006 and 2007 there were several highly publicized stories of cancer patients who had experienced delayed diagnosis or treatment and who had died. This was corroborated by a national survey that showed that 20 per cent of cancer patients experienced long waiting times. In response, the Danish prime minister announced in 2007 that cancer should be treated as an acute condition. Subsequently, the government and the regions agreed to introduce mandatory pathways for all cancer types by the end of 2008.

The process of 'comparing for policy making' is not a neutral but a highly politicized activity and the literature on policy learning identifies different dimensions of this complexity (Klein 2009; Marmor, Freeman and Okma 2005; Russell et al. 2008), as follows:

- The process of policy learning itself is selective and more often than not reflects the specific, domestic agendas of policy makers. For example, historically, the introduction of hospital funding based on Diagnosis Related Groups (DRGs) was most likely in countries where long waiting lists highlighted the shortcomings of existing services (Gilardi, Füglister and Luyet 2009). Here, the experience with DRGs from other countries suggested that DRGs led to increases in efficiency. Policy learning from other countries is often concerned with finding additional arguments for a political decision.
- Best practices are deeply embedded in specific national, social, economic and political contexts and therefore cannot be transferred easily. Indeed, the literature suggests that

health policies are highly context-dependent (Wrede 2011) and follow country-specific paths and reflect existing institutional frameworks in health care and the broader political system (Wilsford 1994). For example, in his influential study of health care reform, Wilsford showed that individual countries display a very different propensity for health policy change: while Germany and the United Kingdom exhibited the right conditions for major reform, the opposite was true in France and the US. Thus, past policy choices may constrain the scope for policy learning (Marmor, Freeman and Okma 2005). For example, although primary health care has been the central focus of health reforms for more than two decades across Europe, countries have implemented very different national models (Groenewegen et al. 2015). In some countries, single-handed practices dominate, while in others, larger practices with multiple professional groups are the norm. This is partly explained by differences in policy goals, in political institutions and in the structure of health systems. In countries with a stronger focus on developing the workforce in primary care and more comprehensive primary care delivery, the number of different multi-professional groups working in primary care is higher. This also means that the relative success of each best practice is highly conditional and depends on the context and setting. Any transfer is likely to be partial and requires some adaptation.

What are the implications of these political factors for the researcher undertaking comparative health research? The literature suggests that researchers must be aware of the limitations of research for policy. They should recognize that the most desirable comparative research design for policy makers may not necessarily be the most fruitful analytically. Researchers also need to be sensitive to the specific contexts and conditions under which best practices may be considered as 'best'.

The methodological challenges of comparative health research

Sampling: Choosing cases

The first challenge is related to sampling. Sampling requires clarifying the rationale for comparison. What is it that comparison is supposed to explain? Individual studies should focus on either differences or similarities, depending on what it is they aim to analyse and/or explain. For example, a study looking at New Public Management and the introduction of market mechanisms like competition among hospitals, incentive payments for doctors and systems for controlling the quality of health services needs to carefully choose its cases. The same study cannot both analyse convergence towards marketization in health care reforms and also the differences in the substance of corresponding health policies. This is because the choice of countries as cases is shaped by a specific purpose.

Sampling is thus about choosing suitable countries or 'cases' for comparison – that is, cases from which one can learn most in terms of what the study aims to analyse and explain. The choice of cases is closely tied to the underlying theoretical framework of a study (Ebbinghaus 2005; Yin 2017). For example, the widespread reference to New Public Management in health reforms may reflect processes of policy learning. Relevant theories suggest that such cross-country learning is most likely where there are similarities in the mode of health care delivery between countries. Thus, England and Sweden, with their tax-funded national health systems, can be used as comparators (Blank, Burau and Kuhlmann 2017).

In contrast, if the focus of attention is on analysing why New Public Management in health care has been implemented in very different ways across European countries, it would be more appropriate to include countries with contrasting or dissimilar health systems (Kuhlmann et al. 2013; Pavolini 2015). Institutionalist theories suggest that differences in policy output reflect differences in the institutional setting. However, both research strategies require that the cases chosen are comparable in the first place and the literature identifies different strategies to achieve this. From a variable-oriented perspective, Lijphart (1975) defines comparability as a strategy whereby the theoretically insignificant 'background variables' are held constant. This means choosing countries with comparable levels of economic wealth, with stable democratic political systems and with developed welfare states for a study. From a context-oriented perspective, comparability is established by analysing thoroughly the specific contexts in which the individual cases are embedded, in order to identify the similarities (and differences) among them (Mangen 2014; Wrede 2011).

Equivalence: Ensuring comparability

A second challenge relates to the notion of 'equivalence': this can be understood as identifying comparable units for cross-country comparison. These can range widely and can be anything from the roles of specific health workers to professional practices, disease patterns, health services, health policies or health outcomes. The aim for cross-country comparison should be comparing 'apples with apples' rather than 'apples with pears' (see Øyen 2004). The question arises at the research planning phase. However, comparing 'apples with apples' rather than 'apples with pears' is less straightforward than it appears. The units for comparative health research can be anything from specific health workers to professional practices, disease patterns, health services, health policies or health outcomes.

Identifying such units of comparison across countries is complicated as it involves being aware not only of differences in the use of language, but also differences in the specific cultural meaning and the related function of such units (Wrede et al. 2006). In the literature, this is referred to as the difference between 'formal' and 'functional' equivalence. For instance, units that have similar cultural meanings (and functions) may have different names; conversely, units with the same name may have very different cultural meanings (and functions). Health care is culturally embedded within society (Wrede 2011), as highlighted by Box 22.2.

Box 22.2   Formal versus functional equivalence: The case of the hospital

Although the English term 'hospital' can be translated directly into other European languages (as *hôpital* in French, *Krankenhaus* in German, or *sygehus* in Danish), this disguises differences in cultural meaning and function. For example, English hospital trusts are providers of specialist health care and cover both inpatient and outpatient services, whereas their German counterparts focus on inpatient specialist care only. This reflects the fact that the majority of outpatient specialist care is delivered by office-based specialists.

To secure the validity of a piece of comparative research, it is essential to identify similar units for comparison. It is, however, a complex process requiring translation of both words and meanings and an acknowledgement of the social construction of concepts (Barbour 2010). One way of taking account of linguistic and cultural differences while ensuring comparability is to work with 'functional equivalents'. This means the researcher makes a choice of the unit of analysis on the basis that its substantive functions are comparable. For example, a British–German comparison of hospital care could use the unit 'inpatient specialist care' as a focus of study. Wrede and colleagues (2006) go one step further and develop a comprehensive approach to integrating sensitivity to differences in cultural contexts in comparative health research. The so-called 'decentred approach' suggests that expertise is always distributed and recommends that ideally research should be conducted by a research team with researchers from different countries. The research team has to engage in intensive collaboration that extends to all stages of the research process. This includes formulating the initial research interest, defining key conceptual terms, analysing the research results and comparing across-country cases.

Managing complexity: Processing and interpreting data

A third challenge of comparative health research is to manage the quantity, diversity and complexity of the data collected in a systematic and theoretically meaningful way. This must be achieved through all the phases of the research from data collection to data processing and interpretation where more than two countries are included. It is especially important to process the material emerging from comparative health research in a systematic way by specifying clearly what material is relevant and in what way. This is about labelling and categorizing but is more than a technical exercise. Instead, processing comparative research material is at the centre of the interpretation itself. To be done systematically, analysis must be theory-led. The analysis has to reflect the specific hypotheses that are expected to explain differences or similarities across countries.

The use of ideal types

One method used for data collection and interpretation is to cluster explanatory factors into 'ideal types'. In general, these are constructs that can be understood as the basic variants of a particular phenomenon, such as a health system. They have been a particularly important tool in meso-level comparative health research (Burau, Blank and Pavolini 2015). For example, a commonly used typology of health systems defines them as representing specific sets of institutional characteristics. A typology can be used to explain variations in health policies across different countries. It can be based on variations in how health care is funded and can correspond to differences in the organization of health care provision (OECD 1987). It distinguishes three basic models of health systems:

- The national health service model with funding out of general taxation
- The social insurance model with compulsory social insurance funded out of employer and employee contributions
- The private insurance model funded by individual and/or employer contributions.

The underlying assumption of this typology of health systems is that the public funding of health care, or lack of it, is the defining characteristic of the extent of state involvement in health care. Thus, Essen (2009) uses the typology to explain specific variations in the politics and policies of new hospital funding systems in three European countries. The ideal type model of health systems helps not only to describe and categorize the organization of health care, but also to explain why countries respond to health problems in certain ways. In consequence, the analysis moves beyond the specificity of individual countries towards more insight into health systems in general.

The limitations of typologies

Using typologies is not without its problems, many of which arise from the ambiguous relationship between ideal types and real systems. Ideal types of the health system are abstractions drawn from actual health systems and are meant to help in understanding the organization of health care. Typologies aim to simplify reality but, in doing so, they may limit understanding. In Singapore, for example, health care funding comes from private sources in the form of personal savings accounts, although payment into such accounts is mandatory. The health system of Singapore therefore fits poorly into the typology of health systems referred to above. In this case, the typology raises more questions than it answers (see Blank, Burau and Kuhlmann 2017).

Another danger is that analyses become divided by individual ideal types and do not effectively compare across different countries. An example is the international literature on health professions, which has long been based, more or less explicitly, on a typology centred on the Anglo-American professions, which are seen as autonomous from the state (Kuhlmann et al. 2013). Its limited explanatory power has led to a focus on conflict in studies of medicine and management (Numerato, Salvatore and Fattore 2011).

In comparative health research, there is an underlying tension between uniqueness and generalization. Typologies are highly problematic but are nevertheless essential (Freeman and Frisina 2010). Broad-brush characterizations often do not hold up when confronted with the complex detail of actual arrangements. Yet the dilemma is that once one departs from such characterizations, research can become merely descriptive, which militates against identifying clear and all-encompassing contrasts. Thus, classification is at the heart of comparative health studies, which is illustrated further in Case Study 22.1.

CASE STUDY 22.1

Comparative health research in practice

The following discussion is based on a comparative study of primary care in Denmark and New Zealand (Tenbensel and Burau 2017). The initial interest in the study arose from the following puzzle. Governments can be expected to have a strong interest in governing primary care: general practitioners are often the first point of contact for patients, and in many countries general practitioners also have a gatekeeping function in access to specialized hospital care. Yet primary care is notoriously difficult to govern: the majority of general practitioners are independent, private entrepreneurs who are contracted to provide services in publicly funded health care systems. The aim of the study was two-fold: to identify the specific instruments to govern primary care in Denmark and in New Zealand and to explain the differences between the strategies in the two countries. The study used two sets of theories: performance governance and comparative health policy. Performance governance is about designing mechanisms for collecting and interpreting information on performance as well as to harness this for the broader task of assessment and control. Instruments can vary. They may be hierarchical (top-down) and involve the direct use of state authority; they may draw on market mechanisms and entail 'pay for performance'; or they may rest on professional networks that entail collegial processes. The study drew on the literature on comparative health policy to account systematically for the differences in choice and mix of instruments. The focus was on three institutional dimensions of primary care governance: the institutional context of primary care, governance processes and governance problems.

The research questions and the choice of theoretical framework had implications for the design of this cross-country comparative study. The effect of institutions is relatively easy to identify where institutions are different, and this study focused on Denmark and New Zealand, where the institutional arrangements for primary care governance appeared to differ.

(Continued)

(Continued)

The countries are similar in certain key respects. Both are small countries, where many of the complexities associated with larger countries are not pertinent. The two countries have health systems that are predominantly funded by taxes and have implemented reforms influenced by theories drawn from New Public Management ideas. Despite these broad similarities, Denmark and New Zealand exhibit major differences in the types of instrument adopted for performance governance. In Denmark, the approach is cautious and can be characterized as 'softly hierarchical', reflecting a combination of network and hierarchical instruments, but without the deployment of sanctions. This contrasts with New Zealand, where the approach is more assertive and where the instruments have been characterized by a combination of top-down control and market-like incentives.

To examine how instruments of performance governance in primary care had been shaped by different institutional arrangements required a two-part analysis:

- An analysis of the structures of primary care governance in the two countries
- A case study of the instruments of performance governance in primary care.

For the case study, comparable units of analysis had to be chosen to deal with issues of equivalence. Despite differences in the organization of primary care, general practitioners are at the centre of primary care provision. The research focused on a literature review of policy documents that were directed at performance governance of general practice. This covered documents such as health care legislation and trade union agreements.

As with most comparative research, complex data had to be collected, processed and interpreted. The study used a theoretical framework that combined the institutional dimensions of primary care governance and the instruments of performance governance to order the material from the two countries.

Conclusion

In attempting to carry out a piece of comparative research, a number of choices have to be made in terms of strategy and this chapter has aimed to provide a structured approach to making those choices and to negotiate the pitfalls of a complex field. First, a choice must be made about the unit for comparison across countries. It has been suggested that there should be functional equivalence in what is being compared. Second, in choosing the countries in a study, the best strategy is to compare countries that have some broad similarities. Here, typologies or ideal types are a useful device, although one that should be used cautiously as real systems rarely conform fully to a concept that is based on an abstraction. Third, the researcher should then decide whether, in making comparisons, their strategy is to look for lines of difference or lines of similarity. They should also decide whether the study they are undertaking is exploratory, explanatory or evaluative. Finally, any analysis of similarity or difference should be theory-led; that is, the researcher should identify a general proposition or hypothesis about the way in which policies, organizations, groups or individuals function that they are seeking to explain.

Exercise 22.1   Comparing health care expenditure and cost containment policies

In principle, health policy in most developed capitalist democracies has been based on achieving three goals: the provision of high-quality services; equal access for all citizens to health care; and cost-efficient provision (Blank, Burau and Kuhlmann 2017). In the first two decades following the Second World War, health policy initiatives were particularly concerned with the first two goals. Since the 1970s, cost-efficiency and containment have become dominant across countries. With this in mind, examine the OECD's data on the total expenditure on health as a percentage of GDP (see Table 22.1) and answer the following sets of questions.

TABLE 22.1   Total expenditure on health as a percentage of GDP

	1980	2016
Austria	7.4	10.4
France	7.1	11.0
Germany	8.7	11.3
Italy	7.7*	8.9
Netherlands	7.5	10.5
New Zealand	5.9	9.2
Spain	5.4	9.0
Sweden	9.1	11.0
United Kingdom	5.6	9.7
United States	8.7	17.2

*Figure for 1985

Source: OECD (2017)

Looking at the figures for 2016, rank countries in order of the percentage of GDP spent on health care.

- What is the difference in percentage points between the country at the top and bottom of the list?

(Continued)

(Continued)

- Are countries spread evenly or do they cluster into separate groups? Are there any clear outliers?

Looking at the development of health care expenditure between 1980 and 2016, rank countries in order of the relative increase in percentage of GDP spent on health care.

- What is the difference in percentage points between the country at the top and bottom of the list?
- Are countries spread evenly or do they cluster into separate groups? Are there any clear outliers?

Using your analysis of OECD health expenditure data, list those observations you find particularly interesting, striking and/or surprising. Use this as a basis for formulating two or three research questions, which you feel require further comparative analysis.

With your questions for comparative research in mind, read the summaries in Table 22.2 of the health systems in Germany England and Sweden. Based on the summaries, make a list of the factors relating to the organization of health care and the state which facilitate and mitigate against successful cost containment, respectively.

TABLE 22.2   The health care systems in Germany, England and Sweden

	Germany	England	Sweden
Funding	• Access to health services mainly on the basis of social insurance membership	• Access to health services on basis of social citizenship	• Access to health services on basis of social citizenship
	• Funding primarily through social insurance contributions raised by statutory, non-profit insurance funds, complemented by taxes and co-payments	• Funding through general taxation raised by central government	• Funding through income tax raised by regional governments
	• Allocation of funding based on contracts between insurance funds and providers through various mechanisms; federal legislation as framework	• Allocation of funding based on national global budget and through local budget allocations embedded in a central framework	• Allocation of funding based on regional global budget but through a variety of mechanisms

	Germany	England	Sweden
Provision	• Hospitals in public, non-profit or private ownership; service delivery based on contracts; control jointly by insurance funds and providers	• Hospitals are independent non-profit trusts; service delivery on basis of contracts, embedded in centralized structures with performance management and planning	• Most hospitals are run by regional governments; service delivery subject to national framework and monitoring
	• Hospital doctors are salaried employees, office-based doctors work as independent contractors	• Hospital doctors are public employees, GPs work as independent entrepreneurs in public primary care trusts	• Most hospital doctors and GPs (working in health centres) are public employees
	• Decisions about medical technology are part of budget negotiations between insurance funds and providers	• Decisions about medical technology made by regional government agencies based on local applications within central framework	• Decisions on medical technology made on a case-by-case basis by regional governments

With your insight into the factors making for more/less successful health care cost containment in mind, re-read the research questions you have formulated and address the following issues:

- Which one research question do you think is the most important, and why?
- Which two countries would it be most useful to compare to answer your research question, and why?
- What additional aspects of the institutional context for health care provision would you look at in each of the countries you have chosen, and why do you think these are important in answering your research question?

Recommended further reading

This introductory comparative text analyses key issues in health policy from a research viewpoint and assesses how far policy problems and responses in different countries have common or diverse origins:

Blank, R. H., Burau, V. and Kuhlmann, E. (2017) *Comparative Health Policy*, 5th edition. Basingstoke: Palgrave Macmillan.

This article discusses the strengths and weaknesses of different approaches to understanding the country-specific contexts of health care and health policies:

Freeman, R. and Frisina, L. (2010) 'Health care systems and the problem of classification', *Journal of Comparative Policy Analysis*, 12: 163–78.

This chapter discusses different critical approaches to comparative health policy and the implications that less theory-driven approaches have for the research process:

Wrede, S. (2011) 'How countries matter: Studying health policy in a comparative perspective', in I. L. Bourgeault, R. Dingwall and R. de Vries (eds), *Sage Handbook of Qualitative Methods in Health Research*. London: Sage.

References

Barbour, R. S. (2010) 'Using qualitative methods in comparative research', *Salute e Società*, 9: 65–79.

Blank, R. H., Burau, V. and Kuhlmann, E. (2017) *Comparative Health Policy*, 5th edition. Basingstoke: Palgrave Macmillan.

Burau, V., Blank, R. B. and Pavolini, E. (2015) 'Typologies of healthcare systems and policies', in E. Kuhlmann, R. H. Blank, I. L. Bourgeault and C. Wendt (eds), *The Palgrave International Handbook of Healthcare Policy and Governance*. Basingstoke: Palgrave Macmillan.

Burau, V., Carstensen, K., Lou, S. and Kuhlmann, E. (2017) 'Professional groups driving change toward patient-centred care: Interprofessional working in stroke rehabilitation in Denmark', *BMC Health Services Research*, 17: 662.

Clasen, J. (2014) 'Defining comparative social policy', in P. Kennett (ed.), *A Handbook of Comparative Social Policy*, 2nd edition. Cheltenham: Edward Elgar.

Dobbin, F., Simmons, B. A. and Garrett, G. (2007) 'The global diffusion of public policies: Social construction, coercion, competition, or learning', *Annual Review of Sociology*, 33: 449–72.

Douw, K., Nielsen, C. P. and Pedersen, C. R. (2015) 'Centralising acute stroke care and moving care to the community in a Danish health region: Challenges in implementing a stroke care reform', *Health Policy*, 119: 1005–10.

Dunne, R. (2002) 'Will extra billions cure NHS ills?', *BBC News*. Available at: http://news.bbc.co.uk/1/hi/health/1935417.stm

Ebbinghaus, B. (2005) 'When less is more: Selection problems in large-N and small-N cross-national comparisons', *International Sociology*, 20: 133–52.

Essen, A. M. V. (2009) 'New hospital payment systems: Comparing medical strategies in the Netherlands, Germany and England', *Journal of Health Organization and Management*, 23(3): 304–18.

Freeman, R. and Frisina, L. (2010) 'Health care systems and the problem of classification', *Journal of Comparative Policy Analysis, 12*: 163–78.

Gilardi, F., Füglister, K. and Luyet, S. (2009) 'Learning from other: Diffusion of hospital financing reforms in OECD countries', *Comparative Political Studies, 42*(4): 549–73.

Goodman, C. S. (2014) *HTA 101: Introduction to Health Technology Assessment*. Bethesda, MD: National Library of Medicine (US).

Groenewegen, P. P., Heinemann, S., Greß, S. and Schäfer, W. (2015) 'Primary health care in 34 countries', *Health Policy, 119*(12): 1576–83.

Jefferson, T., Cerbo, M. and Vicari, N. (eds) (2015) *Structured Telephone Support (STS) for Adult Patients with Chronic Heart Failure (Core HTA)*. Rome: Agenas – Agenzia nazionale per i servizi sanitari regionali. Available at: http://meka.thl.fi/ViewCover.aspx?id=305

Kirkpatrick, I., Jespersen, J. P., Dent, M. and Neogy, I. (2009) 'Medicine and management in a comparative perspective: The case of Denmark and England', *Sociology of Health and Illness, 31*(5): 642–58.

Klein, R. (2009) 'Learning from others and learning from mistakes: Reflections on health policy making', in T. R. Marmor, R. Freeman and K. G. Okma (eds), *Comparative Studies and the Politics of Modern Medical Care*. New Haven, CT: Yale University Press.

Kuhlmann, E., Burau, V., Correia, T., Lewandowski, R., Lionis, C., Noordegraaf, M. and Repullo, J. (2013) '"A manager in the minds of doctors": A comparison of new modes of control in European hospitals', *BMC Health Services Research, 13*(1): 246.

Lijphart, A. (1975) 'The comparable-bases strategy in comparative research', *Comparative Political Studies, 8*(2): 158–77.

Lou, S., Carstensen, K., Møldrup, M., Shahla, S., Zakharia, E. and Nielsen, C. P. (2017) 'Early supported discharge following mild stroke: A qualitative study of patients' and their partners' experiences of rehabilitation at home', *Scandinavian Journal of Caring Sciences, 31*: 302–11.

Malgieri, A., Michelutti, P. and van Hoegaerden, M. (eds) (2015) *Handbook on Health Workforce Planning and Forecasting: Methodologies across EU Countries*. Joint Action Health Workforce Planning and Forecasting. Bratislava: Ministry of Health of the Slovak Republic.

Mangen, S. (2014) 'Cross-national qualitative research methods: Innovations in the New Millennium', in P. Kennett (ed.), *A Handbook of Comparative Social Policy*, 2nd edition. Cheltenham: Edward Elgar.

Marmor, T. R., Freeman, R. and Okma, K. G. H. (2005) 'Comparing perspectives and policy learning in the world of health care', *Journal of Comparative Health Policy Analysis, 7*(4): 331–48.

Numerato, D., Salvatore, D. and Fattore, D. (2011) 'The impact of management on medical professionalism: A review', *Sociology of Health and Illness, 34*(4): 626–44.

OECD (1987) *Financing and Delivering Health Care: A Comparative Analysis of OECD Countries*. Paris: OECD.

OECD (2017) *OECD Health Statistics: Health Expenditure and Financing*. Paris: OECD.

Okma, K. G. H., Cheng, T. M., Chinitz, D., Crivelli, L., Lim, M. K., Maarse, H. and Labra, M. E. (2010) 'Six countries, six health reform models? Health care reform in Chile, Israel, Singapore, Switzerland, Taiwan and The Netherlands', *Journal of Comparative Policy Analysis: Research and Practice*, 12: 75–113.

Øvretveit, J. (1998) *Comparative and Cross-cultural Health Research: A Practical Guide*. Abingdon: Radcliffe Medical Press.

Øyen, E. (2004) 'Living with imperfect comparisons', in P. Kennett (ed.), *A Handbook of Comparative Social Policy*. Cheltenham: Edward Elgar.

Pavolini, E. (2015) 'Marketization and managerialization of health care policies in Europe in a comparative perspective', in T. Klenk and E. Pavolini (eds), *Restructuring Welfare Governance: Marketization, Managerialism and Welfare State Professionalism*. Cheltenham: Edward Elgar.

Probst, H. B., Butt, Z. and Andersen, O. (2012) 'Cancer patient pathways in Denmark as a joint effort between bureaucrats, health professionals and politicians: A national Danish project', *Health Policy*, 105(1): 65–70.

Rechel, B., Thomson, S. and van Ginneken, E. (2010) *Health Systems in Transition: Template for Authors*. Copenhagen: WHO Regional Office for Europe.

Rose, R. (2000) 'What can we learn from abroad?', *Parliamentary Affairs*, 53: 628–43.

Russell, J., Greenhalgh, T., Bryne, E. and McDonnell, J. (2008) 'Recognizing rhetoric in health care policy analysis', *Journal of Health Services Research and Policy*, 13(1): 40–6.

Saltman, R. B. (2012) 'The role of comparative health studies for policy learning', *Journal of Health Politics, Policy and Law*, 7(1): 11–13.

Schmid, A., Cacace, M., Götze, R. and Rothgang, H. (2010) 'Explaining health care system change: Problem pressure and the emergence of "hybrid" health care systems', *Journal of Health Politics, Policy and Law*, 35: 455–86.

Scott, C. D. (2011) *Public and Private Roles in Health Care: Experiences from Seven Countries*. Buckingham: Open University Press.

Tenbensel, T. and Burau, V. (2017) 'Contrasting approaches to primary care performance governance in Denmark and New Zealand', *Heath Policy*, 122: 853–61.

Tuohy, C. H. (2012) 'Reform and the politics of hybridization in mature health care states', *Journal of Health Politics, Policy and Law*, 37(4): 611–32.

Vassy, C. and Keller, R. (2011) 'Cross national qualitative health research', in I. L. Bourgeault, R. Dingwall and R. de Vries (eds), *Sage Handbook of Qualitative Methods in Health Research*. London: Sage.

Wendt, C. (2015) 'Healthcare policy and finance', in E. Kuhlmann, R. H. Blank, I. L. Bourgeault and C. Wendt (eds), *The Palgrave International Handbook of Healthcare Policy and Governance*. Basingstoke: Palgrave Macmillan.

Wilsford, D. (1994) 'Path dependency, or why history makes it difficult but not impossible to reform health care systems in a big way', *Journal of Public Policy*, 14: 251–83.

World Health Organization (2013) *Research for Universal Health Coverage*. Geneva: WHO.

Wrede, S. (2011) 'How countries matter: Studying health policy in a comparative perspective', in I. Bourgeault, R. Dingwall and R. de Vries (eds), *Sage Handbook of Qualitative Methods in Health Research*. London: Sage.

Wrede, S., Benoit, C., Bourgeault, I. L., van Tejlingen, E., Sandall, J. and De Vries, R. (2006) 'Decentred comparative research: Context sensitive analysis of maternal health care', *Social Science and Medicine*, *63*: 2986–97.

Yin, R. K. (2017) *Case Study Research and Applications: Design and Methods*. London: Sage.

23

Interdisciplinary Research in Health Care

A. PAUL WILLIAMS AND JANET M. LUM

Chapter objectives

- To discuss what is interdisciplinary research in health care
- To clarify why interdisciplinary research in health care is important
- To outline the key challenges and benefits to conducting interdisciplinary research
- To highlight the importance of including academic and non-academic researchers in the research process.

Introduction

In this chapter we consider the theory and practice of interdisciplinary research focusing on health care. Although definitions and approaches in interdisciplinary research may vary, such research typically moves beyond the classic notion of the solo researcher who independently engages in scholarly activities aimed at investigating questions of interest within a single academic discipline or field of knowledge. Instead, collaborative teams of researchers trained in different disciplines or fields, often alongside non-researcher partners and end-users such as policy makers, providers and consumers, address more complex questions spanning disciplinary boundaries. For example, while a clinical researcher might investigate the impact of a particular risk factor, such as smoking on the likelihood that older persons will experience dementia, interdisciplinary teams with expertise in gerontology, nutrition, social work, physical therapy and sociology, are better equipped to investigate the impact of multiple factors, such as gender, class, food, exercise, social engagement and loneliness, as well as smoking, not only on the likelihood of experiencing dementia, but on the ability of older persons and their family carers to 'live well' with dementia on a day-to-day basis.

This chapter is presented in four sections. In the first section, we offer a brief introduction to interdisciplinary research, what it entails, why it is important, and how it parallels a corresponding shift in health care delivery away from solo practice to more collaborative forms of team practice. In the second, we consider the key challenges and opportunities of interdisciplinary research. These include the time and effort required to ensure that team members work collaboratively across disciplines rather than remaining within their disciplinary 'silos'. In the third section, we offer two case examples of research projects conducted by the authors illustrating the utility, and some of the challenges, of using interdisciplinary team approaches to investigate complex questions in the increasingly important field of community-based care for older persons. In the fourth, we conclude that a shift from the classic notion of the 'solo researcher' to the more contemporary idea of 'interdisciplinary team research', while posing challenges, also offers exciting new opportunities to address complex health care challenges in creative and innovative ways.

What is interdisciplinary research?

Interdisciplinary research is one of a family of related research approaches, including multidisciplinary research and transdiciplinary research, all of which emphasize collaboration and joint working across different disciplines or fields of knowledge, albeit to different degrees.

In multidisciplinary teams, researchers engaged on common problems may still work relatively independently by examining different aspects of the topic from their particular disciplinary perspective. Findings may then be synthesized at the end of a project or published independently to add to a cumulative body of knowledge. As Middleton (2011) observes, while successful solutions to complex problems, such as climate change, must be formulated across many disciplines, including natural science, engineering, social science and the humanities, researchers on multidisciplinary teams may still not be familiar with what other team members do, or how they contribute to the larger whole.

By comparison, interdisciplinary team research anticipates more active collaboration and joint working throughout the research process. Interdisciplinarity analyses, synthesizes and harmonizes links across disciplines into a coordinated and coherent research enterprise. It is:

a mode of research by teams of individuals that integrates information, data, techniques, tools, perspectives, concepts, and/or theories from two or more disciplines or bodies of specialized knowledge to advance fundamental understanding or to solve problems whose solutions are beyond the scope of a single discipline or area of research practice. (Committee on Facilitating Interdisciplinary Research, Committee on Science, Engineering, and Public Policy 2004: 2)

Definitions of interdisciplinary research also emphasize the importance of a shared conceptual and methodological framework. As Aboelela and colleagues (2007: 341) say: 'The research is based upon a conceptual model that links or integrates theoretical frameworks from [the different] disciplines, uses study design and methodology that is not limited to any one field, and requires the use of perspectives and skills of the involved disciplines throughout multiple phases of the research process'. Such shared understandings encourage researchers to learn from each other, to think of complex problems in new ways, to devise novel research approaches and measures, and to communicate research findings broadly across disciplines and fields.

Transdisciplinary research is also worth mentioning since it points to the continuing evolution of research collaborations. While multidisciplinary and interdisciplinary research often work within established fields of knowledge, transdiciplinary research aims to develop new fields based on a synthesis among different disciplines (Choi and Pak 2006; Sommerville and Rapport 2002). For example, the Harvard Transdisciplinary Research in Energetics and Cancer Center (2018) – a new field in itself – defines transdisciplinary research as 'research efforts conducted by investigators from different disciplines working jointly to create new conceptual, theoretical, methodological, and translational innovations that integrate and move beyond discipline-specific approaches to address a common problem'.

Why interdisciplinary research matters

Interdisciplinary collaborations (and possibly transdiciplinary research in the future) are increasingly important and prevalent in health care research. A major factor advancing this approach is the rise of multiple chronic health and social needs in ageing societies. Across the industrialized world, more people are living longer and, for the most part, healthier lives. Nevertheless, as they age, people are more likely to experience combinations of illnesses and disabilities (often referred to as 'multi-morbidities') which, by definition, cannot be cured in hospitals on a short-term episodic basis, but must be managed over the long-term where people live day-to-day. Here, instead of treating well-defined illnesses or medical conditions one at a time using highly specialized expertise and technology (examples include heart surgery, joint replacements and eye surgery), health care researchers, often alongside research end-users such as providers and policy makers, have to grapple with the complexities of caring for growing numbers of older persons with multiple ongoing health challenges, such as dementia, diabetes and heart disease, in addition to social challenges such as poverty, isolation and depression. Evidence points to the importance of gender, socioeconomic status and cultural background not only in determining who will experience complex health and social needs but to what degree. It also shows that access to a range of community-based supports is needed to maintain individuals (and their family carers) as independently as possible, for as long as possible, in their own homes.

Recent work by the World Health Organization (2015) illustrates the multidimensional, interdisciplinary nature of such challenges. It identifies a constellation of factors influencing healthy ageing, including 'individual' factors such as genetics, personal behaviour such as smoking and exercise, and disease, including heart disease, cancer and dementia, as well as 'environmental' factors such as housing, assistive technologies, social facilities and transportation. The World Health Organization (2007) also applies the concept of healthy ageing in the specific context of cities, the geographic location where most people live and work. In its *Global Age-Friendly Cities* project, it concluded that cities can enhance the wellbeing of ageing populations through urban-specific initiatives such as more accessible outdoor spaces and public buildings, age-friendly transportation networks and housing, and enhanced opportunities for civic engagement and employment.

As a result of inherent limits to their training and resources, solo researchers, or even groups of researchers within a single discipline, may of necessity limit their investigations to a particular aspect of such complex realities. For instance, experts in engineering and information technology may highlight ways in which computers, 'smart' appliances (such as stoves and refrigerators), and sensors which track activity can assist older persons to live independently in their own homes and apartments but leave aside important questions related to access, costs and affordability, as well as issues concerning the implications for privacy and social isolation. Similarly, dietitians may do valuable research into the components of a healthy diet, but will not be able to consider fully how older persons with physical or cognitive deficits living in poverty, with no family members to help them, can afford healthy foods, get out to buy groceries, or carry out related household tasks such as preparing meals, washing up and putting out the garbage. In such contexts, interdisciplinarity offers clear advantages. Not only can research teams examine various aspects of complex problems concurrently, they can also begin to sort out how these aspects are interrelated. In addition to seeing the individual trees, interdisciplinary teams thus offer a greater potential to see the entire forest.

Interdisciplinary research of this kind reflects, and is supported by, an increasing push towards interdisciplinary education, training and practice at the undergraduate and graduate levels in universities around the world. The aim is for future researchers to have a basic understanding of other disciplines and the importance of joint working beyond their own disciplinary base. This follows from the principle that challenges such as climate change and ageing are extraordinarily complex, and that interdisciplinary inquiry holds the key to 'big picture' thinking as well as innovative and creative breakthroughs (Pourbohloul and Kieny

2011; Science Europe 2012). Students are now learning how to frame research questions that extend beyond their primary area of expertise, and to recognize the contributions that other disciplines can make. While in the past, students in the health sciences tended to be trained within their own disciplinary 'silos' – for example, in faculties of medicine, nursing, and rehabilitation – new entities such as interdisciplinary schools of health sciences and interdisciplinary health programmes are now emerging in universities in Canada and internationally.

Health care research leaders and funders increasingly expect interdisciplinary research. This expectation is a consequence of escalating health care costs, and growing calls for enhanced transparency, accountability, person-centred care and value-for-money. Collaborations and cross-pollination across health disciplines and beyond are seen to offer the potential to challenge prevailing discipline-based hierarchies of knowledge, and they have the capacity to craft out-of-the-box solutions that work for end-users and sustain stretched health care systems. In Canada, the Canadian Academy of Health Sciences (2005), established in the early 2000s, brought together leaders in six health sciences disiplines to assess the environment for conducting and promoting interdisciplinary health research (Hall et al. 2006). It concluded that interdisciplinary teams were essential for addressing complex public-health issues, such as breast cancer, obesity and avian influenza. It also noted that the Canadian Institutes of Health Research (CIHR), Canada's national research funder, funds interdisciplinary training programmes, grants for emerging interdisciplinary teams, and grants for interdisciplinary capacity enhancement (Hall et al. 2006).

Interdisciplinarity also offers greater potential to make research more relevant to policy makers addressing real-world challenges such as the supply of health human resources. In the past, researchers typically worked on a profession-by-profession basis to estimate how many doctors or nurses or rehabilitation therapists were required to meet future demand. This was based on what they currently do. Supply issues are now seen as more complex. Home and community care involve a range of practitioners. As well as the dominant health care professions (such as nursing and medicine), other health care professions (such as pharmacy and rehabilitation), and various occupational groups (such as unregulated health support workers) provide care. Unpaid family carers are a critical source of support too. Instead of considering each of these different providers one at a time, interdisciplinary research teams could aim to understand how different providers now interact and how they can substitute for one another. Non-professionals in the community can carry out tasks done by regulated health care professionals in hospitals. Fewer regulated professionals may be required in future if unregulated health workers carry out procedures. Indeed, family carers already perform many routine tasks, such as administering medications. More health care workers may be required in the community to carry out essential tasks such as personal care and household tasks and meals for those unable or unwilling to fill the growing 'care gap' (McNeil and Hunter 2014). When faced with such complex problems, interdisciplinary teams will be essential to 'connect the dots'.

Movement towards interdisciplinary research is also accelerated by the 'digital revolution' in areas such as 'e-health'. According to the World Health Organization (2016: 11), 'eHealth is the cost-effective and secure use of information communication technologies (ICT) in support of health and health related fields, including health-care services, health surveillance, health literature, and health education, knowledge and research'. E-health has the capacity to generate vast amounts of health-related data, potentially leading to new and more holistic understandings of health, new innovations in the field of health and social care, and new relationships between providers and more educated and empowered consumers. Technological advances may offer powerful administrative tools to simplify user interactions with the health care system. Information management and communication tools may permit patients to be more informed partners. Assistive technologies such as home modifications, communications equipment and sensors can help people with ongoing health and social needs to manage better, and for longer, in familiar home settings with a greater degree of autonomy and control. Such developments also push towards broader definitions of interdisciplinarity that can integrate the 'lived experience' of patients, clients, consumers and caregivers.

In England, the National Institute for Health Research (NIHR) now promotes 'patient and public involvement and engagement' as a means of ensuring that health research is as effective and as relevant for patients as possible. It publishes a guide encouraging patients, service users, carers or lay persons who are enthusiastic about health research and willing to communicate that to patients and the public as well as health care professionals to become 'patient research ambassadors' (NHS England 2018). Opportunities include raising awareness of research to patients and the public and becoming a 'lay champion' in areas like dementia, cancer or diabetes (NHS England 2018; Ontario Ministry of Health and Long-Term Care 2015; Paparella 2016).

The challenges of interdisciplinary research

While offering more robust capacity for investigating new and more complex problems, interdisciplinary research also presents challenges, three of which we highlight below.

Teams versus teamwork

Teamwork is often cited as a positive aspect of the research process but is a challenge to implement – not least because it requires leadership. Collaborative teamwork is based on building strong working relationships among team members to ensure that all views and perspectives are heard. It is critical that disciplinary hierarchies and power asymmetries are not superimposed on the research agenda. For example, a common point of contention when conducting interdisciplinary research relates to methodology: what data are collected, and how they are collected, synthesized and analysed (Tobi and Kampen 2018). The perceived value and credibility of different approaches can reflect disciplinary cultures and established power hierarchies. In health care research, as in health care practice, clinical perspectives still tend to dominate. Randomized controlled trials (RCTs) – where research participants are randomly assigned to receive a 'new' treatment or, as a control, a placebo or the 'old' standard treatment – are still frequently presented as the 'gold standard' for health care research even though they may not be applicable to complex realities outside the hospital walls. As we have seen, in fields such as community-based care for older persons, multiple factors within and beyond health care can affect wellbeing and independence, making it difficult, and often counterproductive, to isolate any one factor. Moreover, outcomes are hard to quantify. Regardless of the quality and appropriateness of care, older persons will inevitably decline and die.

Ethical challenges can come into play since it may not be acceptable to withhold a potentially valuable programme or service from a vulnerable person who could potentially benefit from it for the sake of an experiment. Such challenges are further complicated as pressure grows to integrate the 'lived experience' of research 'subjects', in this case older persons and family carers, into the design and conduct of health care research. Historically, their perspectives have been ignored.

Time and resources

A second key challenge relates to the time and resources required to recruit and manage diverse interdisciplinary teams. While researchers from a particular disciplinary background may make similar assumptions about research objectives, protocols, methods, ownership of intellectual property, interdisciplinary teams will often have to work hard to build consensus at each point through the research process. Deciding where and when research findings should be published can be particularly contentious. Most of the influential health care journals (including the *New England Journal of Medicine* and *The Lancet*) still tend to be discipline-focused. Aboelela and colleagues (2007), in their study of the factors that contributed to the success of interdisciplinary work, found that those most often mentioned were communication, leadership and trust. An explicit institutional commitment to interdisciplinarity and sufficient resources were also required to ensure that team members continued to collaborate rather than fall back onto familiar 'turfs'.

What counts as legitimate research

This leads to a third challenge. While researchers themselves may be enthusiastic about interdisciplinary research, some funding agencies, journals and peer reviewers may still expect to see well-defined questions addressed using established methods. In Canada, for example, health care research, including much clinical research, is funded by one agency, the Canadian Institutes for Health Research (CIHR). Social science research, however, is funded by another agency, the Social Sciences and Humanities Research Council (SSHRC), which will not consider health care research *per se*. Such funding streams can leave inter-disciplinary research teams in a dilemma regarding how to 'frame' projects to meet funding requirements. Evaluative mechanisms to judge the quality of interdisciplinary research are still the exception rather than the rule, and, as noted, high-impact journals tend to focus on particular audiences.

For their part, many universities, while claiming to support communication and collab-oration across fields of study, are still organized along traditional disciplinary lines, such as the faculty of medicine, faculty of social work and the faculty of engineering. As Brewer (1999) noted, the world has problems, but universities have departments. In addition, interdisciplinary research is sometimes viewed with scepticism. It is seen as lacking aca-demic rigour, legitimacy and credibility following the view that 'someone who is a master of several disciplines is a master of none'. Research and ethics committees can reinforce divisions by requiring that research proposals be submitted to the researcher's disci-pline-specific review panel, on the grounds that peers are most familiar with approaches and concerns within disciplines. As the Canadian Academy of Health Sciences concluded in its initial report, 'the discipline-bound structure of most Canadian universities implies that what is valued within academic culture is the independent scholar from a singu-lar discipline. Today, the persistence of long-held academic traditions and administra-tive processes make sustainable interdisciplinary training and research a still-distant goal' (Hall et al. 2006: 767).

Nevertheless, there is growing momentum towards interdisciplinary health care research, precisely because it offers new and exciting opportunities to address complex problems. As noted earlier, more universities now offer interdisciplinary academic programmes and degrees. In contrast to traditional faculties, such as medicine and nursing, schools of health sciences and public health can span multiple health disciplines as well as non-health fields such as business, engineering, economics and policy sciences. Similarly, major research fund-ing agencies, such as the National Institutes of Health (NIH) in the United States, the Seventh Research Framework Programme in the European Union, the Canadian Institutes of Health Research (CIHR) and the World Health Organization (WHO), now actively promote interdisciplinary health research as a means of addressing increasingly complex health challenges.

From research to policy action

An additional challenge, touched on briefly above, relates to making research findings acces-sible and relevant to research end-users, including growing numbers of private commercial businesses.

In Canada and many other countries, universities have become more active players in the 'commercialization' of research findings, often promoting start-ups or spin-off companies, and the translation of intellectual-property into commercial products to access new revenue streams. In turn, university researchers may be increasingly bound by the concept of 'return on investment' that can push them towards projects which are tightly focused, highly managed and driven by clearly defined outcomes, or products which can be sold for a profit. Since industries are less concerned with how such work is accomplished, as long as the job is done, research teams may have an incentive to refocus their work within traditional disciplinary silos.

Particularly when funded by private businesses, researchers may face pressures to avoid topics which antagonize commercial interests, or even suppress research evidence that is unfavourable to those interests. Cigarette smoking is a case in point. Until recently, substantial scientific evidence linking lung cancer to cigarette smoking was publicly denied by the tobacco industry-funded research. They argued that there was no conclusive, statistically significant or scientifically established causality between smoking, cancer and ill health (Bates and Rowell n.d.). Currently, there is a similar debate regarding the link between sugar and both obesity and Type 2 diabetes.

In such circumstances, it may be especially challenging to 'sell' interdisciplinary research which takes the 'broader view' or gives voice to those who are not powerful players in commercial markets. For example, narratives that underscore the importance to older persons of low-cost, low-tech supports for daily living, such as meals, transportation and friendly visits, may be less appealing to potential commercial investors than narratives that highlight the importance of specific high-cost, high-tech products such as 'breakthrough' medical technologies and drugs where immense profits are possible.

Nevertheless, judgements about what kinds of research are valuable and what can be considered the weight of 'evidence' are changing, particularly among decision makers in the health sector. Governments now face increasingly complex problems with ageing populations which have no 'cure'. In this context, qualitative research is particularly valuable. The methodology of compiling broad narratives, including the voices of historically under-represented groups, such as older persons and family carers, is gaining support in public policy circles. Paul Thomas (2006: 44) argues: 'To promote deeper understanding of what the numbers mean, public organisations need to be able to "tell their stories". ... Storytelling should not be dismissed as merely self-serving anecdotes. Stories serve to put measures in context and to provide explanations.' Thomas adds that although performance stories will never achieve the status of scientific proof, over time they can identify patterns of response that provide credible evidence. Compiling a body of similar narratives can strengthen the conclusion that supportive interventions have had a substantial impact on the health outcomes for older people as well as for the health care system (Tobi and Kampen 2018).

Below we offer two examples of funded research conducted by the authors which illuminate both challenges and opportunities of interdisciplinary research.

When home is community

Accessible housing is now widely acknowledged as essential to the wellbeing and independence of older persons. However, in Canada there has been relatively little investigation of what type of housing is suitable for particular groups. For older people with chronic health and social needs, a combination of housing with a range of non-medical supports for daily living, such as meals, personal care, transportation and social engagement, is needed.

When Home is Community (Lum, Ruff and Williams 2005) was an interdisciplinary research project engaging academic researchers and graduate students from two universities in the faculties of arts and medicine. It also included non-researcher partners, including care managers from three community service agencies, administrators from Toronto Community Housing (Canada's largest provider of non-profit, Rent-Geared-to-Income (RGI) social housing), and older people themselves. The aim was to compare the outcomes for older people living in 'supportive housing' (RGI apartments *with* coordinated access to needed community supports), against those of older people living in geographically proximate 'social housing' (RGI apartments *without* coordinated access to community supports). Internationally, supportive housing has been called retirement villages and hostels in Australia, sheltered housing in the United Kingdom, and assisted living in the United States.

In this project, team members had already participated in an established network that promoted research and knowledge transfer for community-based care in the *Canadian Research Network for Care in the Community* so joint working was already supported. The network provided a pool of potential team members with diverse perspectives who nonetheless shared a mutual understanding of, and commitment to, policy-relevant interdisciplinary research and evidence-informed decision-making. This paved the way to smooth and equitable working relationships. Nonetheless, considerable time and effort were invested to build consensus on the design and conduct of the research. In particular, non-researcher partners wanted to ensure that the project would investigate 'top-line' impacts. This term referred to outcomes that improved the quality of life and independence of older people in their day-to-day lives. 'Bottom-line' impacts were considered as those related to the cost-effectiveness of care and the sustainability of the health care system.

Methodology was an issue. The academic researchers used quantitative data to document 'what' services were used by older people in social housing and the cost, compared to the costs of those services in supportive housing. The community-based research partners stressed the importance of qualitative interviews that probed the 'life narratives' of older people to understand 'why' they made the choices they did, and 'how' different ways of accessing non-medical community supports affected their wellbeing, as well as their use of hospitals and other health care services. As a result, we combined quantitative costing and service utilization data with qualitative in-depth interviews with 226 seniors living in three pairs of supportive housing and social housing buildings located close to each other. The interview process, including recruitment of interviewees, was facilitated by community meetings

(Continued)

(Continued)

in these buildings to explain the nature of the research and its aims, and to invite input from a range of participants.

Our non-researcher partners wished to integrate 'lived experience' more fully into the research process and the project findings provided unanticipated insights that challenged conventional wisdom. The older people interviewed said that the factors that mattered most in their day-to-day lives were 'lower level' non-medical services such as vacuuming, laundry, cleaning, grocery shopping, cooking and personal hygiene. These services allowed them to continue to live safely and independently without becoming isolated. This was despite the fact that many of the older people interviewed faced multiple health and social challenges, that on paper at least, put them 'at risk' of illness and institutionalization. Services worked best when care managers helped to identify, access and coordinate them. For supportive housing, the interviews showed that what people wanted was reassurance from care managers that services were there and that they could access them when needed. Fewer services were used than anticipated when the choice was left to users. In contrast, individuals in social housing, where there was no such input from managers, asked for services even when they did not immediately need them as a way to insure against future needs.

The use of costly emergency services showed a similar pattern: when faced with an emergency, residents in supportive housing called the 24-hour on-site emergency response number, with the aim of getting help immediately in their own apartments. Those in social housing were more likely to call 911 (the equivalent of 999 in the UK), increasing the likelihood of a costly, and potentially avoidable, hospital admission. In sum, the findings from this interdisciplinary project suggested that managed access to non-medical community supports avoided the use of more costly medical care and contributed to health system sustainability by moderating costs. It was not a cost add-on.

Balance of care research

This research asked the question: why can many older persons with relatively high needs age successfully at home, while others with similar or lower needs require residential long-term care? Building on groundbreaking study conducted by researchers at the Personal Social Services Research Unit, University of Manchester, England (Challis and Hughes 2002; Clarkson, Hughes and Challis 2005; Hughes and Challis 2004; Tucker et al. 2008), we hypothesized that the likelihood of an older person losing independence and ending up in a residential care bed was not simply a matter of their individual needs, as conventional wisdom would suggest, but was heavily dependent on local system capacity to provide essential non-medical, community-based supports for daily living. Where support was readily accessible, the 'tipping point' for residential long-term care would be higher. Even with high levels of need, older people could age successfully at home. Conversely, where community-based supports were less readily available, the likelihood of residential care placement increased (Williams et al. 2009).

CASE STUDY 23.2

We assembled an interdisciplinary team including researchers from three universities with expertise in health care, public policy, social work, as well as senior home care administrators familiar with supports available at the local level. We also recruited and relied heavily on an 'expert panel' of experienced front-line care coordinators who provided valuable insight into the 'on the ground' reality as well as knowledge of available home and community care services. To ensure that different perspectives were heard, expert panelists were recruited from organizations across the care continuum in home care, hospitals and residential long-term care.

As usual in this type of research, considerable time and effort were invested in negotiating the roles and responsibilities of members, agreeing on methods, and getting ethics approvals from a number of separate provider agencies and organizations. This was a time-consuming and complex task. However, team members and reviewers had confidence in the study methodology as it had been tested elsewhere. They were reassured that the research would not pose significant risks to participants and would provide beneficial insights and outcomes for older people, their care providers and policy makers.

A key finding was that between a third and a half of all older persons then waiting for a residential long-term care placement could potentially be safely and cost-effectively supported in their family residences or in supportive housing. This conclusion was based on our quantitative analysis of home care assessment data together with the qualitative insights of our expert panellists. We found that many older people 'defaulted' to residential care wait lists due to a lack of coordinated access to community-based services at the local level. This problem reflected an inadequate system of supportive services rather than a problem of individual needs *perse*. Our front-line experts stated that there was the flexibility to achieve viable solutions. For example, if poor nutrition was quickening decline, community-based solutions could include assistance with grocery shopping, in-home help to prepare nutritional food, meals-on-wheels where prepared foods could be delivered to the home, or congregate dining, where individuals could share meals with others at community centres.

In terms of methodology, we concluded that our decision to engage with non-researcher practitioners as active members of our team substantially improved our visibility and 'street credibility'. The research methodology and findings gained a wide audience beyond academia, particularly among local health care planning bodies and provider agencies. This, in turn, led to invitations to reproduce the research in other localities. To date, our team has conducted Balance of Care projects in 12 of 14 health care regions of Ontario, Canada's largest province, establishing a wide base for comparative analysis.

Conclusion

In this chapter, we have provided readers with a brief introduction to the theory and practice of interdisciplinary research. This approach to doing research has considerable potential. It involves active collaboration among researchers from different disciplines and fields of knowledge. It can include a range of participants: consumers, practitioners and policy makers who can learn from one another, see complex problems in new ways, devise innovative methods and measures, communicate findings to wide audiences and put conventional wisdom to the test. Such approaches appear particularly valuable in addressing complex issues such as climate change and ageing, where many different disciplines and fields of knowledge can make valuable contributions, and where there is no one single solution.

Of course, there are real challenges, including the time and effort required to encourage researchers from different disciplines and fields of knowledge to work together as a team, and to convince universities, funding agencies and reviewers of the value-added of this cross-boundaries approach. Indeed, as we have observed, there may also be factors such as the increasing push to commercialize research findings, which in turn can push researchers to investigate well-defined problems with clear outcomes as opposed to more messy and complex health issues.

Nevertheless, there appears to be growing momentum towards interdisciplinary research from funders, supported by a rise in interdisciplinary education in universities, both aimed at encouraging a culture of collaboration and joint working. As our own experience suggests, such research is particularly well suited to understanding complex 'big picture' issues such as ageing. In addition, there are constructive ways of mitigating challenges and ensuring that the benefits of interdisciplinary research outweigh the costs. These include calling on existing networks of researchers and research end-users with a shared commitment to joint working and building on proven methodologies which go beyond a narrow disciplinary base.

Exercise 23.1 Planning for age-friendly communities

With increasingly vocal demands from older persons to be able to live at home as independently as possible, for as long as possible, you have been tasked by a regional health authority in a predominately rural area in Canada to plan for age-friendly communities. Because young people tend to leave such communities to follow education and jobs in cities, rural communities tend to age faster than those in urban areas. In addition to supporting the quality of life and independence of older persons and family carers, the health authority is concerned with moderating health care costs by reducing avoidable use of hospital emergency rooms and the numbers of Alternate Level of Care hospital beds. These are beds occupied by individuals, including many older persons, who no longer require hospital care but cannot be discharged because of a lack of community-based care options.

This exercise is designed to make you think about how to design a research project drawing on interdisciplinary expertise. While the material contained in this chapter may help you consider many of the issues, you may wish to access additional material from a library or the internet to write a formal research proposal.

- *The 'what' and the 'why'*: Identify the objective of the research and the complexity of issues related to this objective. Why does interdisciplinary research make sense in this context? What disciplines will you draw upon?
- *The 'who'*: Think about the range of people to include on the research team (older people, family carers, voluntary agencies, community service providers, housing providers, health professionals, non-professional health providers, public sector policy analysts). Consider the older person's ageing trajectory so that your research will reflect the varying needs of people as they age. Since you are also looking at broader community factors, you may also wish to consider including personnel from the local libraries, grocery stores, schools, community centres and banks, and the role they can play in facilitating 'age-friendly' communities.
- *The 'how'*: How will you gather your data? What data/information are important to gather? Observation? Questionnaires (in person or online or mail)? Focus groups (privacy may be an issue for some older people)? Key informant interviews? A combination of these instruments? Is there a methodology that has been used elsewhere successfully that you can adapt? How will you bring together the analysis of different kinds of data? Qualitative data? Quantitative data?
- *The context*: What background information/data will you gather? Statistical population data in the area you are studying will be helpful to track future trends, such as a declining youth population that will accelerate an ageing community. How does the population distribution in this area compare with the population distribution in other areas (other rural or urban areas)?
- *Analysis*: What forms of analysis will be appropriate?
- *Resources*: How will you cost your proposal? What resources will you need?
- *Time management*: Plot the different research activities over time and in relation to resources. At each stage, remember to set aside sufficient time to create a common analytical framework and to build consensus among project team members for joint interpretation of the findings.
- *Knowledge mobilization*: How will you present your findings? How will you translate your research into policy action? To whom? In what format? If you are considering a publication, who will you include as co-authors? Consider a community 'town hall' meeting, a website publication, and articles in local and national newspapers. Consider an event and invite local and regional politicians and their policy assistants.

Recommended further reading

This article examines the cultural and structural characteristics of government, industry and academia in Canada to identify the factors that help or hinder interdisciplinary health research. The paper also suggests how universities best support/enhance interdisciplinary health research to benefit science and to meet the needs of industry and government:

Hall, J. G., Bainbridge, L., Buchan, A., Cribb, A., Drummond, J., Gyles, C., Hicks, T. P., McWilliam, C., Paterson, B., Ratner, P. A., Skarakis-Doyle, E. and Solomon, P. (2006) 'A meeting of minds: Interdisciplinary research in the health sciences in Canada', *Canadian Medical Association Journal*, *175*(7): 763–71.

This book offers a comprehensive and systematic presentation of the interdisciplinary research process and the theory that informs it:
Repko, A. F. and Szostak, R. (2016) *Interdisciplinary Research: Process and Theory*, 3rd edition. Thousand Oaks, CA: Sage.

This provocative monograph examines performance measurement as practised by governments in Canada, the United States, Australia and New Zealand. His discussion informs interdisciplinary research by demonstrating that any one particular set of measures will always be partial, contextual and not necessarily objective:
Thomas, P. G. (2006) *Performance Measurement, Reporting, Obstacles and Accountability: Recent Trends and Future Directions*. Canberra: The Australian National University EPress.

This article is helpful in setting out a methodology for an interdisciplinary framework:
Tobi, H. and Kampen, J. K. (2018) 'Research design: The methodology for interdisciplinary research framework', *Quality and Quantity*, *52*: 1209–25. Available at: https://link.springer.com/content/pdf/10.1007%2Fs11135-017-0513-8.pdf

References

Aboelela, S. W., Larson, E., Bakken, S., Carrasquillo, O., Formicola, A., Glied, S. A. and Gebbie, K. M. (2007) 'Defining interdisciplinary research: Conclusions from a critical review of the literature', *Health Services Research*, *42*(1): 329–46.

Bates, C. and Rowell, A. (n.d.) *Tobacco Explained: The Truth about the Tobacco Industry...in Its Own Words*. London: Action on Smoking and Health. Available at: www.who.int/tobacco/media/en/TobaccoExplained.pdf

Brewer, G. D. (1999) 'The challenges of interdisciplinarity', *Political Sciences*, *32*(4): 327–37.

Canadian Academy of Health Sciences (2005) *The Benefits and Barriers to Interdisciplinary Research in the Health Sciences in Canada: Framework Document*. Ottawa: CAHS. Available at: http://cahs-acss.ca/wp-content/uploads/2015/07/2006-01.assessment.pdf

Challis, D. and Hughes, J. (2002) 'Frail old people at the margins of care: Some recent research findings', *British Journal of Psychiatry*, *180*(2): 126–30.

Choi, B. C. and Pak, A. W. (2006) 'Multidisciplinarity, interdisciplinarity and transdisciplinarity in health research, services, education and policy: 1. Definitions, objectives, and evidence of effectiveness', *Clinical and Investigative Medicine*, *29*(6): 351–64.

Clarkson, P., Hughes, J. and Challis, D. (2005) 'The potential impact of changes in public funding for residential and nursing-home care in the United Kingdom: The residential allowance', *Ageing and Society*, *25*(2): 159–80.

Committee on Facilitating Interdisciplinary Research, Committee on Science, Engineering, and Public Policy (2004) *Facilitating Interdisciplinary Research*. National Academies. Washington, DC: National Academy Press. Available at: https://nsf.gov/od/oia/additional_resources/interdisciplinary_research/definition.jsp

Hall, J. G., Bainbridge, L., Buchan, A., Cribb, A., Drummond, J., Gyles, C., Hicks, T. P., McWilliam, C., Paterson, B., Ratner, P. A., Skarakis-Doyle, E. and Solomon, P. (2006) 'A meeting of minds: Interdisciplinary research in the health sciences in Canada', *Canadian Medical Association Journal*, *175*(7): 763–71.

Harvard Transdisciplinary Research in Energetics and Cancer Center (2018) *About Us: Definitions*. Boston, MA: Harvard T. H. Chan School of Public Health. Available at: www.hsph.harvard.edu/trec/about-us/definitions/

Hughes, J. and Challis, D. (2004) 'Frail older people – Margins of care', *Review of Clinical Gerontology*, *14*(2): 115–64.

Lum, J. M., Ruff, S. and Williams, A. P. (2005) *When Home is Community: Community Support Services and the Well-being of Seniors in Supportive and Social Housing*. Toronto: Ryerson University and University of Toronto. Available at: www.ryerson.ca/crncc/relatedreports/#supportive

McNeil, C. and Hunter, J. (2014) *The Generation Strain: Collective Solutions to Care in an Ageing Society*. London: Institute for Public Policy Research. Available at: www.ippr.org/publications/the-generation-strain-collective-solutions-to-care-in-an-ageing-society

Middleton, B. A. (2011) 'Multidisciplinary approaches to climate change questions', in B. LePage (ed.), *Wetlands*. Dordrecht: Springer.

NHS England (2018) *Developing Patient Centred Care*. London: NHS England. Available at: www.england.nhs.uk/integrated-care-pioneers/resources/patient-care/.

Ontario Ministry of Health and Long-Term Care (2015) *Patients First: A Proposal to Strengthen Patient-centred Health Care in Ontario*. Toronto: Queen's Printer for Ontario. Available at: www.health.gov.on.ca/en/news/bulletin/2015/docs/discussion paper 20151217.pdf

Paparella, G. (2016) *Person-centred Care in Europe: A Cross-country Comparison of Health System Performance, Strategies and Structures*. Oxford: Picker Institute Europe. Available at: www.picker.org/wp-content/uploads/2016/02/12-02-16-Policy-briefing-on-patient-centred-care-in-Europe.pdf.

Pourbohloul, B. and Kieny, M. (2011) 'Complex systems analysis: Towards holistic approaches to health systems planning and policy', *Bulletin of the World Health Organization*, *89*: 242.

Science Europe (2012) *Science Europe Position Statement – Horizon 2020: Excellence Counts*. Brussels: Science Europe. Available at: www.scienceeurope.org/wp-content/uploads/2014/05/SE_H2020_Excellence_Counts_FIN.pdf

Sommerville, M. A. and Rapport, D. J. (eds) (2002) *Transdisciplinarity: Recreating Integrated Knowledge*. Montreal: McGill, Queens University Press.

Thomas, P. G. (2006) *Performance Measurement, Reporting, Obstacles and Accountability: Recent Trends and Future Directions*. Canberra: The Australian National University EPress.

Tobi, H. and Kampen, J. K. (2018) 'Research design: The methodology for interdisciplinary research framework', *Quality and Quantity*, *52*: 1209–25. Available at: https://link.springer.com/content/pdf/10.1007%2Fs11135-017-0513-8.pdf

Tucker, S., Hughes, J., Burns, A. and Challis, D. (2008) 'The balance of care: Reconfiguring services for older people with mental health problems', *Aging and Mental Health*, *12*(1): 81–91.

Williams, A. P., Challis, D., Deber, R., Watkins, J., Kuluski, K., Lum, J. M. and Daub, S. (2009) 'Balancing institutional and community-based care: Why some older persons can age successfully at home why others require residential long-term care', *Healthcare Quarterly*, *12*(2): 95–104.

World Health Organization (2007) *Global Age-friendly Cities: A Guide*. Geneva: WHO. Available at: www.who.int/ageing/publications/Global_age_friendly_cities_Guide_English.pdf

World Health Organization (2015) *World Report on Ageing and Health*. Geneva: WHO. Available at: http://apps.who.int/iris/bitstream/10665/186463/1/9789240694811_eng.pdf?ua=1

World Health Organization (2016) *Global Diffusion of eHealth: Making Universal Health Coverage Achievable*. Report of the Third Global Survey on eHealth. Geneva: WHO. Available at: http://apps.who.int/iris/bitstream/handle/10665/252529/9789241511780-eng.pdf;jsessionid=772522CF036563085FA8EABE38D96393?sequence=1

24

Mixed Methods in Health Research

JONATHAN TRITTER

Chapter objectives

- To consider the advantages and disadvantages of using mixed methods in health research
- To examine the consequences of employing mixed methods for project planning and management
- To discuss how the challenges raised by mixed method research in health may be met
- To consider in what ways research teams in particular may address the issues posed by mixed methods.

Introduction

The key aim of this chapter is to examine the benefits and limitation of mixed methods research in health care and the implications this has for project planning and management. Increasingly, those who fund research and publishers of professional journals require health research that is based on data collected using different methods and typically draws on expertise from both the biomedical and social sciences. A project may draw on physiological measurement and epidemiological data, as well as data that explore people's understanding of their illness – collected, for example, from illness diaries or narratives. The chapter describes mixed methods research, outlines the strengths and weakness of mixed methods research, and considers the implications for research design and project management. The chapter explores some of the reasons for adopting mixed methods in research and illustrates a number of typical research designs. It identifies some of the difficulties that can arise and suggests ways of meeting the challenge. Fundamental to this is careful forethought and a strategic approach to research. The key challenge faced by researchers is the nature and type of data most appropriate to explore specific research questions. Different types of data generate different kinds of understanding and increasingly multiple forms of data are needed to understand and issue. This requires more complex, but integrated, methodological approaches. Research designs need to consider how to coordinate the design of research instruments, analytical approaches should be chosen that are driven by common problematics and ensure the appropriate methodological expertise is included in a research team.

Mixing methods: Some typical approaches

Beginning with qualitative inquiries

As earlier chapters have discussed, different research methods are associated with different kinds of research questions. However, the same method may serve different purposes depending on the order that it is applied within a research project. Often research in an area about which little is known begins with an open approach that seeks to identify relevant issues or topics. Exploratory research rarely has explicit questions or a hypothesis to be tested. Instead, these are developed in the initial phase using a qualitative method such as observation, in-depth interviews or focus group discussions. Such an approach should yield the key dimensions that can then be used to frame the later stages of the project – stages that will adopt other methods.

For example, we know from epidemiological studies that asthma has become more prevalent, and the incidence is increasing among children (Ellwood et al. 2017). In order to understand the experience of children with asthma at different ages, say in secondary schools, initially research might begin with observing playground activities or physical education lessons. Another approach might be to convene a number of focus groups to include children of the same age for a discussion of how they think asthma affects their life in school. Each strategy would yield different information, but both approaches provide a way of identifying key issues for research participants. Other methods could be used to measure these more precisely. Whatever methods are adopted, researchers deploying these approaches need to have relevant expertise; mixed methods research is typically adopted by collaborating teams of researchers who bring different methodological expertise to bear on a common problem.

Interviews or focus group discussions can also help to develop and refine research instruments. For example, the focus group discussion could be used to identify five key areas where children felt their school experience was affected by asthma. These could provide a basis for an unstructured interview topic guide or be used to design items in a questionnaire. A project that begins with a qualitative method ensures that research is grounded in the experience of those who are the object of study. Research that builds on the health needs expressed by a population group being studied is especially relevant when the aim is to evaluate or develop health services. It has been argued that the increased policy emphasis on user involvement in research (Conklin, Morris and Nolte 2012) and on patient and public participation in health policy (Tritter and McCallum 2006) may privilege studies that involve service users.

Laying the groundwork with quantitative methods

A project may begin with a quantitative study by undertaking a survey of a sample population to establish the frequency of a certain phenomenon. Using the example of asthma from above, a survey could be used initially to identify the number of children with asthma in secondary schools in a given area. The data could then be used to provide a sampling frame to identify a sub-sample for further investigation. We might be interested in how children of different ages in different schools experienced and managed their illness. We could use the survey data to identify a sub-sample of children that was then stratified according to age, school and gender and use this to invite children to a focus group or interview. The second qualitative phase of the research would explore the meaning of illness for these children – a very different type of research question than simply establishing prevalence.

The ethnography and case study approach

Ethnographic and case studies are dependent on using mixed methods. Ethnography relies on observation as an essential aspect of its methods toolkit, but this is typically augmented by interviews, focus groups and sometimes surveys. Similarly, case study research is premised on collecting multiple forms of data (Yin 2018). This may include a critical review of documents and policies produced by the case-study organization, observation of key meetings and interviews with a range of staff. For both of these instances, the convergence of multiple sources of evidence is the key to obtaining more rounded and, arguably, more valid findings – as increasingly endorsed in the multitude of research texts on mixed methods (see, for example, Cresswell 2015; Pope, Mays and Popay 2007; Tashakkori and Teddlie 2010).

Research design and mixed methods

The various ways that different kinds of research methods can be combined has been outlined. The order and combination of methods must be planned carefully to accrue maximum benefit, generate the greatest research validity and be undertaken by researchers with appropriate expertise and competence. Simply applying a range of methods to a research problem – a shotgun approach – is likely to yield little additional benefit. The particular research problem or question must be determined first. It is only after such decisions are made that actual methods and research instruments can be defined, evaluated and adopted.

An important consideration in a mixed-method research design is the intended relationship between the types of data to be collected. Most designs rely on data collected at an early research phase influencing subsequent phases, through the definition of a sample or the development of a research instrument. A further vital issue is how different kinds of data collected from different sources can be integrated analytically. Furthermore, it is important to consider at an early stage how research findings that draw on different forms of data will be presented in a final report.

Triangulation

The use of multiple sources of data is one of the principles behind the notion of triangulation. Triangulation, a navigational term based on using two bearings to locate an object, has been used in a number of ways in the social sciences. The primary use of triangulation is as a term suggesting the aggregation of data from different sources as a way to validate a particular truth, account or finding (see Denzin 1970). A second form of triangulation is premised on the application of multiple methods to a particular research problem in order to generate a greater understanding of a particular phenomenon – it can be seen from a number of different perspectives, each of which is defined by a particular method. Triangulation is used in the latter sense here. Collecting different kinds of data (for example, first-person accounts of an experience, observational video, survey data from participants and focus groups with participants) provides the opportunity to build a holistic understanding of the object of study. It does not attempt to privilege one account over another. The account given of a phenomenon through different methods will be based on a particular theory and the structure and meaning provided by that perspective (see Silverman 2011).

The application of a coordinated analysis of a common data set using a range of different analytical perspectives is another aspect of triangulation. This might involve a series of interview transcripts being analysed independently by three scholars: a sociologist, political scientist and psychologist. The findings from the three different analyses of the same data set, when brought together, might reveal more than the application of any single analytical framework. Similarly, a number of researchers in a project team could agree a common coding framework and then independently apply this to all of the data before meeting to reach a consensus on the findings and discussion of the interpretation; this generates far more valid and robust results.

Towards a more holistic approach to health

The impact of lifestyle and the importance of patient participation in decisions about health care are now recognized as key aspects in ensuring good health. It is also acknowledged that chronic conditions and recovery from trauma or illness can be managed more successfully with patient and carer participation. No longer can health outcomes be simply understood as the product of medical intervention or pharmaceutical treatment alone. How patients access services, the ways they participate in decisions about treatment and the social context in which they are treated, live and work are all important factors that explain health outcomes. The implication of this 'holistic' model of health for research is that a number of different disciplines and research methods are required to adequately study the impact of health and illness.

For instance, smoking is associated with between 5 million and 10 million deaths worldwide annually (Jha and Peto 2014). Smoking changes the metabolism and retards healing. Therefore, smoking cessation is important from a public health perspective, and is also recommended as part of the 'treatment' for many medical conditions from asthma to coronary heart disease (Mackay and Eriksen 2002). But there is no way to 'prescribe' smoking cessation, or to understand the meaning of smoking, without considering the social context and the lifestyle of the patient (Copeland 2003).

Another factor leading to a more holistic view of health, and, *inter alia*, the importance of research using mixed methods, is the recognition of the impact of long-term, chronic conditions on health expenditure (Prince, Wu et al. 2015). This has placed greater emphasis on the potential benefit of professional/patient partnership on day-to-day self-management. The adoption of the Expert Patient Programme by the National Health Service is one example of this (Department of Health 2001). This programme became an independent charity Self-Management United Kingdom in 2014. The programme is a development from an earlier initiative developed at Stanford University in the United States and more than 120,000 patients in the United Kingdom have participated in courses to support them to manage their own condition (www.selfmanagementuk.org).

This broader view of health has in turn contributed to an interest in, and acceptance of, patient narratives as an important method and type of data in designing health services. Patient narratives take many forms, but in general they provide a temporal framework for the patient experience and help people to explore the impact, meaning and understanding of their illness experience and how this affects broader social networks and lived experience (Bury 2001; Frid, Ohlin and Bergbom 2000; Kleinman 1988). The use of patient narratives and the study of patient pathways or journeys through the illness and treatment process put further pressure on health care to be more human and holistic (Carlick and Biley 2004). Furthermore, acknowledging the value of qualitative research in health in terms of providing access to the patient experience is potentially an effective mechanism for increasing patient satisfaction and their willingness to follow medical advice. This may be one factor behind the increasing acceptance of qualitative methods among physicians.

At a more macro policy level, the Wanless (2004) report on future health strategy in the United Kingdom urges the government and the NHS to pursue a 'fully engaged scenario' in order to mitigate the impact of chronic illness, and to ensure that all members of the public feel responsible for their health and are encouraged to act in ways that work with, rather than against, clinicians. This is a challenge for the researcher as it implies a reconceptualization of 'health work' as an activity that takes place both outside and inside clinical settings.

The consequences for researchers of a holistic approach

The implication for researchers is that research methods suited to exploring lifestyle and the experiential aspects of health care, as well as classic epidemiological data about incidence, morbidity and mortality, are required. Researchers must also consider various types of theoretical and conceptual frameworks to explain their findings. Clinical knowledge must be integrated with social science expertise as well as other disciplines, such as history and statistics, in order to explore and understand contemporary health care. Such an approach to research in health care is challenging as it goes against historical hierarchies of knowledge in medical care. Researchers must now attempt to draw in the range of health professionals who are concerned with diagnosing, treating and caring for people. These factors indicate increased complexity in the research process and underline the importance of good research management if high-quality work is to be undertaken (O'Cathain, Murphy and Nicholl 2008).

Research credibility

For research to have an impact on policy, on practice and on the thinking of professionals and academics, the findings must be credible. Many factors affect credibility, such as the research methods used, the findings and outcomes from research, the reputation of researchers, the status of the funding body and the peer review process. The most fundamental factor is the first: the logic of the design, the management and process of the research, the methods used to collect data and their link to research questions, and acceptance of the analytical framework adopted. These will all affect the perceived validity of the findings. The degree of fit or triangulation between the findings when using different methods is an important mechanism for ensuring acceptance of research findings.

Multiple forms of data derived from different methods, but analysed and interpreted in an integrated fashion, are now seen to yield greater validity. However, in biomedical circles, as noted elsewhere in this volume, the randomized controlled trial (RCT) is still seen as representing the most powerful form of research evidence. The RCT yields quantitative statistically validated results but, as suggested in Chapter 2, it constructs physiological and social factors in a very particular way. The lack of recognition of epistemological differences is at the heart of some of the difficulties in integrating qualitative and quantitative data.

The credibility accorded different kinds of data is a reflection of different disciplinary cultures. The dominance of quantitative data and the RCT is in part a consequence of their centrality to epidemiology and medical training that draws on bioscience. This creates a culture in which issues of sampling, the representativeness of a sample and generalization are central to the evaluation of research findings. These criteria are antithetical to qualitative methods and interpretive data analysis. It is worth noting that in health care many of the decisions are made by a managerial or policy elite who may not be clinically trained. In the past, the longstanding bias of decision makers for 'hard' quantitative data with numerical measures of outcomes and effects is well known (Bowling 2014). This has undermined the opportunity for qualitative and mixed-method research to make a significant impact on health planning and policy, although it is worth noting that there were significant exceptions. For example, the early work of Stacey on the care of children in hospitals as well as other studies have made a significant impact on policy making to the benefit of patients (Hall and Stacey 1979; Stacey et al. 1970).

Despite this dominant tradition, there is growing appreciation of the value of other methods and multiple-methods research. Dixon-Woods, Fitzpatrick and Roberts (2001) and Donovan, Brindle and Mills (2002) argue that qualitative, and quality of life, measures should be integrated into RCTs, while Bartlam and colleagues (2016) argue for adopting mixed methods within RCTs. It is also apparent that, increasingly, articles published in health journals adopt a mix of methods. Similarly, it has been recognized that multiple methods are likely to maximize the opportunities to present a study and research findings as legitimate and valid. This will enable a tailoring of the findings and a presentation of the research design that is more appropriate and acceptable to those who draw on research. Indeed, many research funders actively encourage the inclusion of health economists and epidemiologists with clinical researchers, and more recently have recognized the strength of research collaborations between the social and medical sciences (see, for instance, Øvretveit 2009).

Mixed methods research in practice

An example of a project highlighting the benefits of mixed methods research is *Developing and Evaluating Best Practice in User Involvement in Cancer Services*, which was part of the United Kingdom Health in Partnership initiative that the author led between 2000 and 2003. It provides a good example of a collaborative project that used a variety of methods and relied on the participation of a range of organizations, as well as managers, health professionals, service users and academic researchers from a number of disciplinary backgrounds. The project was funded by the Department of Health over a three-year period, and was based at Avon, Somerset and Wiltshire Cancer Services. Two universities, the West of England and Warwick, and two voluntary organizations, the Bristol Cancer Help Centre and Cancerlink Macmillan, collaborated in the project, as did a number of NHS Hospital Trusts.

(Continued)

CASE STUDY 24.1

(Continued)

Drawing on the different expertise of the academic, voluntary sector and health service partners, the project aimed to identify how user involvement was understood and practised within one cancer network. Specifically, it aimed to:

- Identify the variety of definitions of user involvement and methods that had been used by different health organizations and multidisciplinary cancer teams
- Develop a consensus statement on user involvement in cancer services that could be supported by a range of stakeholders
- Explore the impact of user involvement on both providers and users
- Document the influence of user involvement in training and support programmes
- Identify facilitators and barriers to success in user involvement activities and find examples of good practice.

The research team adopted different research methods to fulfil these aims and research tasks were disaggregated into five phases, which are described in the main text.

Mapping user involvement activities across the network

The first task was to undertake a mapping exercise of existing mechanisms for user involvement in cancer services in the region. We focused on activity in the health service and the cancer voluntary sector, but also collected data from hospices and local government. Focus group discussions were used to construct two questionnaires: one for the voluntary and one for the statutory sector. These were then piloted extensively. In late 2000, the statutory questionnaire was administered to 65 individuals with a 68 per cent response rate. In early 2001, 70 local voluntary organizations providing support services were sampled from a database and the questionnaire administered in January 2001. The response rate was 57 per cent. From the data, a range of different definitions of user involvement was identified. The analysis also showed the scope of user involvement and provided examples of implementation across the cancer network.

Consensus development around user involvement

In the second phase, we undertook a formal consensus development exercise applying to both a two-stage Delphi exercise and the nominal group technique to obtain information. Bowling (2014) describes these techniques (see also Daykin et al. 2002). She sees the Delphi technique as an efficient way of getting information from a large number of people. A postal questionnaire asking open-ended questions on a topic is sent to a range of experts who give answers anonymously. Their responses are recycled into a questionnaire and participants are asked to rank their level of agreement with the ranking. In the nominal group, or expert panel, process, a small number of experts (around 12) decide their individual views on a topic or health intervention by ranking factors on a Likert scale from 0 (never use) to 9 (always use). At a subsequent meeting and sometimes after reading additional literature, the results are summarized, discussion takes place and panel members re-rank their views. In the cancer project, the techniques were used to agree a consensus statement on best practice in user involvement in cancer care. We drew on the expertise of 367 individuals from key stakeholder groups, such as cancer doctors, managers, general practitioners, cancer nurses, users, cancer voluntary organizations and academic researchers. Our final statement identified nine key aspects that all participants agreed were central to user involvement.

Interviews with users about their experience of involvement

In the third phase, we undertook interviews with users about their understanding, experience and satisfaction with user involvement. Our sample of 37 users of cancer services included three groups: those with experience of user involvement; those who had taken part in a training programme alongside health professionals; and those with no experience. The interviews allowed us to explore factors that contributed to users' conceptions of what it meant to be involved and their level of satisfaction.

A survey of users' willingness to be involved

In the fourth phase based on the above interviews, a questionnaire was developed to survey users' attitudes towards involvement and their willingness to contribute to the evaluation and development of cancer services in the future. A random sample of 700 users that met particular inclusion/exclusion criteria was extracted from cancer registry data. The accuracy of the data was checked against patient records and, with approval from clinicians, 388 users were surveyed in the summer of 2002. The response rate was 67 per cent. The survey was the first to give an indication of the proportion of cancer patients who were willing to be involved in service development, and the factors that affect willingness to participate, such as demographic characteristics, cancer type and the level of satisfaction with care received. Based on a verified random sample of 388 surviving cancer patients drawn from the Regional Cancer Registry database in January 2002, 19 per cent had some experience of contributing to service development. Of these, 71 per cent said they would be willing to be involved again. Almost half (49 per cent) of those who had no experience said they would be willing to participate in the future (Evans et al. 2003).

Selected case studies of a cancer multidisciplinary team in three trusts

The fifth phase of the study aimed to understand the differences in the interpretation, attitude and experience of user involvement within different trusts, and within the multidisciplinary teams responsible for treating different types of cancer. We conducted case studies in three trusts, one in each of the health authorities covered by the cancer network and with varying levels of user involvement. In each setting, we looked at the multidisciplinary teams delivering services to people with the same range of cancers – breast, colorectal, lung and prostate cancer – as well as palliative care. Key providers and managers were interviewed to establish policy, rationale and practice and those data were used to evaluate the user involvement system against criteria developed in the earlier stages of the project and from the literature.

Project management

This project also highlighted the importance of project management in mixed methods research. Members of the team came with different research and methodological experience and were employed by different organizations outside the project. Specific roles were established within the team to ensure appropriate expertise, management and support for researchers and administrative staff associated with the project. We set up a steering group to include service users. Following advertisements in local media and surgeries and clinics, two users agreed to serve although only one stayed throughout the project. We paid a monthly fee to users to cover reading and preparation, and an additional fee for attending the steering group and associated travel costs. Time was allowed for discussion with cancer service users before and after meetings to keep them well briefed.

Much of the research in health necessarily involves working collaboratively in a clinical context and with clinical colleagues. A major benefit of working in a clinical setting is the access it brings to health care professionals and to patients and patient data that would otherwise require lengthy negotiation. In particular, access to medical staff and medical networks can bring great benefits to the research process. From negotiating research ethics committees to gaining agreement from staff to participate in interviews or identify potential respondents, medical personnel add legitimacy to a research team. These benefits are often directly related to the seniority as well as the discipline of the staff member. In health care settings, status differentiation still runs along professional lines. For example, having the senior cancer consultant and ex-director of the Oncology Centre working in one of our projects helped to identify the names and location of key clinical managers within the eight area hospitals in the study. His experience of working in the local area for 20 years and his high profile in cancer care nationally helped to ensure that the team were well prepared when seeking access, as well as providing credibility to the project.

The challenges of adopting a mixed methods paradigm

The experience of working on a multidisciplinary project suggests that a number of common difficulties and challenges arise when working across different institutional and disciplinary cultures.

Balancing the research team

In developing a research proposal, balancing the composition of the project team with the requirements of the research design is one of the primary objectives. Projects that adopt mixed methods are likely to incorporate researchers from a range of disciplines. The specialization of individuals in particular methods may be a key justification for their inclusion in a research team. However, this can lead to a series of separate mini-research projects, each of which has been conducted independently. Such an approach may serve as a barrier to a common conceptualization of the research problem and the opportunity to adopt an integrated approach to the analysis and the interpretation of data. The benefits of using different methods and data through triangulation may be lost and this in turn may undermine the validity of the research findings.

The challenge for research management

The difficulties of research management are likely to be increased when research teams come from different institutions and/or there is a separation of research responsibilities. Inevitably, members of research teams who have had little history of working together and are drawn from different disciplinary backgrounds and work contexts will have different experiences and expectations of how to conduct research. Furthermore, applied research may be based on collaboration with staff who have little experience of research. Their expectations may be very different from those of the project team and funders. Lack of knowledge about work cultures, responsibilities and styles of working can lead to confusion, disagreements and inefficiency. Good project management, regular team meetings and investment of time in creating a common conceptualization of the whole project, the contribution of each objective to the project as a whole and their relationship to each other, are the best way to avoid fragmentation.

Many projects establish an advisory group as an aid to project management. Typically, such groups include representatives of stakeholders such as user groups, funding bodies, statutory authorities or independent experts with particular skills. These can be useful sources of advice and data for a project but can also add layers of communication that increase the administrative workload and may slow down decision making. It is important to establish roles and responsibilities at the start. Furthermore, the research team should be clear on what they want from an advisory group and prepare well for meetings.

Writing up results by research teams

The process of writing up and the attribution of authorship vary significantly between disciplines. For example, it is common in scientific disciplines for authorship to include the entire research team, while in the social sciences team members are credited in the text but do not necessarily appear as authors. As other chapters in this book point out, issues of authorship can cause unhappiness and conflict, so they are best tackled early. For a long-term project, items written late in the life of a project may cause particular difficulties. Junior members of the team may have left to take up other posts. Certain kinds of funding may not include time to write up findings for publication. Wherever possible, this should be costed and written into research proposals – as discussed further in Chapter 26.

Generating a common approach in mixed research projects

The issues raised above highlight the different forms of collaboration in research and also suggest the importance of working through differences in perspective and arriving at a consensus on an approach that is acceptable methodologically to all team members. The resulting research will be far more integrated and coherent and have greater potential to yield methodologically interesting results. However, collaborative research adopting mixed methods requires a great deal of time and contact early on in the project in order to learn about and from the different members of the research team.

Research that has an international aspect, because the study either draws data from different countries or involves researchers from different national backgrounds, presents particular challenges. Language differences themselves may make communication or comprehension difficult. If data are sourced in different languages, the costs of translation must be taken into account. Translation may hide rather than reveal different underlying cultural assumptions.

Conclusion

The use of a range of methods in a single research project is becoming the dominant paradigm in health research. Indeed, many of the chapters in this book illustrate these themes and Chapter 22 is devoted to the challenge of comparative research. Using mixed methods and working with colleagues both nationally and internationally can be achieved in small-scale as well as larger projects. There are both benefits and pitfalls and, as the research process becomes more complex, managing and planning the process becomes a major task.

In terms of using a number of methods in a single project, as argued in this chapter, it is extremely important to consider the purpose and value of employing particular methods when planning a project and to ensure appropriate expertise within the research team. The epistemological status of the data collected, that is the nature of data and the kind of knowledge produced, should also be considered. Where different methods are used, the purpose and added value to understanding should be examined carefully. A crucial decision to be made is the order of data collection using different methods. As has been demonstrated here and in other chapters, there may be an argument for first using a qualitative method, such as a focus group or in-depth interviews, to explore the concepts and understandings of the research participants. The insights gained may then be incorporated into a questionnaire to test the generalizability of a hypothesis or frequency of occurrence. However, there may also be an argument for an initial questionnaire to explore the frequency of a particular phenomenon, followed by, for example, in-depth interviews to investigate a different aspect of the phenomenon. A variety of combinations is possible, but it is vital that the reason for using a particular combination of methods and the associated value added are clear and that they fall within the available budget. An exercise to facilitate further understanding of some of the issues raised in this chapter is now included.

Exercise 24.1   Mixed methods research application to develop support for people with dementia and their carers

Dementia, 'a clinical syndrome of cognitive decline that is sufficiently severe to interfere with social or occupational functioning' (Chertkow et al. 2013: 52), is a significant and growing challenge globally and in the United Kingdom. Worldwide over 46.8 million people live with dementia (Prince, Wimo et al. 2015) and an estimated 767,000 in the UK, although this is predicted to increase to 872,000 by 2020 (Ahmadi-Abhari et al. 2017: 1). While both the cause of dementia and the level of impairment varies, the vast majority of care for people with dementia is delivered by carers who are typically relatives; there were an estimated 670,000 family carers in the United Kingdom in 2014 (Knapp et al. 2014). You have been asked to develop a proposal to identify the needs of carers for people with dementia in your local area. The findings are intended to be used to develop a package of support for those who care for people with dementia within a particular community.

The exercise is designed to encourage you to think about how to design research using mixed methods. While the material contained in this chapter may help you consider many of the issues, you may wish to access additional material from a library or the internet. If you want to prepare a formal answer, then write a research proposal or protocol.

1. What sort of methods will you use to map the number of carers within the community and identify their characteristics?
    *   Consider the range of possible sources of information, which will include patients, carers, voluntary organizations, health professionals and information leaflets.

(Continued)

(Continued)

- What types of data will you need to use and how should these be collected in order to link to latter phases of the research?

2. How will you select the sources of data that are relevant to ensure you are approaching the mapping process systematically?

- Consider what sort of methods you want to use and your need to generate a defined population and appropriate sampling frame.
- How will you manage generalizability?

3. Once you have mapped the carers and categorized them into salient types, how will you then go on to identify their needs?

- Consider the patient pathway and how you will ensure that your data reflect the needs of carers for people at different points in their journey through dementia? Here you need to consider not just the characteristics of the carer, but also the characteristics of the person with dementia for whom they care.
- How will you account for issues of co-morbidity?
- What forms of coding and analysis will be appropriate?

4. Once you have identified the needs of different types of carers and related these to different types of people with dementia, how will you link these findings back to your initial mapping exercise to ensure that the design of a support programme for carers for people with dementia is appropriate?

5. Can the data you collect be used to estimate the resources needed to provide the support?
- What mechanisms will you use to create a common analytical framework and the opportunity for joint interpretation of the findings?

6. What sort of resources will you need to undertake the research?

7. Can you plot the different activities over time and in relation to resources?

8. How do various types of project meeting fit into this timetable?

9. How will you present your findings and to whom?

10. What would be your plan for dissemination?

11. What are the implications for authorship?

12. How would you begin to cost your proposal?

Recommended further reading

This book engages explicitly with the challenges of integrating data from different data collection methods and the implications this has for the interpretation of results:

Bazeley, P. (2017) *Integrating Analyses in Mixed Methods Research*. London: Sage.

This is an accessible volume that includes chapters on writing up a mixed methods study for publication and evaluating the quality of mixed methods:
Cresswell, J. W. (2015) *A Concise Introduction to Mixed Methods Research*. London: Sage.

This is an interesting consideration of how qualitative and quantitative evidence can be synthesized together and influence clinical practice:
Dixon-Woods, M., Fitzpatrick, R. and Roberts, K. (2001) 'Including qualitative research in systematic reviews: Opportunities and problems', *Journal of Evaluation in Clinical Practice*, 7: 125–33.

This definitive book on the case study as a form of research usefully illustrates how to bring together a range of methods to generate a holistic understanding of specific areas:
Yin, R. (2018) *Case Study Research and Applications: Design and Methods*, 6th edition. London: Sage.

References

Ahmadi-Abhari, S., Guzman-Castillo, M., Bandosz, P., Shipley, M., Muniz-Terrera, G., Singh-Manoux, A., Kivimaki, M., Steptoe, A., Capewell, S., O'Flaherty, M. and Brunner, E. (2017) 'Temporal trend in dementia incidence since 2002 and projections for prevalence in England and Wales to 2040: Modelling study', *British Medical Journal*, *358*: j2856.

Bartlam, B., Waterfield, J., Bishop, A., Holden, M., Barlas, P., Ismail, K., Kettle, C. and Foster, N. (2016) 'The role of qualitative research in clinical trial development: The EASE back study', *Journal of Mixed Methods Research*. Available at: https://doi.org/10.1177/1558689816656740

Bowling, A. (2014) *Research Methods in Health: Investigating Health and Health Services*, 4th edition. Maidenhead: Open University Press.

Bury, M. (2001) 'Illness narratives: Fact or fiction?', *Sociology of Health and Illness*, *23*: 263–85.

Carlick, A. and Biley, F. C. (2004) 'Thoughts on the therapeutic use of narrative in the promotion of coping in cancer care', *European Journal of Cancer Care*, *13*(4): 308–17.

Chertkow, H., Felman, H., Jacova, C. and Massoud, F. (2013) 'Definitions of dementia and predementia states in Alzheimer's disease and vascular cognitive impairment: Consensus from the Canadian conference on diagnosis of dementia', *Alzheimer's Research and Therapy*, *5*(Suppl1): S2.

Conklin, A., Morris, Z. and Nolte, E. (2012) 'What is the evidence base for public involvement in health-care policy? Results of a systematic scoping review', *Health Expectations*, *18*(2): 153–65.

Copeland, L. (2003) 'An exploration of the problems faced by young women living in disadvantaged circumstances if they want to give up smoking: Can more be done at general practice level?', *Family Practice*, *20*(4): 393–400.

Cresswell, J. (2015) *A Concise Introduction to Mixed Methods Research*. London: Sage.

Daykin, N., Sanidas, M., Barley, V., Evans, S., McNeill, J., Palmer, N., Rimmer, J., Tritter, J. and Turton, P. (2002) 'Developing consensus and interprofessional working in cancer services: The case of user involvement', *Journal of Interprofessional Care, 16*(4): 405–6.

Denzin, N. (1970) *The Research Act*. Chicago, IL: Aldine.

Department of Health (2001) *The Expert Patient: A New Approach to Chronic Disease Management in the Twenty-first Century*. London: HMSO.

Dixon-Woods, M., Fitzpatrick, R. and Roberts, K. (2001) 'Including qualitative research in systematic reviews: Opportunities and problems', *Journal of Evaluation in Clinical Practice*, 7: 125–33.

Donovan, J., Brindle, L. and Mills, N. (2002) 'Capturing users' experiences of participating in cancer trials', *European Journal of Cancer Care, 11*(3): 210–14.

Ellwood, P., Asher, M., Billo, N., Bissell, K., Chiang, C.-Y., Ellwoed, E., El-Sony, A., Garcia-Marcos, L., Mallol, J., Marks, G., Pearce, N. and Strachan, D. (2017) 'The global asthma network rationale and methods for Phase I global surveillance: Prevalence severity, management and risk factors', *European Respiratory Journal, 49*(1). Available at: doi 10.1183/13993003.01605-2016

Evans, S., Tritter, J., Barley, V., Daykin, N., Sanidas, M., McNeill, J., Palmer, N., Rimmer, J., Sandidas, M. and Turton, P. (2003) 'User involvement in UK cancer services: Bridging the policy gap', *European Journal of Cancer Care, 12*(4): 331–8.

Frid, I., Ohlen, J. and Bergbom, I. (2000) 'On the use of narrative in nursing research', *Journal of Advanced Nursing, 32*: 695–703.

Hall, D. and Stacey, M. (eds) (1979) *Beyond Separation: Further Studies of Children in Hospital*. London: Routledge & Kegan Paul.

Jha, P. and Peto, R. (2014) 'Global effects of smoking, of quitting, and of taxing tobacco', *New England Journal of Medicine, 370*: 60–8.

Kleinman, A. (1988) *The Illness Narratives*. New York: Basic Books.

Knapp, M., Black, N., Dixon, J., Damant, J., Rehill, A. and Tan, S. (2014) *Independent Assessment of Improvements in Dementia Care and Support since 2009*. London: Policy Innovation Research Unit and NIHR School for Social Care Research.

Mackay, J. and Eriksen, M. (2002) *The Tobacco Atlas*. Geneva: World Health Organization.

O'Cathain, A., Murphy, E. and Nicholl, J. (2008) 'The quality of mixed methods studies in health services research', *Journal of Health Services Research and Policy, 13*: 92–8.

Øvretveit, J. (2009) 'The contribution of new social science research to patient safety', *Social Science and Medicine*, *69*(12): 1780–3.

Pope, C., Mays, N. and Popay, J. (2007) *Synthesizing Qualitative and Quantitative Health Research: A Guide to Methods*. Maidenhead: Open University Press.

Prince, M., Wimo, A., Guerchet, M., Ali, G.-C., Wu, Y.-T. and Prina, M. (2015) *World Alzheimer Report 2015. The Global Impact of Dementia: An Analysis of Prevalence, Incidence, Cost and Trends*. London: Alzheimer's Disease International.

Prince, M., Wu, F., Guo, Y., Robledo, L., O'Donnell, M., Sullivan, R. and Yusuf, S. (2015) 'The burden of disease in older people and implications for health policy and practice', *The Lancet*, *385*(9667): 549–62.

Silverman, D. (2011) *Interpreting Qualitative Data: Methods for Analysing Talk, Text and Interaction*, 3rd edition. London: Sage.

Stacey, M., Dearden, R., Pill, R. and Robinson, S. (1970) *Hospitals, Children and their Families*. London: Routledge & Kegan Paul.

Tashakkori, A. and Teddlie, C. (2010) *Handbook of Mixed Methods in Social and Behavioural Research*, 2nd edition. Los Angeles, CA: Sage.

Tritter, J. and McCallum, A. (2006) 'The snakes and ladders of user involvement: Moving beyond Arnstein', *Health Policy*, *76*(2): 156–68.

Wanless, D. (2004) *Securing Good Health for the Whole Population*. London: HMSO.

Yin, R. (2018) *Case Study Research and Applications: Design and Methods*, 6th edition. London: Sage.

25

Online Research in Health

DENIS ANTHONY

Introduction

This chapter shows some of the ways to use online resources in health research. It looks not only at internet-based data sources but also more widely at some of the clinical databases to illustrate the advantages and limitations of using these for research. In general, using internet-based resources can make health research quicker and less labour intensive with rapid access to data and references. It can also provide tools to carry out data collection and analysis. However, researchers may have to learn how to use the tools available and not all health data are available to researchers. Some clinical databases are closed systems for reasons of patient confidentiality. These systems may be web-based but are on intranets rather than on the public internet with wider access – such as those that are part of hospital information and support systems (HISS).

The chapter draws on examples of my own work and that of colleagues with whom I have collaborated in research. These are not necessarily the best, and certainly not the only, examples, but they are studies where I have had access to the data and am aware of the difficulties that can be encountered in both identifying useable data and interpreting such data. Articles on methodology and methods often take the view that if general principles are followed, then research is straightforward and choices obvious. This is not always the case.

In practice, researchers may follow appropriate methods, but meet with obstacles and they must find ways around problems. Failures in the early stages can often lead to finding ways forward that work better. For example, one of my doctoral students was given permission to use the mailing list of the Tissue Viability Society as a way to reach nurses and other health professionals who were considered experts in dealing with wound care. This seemed sensible but there were few responses to his requests to participate in a research project. He then looked at all the webpages of all the health trusts in the UK to find a named person who dealt with this aspect of care and sent them an individual invitation. This approach was more effective in obtaining respondents who were willing to take part.

At the start of all research the researcher needs to assemble the background information. This usually includes searching the internet so I will explore this next.

Tools for research online

The internet can be used for a variety of research tasks. This section aims to identify the possibilities together with some of the advantages and pitfalls.

Using search engines

While for many people searching the internet is synonymous with Google (which has roughly three-quarters of market share), there are other options. Commercial search engines, including Yahoo and Bing, may also be used to search the internet. Wikipedia currently lists 14 general search engines, of which 10 are multilingual or English-language based. There are also many specialized search engines, such as gopubmed for searching publications, pubmed, the freely available gateway to Medline, which is the United States National Library of Medicine® bibliographic database, and Health Line (www.healthline.com/), another source for health information.

Researchers should be aware that different results may be obtained from a search using the same terms but in different search engines. One reason for this is advertisers can pay in some systems to appear higher in the list of results shown. This is referred to in the jargon as 'bubbling'. The search engine is set to guess what a user may want based on their search history and other factors, such as their geographical location. This is a disadvantage for the researcher as it may serve to reinforce their viewpoint as they will be shown only material that fits their search profile. This will exclude items they are likely to disagree with, or these may be listed but given a lower priority. Hence, the user is kept in a bubble – the origin of the term, 'bubbling'.

An alternative search engine for general searches is duckduckgo (https://duckduckgo.com/) that does not track users. It never keeps data on users and does not show adverts. It therefore avoids 'bubbling'. Other general search engines include Yahoo (https://uk.yahoo.com/) and Bing (www.bing.com/). You will get different results from each engine, so it may be worth using an alternative search engine if you do not find what you want. Both Yahoo (as stated on its website) and Bing employ bubbling (see www.tawannadillahunt.com/wp-content/uploads/2015/03/SESAndSearchv8-final.pdf).

Bibliographic databases

Some of the most useful online resources are bibliographic databases. These include databases that relate to specific health professions. For medicine, pubmed gives free to access to the National Library of Medicine (www.ncbi.nlm.nih.gov/pubmed) and for nursing and allied professions, the Cumulative Index to Nursing and Allied Health Literature (CINAHL) is available on subscription. Students or members of staff in a United Kingdom university and those who work in the National Health Service or other health services are likely to have access to subscription services for CINAHL, so ask your librarian to assist. For example, if a researcher wanted to update themselves on a given topic, such as the effects of using cannabis to treat people with schizophrenia, including both its use and the withdrawal effects, there will be a database to identify all relevant studies. These studies can be read and the researcher can come to a view based on the evidence.

However, for any given topic, students should first check whether a systematic review of the literature has already been undertaken. This can be done by accessing the Cochrane Collaboration (www.cochrane.org/) which is a specialized database for completed systematic reviews. Consulting this prior to doing a review can save time and labour for the researcher. Chapter 4 also considers how to do systematic reviews.

Reference management systems are a useful tool to file and order multiple references. EndNote, RefMan and Procite are examples of reference management systems. The system I use is EndNote, but all systems are comparable. It is possible with these systems to access Medline, CINAHL or many other databases and to download references directly in a format the reference management system can read. The university or hospital library will probably have a resource guide showing how to access these systems.

Using clinical databases

Data that used to be held on paper records in hospitals and clinics are now normally kept electronically in a database. While such data are collected by clinicians for clinicians, they are also a potential source of interest for researchers. These data sets are potentially huge, but the researcher should be aware that data that has already been collected may not be in a form that suits their purpose exactly. It may not be as accurate as they would like either. For example, data may be missing in a data set for reasons unknown. Nevertheless, the researcher may have to accept such data as the best that are available.

Data that are collected prospectively – that is, as a study develops – are more accurate and reliable as the conditions for collection can be controlled more easily. For example, randomized controlled trials (RCTs) collect data prospectively. This allows the cases to be selected from a population through randomization and the items recorded and standardized during an ongoing trial. However, prospective studies are expensive and, in some situations, not possible. The analysis of an existing data set may be the only way forward. Chapter 14 discusses these issues further.

Data collected for clinical purposes are termed 'epidemiological' data. That is, they have the potential to tell us about patterns or trends in the incidence of illness, treatments and outcomes in populations. However, such databases, although potentially useful, are tricky to analyse. Looking at raw data is problematic. It is often possible to see patterns, but are these patterns real or a creation of the researcher? Further exploration may show the apparent relationships are a mirage, as will be shown in Case Study 25.2 towards the end of this chapter.

Prospective data are also easier to analyse. For example, in an RCT, it can be assumed that both groups start with no significant differences. Therefore, any difference that is found at the end of the study may be attributed reasonably to the intervention. This is never true of epidemiological data which are correspondingly much harder to analyse as we cannot assume groups are similar and have to account for such differences.

If clinical data are to be used for research, ethical approval to proceed will probably be required. There is a grey area if the work is considered service development rather than research as the former may not require scrutiny by an ethics committee. But if the work is not considered research, it may prove difficult to get it published as research. As a rule, if I want to use data from such systems I always ask the relevant ethics committee for their advice. The committee may decide ethical review is not needed, but they will want to make that decision, so always ask them.

Even if approval has been given to access clinical data, records will have to be anonymized if they are to be used in a research project and details kept in a secure place. Depending on the study design, there can be further problems. For example, if a patient's pathway is to be followed through different stages of the care system, an identification marker will be needed to track the patient's progress. The mechanism used for identification must be unrelated to patient's hospital number and must be specially created.

A further common problem is then getting the data into a usable format. Some systems for analysis expect the data to be inputted first into proprietary packages like Excel for further analysis by IT staff or others. Even if a researcher is not using Excel, it can nevertheless be helpful to do so as many packages read Excel formats. However useful these systems may be for analysis, I have had to sometimes write computer programs to change one format into another for ease of use.

Sometimes clinical databases are the only ethical source of research data. Imagine you wanted to see if tobacco smoke was harmful to humans. Would you set up an RCT where half of the population were given tobacco to smoke while a control group did not receive it? Or would you look at cancer and other disease rates among smokers compared with non-smokers? Clearly, taking the epidemiological route is more sensible and ethical. As smokers are different from non-smokers in a variety of ways (such as in relation to gender, ethnic group, age, social class and education level), you need to account for the differences in some way, but there are methods such as regression analysis and different techniques that will allow this to be done (Vanderos et al. 2013).

Employing the internet to collect and analyse data

Using on online surveys

There are several systems to support the use of surveys electronically. A commonly used system is SurveyMonkey (www.surveymonkey.com/). This is a commercial product, but for small surveys (up to 10 questions and up to 100 respondents) it is free to use so can be employed for training purposes at no cost. Online course systems like Blackboard also have e-survey facilities embedded within them.

Online surveys need the same attention to detail as traditional paper-based surveys. The design of the survey needs to address issues such as the size of the questionnaire. You will need to have sufficient relevant items to answer your research questions. There can be a temptation to ask anything that might later be useful. However, too many questions will put people off and give a low response rate. Furthermore, if the items do not directly address the research question, it is unlikely the results from these items will be useful or used.

A response to a survey question may be closed or open. Open responses are useful to collect qualitative data. Closed responses can be analysed by statistical methods that may be descriptive – such as mean or median values, measure of dispersion like standard deviation or inferential. Inferential tests can include group differences. For example, they can establish if the control group is different from the treatment group. Correlation studies explore whether one variable is correlated with another – which does not necessarily mean one causes the other as they both may be related to a third variable. Regression analysis is where variables are used to predict some outcome that may be continuous – blood pressure or serum glucose, for instance – or binary, offering two choices only, such as died/did not die.

Closed questions can have single or multiple responses. Thus gender (male/female) or ethnic group (using the UK census definitions) will be closed with a single response. However, a question on, say, where a respondent saw health information (TV, radio, press, websites or social media) may have multiple responses as the information could have been seen on more than one platform. Online surveys typically have a variety of open and closed items. Open items may be free text. Closed items can force one response only or allow several responses with tick boxes or a similar device. Using free text to allow respondents to give closed responses is ill advised for several reasons, not least as it gives more work to the respondent and responses may not be subject to consistent categorization.

If SurveyMonkey or other online survey tools are being used, these can be exported to an Excel file. Data can be analysed in Excel or other spreadsheet packages that read Excel files. However, these are not ideal for serious statistical use. Using SPSS and other statistical packages, which can input Excel files, will analyse data more powerfully. Where a single response from a closed question is found, it will be put into one variable, but multiple responses will be placed into as many variables as there are possible responses. The data can normally be imported as numerical values (for instance, 0 for male and 1 for female) or labels (such as 'male' and 'female'). In most cases it is easier to import numerical values into a package and use the labelling facility (as found in SPSS, for example) to allow these numbers to be presented as meaningful outputs in reports and graphs (see Chapters 17 and 18).

Using the e-Delphi method

The Delphi method is a process whereby a group of experts is used to generate new ideas on a topic. It was first employed to estimate the number of atom bombs the Russians would have needed to destroy United States industry (Dalkey and Helmer-Hirschberg 1962). It is now used widely in health research and some examples are given below. The process is typically conducted in three rounds:

- Round 1: Experts are invited anonymously to contribute their ideas on the subject in question and these individual responses are then summarized and circulated among the panel, typically in the form of a questionnaire.
- Round 2: Panel members then individually rank their level of agreement with each statement and these individual responses are then summarized and circulated to the panel with a repeat questionnaire.
- Round 3: Panel members are given the opportunity to revise their opinions in the light of the findings of the previous round and these results are again summarized and fed back to the panel.

Early Delphi used surface mail to send questions and get responses. Now it would be more usual to employ email or e-surveys (Holloway 2012).

A classic example of using online methods to conduct a Delphi study was the Diagnostic Instruments for Autism in Deaf Children's Study (DIADS) conducted by the University of York, Leeds and York Partnership NHS Foundation Trust, Newcastle University and the University of Manchester (Wright et al. 2018). Delphi was selected partly because the experts were few in number and spread across the globe, making meetings in person difficult. There are other benefits in using online Delphi: the anonymity of responses can be preserved so that any bias due to perceived status, for example, can be removed. In the autism study, SurveyMonkey was used to collect data and the results were then transferred to SPSS for analysis.

Online ethnography

Ethnographic methods can be adapted to study cultures using computer-mediated social interaction (Wikipedia 2017). As with conventional ethnography, the researcher may be a participant or not (a 'lurker' in online parlance) in the community under study. Communities may be Facebook groups, email lists or online gamers, for example. The researcher needs to be mindful that the *persona* demonstrated online may have little resemblance to the real-life person who creates it.

Web-based experiments (Wikipedia 2018b) have been used in a variety of disciplines, including psychology. One advantage is access to subjects across the globe, but disadvantages include greater difficulty in establishing control over the selection of participants or even knowing whether a participant exists. Examples of the use of this research method have included sound perception and attitudes of jurors to expert witnesses, which both may have relevance for health.

Tools for content analysis and network analysis online

Just as paper studies employ content analysis to develop items and themes from data collected, online content analysis uses data from the internet. The methods employed for online data are essentially those used for paper material. One difference is scope. A paper copy has a specific boundary, for example an article in a paper or an interview transcript. Online material is less easy to define as there may be links from one page to another or threads in discussions. Thus, a researcher must be clear about the unit of data being analysed. For example, this may be a website or a webpage or an email list or bulletin board. A drawback is that all the items listed can change rapidly. It is therefore necessary to say when the data were collected by noting the date of collection.

While online data can be analysed by hand or entered into a qualitative analysis package such as NVivo, there are additional advantages for data that are already in digital form. The data can be analysed by machine methods. For instance, the researcher can label a set of data and use this to train a machine learning algorithm. Thus, the existing social media data set that was associated with HIV and coded by an HIV domain expert, employed four types of machine learning to learn patterns associated with HIV risk behaviour (Young, Wu and Wang 2017). A dictionary method is where the researcher selects keywords for each category and then the machine uses these to classify each text into a category – as in the case of prescription opioid keywords identified in tweets and machine learning employed to detect the illegal use of such drugs, as described in more detail below (Mackey et al. 2017).

Social network analysis (Wikipedia 2018a) investigates social structures through the use of networks and graph theory. It is widely employed in sociology and is increasingly used in psychology. Examples include signed graphs to show good and bad relationships between humans. Positive edges between nodes, which are linked to each other in strength and direction, indicate alliance or other positive relationships (such as dating) or show hatred and other negative relationships. The purpose is to predict the evolution of the overall relationship pattern. For example, a group may be *unlikely* to change their views and hence opinions of others, or they are predicted as *likely* to change their views.

Using social media for research

Social media is used extensively to disseminate health information on matters of personal health and especially in relation to promoting and researching public health. It will continue to be a useful tool to access groups that are otherwise hard to reach, but also to gather information that may be useful for policy makers. For example, as will be seen, social media can be used to track infectious disease outbreaks and prevent the spread of infection.

An example of research using social media is the study by Mackey and colleagues (2017) of the use of social media in marketing controlled substances online. They analysed 619,937 tweets containing the keywords codeine, percocet, fentanyl, vicodin, oxycontin, oxycodone, and hydrocodone over a five-month period and found that a small proportion (< 1 per cent) were identified as marketing the sale of controlled substances online. They concluded that it was possible to identify illegal online sellers of controlled drugs using this method. While the numbers of tweets were huge and the number appearing to engage in criminal activity a very small proportion, unsupervised machine learning (where the computer is not given the rules for working out a solution) reduced the number down to a more manageable and focused quantity that could be further analysed by other methods involving human researchers.

Tweets were also used to estimate numbers with Dengue Fever, a mosquito-borne viral disease, with an estimated annual incidence of 390 million infections, and to forecast the likely spread over a period up to eight weeks with high accuracy at both country and city level (Marques-Toledo et al. 2017). The level of public concern over the spread of the Zika virus in the areas affected in Brazil was also evaluated by analysing tweets, Google Trends, Google News, YouTube and Wikipedia search queries (Bragazzi et al. 2017). The majority of queries concerned the symptoms of the Zika virus, its vector of transmission and its possible effect on babies, including the onset of microcephaly. These same social media outlets were also employed to disseminate health information to those who were seeking information on the disease.

Specialist tools available online

There are a number of online tools available for the health researcher that can be downloaded, although they are also available on paper. For example, there are several risk assessment scales available for download to study a range of conditions such as pressure ulcers (for example, Waterlow, Glamorgan, Braden), coma (for instance, the Glasgow coma scale) and many other conditions. There are also health questionnaires such as the RAND 36-Item Short Form Health Survey or the shorter SF-12 Health Survey, both widely used in health research. These are freely available for users.

A number of other electronic tools are also available on the internet that are freely available for specialized tasks. An example already cited in the book is the tool for systematic reviewing. Just looking at this one topic, there are several online resources. One of these is the Rayyan systematic review web-based system that is free (Ouzzani et al. 2016). This gives each reviewer access to the reference list. They are then able to upload the full studies, as shown in Figure 25.1.

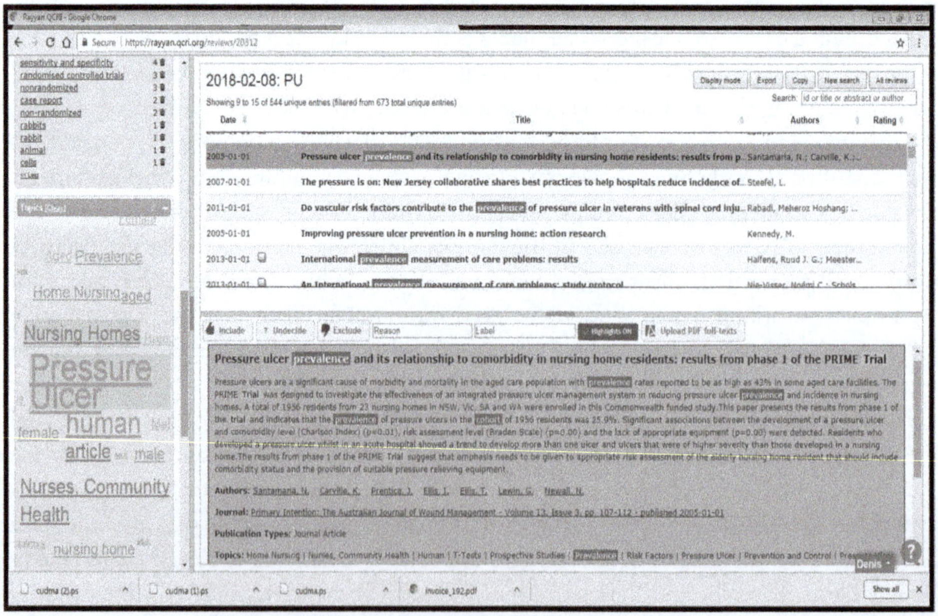

FIGURE 25.1   Rayyan showing a list of uploaded articles

Reviewers can be blinded to the results of other reviewers. The purpose of Rayyan is not to automate the process of reviewing, but to streamline the workflow and allow easier collaboration between reviewers. It enables each paper to be downloaded only once onto a shared registry. Papers can be filtered with a variety of methods, including MeSH keywords. A similarity analysis is inbuilt that allows papers to be placed on a cluster graph based on distance metrics, which measure how close one article is to another in relation to such aspects as title and abstract content and authors.

Another example is the RevMan downloadable software from the Cochrane Collaboration that is used for preparing and maintaining Cochrane Reviews. Prospero (www.crd.york. ac.uk/PROSPERO/) is a web-based system where prospective systematic reviews are described and can be added to by prospective reviewers.

It is impossible to list all the available software and materials that might be employed in a research study. If you need something, look in one of the general or subject-specific search engines or go to a site known to have your interest as a topic. For systematic reviews, the Cochrane Collaboration would be a sensible place to start. Other places to look include medical charities such as Arthritis Research UK (www.arthritisresearchuk.org/) or the Alzheimer's Society (www.alzheimers.org.uk/). I use Wikipedia frequently (https://en.wikipedia.org/wiki/Main_Page), although some academics frown on its use as it is not peer reviewed. However, in my experience it is at least as accurate as any other publication and is extremely extensive. Most errors are corrected quickly by online editors or bots (small computer programs that scour the web cleaning up minor errors such as grammatical or spelling errors).

Video conferencing

It is expensive to meet face to face, especially if collaborators are geographically remote. An alternative is video conferencing. This may be utilized in dedicated suites found in universities and other large organizations. However, cheap, and even free, video conferencing is available and can be employed on standard PCs, laptops, tablets and smart phones. Skype is a commonly used system that allows free video conferencing between two users. Upgrading to a paid subscription allows additional facilities such as multiple users (more than two) being able to video conference. Whichever system is used, other conference attendees will need to have the relevant software installed.

Video conferencing can be used to give seminars and to collect research data. For instance, a clinician may be shown a patient to make an assessment that may later become data in a study. Examples include showing a wound to a tissue viability nurse. Video conferencing methods can also be used to conduct online interviews or online focus groups. Online meeting organizers such as doodle (https://doodle.com/) also have a place in research. They can be used to arrange a best date/time for all conference attendees and Eventbrite (www. eventbrite.com) provides a forum for selling (or giving for no charge) tickets of conferences or seminars (or any event).

Using online storage

Many research files are large and sending by email is not appropriate or even possible in certain cases. There may also be other files and papers that researchers want to share and there are several options for storing large files on the internet. File transfer protocol (ftp) is one option. Created in 1971 and running on a predecessor to the internet, it is a mature technology. It ran on Network Control Program (NCP), but now allows a user to transfer files across the internet. These sites can be password protected so only those with relevant permission can access or deposit data. While the protocol underpinning ftp has been around for nearly half a century, there are modern 'clients' or programs that allow access to ftp sites that are web-based. Indeed, it is possible to access ftp sites within most web browsers, with password permission. There are alternatives to ftp such as Dropbox (www.dropbox.com), which performs a similar task by allowing distributed access to files to users around the globe. Dropbox uses a premium business model: users are given a free account with a set storage size (currently two gigabytes), but have to upgrade to a subscription service beyond that storage capacity.

Three case studies now follow that illustrate the use of online research in health.

CASE STUDY 25.1

Community interventions for health

The Community Interventions for Health (CIH) programme was a public health intervention in three countries: Mexico, India and China (Dyson et al. 2015). It had a methodology team based in the United States and the principal investigators and the statistician were based in the United Kingdom. While face-to-face meetings were arranged throughout the study, there was a need to have a place to store data. These data sets were large, as there were over 36,000 participants – 6,000 in the community, 12,000 schoolchildren, 16,200 employees in various workplaces and 2,400 in clinical centres. Data on each subject were substantial (questionnaires on diet, physical activity and tobacco and clinical measurements such as blood pressure, height, weight and serum values). In a second stage, data were collected again on a similar number of different participants in the same areas after interventions designed to improve risk factors for health. In all, the study therefore included around 72,000 participants.

Sending data by email was not an option. The files were far too large. Furthermore, there were separate files on each of the four areas (community, workplace, schools and clinical sites) and in some cases more than one file (for instance, one for a survey, another for serum values) and there were additional files for process evaluation and scans of the geographical area. Then all the files were repeated on follow-up.

All data were anonymized. Each country site had access to an ftp site. These were organized with separate folders for each site, area and timeline (pre- or post-intervention).

Having security with password protection was a priority for, although the data were anonymized, the research team did not want public access to the data until it was fully cleaned and fit for purpose. By cleaning, I mean removing obvious errors and thorough checking to ensure the data were consistent. For example, if one country had additional questions (to address local issues) not asked in the other sites, a combined data set would not include them. My job was to combine all the data from the different sites into SPSS files and perform the analyses. Fortunately, SPSS has effective methods for merging files. We used the ftp site that has a useful way of locking the data. At a certain point, when data had been checked and cleaned as far as was practical, the files were locked so they could not be edited or replaced. This meant any future analysis of data, which was publicly available, would use the same data sets. There is an ongoing analysis of our files by the Bill and Melissa Gates Foundation, where the aim is to establish whether the results reported by us are reliable.

This study shows how online methods allow the various research groups to share data, but also facilitate greater transparency by allowing external audit.

Clostridium Difficile and religion

A report was made to me by clinical staff in a city in the Midlands in the United Kingdom that Muslim patients did not seem to be getting the Clostridium Difficile infection. This was of great interest as C Difficile was a serious problem in the local hospital and indeed across the country at the time. Anything that might reduce the risk would be valuable. Could it be the diet of Muslims that protected them or was ritual washing a protective factor?

The IT section at the hospital provided me with a file that included the variables: gender, age, religion, ethnic group and whether the patient developed Clostridium Difficile-Associated Diarrhoea (CDAD). This file was not in a format that could be directly imported into SPSS but with a bit of work, employing Excel as an interim package, we were able to get the data into the right format and analyse it.

What was immediately obvious was that Muslim patients did get CDAD but at a much lower rate than other religions. There are several infections that appear to be affected by ethnicity. For example, white females have been more susceptible to rubella than black females (Kotzen and Mets 1988) so there was a possible link.

The sample size for the study was large – 208,604 patients, 2,476 of whom had been diagnosed with CDAD during their hospital stay, so the study was well powered. This suggested that, if there was a significant effect, it was highly likely we would see it. The advantage of using existing databases is their size. Prospective studies have smaller numbers.

Background demographic

The majority (79 per cent) of CDAD cases were inpatients aged more than 65. Although Asian patients make up 13 per cent of the hospital's patients, only 7 per cent

(Continued)

CASE STUDY 25.2

(Continued)

of patients aged over 65 years were Asian. Among Asians in Leicester, on which the study was focused, Muslims are younger than the majority Hindu population. In 1972, Hindus arrived in large numbers after Idi Amin expelled all Asians from Uganda. Muslim migrants are more recent, and this explains why they are younger as a group.

Method

We decided to undertake a multivariate analysis of the populations concerned, with religion as a given factor. This allowed us to examine a range of variables in measuring CDAD against religion and to take into account age, gender and any other factors that could be relevant to developing CDAD. Then, if there was a difference remaining, it could be real – although only if you have accounted for all the relevant factors. Using the statistical technique binary logistic regression, we were able to see if it was religion or age or both that explain the lower rate of infection in Muslims in Leicester. Binary logistic regression gives a binary outcome (yes/no, disease/ no disease, died/did not die) and includes several explanatory variables, such as religion, age and gender. Here our binary outcome was CDAD (yes/no).

Findings

Once SPSS is running, the analysis is relatively simple, and it showed that all the differences for C Difficile between Muslims and other religions was entirely explained by their age. There was no protective factor, it was just that Muslims in Leicester tend to be younger and less likely to have CDAD on that basis (Tanner et al. 2008).

This is similar to another study I undertook with colleagues in Burton, also using existing data from their HISS system, where it was seen with raw data that people of Pakistani origin were less likely to develop pressure ulcers. There are studies that show differences among ethnic groups with respect to these ulcers, though the studies are not of high quality. We found again age was the relevant factor. Older people of Pakistani heritage were as likely to develop pressure ulcers as any other ethnic group (Anthony et al. 2002).

Systematic review of pressure ulcer prevalence and incidence

I am currently engaged in a systematic review. The idea came from an interest in pressure ulcer incidence and prevalence in care homes and nursing homes. All components of the study are done online or use software.

There are many systematic reviews of hospital patients in intensive care units (Keller et al. 2002; Shanin, Dassen and Halfen 2008), paediatric units (Kottner, Wilorn and Dassen 2010) and acute care (Tubaishat et al. 2017). Moore, Johanssen and van Etten (2013) looked at the incidence in all care settings (hospitals, hospices, children,

CASE STUDY 25.3

community and care homes), but the study covered only Ireland, Denmark, Sweden, Norway and Iceland. In this study, the long-term care incidence was 6.6 per cent (95 per cent confidence interval 3.1–8.4 per cent), albeit in only five long-term sites – none of them in the United Kingdom.

Method

Our first task was to find out if there were systematic reviews of incidence and prevalence of pressure ulcers in care homes or nursing homes. Systematic reviews are very time-consuming and expensive. A good review is often worth the money as it identifies all studies of quality, summarizes them, assesses the level of quality and is able to form the basis for detailed guidelines or clinical pathways. Thus, National Institute of Health and Care Excellence (NICE) guidelines in the United Kingdom are typically based on systematic reviews.

Literature review

There are online resources where we can look for systematic reviews. The best known is the Cochrane Collaboration. We entered some search strings that would be expected to locate systematic reviews of pressure ulcer incidence and prevalence in care and nursing homes. We found none. This does not mean none exists, but if such a study had been conducted it would probably be found in Cochrane (see also Chapter 21 and other chapters in this book).

Clearly, if another team was planning to do such a study and had submitted its protocol, we would be ill advised to continue with our plan, so we looked on Prospero.

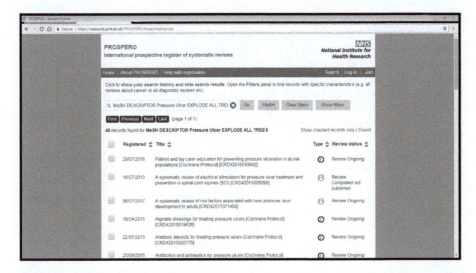

Figure 25.2 Prospero register of systematic reviews

(Continued)

(Continued)

We searched on the MeSH keyword 'pressure ulcers'. This gave only 40 results, as shown in Figure 25.2. So we looked at all the titles of the research, rather than refine our search as surely any relevant protocol would have this MeSH heading.

None covered the ground of our proposed study, so we went ahead and placed a new protocol on Prospero. This involved registering with Prospero, but this is simple and free. A portion of the protocol is seen in Figure 25.3.

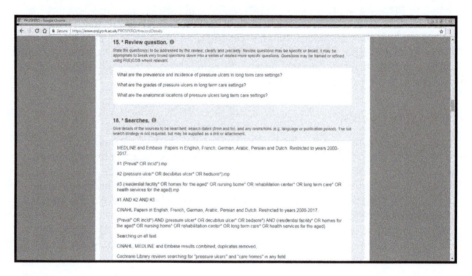

FIGURE 25.3 Part of a systematic review proposal

We did an exploratory search using the search criteria and databases in the protocol and found several hundred papers that fitted the initial inclusion criteria. Many of these were in German or Dutch. Often reviews are limited to English and normally with prevalence reviews this would be adequate. For, unlike reviews of treatments where one ground-breaking study might change the evidence base, one more or one less prevalence figure is unlikely to make much difference. But the papers in German or Dutch were largely studies with primary data and those in English (mostly based in the United States) used secondary data from databases collected by insurance organizations. We did not feel we could ignore the primary studies, so we invited colleagues from Germany with specific experience in the field to join the team. We communicated by email and Skype to develop the design for our study.

With co-researchers in two cities in England and a further site in Germany it was useful to create a common repository for the papers and some way of organizing and coordinating our review. We shall use the Rayyan system. In this system, two reviewers will be blind to both the selection of papers and the assessment of quality of selected papers. Quality will be evaluated using the Joanna Briggs Institute Critical Appraisal Instrument for Studies Reporting Prevalence Data (Munn et al. 2017).

Overview

To accomplish the proposed study, I did not have to leave my home. I could contact all the potential collaborators by email/Skype/telephone. I could find out if the study had already been done by looking online at Cochrane and even see what was planned by looking in Prospero. I could obtain abstracts of potential papers via bibliographic databases. I could access full papers of articles that looked interesting.

I can apply for funding online (in fact in most cases you cannot apply any other way). In due course, if the study goes ahead, I will be able to conduct the reviews collaboratively (with blinding) and rate studies using Rayyan. I found all the tools for assessing papers and those for evaluating search strategies on the web. A final paper can be submitted online and reviewers of the paper will review it online, although they may print it out as paper still has some advantages, such as you can take it to the beach, read it in the bath and write all over it.

Conclusion

There has been a revolution over the last 20 years in the way health research is conducted. The technology has been around for rather longer, but health is broadly in line with most disciplines in terms of adoption. It first adopted computing, and then took on board distributed computing – that is, computers connected in a network with the ability to access information at your computer from other computers online.

Online resources have made collaborative research easier and more efficient in terms of human capital and financial costs. In some cases, online methods allow new techniques to be exploited, such as machine learning. Some online research methods used in sociology, psychology and other disciplines seem to have been little used in health research, but they may be particularly useful in nursing, midwifery and the allied health professions.

Exercise 25.1 Evaluation of a risk reduction scheme for paediatric pressure ulcers

You have been asked to evaluate a risk reduction scheme for paediatric pressure ulcers. The scheme has been running for a year in four paediatric (including neonatal units) hospitals in the United Kingdom. Data have been collected by the tissue viability nurse at each site and entered into a spreadsheet. The data consist of demographic data on the children (such as age and gender), items of the risk tool, and clarify whether the child developed a pressure ulcer and, if so, the grade and

(Continued)

(Continued)

location. What online methods might you employ to undertake this work? The aim is to identify methods from this chapter that could be useful.

Consider what data are available and how to get the data into a form you can analyse. Consider how you will write your report. Do you need to review the literature and, if so, where should you look? Can you find a review that already exists? What methods will you employ to analyse the data?

Recommended further reading

There are more recent books on statistics, but the chapter on manipulating data from the internet and elsewhere remains very useful:

Anthony, D. M. (2011) *Statistics for Health, Life and Social Sciences*. Copenhagen: BookBoon (Ventus Publishing Aps). Available at: https://bookboon.com/.

This book covers a wide range of social media and the lessons are transferable to health:

Lance, K. (2017) *#GetSocialSmart: How to Hone Your Social Media Strategy*. CreateSpace Independent Publishing Platform.

This book considers social media and big data with a specific focus on health, covering such areas as communicating with the community in epidemics, using social media to change behaviour and managing the huge data sets generated in social media:

Syed-Abdul, S., Gabarron, E. and Lau, A. (2016) *Participatory Health Through Social Media*. Cambridge, MA: Academic Press.

This is an excellent text on the Delphi technique specific to nursing research, but is also relevant to wider health research:

Keeney, S., McKenna, H. and Hasson, F. (2010) *The Delphi Technique in Nursing and Health Research*. Chichester: Wiley-Blackwell.

References

Anthony, D. M., Johnson, M., Reynolds, T. and Russell, L. (2002) 'Ethnicity in pressure ulcer risk assessment, with specific relation to the Pakistani ethnic minority in Burton, England', *Journal of Advanced Nursing*, *38*: 592–7.

Bragazzi, N. L., Alicino, C., Trucchi, C., Paganino, C., Barberis, I., Martini, M., Sticchi, L., Trinka, E., Brigo, F., Ansaldi, F., Icardi, G. and Orsi, A. (2017) 'Global reaction to the recent outbreaks of Zika virus: Insights from a Big Data analysis', *PLoS One*. Available at: https://doi.org/10.1371/journal.pone.0185263

Dalkey, N. and Helmer-Hirschberg, O. (1962) *An Experimental Application of the Delphi Method to the Use of Experts*. Santa Monica, CA: RAND Corporation.

Dyson, P. A., Anthony, D., Fenton, B., Stevens, D. E., Champagne, B., Li, L. M., Lv, J., Ramírez Hernández, J., Thankappan, K. R., Matthews, D. R. and Community Interventions for Health (2015) 'Successful up-scaled population interventions to reduce risk factors for non-communicable disease in adults: Results from the International Community Interventions for Health (CIH) Project in China, India and Mexico', *PLoS One*. Available at: https://doi.org/10.1371/journal.pone.0120941

Holloway, K. (2012) 'Doing the E-Delphi: Using online survey tools', *Computers Informatics Nursing*, *30*: 347–50.

Keller, B. P., Wille, J., van Ramshorst, B. and van der Wereken, C. (2002) 'Pressure ulcers in intensive care patients: A review of risks and prevention', *Intensive Care Medicine*, *28*: 1379–88.

Kottner, J., Wilborn, D. and Dassen, T. (2010) 'Frequency of pressure ulcers in the paediatric population: A literature review and new empirical data', *Intnational Journal of Nursing Studies*, *47*: 1330–40.

Kotzen, I. and Mets, J. (1988) 'Rubella sensitivity in young women: An occupational hazard in hospitals', *South African Medical Journal*, *74*: 62–5.

Mackey, T. K., Kalyanam, J., Katsuki, T. and Lanckriet, G. (2017) 'Twitter-based detection of illegal online sale of prescription opioid', *American Journal of Public Health*, *107*: 1910–15.

Marques-Toledo, C. A., Degener, C. M., Vinhal, L., Coelho, G., Meira, W., Codeco, C. T. and Teixeira, M. M. (2017) 'Dengue prediction by the web: Tweets are a useful tool for estimating and forecasting Dengue at country and city level', *PLoS Neglected Tropical Diseases*, *11*(7): e0005729.

Moore, Z., Johanssen, E. and van Etten, M. (2013) 'A review of PU prevalence and incidence across Scandinavia, Iceland and Ireland (Part I)', *Journal of Wound Care*, *22*: 361–2, 364–8.

Munn, Z., Moola, S., Lisy, K., Riitano, D. and Tufanaru, C. (2017) 'Systematic reviews of prevalence and incidence', in E. Aromataris and Z. Munn (eds), *Joanna Briggs Institute Reviewer's Manual*. Adelaide: The Joanna Briggs Institute.

Ouzzani, M., Hammady, H., Fedorowicz, Z. and Elmagarnid, A. (2016) 'Rayyan – a web and mobile app for systematic reviews', *Systematic Reviews*, *5*: 210.

Shanin, E. S., Dassen, T. and Halfen, R. J. (2008) 'Pressure ulcer prevalence and incidence in intensive care patients: A literature review', *Nursing in Critical Care*, *13*: 71–9.

Tanner, J., Anthony, D. M., Johnson, M. R., Khan, D. and Trevithick, C. (2008) 'Clostridium difficile, ethnicity and religion', *Journal of Hospital Infection*, *68*: 90–1.

Tubaishat, A., Papanikolaou, P., Anthony, D. and Habiballah, L. (2017) 'Pressure ulcers prevalence in the acute care setting: A systematic review, 2000–2015', *Clinical Nursing Research*. Available at: https://doi.org/10.1177/1054773817705541

Vanderos, S., Hessel, P., Leone, T. and Avendana, M. (2013) 'Have health trends worsened in Greece as a result of the financial crisis? A quasi-experimental approach', *European Journal of Public Health*, *23*: 727–31.

Wikipedia (2017) 'Cyber-ethnography', *Wikipedia*. Available at: https://en.wikipedia.org/wiki/Cyber-ethnography 2018

Wikipedia (2018a) 'Social network analysis', *Wikipedia*. Available at: https://en.wikipedia.org/wiki/Social_network_analysis 2018

Wikipedia (2018b) 'Web-based experiments', *Wikipedia*. Available at: https://en.wikipedia.org/wiki/Web-based_experiments 2018

Wright, B., Phillips, H., Sweetman, J. and Allgari, V. (2018) *Using Delphi Consensus Methodology with International Experts to Modify Autism Assessment Tools*. Diagnostic Instruments for Autism in Deaf Children's Study, University of York, Leeds and York Partnership NHS Foundation Trust, Newcastle University and the University of Manchester.

Young, S. D., Wu, W. and Wang, W. (2017) 'Toward automating HIV identification: Machine learning for rapid identification of HIV-related social media data', *Journal of Acquired Immune Deficiency Syndromes*, *74*: S128–31.

PART V

Applying Health Research

26

Health Research: Proposals, Planning and Writing Up

JUDITH ALLSOP AND MIKE SAKS

Chapter objectives

- To outline key aspects of constructing a health research proposal
- To discuss the process of planning a health research project
- To consider how best to write up health research.

Introduction

This chapter looks at three aspects of health research: putting forward a research proposal, planning a project and writing up the findings. Writing is a key activity during all stages and the aim of the chapter is to provide some general guidelines and suggestions for practice.

Writing a health research proposal

Writing a research proposal provides a plan for carrying out a research project. This may occur at different career stages and the purpose may vary, but some general principles apply. The types of research proposal in health and other fields include the following:

- Some undergraduate Research Methods courses are completed with a requirement to write a research proposal as an assessed exercise
- Typically, MA/MSc courses include a requirement to complete a small-scale research project for the award of a degree
- To enrol for a PhD or equivalent (such as an MD), candidates will be expected to present an outline proposal
- Research programmes at doctoral and post-doctoral level may be funded by public and private bodies
- More established researchers may bid individually and collaboratively to such bodies to undertake larger-scale commissioned and non-commissioned research.

In the United Kingdom, health research funders include such public bodies as the Economic and Social Science Research Council (ESRC), Medical Research Council (MRC), the National Health Service (NHS) and the National Institute of Health Research (NIHR). Funding is also available from philanthropic charitable bodies such as the Wellcome Foundation, universities themselves and private sector sponsors. Typically, funding is awarded on a competitive basis. If working in health care settings, both professionals and academics are expected to able to assess and submit research proposals either as individuals or as part of a team. Research is a key aspect of developing evidence-based practice, policy and innovation in the health domain.

A research proposal is based on the same principles as those used in planning, and carrying out, a research project. The degree of sophistication that is expected depends on the context of the proposal, but the framework for writing a research proposal follows a predictable pattern, including developing a title, aims and objectives, posing research questions, setting out methods, assessing the resources needed, and presenting a project timetable and a plan for the dissemination of findings. Of course, the level of detail required will vary with the scale and complexity of the project. Typically, applications for a higher degree are based on a two-page outline rather than a fully developed research proposal, as outlined below.

Time should be set aside for preparing a research proposal. Developing a plan for a feasible and sound project that adds to knowledge is an iterative process – a cycle of critical thinking, reading, drafting, reflecting and rewriting to achieve a proposal that is logical and clear. Research that is poorly thought through and that does not in some way add to knowledge is a waste of resources, both for the researcher in terms of time, effort and opportunity cost and the researched who contribute to a project. Where there is competition for sponsorship or funding, the case for careful preparation is even stronger.

Always keep in mind that you are writing for an audience. You will need to be persuasive. This is discussed further below. Those who read a research proposal are making an assessment on three criteria. Will the project add to knowledge? Does it demonstrate competence? Is the proposal feasible in terms of methods and resources and achievable within a given timescale? In the case of an in-course assessment, there can be revisions or, in the case of a PhD, further discussion with the institution concerned. If it is an application for research funding from an external body, there is often a two or three-stage selection process. There will be a preliminary decision about whether a proposal meets the basic standard for further consideration, and then a further competitive round where proposals are appraised alongside other bids in relation to a budget. Here, competition can be intense. Timing – including the topicality of your project – and luck play a part in decisions. If at first you don't succeed, try again.

Obtain and follow the guidelines

A first step in writing a research proposal is to obtain and then follow the guidelines provided to the letter. Despite this obvious point, evidence suggests that a significant proportion of applicants do not. These will fall at the first hurdle. Denscombe (2017) notes that the ESRC rejects 10 per cent of applications on this basis. For research proposals on taught Research Methods courses, PhDs and wider applications for funding, there will be guidelines to follow. In class, group work through short presentations can provide support in thinking through proposals and getting feedback. If these are not available, create your own support – find a writing partner and seek guidance from the prospective institution.

Some common reasons for the rejection of both quantitative and qualitative research papers are the following: the paper was not original; it did not pose a question that could be answered; the method chosen was not appropriate; the research was compromised by practical difficulties; the sample size/number of respondents was inadequate; the statistical analysis or data analysis was unsatisfactory; the data did not warrant the conclusions made; there was a conflict of interest; and, finally, the presentation and drafting were poor. The last reason is simplest to correct – use spell check and grammar check, and where helpful read the text aloud. See Box 26.1 for further articulation of some of these points from the personal experience of the authors/editors.

Box 26.1   Some common reasons why research proposals fail to be approved

As members of multi-centre health research ethics and related committees, we found that the most common reason for referring applications back to the proposer was the failure to provide a clear description of the research in lay terms in the patient information sheet. Poor English, the over-use of technical terms and inadequate explanations of what would be expected of the patient/participant were common faults. Other common reasons for rejection were a failure to obtain statistical advice on data collection and a judgement that a project did not add to knowledge, as it repeated earlier studies. Decisions were subject to appeal and applicants could provide further clarification in writing or in person.

Questions to ask are: Is there something original in the proposal? Does it address a topic that has not been addressed in the same way before? Does the research apply a well-researched issue to a different group, area or institution? Does it use an unusual method? Not all research proposals involve empirical research – that is, gathering data. Working with documents or carrying out a systematic review of literature on a particular narrow topic can also make a major contribution to knowledge, and existing data sets can be examined to address questions that have not been asked before. White (2017) examines how social scientists can develop research questions.

Main elements of a research proposal

Typically, a research proposal in health and other areas will require the following basic elements:

Name, position, qualifications and speciality of the applicant

This sets the scene by providing information on competence.

Contact details

Place of work/study, contact address, landline telephone, mobile and email should be given.

Role in the project

This should state whether the applicant is the sole researcher or part of a team.

Time allocated to the project

This will vary depending on the level of the application. Some institutions indicate time allocations as a guideline of the number of hours predicted in terms of hours per week for the duration of the project. For example, six hours per week for an undergraduate doing a research proposal, 10 hours per week for an MA/MSc dissertation and 25 hours for a PhD.

Other applicants

This is applicable to funded projects. Personal details are required as well as the percentage of time devoted to a project. This is used to calculate costs.

Title of the project

This should be short, succinct and explanatory.

The aims of the research (What is the purpose of the research?)

This section provides an opportunity to outline the main question(s) the research seeks to address. It should be brief as these will be elaborated more fully in the body of the proposal. If you have a particular hypothesis in mind, then it could be stated here. Even a small project can generate a number of 'what', 'how, and 'why' questions. These should be listed. Denscombe (2017) suggests that active verbs are useful. For example, the aim may be to describe the causes and consequences, to criticize or evaluate, to examine a theory or belief, to describe something, to forecast an outcome, to develop good practice or to empower a social group.

The objective(s) of the project

What outcome(s) is expected? Who will benefit? (see Offredy and Vickers 2010 for a practical guide). Some of these points are illustrated in Box 26.2.

Box 26.2   Questions to be asked when drawing up a research proposal

A policy-oriented study could take an innovation such as the periodic revalidation of doctors' competence to practise, which occurs in a number of countries, including the United Kingdom. A comparison could be made between doctors in two primary care practices in an urban area. Some questions could be: What are the professional standards expected, as outlined by the professional body? What organizational mechanisms have been used to assess continuing competence? What is the theory implicit or explicit in these mechanisms? How have mechanisms been implemented by the responsible Regional Officer for the area? How has revalidation been implemented within the two practices? What are the experiences of stakeholders: the appraisers and those appraised? Has any sub-optimal performance been identified? What action has been taken? What have been the costs? Can lessons be learnt?

Background and context (Why is the research important?)

In most research proposals, there is a section to explain the background of the research and provide a context for explaining why the question(s) to be addressed are important and to provide a rationale for the proposal. In the case of the above example, the periodic revalidation of professional competence has assumed a political importance due to instances of poor practice. There is public pressure to ensure that doctors practise safely throughout their career. This now applies to all groups of health professionals and research in this area has become timely. The question of revalidation has been contentious within the health professions, difficult to implement and costly.

Literature review (What do we know?)

Research proposals should contain a *brief* review of the literature. This shows preliminary reading and thinking and the opportunity to demonstrate competence. Do not attempt to be comprehensive. Focus on a few major contributors and highlight different points of view. If possible, refer to concepts and theories applicable to your study – for example, the concept of a profession, professional/state relations and theories of organizational change could be relevant.

Research design, methodology and methods (How will I find answers to the questions? How will I collect data?)

This section relates to how you are going to go about your research (see Chapter 2). Your research proposal can be theoretical, empirical, historical, comparative, policy-focused, a documentary analysis or a systematic review (see specific chapters for guidance). You should say why you have adopted a particular method. If you are using a mix of methods, you should indicate your purpose. Explain how respondents will be selected and recruited and how data will be analysed. Clinical research with human subjects will definitely require ethical approval and a patient information sheet. Other studies may also require research committee approval and information for participants.

Outcomes from the research (What do I expect to find and who will benefit?)

If you are applying for a research studentship funded by the ESRC or most other public or charitable bodies, you will also be asked to explain how the outcomes of the research will benefit society or the economy.

Plans for user engagement

In some research, it will be important to engage with participants before and during the project. This contact can be helpful in identifying problems, designing research tools and supporting the implementation of findings and recommendations. It is a requirement for consideration for research proposals funded by the United Kingdom NIHR initiative, Research for Patient Benefit.

Plans for dissemination of findings and publications

Research proposals require an indication of how the findings will be disseminated. This can take a variety of forms. First, findings should be discussed with participants through oral presentations. This can provide valuable insights into audiences for other forms of output, for instance for service providers or policy makers. Funding bodies will also require written feedback through reports. These should include a brief review of objectives, methods and outcomes. Finally, written outputs or media outputs can be targeted towards particular audiences in a form likely to make the greatest impact – short reports, articles in professional or academic journals and conference papers are ways of reaching a wider audience, as well as using other media outputs.

Timetable (How long will it take?)

A research proposal should include a plan for carrying out different stages of the project. You should make a list of the tasks to be undertaken over the projected period of the research. This should include a period for planning the research. For example, if you intend to do interviews, you will have to decide who to interview and negotiate access. You may need to seek permission from your institution and/or a health service research ethics committee. If you are using a questionnaire, then this instrument must be designed. The planning period requires good time management skills. As will be highlighted in the next section, a Gantt chart – a tool for project management – may be useful and can be downloaded from the internet.

Resources (What will I need?)

Research does incur costs in terms of time and money. An institutional affiliation will reduce personal costs through access to equipment and a library. However, in planning your research you must think through the non-recoverable costs you may incur through travel and living costs and if specialist equipment is required. Such costs need to be included in your research proposal.

Impact (Who will benefit?)

Here a short account can be given of who will benefit from the research. This can cover a number of different constituencies, from health professionals themselves to policy makers and sections of the wider public.

Planning health research

The various aspects of planning research can be illustrated by a research-based masters' dissertation or doctoral thesis.

Schedules and timing

Once a proposal has been agreed, then a plan will need to be developed for accomplishing the research over the following year for a master's dissertation, or three to four years for an MD or PhD (see Dunleavy 2003). An initial step is to draw up a timetable with an end point. The Gantt chart in Figure 26.1 will provide a structure for scheduling project phases and show how they overlap. There can be a difference in scheduling depending on the method employed. In clinical research, a hypothesis is drawn from an existing body of literature and instruments and methods for analysis must be fully developed. With qualitative methods the refinement of research questions in conjunction with an extended literature review may take longer and so may data analysis. All research plans must allow time to obtain research and/or ethics committee approval.

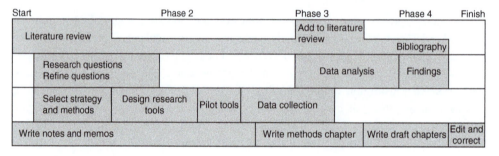

FIGURE 26.1   Research project plan

Source: Gantt chart (adapted from Denscombe 2010)

The Gantt chart provides a typical schedule within which to allocate your time. There are predictable stages in the research process and these are outlined in research texts both generally (see Cresswell 2009; Denscombe 2017) and in the health field specifically (see Polgar and Thomas 2019), which will now be considered in turn. These include a literature review, data collection, establishing access to participants/respondents, collecting and analysing data, describing and interpreting findings and the final stage of writing up, which will be discussed later in this chapter. This can be done in the form of a flow chart with the weeks and months along a horizontal axis and the tasks to be completed along the vertical axis. Allow plenty of time for writing up.

Project management

As indicated above, undertaking research for an academic qualification is a challenge and is an exercise in thinking, planning and problem solving. It is a process led by the student but supported by their supervisor and through collaboration with fellow students. Producing a dissertation, and particularly a PhD, can be a lonely experience, especially if a student has other commitments to work or family. Unexpected problems will arise even in the best planned project. These must be solved pragmatically and quickly. It can also be rewarding to seek out new knowledge, develop expertise and make a contribution to society.

Time management is important

In order to keep on track, write your project title, a list of research questions and a list of chapter headings for a dissertation or PhD and keep these displayed in a prominent place. The constituent parts are shown in Box 26.3. Again, reference to these can help to focus on the main task.

Box 26.3   The structure of a dissertation or thesis

Title: This should be short and descriptive.

Abstract: This concisely sets out the research topic and why it is important, how the research was carried out, what the key findings were and the contribution to knowledge.

List of contents: This includes sections and chapters, tables and figures, and references.

Introduction: This should incorporate your statement of the research questions, the rationale for the research and your claim to make a contribution to knowledge.

Chapter on the literature: This needs to include key concepts and theories, what others have written, and the research methods used together with a critique.

Chapter on background and context: This is part of some studies.

Chapter on research methods: State why the method was chosen, how data were collected, how dilemmas were resolved and what ethical issues were encountered. How was the data analysed?

Chapters on findings with results: This needs to include evidence and discussion.

Chapter discussing findings: This should link back to the aims, objectives, literature and theory.

Conclusion: This is a summary of what the research has added to knowledge and its potential impact on future policy. Reference should also be made to further research that might be conducted.

Develop a work pattern

It is helpful to establish patterns of working. See your supervisor at regular intervals (ideally, monthly), plan ahead and set a target for each meeting with your supervisor. For such meetings bring an agenda and prepare a written account of your activity since the previous meeting or write a memo on emergent themes from the data for discussion.

Update your skills

During this phase of the project, you may find gaps in your knowledge or seek specialist expertise (see Ramkalawan 2005). Statisticians are usually prepared to help researchers or, alternatively, take a course in statistics. You may need to learn how to use SPSS or NVivo or other tools for data analysis.

Keep writing

Writing should be continuous throughout a project. It is an aid to critical thinking and if memos and other documents are labelled and filed away, they can be listed and used during the phase of analysis and writing up. A helpful exercise at this stage is to consider a topic related to your research – say a concept such as Social Capital or a theory such as Normal Process Theory or Nudge Theory. The latter is drawn from behavioural science and uses experimental methods, including randomized controlled trials, to test the efficacy of different techniques to encourage changes in behaviour to promote the common good. 'Nudge' techniques are about framing choices. They include giving cues and signals, introducing small incentives, exerting peer pressure, providing information and/or consulting in different ways. An account of these experiments in public policy can be found in the work of John and colleagues (2011). The approach is an interesting one as it provides an example of a way of comparing and testing small-scale, local-level interventions using a rigorous method.

Keep a diary and use a notebook

A diary can be used to plan ahead by week and month and will provide a record of activity and a prompt for deadlines to be met. A notebook can be used, among other things, for comments and references as well as to record decisions made, ideas and impressions following interviews or meetings. This is particularly important when using qualitative methods when emerging themes can be noted.

The phases of a project

Developing the literature review continues throughout the project, but is more intensive in the early stages and the later stages. The internet is a readily accessible way to begin a search, but information should be checked later against other sources. Libraries provide the most reliable place to search for sources. They have electronic resources and journals can be accessed online with an institutional password. A tip for extending a search is to find one book on a topic, then look around the shelf for others in the same section. The citations given in books or articles can also provide further sources.

In order to keep track of your reading, write short memos on particular topics. For example, to extend your coverage of the literature, you could look up seven references on a theory or concept, reflect on the strengths and limitations and write a critical commentary to discuss with your supervisor. Or find three empirical studies that use a particular study design and methodology and follow the same process. Memos should be labelled and filed away for future reference. Aim to sort your literature review into topics a quarter of the way into a project and assess any gaps in coverage. You can add to it later. It is also important to know when to stop looking for new material.

In the first phase of a study, research question(s) should be refined and decisions made on methodology and methods. Data collection is the core of any research project (Sapsford and Jupp 2006) and three critical decisions are: what methods to use and which instruments to use; how research subjects are to be recruited or texts located; and what resources will be needed to carry out the study.

Some qualitative studies will require the design of an instrument such as a semi-structured interview schedule. Setting up focus groups, selecting key informants, negotiating access and recruiting participants takes time. A question often asked in qualitative research is: how many to interview? Qualitative methods texts suggest this is when interview responses reach 'saturation' – that is, when themes or patterns can be identified. Baker and Edwards (2010) review this issue in a podcast and suggest various indicators, but ultimately, researchers must make their own judgement and be able to justify this, as Chapter 5 indicates. A description of a project with aims and objectives should be drawn up to distribute to participants. This enables them to give their consent. Included in this is the length of time to set aside for the interviews. When preparing for an interview, think through how you will introduce yourself, avoid asking leading questions, and consider how you will conclude (see Edwards and Holland 2013 for a practitioner's account).

A quantitative researcher is likely to argue for a very clear, simple primary question. Preparatory work in this early phase is particularly intensive and critical to the success of the project. Research instruments such as questionnaires must be constructed to include the characteristics or variables the researcher wants to represent and compare. This should be tested through a pilot study. It is worth noting that in quantitative research designing research instruments is time consuming. For example, the questionnaire must be constructed and a pilot carried out to ensure external validity. Chapters 12 and 13 consider issues of sampling and sampling frames and primary and secondary samples. The grounds for inclusion or exclusion in a sample should be included. The size of the population to be interviewed will require a statistical justification – as many as is necessary to generalize to a larger population. A survey can be administered in a number of ways, by post, telephone or the internet. Information on the purpose of a survey must be given and consent obtained.

A researcher should also review and select from existing well-tested measures to suit their project. For example, there are numerous instruments for assessing health status and health-related quality of life that cover a wide range of domains, such as emotional well-being, psychological wellbeing, physical status and functioning and social wellbeing (measured by social networking and support, community integration and engagement in social roles). In a review, Bowling (2005) concludes that, while there is considerable overlap in content, there are also differences between instruments, so researchers should check for fit. Experiments, as described in Chapter 15, also require group recruitment. If the study is a randomized controlled trial, then two groups – an intervention group and a matching control – must be recruited. In these cases, whether recruiting healthy volunteers or patients, a patient information sheet must be given to recruits and their consent to participate must be confirmed.

During this phase, a researcher should record the steps of the process, the decisions made, any difficulties encountered and how these were resolved. This commentary will be the basis of your research methods chapter in the case of dissertations and theses.

Resources

Researchers should assess the equipment they will need and the costs of doing the research. These could include a tape-recorder, transcription and travel costs. For instance, interviews must normally be recorded and transcribed. It has been estimated that one hour of interviewing takes six hours to transcribe (Bryman 2016). For documentary analysis, selections of texts must be made. Transcriptions are the basis for a thematic analysis of the data, which also takes time to develop through a process of trial and error.

It is strongly recommended that a written draft of the methods is produced at this point. This should cover how access was negotiated, how instruments were designed and how these were fit for purpose in addressing the research question. This will provide a basis for your research methods section or chapter.

Data analysis

Data analysis occurs in the second phase of a project. The aim is to describe and then assess each theme or factor related to the research question, to explain its contribution to the investigation and to interpret the significance. With qualitative data, no matter which way observations are collected, they must be reproduced in written form so that core themes and sub-themes within these categories can be identified. The aim is to identify recurrences in data that reflect how phenomena are understood by participants. The literature review, observations and notes taken in the field and sources read contemporaneously will inform the analysis and contribute to the construction of a coding framework. There is a zigzag between theory and data. Themes are identified by reading and re-reading so that the data can be coded systematically through the texts (Denzin and Lincoln 2005). Strauss (1987), one of the founder members of the method of analytic induction, recommends writing memos on concepts and theories to aid interpretation. For example, a memo on a theme arising in early interviews can be identified and related to a theory. This can be tested and accepted or discarded at a later stage in the research.

Coding is way of managing a mass of data by reducing it to a number of interconnected themes to develop a structure that is credible. A coding framework is a method for breaking the text down into component parts. This can be a time-consuming process, although the use of a data analysis package can speed up the process. Systematic differences within themes can also be detected – as, for example, differences in how 'something' is perceived by gender, class, age or ethnicity. This is discussed in Chapter 11, but also see Green and Thorogood (2018).

A researcher can choose to code by hand or use a data analysis package. There are a number of computer-assisted qualitative data analysis software (CAQDAS) packages that assist data management through storing segments of data. Coded sequences can be recovered and ordered into categories, making them easier to manipulate. This replaces the old-fashioned method of scissors and paste. Bryman (2016) concludes that there is no clear market leader for qualitative data analysis programs, but nevertheless he provides a useful introduction to using NVivo. Dedoose (2013) is a more recent arrival. While a data analysis package may sort the data into categories of text, there is still the question of how to select illustrative quotations. Silverman (2015) provides guidance on how to choose quotations.

In a research design using quantitative methods, many of the decisions about data analysis are predetermined as they are integral to the design of an experiment, a sampling frame, a questionnaire and how the latter is pre-coded. The questions included in any structured questionnaire will already be based on implicit assumptions related to the research question and the variables for cross-tabulation to test the hypothesis or research question. Questionnaires, telephone interviews and structured interviews must be logged with dates and responses and reminders. Response rates should be calculated. Aim to achieve at the very least a response rate of over 40 per cent of the population contacted.

Once the data are collected, the next step is to manage the data. In a cross-sectional study using a questionnaire, the data are checked for obvious errors, or 'cleaned', and entered into a data-processing program such as SPSS. This form of research method aims to test theory so that the way the data will be analysed is already implicit in the questionnaire design. The analysis will reduce the data to produce, through quantitative measures, tables, figures and graphs showing the relationship between variables and the results of various statistical tests.

Mixed methods

Using a mix of methods poses additional challenges for writing up results (see Cresswell and Tashahkkori 2007). Authors must make their own decisions on the basis of what they think will make the study comprehensible to readers. In writing up projects that use a mix of methods, the rationale for so doing should be explained in terms of the relevance to addressing the research question and the anticipated benefits. The logic of combining two different methods should be reflected in the design of the research instruments and an account of whether the anticipated benefits were realized should be given in the project (Gorad 2010). See Cresswell and Plano Clarke (2017) for an in-depth discussion of this.

It should be explained why a particular mix has been chosen. The justification for the sequence of methods should also be given and how each method contributes to knowledge. Are the different methods seen as complementary? Is one method being used as a stepping stone to another? How will the findings from different methods be integrated or are the findings contributing through triangulation and presenting different aspects of the same phenomenon? Bryman (2016) suggests that the use of mixed methods may lead to a fuller understanding of a problem, although, inevitably, their use adds complexity, requires additional skills and may increase costs.

Research findings

The last phase of data analysis is to produce findings. These will be based on patterns identified from the data. There is a preliminary stage when the results from the analysis are available in a raw form. These may constitute a number of sections or chapters to a dissertation or thesis. In preparation for writing up a project, preliminary work can be done by selecting themes or domains and ordering text related to those themes. This can be followed by a further analysis of text by sub-themes.

Writing a short paper on each theme and sub-theme, revisiting the literature review and looking for new sources can aid thinking about a theoretically based framework that can be linked to textual quotations. There may be an adjustment to the initial research question during this analysis. Quotations should be representative rather than an outlier unless it is to illustrate a deviant case. It can be helpful to use grids or figures to sum up patterns of association and to indicate their strength. At this point, aim to decide on a structure for the final sections or chapters. This may take time to determine. You will not be able to include everything, so you will have to choose carefully.

How findings are discussed will vary with the discipline, methodology and methods. In quantitative research, findings may be presented through tables and graphs and can be tested for significance. Again, the challenge is one of selection. What should be included and what left out? A general guide for inclusion is the relevance of data to answering the research question and therefore contributing to the argument to be made in the discussion and conclusion. It is important to summarize the content of a table, figure or graph and draw attention to the particular aspect of the contents that is important for addressing the research question and supporting (or providing contrary evidence to) your argument. You must spell out for the reader what you want them to know. Point out the association between tables and link your findings to the research questions and relevant theory. There may well be further theoretically based analysis introduced during the course of the writing up. In qualitative studies, it is also advisable to present data graphically or visually as well as in words. When you are confident that most of the pieces of the jigsaw are in place, you can proceed towards writing up a final draft – the last stage of the research process.

Writing up health research

In writing up your research, preparing a final draft of a health research project usually involves an intensive period of thinking and writing. This takes time, even for the most experienced writer. The quality of presentation and the succinctness of the writing are important. In essence, the writer is looking back and presenting an account for the reader. This should follow a narrative arc with a beginning, middle section and an end. Each chapter should also follow this model. This may seem repetitive, but a conventional structure will help the reader to follow the logic from the research question, through the substantive chapters to the conclusion. You should try to put forward an argument, or thesis, and develop this through the work. Ramage, Bean and Johnson (2016) show how to make and support an argument.

When writing a report of your research, consider your audience. For instance, in a thesis or dissertation consider your external examiners and what they will expect to find. Aim for a clear, logical and persuasive account. Sentences with subject, verb, object structure are the easiest to follow. Take care to avoid language that is discriminatory in terms of gender, race, disability or other social category (see Letherby 2003) and be aware that a number of drafts may be required to achieve clarity and intelligibility. Special attention should be paid to introductions, summarizing existing chapters, signposting future chapters, and the conclusions. Appropriately descriptive chapter headings and subheadings also help to structure the content.

The structure revisited

Box 26.3 above outlined the shape of a dissertation or thesis. Leaving aside the *Title, Abstract* and *List of contents*, the first substantive chapter is the *Introduction*. The final draft of this is best left until the end. By then, your chapters will give a coherent and logical account, supporting an argument that runs through the work.

Introduction

The introduction will say what your study is about, why the question you address is of interest and explain how you carried out the investigation. It should refer to the theories and methods used to address the question and some key findings and why these are important. Do not be concerned about revealing your findings; this is not a detective novel. You should also comment on the contribution your research makes to knowledge. This could be in terms of adding to, or providing a critique of, theory and indicating whether there are implications for policy or practice.

The literature review

This is where research questions can be discussed in greater detail, together with associated theories and substantive studies associated with these questions. Chapter 4 provides useful tips. The final draft is where you can include new studies or areas of literature that proved to be valuable in understanding the analysis or discussion in the substantive chapters of the study. You could conclude the literature review chapter by saying how the literature review shaped your choice of research method.

Research methods

This section or chapter is most effective when presented as a chronological account. You will need to check guidelines on presentation and discuss this with your supervisor. It should explain why a methodology and research design was chosen and what methods were used to collect data, including details of sampling and the recruitment of participants.

The methods chapter should refer to decisions on ethical issues that arose during the research. Reference can be made to obtaining ethical committee approval within the university and/or the health service committee (Long and Johnson 2007); how informed consent was obtained from research participants; what information was provided; and whether there was an opportunity to raise questions.

You should also describe how data were secured to maintain the anonymity of research participants. An account is also required of the methods used for data analysis, as described above. The research methods chapter is also the place to refer back to the research question and any weaknesses in the method. It is better to address any limitations yourself. This can pre-empt criticism and strengthen your claim to have given an honest and rigorous account. In qualitative social science research projects as opposed to more quantitative analyses, it has become a convention to write the research methods chapter in the first person. This is the chapter where you can refer to problems – such as changes of direction, revised research questions, difficulties in recruiting participants – and how these have been solved and lessons learnt.

If qualitative methods have been used, researchers should be reflexive about their own position in the research process. Reflexivity is a concept that refers to the role that the researcher plays in the construction of knowledge at all stages of the research (Bryman 2016). The acknowledgement of subjectivity, and the influence of values, can be seen as a defence against criticism. Particularly in data analysis, evidence is based on selection and the interpretation of meaning. It is therefore a responsibility of the researcher to be as transparent as possible in their account of how data were analysed.

Substantive chapters

When using qualitative methods, as research questions are more open-ended, the structure of the chapters that report on the findings of the research are difficult to predict in advance. Typically, the researcher aims to find out how people account for aspects of social life. The themes and sub-themes within these take place in a two-stage process – it is a process of constructing a narrative within a theoretical structure based on the evidence, but also a creative exercise. Bear in mind that chapters can focus on a particular theme, but should be structured to carry through an argument or develop the thesis in answer to the research question. In qualitative research, the writer constructs an account based on themes drawn from the data. This must be based on evidence from the analysis and illustrated through quotations.

It has been noted by qualitative researchers that constructing a plausible narrative can be 'terrifying', according to Smart (2010). Hitherto, a researcher has learnt how to comment on, and critique, existing texts, but in this case they must create their own account. Sometimes this can lead to 'writers' block' or various kinds of diversionary activity. The advice is to overcome this through free writing – that is, do not try to get the text completely correct; write badly if necessary and then revise. It is also important to be disciplined and set a target for writing a given number of hours a week, and to start to write based on accounts drawn from themes and quotations. Shape and structure will develop as writing is also thinking. At this stage, it is helpful to find someone who will read your drafts – a supervisor or someone who is at the same stage. You may not use all you write but establishing a rhythm can help.

In many respects, biomedical scientific writing is more straightforward. Findings do not have to be drawn out of the data but can be interpreted from numeric data and operate within a very strictly defined set of conventions (Greenhalgh 2014). The creative work has been achieved in setting up an experiment or survey. The core of the project describes:

- The hypothesis or null hypothesis addressed
- The type of study: Either primary (experiment, clinical trial or survey) or secondary (overview, guideline study, decision analysis or economic analysis)
- The study design and method: Experimental (randomized controlled trial, cohort study, case-control study, cross-sectional survey) or a single-case report, which will cover inclusion/exclusion criteria and describe how the outcomes were measured
- The research results or findings.

A characteristic of scientific writing in health research is that the voice of the writer is absent from the text. The researcher presents the work as a series of facts. This serves to underline the scientific nature of the writing, although the author still structures, shapes and selects what is written, what constitutes evidence and how this is presented. The form of writing aims to minimize the likelihood of bias and error, but also preserves the way in which knowledge is structured by scientists. Data are likely to be presented in a formal manner with tables and with tests of statistical significance when analysing data sets. The aim is to reduce the complexity of data, editing down, cutting out words, correcting typographical errors and ordering paragraphs.

Discussion of findings

These should be drafted and redrafted to bring out the argument. Headings and subheadings help to structure the argument. Not all results can be included so stick to the findings or interpretations that relate to the research question. One way of doing this is to begin by restating the research question or hypothesis. Sequence the main findings from the general to the specific. Comment on the significance of each main finding and discuss these in turn, indicating the extent to which the findings confirm or not the proposition put forward. Present evidence to support your findings and, if there are competing explanations, cite these as well. This can strengthen your account.

Conclusion

The conclusion should not simply be a summary but be seen as an opportunity to restate your starting point and draw out ways that your thesis has contributed to knowledge. It is the final chance to make an argument. There is an opportunity to look at the ways in which the research has been innovative or original. You may have shed light on a little-known area or been able to question or confirm existing theories and/or methodologies. You may be able draw out the implications of your work for patients and patients' groups, as well as for policy makers and service providers, and the negative consequences of not taking action if there are recommendations made in your study. The limitations of your study should also be highlighted. It is also useful to point to counter-arguments in addition to the possibilities for further research. Both these serve to pre-empt criticism. Some tips for writing up your essay, dissertation or thesis are included in Box 26.4.

Box 26.4 Tips for writing up

- Check the guidelines for presentation
- Develop an argument that is sustained throughout the work
- Present your work within a clear structure through chapters and/or subheadings
- If in doubt, it is better to assume a lower level of knowledge
- Avoid sexist and racist language and statements that are patronizing to research participants

- Read your work aloud to establish the rhythm and flow of the language. If you falter – alter!
- Leave your work aside for a while so you can take a fresh look later
- Ask someone else – your supervisor, a friend or colleague – to read your work through and make comments.

The final draft

The final draft of your dissertation/thesis will require careful editing. Check again the requirements for presentation and follow them exactly: the form of presentation, length, style of referencing, footnotes, endnotes, bibliography, appendices, time limits for presentation, viva arrangements, and so on. Conventions for presentation vary between the clinical and social sciences and also between disciplines in the health field. A cautious student will check with their supervisor that the form of presentation reflects both the methods used and the orientation of their external examiners before writing up the final version of their thesis.

When reading through, remember that a final draft is about reducing the complexity of data, editing down, cutting out words, correcting typographical errors and ordering paragraphs. Check that the language is persuasive and the English is correct. Remember that a simple sentence structure with a noun, a verb and an object is best. Reading chapters aloud can again be helpful. Footnotes or endnotes, references and the bibliography also need to be correct. Make sure that all the sources that are quoted are referenced, are internally consistent and conform to the format recommended. It is also wise to check that the word length is within limits. Add an abstract and any appendices that provide information on your working methods, such as a questionnaire, a list of people interviewed, sample letters, and an information sheet for participants. This can be time-consuming, and remember that a common regret among research students is that they did not leave enough time for writing.

Conclusion

In conclusion, it is worth reiterating that writing up research, like other stages of health research, has a moral aspect. The researcher has an obligation to follow a rigorous and systematic process in data collection, analysis and writing up. Research subjects will have given their opinions, their time and sometimes access to their bodies for additional procedures, interventions and medications because they believe a project is worthwhile and may help others. Given that being a research participant may have emotional and physical costs, health researchers have an ethical obligation to carry out research as rigorously as they can.

Exercise 26.1   The Normalization Process Theory

This exercise may sharpen your critical faculties in undertaking health research. Normalization Process Theory (NPT) is a set of sociological tools to understand and explain how new processes, through which new or modified practices, become successfully embedded (that is, normalized) and sustained and integrated in health care. Find a primary source that defines the theory. Then look up seven studies that have used the theory and make an argument to support or critique the usefulness of the theory in a case study of your choice. A starting point could be: McEvoy, R., Ballini, L., Maltoni, S., O'Donnell, C. A., Mair, F. S. and MacFarlane, A. (2014) 'A qualitative systematic review of studies using normalization process theory to research implementation processes', *Implementation Science, 9*(2). Available at: https://doi.org/10.1186/1748-5908-9-2

Recommended further reading

In this book, Becker, a master of research and a pioneer in qualitative methods, provides a readable and stimulating account of the writing process based on long experience of teaching doctoral students at universities in the United States:

Becker, H. S. (1986) *Writing for Social Scientists: How to Start and Finish Your Thesis, Book, or Article*. Chicago, IL: University of Chicago Press.

This book provides a guide to the research process and examples of how to write up research using examples. It gives practical solutions based on the student experience:

Bryman, A. (2016) *Social Research Methods*, 5th edition. Oxford: Oxford University Press.

This is a useful practical book to assist those completing their doctoral dissertations:

Dunleavy, P. (2003) *Authoring a PhD: How to Plan, Draft, Write and Finish a Doctoral Thesis or Dissertation*. Basingstoke: Palgrave Macmillan.

This text provides insights and strategies for publishing and has the advantage of being specifically directed towards a health professional audience:

Green, J. and Thorogood, N. (2014) *Qualitative Methods for Health Research*, 3rd edition. London: Sage.

References

Baker S. E. and Edwards R. (2013) 'How many qualitative interviews is enough?' *Eprints*. Available at: ncmr.ac.uk/2273/4/how many interview pdf

Bowling, A. (2005) *A Review of Disease Specific Quality of Life Measurement Scales*, 3rd edition. Buckingham: Open University Press.

Bryman, A. (2016) *Social Research Methods*, 5th edition. Oxford: Oxford University Press.

Cresswell, J. W. (2009) *Research Design: Qualitative, Quantitative and Mixed Methods Approaches*, 3rd edition. London: Sage.

Cresswell, J. W. and Plano Clark, V. L. (2017) *Designing and Conducting Mixed Methods Research*, 3rd edition. London: Sage.

Cresswell, J. W. and Tashakkori, A. (2007) 'Developing publishable mixed methods manuscripts', *Journal of Mixed Methods Research*, 1: 107–11.

Dedoose (2013) *Dedoose Version 4.5: Web Application for Managing, Analyzing, and Presenting Qualitative and Mixed Method Research Data*. Los Angeles, CA: Socio-cultural Research Consultants, LLC. Available at: http://www.dedoose.com

Denscombe, M. (2010) *Ground Rules for Social Research*. Maidenhead: Open University Press.

Denscombe, M. (2017) *The Good Research Guide for Small Scale Research Projects*, 6th edition. Maidenhead: Open University Press/McGraw-Hill.

Denzin, N. and Lincoln, Y. S. (eds) (2005) *Handbook of Qualitative Research*, 3rd edition. Thousand Oaks, CA: Sage.

Dunleavy, P. (2003) *Authoring a PhD: How to Plan, Draft, Write and Finish a Doctoral Thesis or Dissertation*. Basingstoke: Palgrave Macmillan.

Edwards, A. and Holland J. (2013) *What is Qualitative Interviewing?* London: Bloomsbury. Available at: ncrm.ac.uk/2376/1/

Gorard, S. (2010) 'Research design, as independent of methods', *Eprints*. Available at: http://eprints.bham/514/1/Gorard_Handbook of Mixed Methods 2010 pdf

Green, J. and Thorogood, N. (2018) *Qualitative Methods for Health Researchers*, 4th edition. London: Sage.

Greenhalgh, T. (2014) *How to Read a Paper: The Basics of Evidence-based Medicine*, 5th edition. Chichester: Wiley-Blackwell.

John, P., Cotterill, S., Moseley, A., Richardson, L., Smith, G., Stoker, G. and Wales, C. (2011) *Nudge, Nudge, Think, Think: Experimenting with Ways to Change Civic Behaviour*. London: Bloomsbury Academic.

Letherby, G. (2003) *Feminist Research in Theory and Practice*. Buckingham: Open University Press.

Long, T. and Johnson, M. (2007) *Research Ethics in the Real World: Issues and Solutions for Health and Social Care Professionals*. Philadelphia, PA: Elsevier Health Sciences.

Offredy, M. and Vickers, P. (2010) *Developing a Healthcare Research Proposal: An Interactive Student Guide*. Chichester: Wiley-Blackwell.

Polgar, S. and Thomas, S. A. (2019) *Introduction to Research in the Health Sciences*, 7th edition. New York: Elsevier.

Ramage, J., Bean, J. and Johnson, J. (2016) *Writing Arguments*, 10th edition. New York: Pearson.

Ramkalawan, T. (2005) 'Training for research', in A. Bowling and S. Ebrahim (eds), *Handbook of Health Research Methods: Investigation, Measurement and Analysis*. Maidenhead: Open University Press.

Sapsford, R. and Jupp, V. (eds) (2006) *Data Collection and Analysis*, 2nd edition. London: Sage.

Silverman, D. (2015) *Interpreting Qualitative Data: Methods for Analysing Talk, Text and Interaction*, 5th edition. London: Sage.

Smart, C. (2010) 'Disciplined writing: On the problem of writing sociologically', *Eprints*. Available at: ncrm.ac.uk 828/disciplined writing pdf

Strauss, A. L. (1987) *Qualitative Analysis for Social Scientists*. Cambridge: Cambridge University Press.

White, P. (2017) *Developing Research Questions: A Guide for Social Scientists*. Basingstoke: Palgrave Macmillan.

27

Disseminating and Evaluating Health Research

MIKE SAKS AND JUDITH ALLSOP

Chapter objectives

- To underline the importance of disseminating health research
- To examine the various means of disseminating research
- To highlight the need to evaluate health research
- To explore the process of research evaluation.

Introduction

The third edition of *Researching Health* has now reached its conclusion, following its exploration of a variety of qualitative, quantitative and mixed methods, and the various issues that they raise, which were introduced in the opening chapter of the book. But before this edited volume does so, there are two further areas that it is vital, from the viewpoint of the readership, to cover in more depth – that of the dissemination of health research and the evaluation of such research. Each of these critical fields will now be covered in turn.

Dissemination

In Chapter 26 it was highlighted that there is an increasing need to include in research proposals a plan for disseminating the research findings. This is vital as some commentators (see, for instance, Bowling 2014) argue that health researchers have a duty to ensure that the evidence from well-designed investigations is disseminated in ongoing fashion during the conduct of their work, particularly where there are implications for treatments or service development. In this context, dissemination is a process of sharing information and knowledge to improve the accessibility of research to those we are attempting to reach (Rivas and Pandya-Wood 2014). This is a key element of developing a strategy for health research.

Oral forms of dissemination

It was noted that, most importantly, health research should be discussed through presentations with participants and other external audiences, such as service personnel or policy makers, as well as in the form of academic and related conference papers. This not only enhances the likely practical impact of the research, but also involves getting feedback on the research and making refinements to the theoretical, methodological and empirical aspects of the research. Often, such presentations form part of the 'first wave of dissemination', although they will also be important after the research is completed (Rivas and Pandya-Wood 2014).

Interim workshops during the research might be included in this 'first wave' too as they enable feedback that could more fundamentally shape evolving aspects of the research. The value of such dissemination and feedback events is underlined by Case Study 27.1.

CASE STUDY 27.1

Regional workshops for the health support worker research project

The Health Support Worker Steering Group, chaired by one of the editors of this volume, reported back to the United Kingdom (UK) Departments of Health, in 2000. This Group, of which the other editor was a member, was funded and tasked by government with (a) examining the roles, functions and responsibilities of support workers employed in health care settings and (b) making recommendations to the four national Health Departments about the extent of regulation which might be appropriate in the interests of public protection and the practical means of providing it. One of the main means of informing the research – apart from a literature review, the distribution of a UK-wide questionnaire to collect qualitative and quantitative data from chief executives in the health and care sector, focus group discussions with interest groups and in-depth interviews with influential figures in the field – was through regional workshops (Saks et al. 2000).

The six advertised regional workshops, involving some 150 key participants such as carers, service users, service providers and unions, were held in medical education centres in Belfast, Birmingham, Cardiff, Edinburgh, Leeds and London. They provided a vehicle for disseminating the interim results of the study under 'Chatham House' rules through short presentations by members of the project team. The workshops also critically promoted discussion of emerging scenarios, capturing the often different views of stakeholders in England, Northern Ireland, Scotland and Wales. The views were a key strand feeding into the final report, which highlighted the current safeguards and risks for health support workers. They recommended:

- Improving the direction and guidance to employees
- Enhancing the active management/supervision of support workers
- Placing greater responsibility on employers/agencies
- Further informing service users about their rights and appropriate standards
- Enhancing the training and qualifications of support workers
- Introducing in stages a basic register for all health support workers.

Some of the recommendations were controversial within the workshops, such as the recommendation of a mandatory register, and are still even now under discussion by the parties concerned, but the workshops and the final report were very important in providing pointers for policy options (Saks and Allsop 2007). This was especially so given that such workers still remain relatively invisible to policy makers, not just in the UK, but globally, despite being by far the largest proportion of the health care labour force (Saks 2020, forthcoming).

Oral presentations may also be important for unfunded research conducted by individuals and small teams, which may take place at the national, international, or indeed local as well as regional level. New forms of technology may be involved in the process of dissemination through Facebook, Twitter and other forms of social media. Many researchers aim to attract attention to research outcomes through radio and television since this may help to ensure further translational activity for the research concerned. If the implementation of the findings is to occur, then researchers need to frame their results in a clear and accessible way in terms of style and content (Bastow, Tinkler and Dunleavy 2014).

Dissemination through publication

The typical way for researchers in any context to publicize their research findings as part of what has been defined as the 'second wave of dissemination' (Rivas and Pandya-Wood 2014) is through publications, with English being the main *lingua franca* outside national boundaries. At the most fundamental level, those undertaking funded projects through such organizations as government research councils or private benefactor bodies will normally be required to produce a report on their research. Here a short and well-structured Executive Summary written in terms understandable by a lay person can be most effective in disseminating key points about such matters as the aims, objectives, design, methods, results, limitations and implications of the research (Bowling 2014). This provides a good basis – as will that of an abstract for a final year undergraduate or postgraduate dissertation – for constructing press releases from which articles in the local and national press may be derived for defined target audiences. Here, as with oral presentations, the marketing offices of the organization concerned may be very helpful in putting messages out into a wider domain – not least in the university sector, where it is important to avoid tensions between the administration and researchers (Saks 2015).

Researchers tend to place most emphasis on scholarly publications to promote and implement their research findings, although newsletters, popular and professional magazines from *Men's Health* to the *Nursing Standard* should not be ignored as a source of influence. However, scholarly publications are very important to researchers as they provide measurable kudos in national and international institutional league tables and research exercises, leading directly or indirectly to increased funding opportunities. They also may be part of the requirements for funded research projects and at the very least they will enhance the *curriculum vitae* of researchers themselves in the job market as a status credential (Rawat and Meena 2014).

Along with research reports and institutionally held dissertations in university libraries, the main outlets for publication in health research are book chapters, edited book collections, specialized academic monographs and articles in scholarly journals, together with abstracts published online or in hard copy arising from conference proceedings. These are not mutually exclusive. Part of a research report, for example, can be published as a journal article with the permission of the funding sponsors and there may well be an expectation by funders that the findings are disseminated to a broader audience through the written word. In this respect, it is also important to appreciate that for various reasons funding bodies in health and other areas may embargo research. Researchers should ensure that their funding contract includes a proviso that permission to publish must not be unreasonably withheld. Hannaway (2008) underlines the significance of this in showcasing the gatekeeping politics of biomedical research. In terms of the lack of mutual exclusivity, sections of completed dissertations may also be published in a modified or unmodified form, if this has not already been undertaken before any *viva voce* examination. The process of publication is assisted by the fact that many outlets are now available on the internet – with a profusion of e-journals and e-books as well as the previously mentioned accessibility of conference proceedings online.

Academic books

In terms of academic books in the health field, these are typically sourced by publishers themselves unless a self-publishing route is being pursued. In the former case, proposals spanning several pages should be submitted in a standard template (which is usually available on the publishers' websites) to a relevant publishing house. Proposals should give an indication of such aspects as the aims and scope of the volume, its chapter-by-chapter contents, potential rival texts, the target audience and the market, including any unique selling points. Often, for new authors, publishers will require sample chapters or indeed the whole manuscript in some cases, for which a finalised dissertation might suffice in the first instance. Where the book is edited or co-edited, potential chapter contributors will typically be approached individually by the editor or editorial team, followed by a commissioning arrangement. The key to the process is getting your proposal or work read, so it is important to look into the kinds of books publishers produce to establish relevance. The proposal will typically go out to referees for assessment, as will the final manuscript, after which adjustments may be required before a publishing contract is issued.

Thought might also be given in the book publishing world to employing an agent (see Owen 2018 for a list of these), although financial returns for academic books are typically small, except for the most well-known authors, as not many copies are likely to be sold beyond library sales. The main focus in academic book publishing is on prestige, although there is some money to be made in high-volume sales of standard university student texts with mass markets. As regards publishers, the most prestigious for monographs tend to be the university presses, such as Yale University Press and Oxford University Press, which both have lists in medicine and health, and large-scale, more commercial publishers like Routledge and Sage, which have parallel interests and strong international networks to promote sales.

Dissemination through scholarly journals

For most health-related disciplines, reports and articles in scholarly journals are the most highly rated form of research output. A very small illustrative selection of the most prestigious journals in health, among the many hundreds on offer globally, is set out in Box 27.1.

Box 27.1   Some examples of high-profile international health journals

American Journal of Ophthalmology

British Medical Journal

Health: An Interdisciplinary Journal

Health and Community Care

International Journal of Health Services

International Journal of Public Health

Journal of Advanced Nursing

Journal of American Medical Association

The Lancet

New England Journal of Medicine

Social Science and Medicine

Social Policy and Administration

Sociology of Health and Illness

As will be seen, some health journals have a single disciplinary or professional focus, while others are multidisciplinary and/or interdisciplinary. It is therefore important to make the right choice for the focus of your paper and to read the journal criteria for accepting papers on the relevant websites very carefully as these vary considerably.

As with the submission of book proposals, the requirements for journal publication are also relatively transparent. However, the filtering process, particularly in highly rated journals, is, if anything, even more rigorous. Hargens (1988) estimated that between 50 per cent and 80 per cent of articles submitted to journals in the social sciences were rejected. Some journals give information on their rejection rate on their website. The commonest reasons for rejection of quantitative and qualitative articles are broadly similar (see Greenhalgh 2014 for further discussion). These can be grouped into three main areas relating to all types of method: authors did not give enough information on the methods used; authors failed to provide an explanation of how data were analysed; or authors failed to write clearly and concisely, drawing out the findings in the conclusion. For further clarification of some of these points from the personal reviewing experience of the editors, see Box 27.2.

Box 27.2 Common reasons for journal rejection of quantitative and qualitative research

Papers submitted to journals tend to be rejected for many reasons, including:

- The paper was not sufficiently original
- The paper did not fit the journal house style, including in length
- It did not pose a question that could be answered
- The method chosen for analysis was not appropriate
- The research was compromised by practical difficulties
- The sample size/number of respondents was inadequate
- The statistical analysis or data analysis was insufficient
- The data did not warrant the conclusions made
- There was a conflict of interest involved with the author(s)
- The paper was poorly drafted and not clearly written
- The article concerned was inadequately referenced
- The links between data and the findings/conclusion was unclear.

Researchers can limit the likelihood of rejection of their work by ensuring they select an appropriate journal for the research, doing spelling and grammar checks, reading the text out and asking a valued colleague in a similar academic field for feedback before submission.

Avenues to publication for journals are controlled by a variety of producers who apply filters and can block access. In this case, it is not the commissioning editors or the board of a publishing house who make judgements, but the journal editors. The decision by a journal to accept or reject an article is made through a graduated system of responses. The editor of a journal may decide simply to 'desk reject' a paper without sending it out to reviewers if it manifestly does not fit the brief. If it does go out to referees for comment, it may be referred back by the editor for minor or major revisions before the acceptance or rejection stage.

However, there are many other journals to select from if the initial submission is rejected. In terms of dissemination, Elsevier alone has over 700 journals in its stable, many of which are in the health arena. Those submitting papers often start with the highest profile journal in their field and work their way down the pecking order until their article is accepted. A critical factor here – apart from subject specialization, the philosophy of the journal and the resonance of the membership of the editorial board – is the journal's impact factor. If the impact factor is high, the article is likely to have a greater number of citations. This not only aids dissemination in the scholarly community but is an indicator of prestige. Researchers submitting papers to top journals should note that rejection should not necessarily be regarded negatively. Learning from reviewer feedback can provide a positive impetus for improving the paper.

Ethical issues and the limitations of dissemination

From an ethical perspective, we should be clear that the main purpose of disseminating health research through publication or other means should ideally be to further the interests of patients or advance the wider public interest (Saks 2012). In this vein, there is an obligation, particularly on field researchers, to publish findings even if these are negative. There has long been concern that there is a publication bias in clinical trials, that there is a long time-lag between a trial and publication, that drug trials are over-represented and that negative results are hard to publish (see, for instance, Chalmers 1990; Chalmers and Matthews 2006; Godlee 2012). The relative absence of the latter may be for many reasons, including that neither journals nor researchers think it worthwhile to publish other than positive results. Cynically, there may sometimes be career promotion and future funding issues at stake (Rivas and Pandya-Wood 2014) or commercial interests from pharmaceutical companies or elsewhere (as highlighted by Goldacre 2013). Yet negative findings also add to knowledge, along with the positive findings that come out of health research, and these can also help to save lives.

Alongside this, it is also necessary to place the limitations of the dissemination of health research in perspective. The dissemination of health research findings will not necessarily in themselves always be enough to effect helpful changes in practice by health practitioners on the ground, by the public in their health behaviour or by politicians in health policy making. The complexities involved here have been well highlighted in the translational literature – not least in analysing the barriers to the implementation of health research in the natural sciences and how these might be overcome. This is highlighted by Brownson, Colditz and Proctor (2018) in a number of areas, from the classic cases of delays in the adoption of insulin and penicillin onwards. However, even though education and audit may not effectively reinforce changes in existing health practices and policies, the dissemination of health research findings is a vital component of the process, alongside such factors as interpersonal contact with respected others and financial incentives (Bowling 2014). Here it should be stressed that change will only be worthwhile if the findings disseminated are sound; that is, if they can be positively evaluated. This brings us to the next section of this chapter – the important subject of the evaluation of health research.

Evaluation

Just as with dissemination, there are many different forms of evaluation. But what is evaluation? Generally, it can be defined as the systematic assessment of the design, implementation or results of an initiative to assist learning or decision making (Poth et al. 2012). One type of evaluation involves assessing whether appropriate forms of methodology and methods have been used in the research and underpin the findings. In the case of the assessment of a research proposal, it will also be important that the framework for the research, including the research question, has the potential to add to knowledge. The evaluator(s) will assess the conduct of the project and, on this basis, decide whether to accept a proposal, award a qualification, fund a project or publish an output. Another type of evaluation in the health arena is where the researcher is more focused on evaluating the effect or outcome of a policy change or intervention. This is often commissioned by local or national government, or a private agency (see also Chapter 22 on types of policy evaluation).

Both forms of evaluation are represented in the various chapters in this book. The latter particularly involves assessing the evidence produced and using the findings to guide relevant policy makers and practitioners on further action and future resource allocation (Parsons 2017). This form of evaluation is more challenging as the researcher has less opportunity to shape the research question and the context for the research is likely to be more complex, with variations in context. Furthermore, researchers are accountable directly or indirectly to a wider constituency, including government project managers, analysts and civil servants, and consultants with a range of commissions in the private sector. In turn, this type of research will very likely be evaluated by external experts to ensure that findings have been validated and have genuinely established good practice.

What is evaluated will vary from the assessment of the latest technological innovations to interventions in hospital and community care. The tools used to conduct the evaluations have their own pitfalls, as illustrated in this book by Chapter 10 on action research, Chapter 18 on the New Public Management and Chapter 22 on comparative health research. There are also other pitfalls which will need to be avoided or at least mitigated in the complicated area of evaluating policy change, such as the excessive absorption of time (Kara 2012) and uses and abuses of bibliometrics in the analysis (Gingras 2016). Why we evaluate ranges from efforts to increase accountability to endeavours to facilitate the development and growth of knowledge (Chelimsky and Shadish 1997). Evaluation more invidiously can be used as a device to legitimate decisions as rational and objective when they are in fact politically contentious. This needs to be avoided from an ethical viewpoint (Parsons 2017). Who, though, are the evaluators in health research and what do they examine?

Evaluators and what they look for

Evaluators are there to make judgements about the quality of the product and the investment of resources, whatever the output. How this is assessed will vary, but usually certain criteria are specified by the organization or person looking to evaluate an output or policy. These are elaborated institutionally in the examples in Boxes 27.3–27.6 set out in the pages that follow.

Mapping groups of evaluators in researching health

Evaluation, like dissemination, may occur at a variety of levels. In terms of decision-making, evaluators in the health field may be, for example:

- Academic researchers analysing primary and secondary research materials in constructing a manuscript for publication
- Policy makers assessing reports on the effect of a particular policy or how a policy has been implemented. They may wish to find out where the next policy development should occur – for example, in delivering a service.
- Professional practitioners sifting through relevant health publications to decide on the best treatment regimes for patients
- Users of health services seeking to inform themselves about the most appropriate treatment options for a condition or intervention
- Undergraduate or postgraduate students interpreting research papers in constructing dissertations and other projects.

At the highest organizational level, an evaluator may sit on a national or international research committee, judging research submissions against others in bids for considerable amounts of funding. Others may be journal editors, members of the editorial boards or referees for papers for major health journals and internal or external examiners for university doctoral theses. The individuals carrying out these roles will be guided by specific criteria for the task. Typically, decisions are made by a panel of members and experts or specialists will be invited to give their opinion in writing to provide a form of peer review. In the UK and elsewhere, the trend has been towards an ever closer specification of assessment criteria for an evaluation with greater transparency about the process. Examples of the criteria can be given as follows.

Box 27.3   Evaluation criteria for assessing the quality of research outputs for panel members of the United Kingdom Research Excellence Framework

The Research Excellence Framework (REF) is a process by which the UK government allocates funding for research in universities, on a periodic cycle of approximately every six years, following submissions from individual universities. Discipline-based experts, including those in a number of health subjects, are recruited to panels to make judgements about the quality of research outputs and the research environment since the previous assessment.

The broad criteria for evaluators in the latest REF in terms of research outputs were to assess the published output of articles, books, reports and other media in terms of the *rigour* of the research, its *originality* and its *significance* (Research Excellence Framework 2012). This approach has been adopted by other countries and, as a consequence, has led to a clearer articulation of what is expected of researchers and what constitutes 'quality' in research.

The greatest emphasis in demonstrating *rigour* is given to showing that the methodology and methods are appropriate for a project, providing a rationale for the design so that the reader can interpret the research journey taken, and articulating the basis of the findings and their contribution to knowledge. Reviewers will expect a justification for the choice of methodology and method, a clear and honest account of the research process, with a consideration for ethics and relations with participants. Findings should be justified on the basis of the evidence shown and clarity in the writing up is seen as part of being rigorous.

In terms of *originality*, this can be taken to be new knowledge, new directions or, in clinical research, findings that strengthen a claim or test a hypothesis. Evaluators are chosen because they are seen as experts – they know the literature and the state of knowledge within a disciplinary field. Borderline decisions are generally made following discussion within a group against the stated criteria. Evaluators are expected to justify why they say an output is original.

The criterion of *significance* is the most subjective of the three criteria. The importance of a research output will depend on its perceived relevance to the discipline concerned and the benefits to society in terms of the contribution to knowledge or to social life. Again, the rationale given for decisions and group decision making can increase credibility. A well-thought-out dissemination strategy with participant involvement can strengthen a claim for the research output to have been significant for a wide audience.

Where there are multiple criteria, these are given numeric values to achieve an overall grade for the outputs submitted for each researcher. This is then put alongside other criteria as the basis for a departmental and institutional profile and, finally, provides a justification for the award of resources. It provides a mechanism for competitively assessing a hierarchy of quality in a situation of scarce resources. Institutions with departments that are found to have higher-quality outputs can and do receive much more funding for research.

Box 27.4 Research evaluation criteria for committee members of the United Kingdom National Institute for Health Service Research (NIHR) Research for Patient Benefit scheme

The National Institute of Health Research (NIHR) Research for Patient Benefit scheme is a national programme that funds research in the UK through eight Regional Advisory Panels made up of clinicians, methodologists (including statisticians), academic researchers and allied health professionals with an applied health research track record affiliated to cognate institutions. Inspired by patients and practice, this scheme aims to generate research evidence to improve, expand and strengthen the way that health care is delivered for patients, the public and the National Health Service.

The overall criteria used by evaluators on the assessing panel in making recommendations about the applications for funding are as follows:

Quality of the research proposed

- Is this an important research question?
- Is the proposed methodology robust and based on a sound scientific rationale?
- Will the proposed methodology answer the research question?
- Has the research involved service users at relevant stages of the project?

Significance and potential benefit to social care and users of services

- What is the trajectory to social care benefit?
- What is the likelihood this will lead to benefit?
- What is the likely scale of impact?

(Continued)

(Continued)

Value for money provided by the application

- Given the likelihood of achieving benefit, is this proposal costed in the right funding tier?
- Given the likely scale of impact, does it provide value for money?

Box 27.5   Assessment criteria for referees for the international journal *Social Science and Medicine*

The journal *Social Science and Medicine* publishes the following types of individual paper contributions:

- Peer-reviewed original research articles and critical/analytical reviews in areas of social science research relevant to health up to 9,000 words including abstract, tables, and references as well as the main text.
- Peer-reviewed short reports of research findings on topical issues or published articles of 2,000 to 4,000 words.
- Submitted or invited commentaries and responses debating, and published alongside, selected articles.

On the website of *Social Science and Medicine* (www.elsevier.com/locate/socscimed), more detailed information on the evaluation criteria for paper submissions is given. As for many other journals, they include areas such as:

- Ethical considerations being followed
- Declaration of conflicting interests being appropriate
- Work having not been previously published
- Papers not being considered for publication elsewhere
- The use of inclusive language
- Concise and informative title to assist information retrieval
- An abstract with keywords for indexing purposes
- Full details of the research methods used
- Prescribed referencing style.

The papers are initially considered by the editor then, if suitable for the journal, are sent out for double-blind review to a minimum of two independent expert referees. The names and affiliations of the authors of the papers are hidden. Having received the subject-specialist reviews of the referees on content, the editor is responsible for the final decision on the acceptance or rejection of a paper in the evaluatory process.

Box 27.6 Typical PhD examination criteria

Although the specifics vary from university to university, examiners are typically asked to evaluate the PhD thesis in terms of such features as:

- Confirmation that it is the student's own work
- Representing a substantial original contribution to knowledge
- Demonstrating the exercise of independent critical ability
- Exhibiting a satisfactory standard of expression
- Ensuring the coherence of its structure.

Usually, the PhD thesis word limit is up to 80,000 words. The candidate who has written the thesis is normally examined in the UK in a *viva voce* with an internal examiner (as a moderator) and one or two external examiners, who are selected for their expertise and experience. This is the most common format, although there are variations. More public forms of examination and assessment at a distance take place in some other countries.

The examiners make a joint report and are invited to agree one of the following recommendations for the student to the university concerned:

- Award of the degree without further conditions
- Award of the degree subject to revisions
- Resubmission of a revised thesis for examination
- The award of a different type of degree (such as an MPhil)
- No award of a degree.

Importantly, all these top-level institutional roles involve evaluation through an expert interpretation of papers and other research outputs. These parallel the skills required by individual academics, postgraduate and higher level undergraduate students, and managers in appraising health research literature in everyday settings.

An illustrative case of evaluation: Reviewing research papers

We shall focus our discussion of evaluation here particularly on critically appraising research papers as an illustrative case. This will help to join up further this section with that on dissemination which preceded it. Earlier chapters in Part I of the book stressed the importance of stating clearly in a paper the research question to address, why the question under investigation is significant and how addressing it will add to knowledge. This provides an argument for carrying out, and presenting the findings of, the research.

Following these introductory remarks, a succinct review of the literature is important as it can show how the research question has been investigated by others. In establishing the viability of the research question, it is helpful for the author(s) explicitly to identify the particular theoretical approach taken, the key concepts used and the substantive areas of investigation to date. This provides a basis for justifying the theoretical and methodological framework chosen for the research. It is also important that the type of design used for the research is outlined and why particular methods have been selected. A description of how the research has been carried out is also necessary. How the data were collected and analysed is critical – and should be described in detail. Anyone reading a research paper should look for these elements in order to evaluate it. The author(s) should always be prepared to be open and honest about the problems they encountered and how these were addressed. This provides a context for the research, while the evidence for the main findings should be assessed in relation to the question posed – based on clearly articulated counterfactuals and an open approach to disconfirming evidence. Here negative findings are as important as those which confirm what is already known.

In this book we have asked our contributors to provide advice on how to read critically different types of qualitative and quantitative research. There is no need to reiterate this advice as it is included in each of the chapters on specific methods (the reader should refer back to these as necessary). There are a number of texts on evaluating research more generally (see, for example, Clarke 1999), including in academic journals in health and other areas (see, for instance, Greenhalgh 2014; Pyrczak 2017). However, it is probably most helpful here to pull together selectively the more important suggestions for reading health research offered by contributors in Parts II and III of this book.

For *qualitative research*, it is especially crucial that the elements below are covered when evaluating health research papers:

- The strategy used for drawing a sample should be made explicit and related to the research question
- Despite smaller numbers of participants in such research, saturation is reached
- Any present/historic documents used are aligned with the researcher's purpose
- The data collected from unstructured interviews is rich enough to bring the study to life
- Sufficient detail is given on fieldwork undertaken in participant observation
- Context and interaction are taken into account when employing focus groups
- In action research, the relationship of researcher and participants is considered
- The researcher counters the intrusion of subjectivity in analysing qualitative data.

For *quantitative research*, it is particularly vital that the following matters are addressed when evaluating health research papers:

- The sampling design is appropriate for providing answers to the research question
- The sample size is large enough to permit precise estimates of key parameters
- The response rate is high enough to have confidence about representativeness
- The participants are appropriately selected/blinded for randomized controlled trials
- Experimental methods are justified as being most suited to the research question
- The consequences of doing nothing are explored in health economics research
- In economic analysis, relevant benefits and costs are identified, measured and valued
- The confidence level at which statistical significance is set should be appropriate
- In statistical analysis, measures of spread should be given along with those of the average.

More generally, as discussed in Part IV of the book on issues in health research, it is critical that reassurance is also sought on the following when evaluating health research papers:

- The study has been approved by an ethics committee and has participant consent
- Participants have been suitably involved in all stages of the research
- Appropriate attention is given to questions of validity, reliability and generalizability
- Different methods of data collection are triangulated where they are used
- The value of mixed methods and interdisciplinary work is acknowledged as relevant
- The limitations as well as the strengths of the study are noted and addressed
- Units in countries with broad similarities are typically studied in comparative research
- Opportunities are taken to use online research methods in health where appropriate.

The difficulties and opportunities provided by evaluation

As indicated above, evaluation can be complex and the evaluation of the effectiveness of policy innovation presents special problems. In some areas, methodologies and methods have been developed to evaluate treatment innovations and these have been referred to in various chapters. For instance, the National Institute for Health and Care Excellence (NICE) in the UK has a methodology to evaluate the medicines and treatments that should be funded in the National Health Service. However, the complexities are exemplified by the introduction of the periodic revalidation of doctors in the UK. This policy has been accepted and, in some settings, has brought some tangible benefits in terms of regulatory oversight of performance. However, due to the many factors involved and differences in patterns of organization, it is difficult to establish cause and effect as regards outcomes. Context matters. Revalidation as it was designed has been easiest to implement in quite large health care organizations (like NHS trusts) where the capacity and capability for clinical governance already existed or could be provided, and where most doctors have a fairly straightforward employment relationship as salaried employees (Tazzyman et al. 2017). The difficulties in evaluation are also highlighted in Chapter 18 in relation to research on the impact of health care managers on the efficiency and effectiveness of the delivery of health services.

More generally, Byrne (2013) observes that it is strictly impossible – despite our best efforts to discover universal empirical regularities – to establish absolutely the causal effect of any intervention in the modern social world in health or other fields, even using much extolled randomized controlled trials. This is because this world is complicated and subject to change. Nonetheless, Byrne believes that we can develop generalizable knowledge beyond single instances if we recognize the importance of context and the significance of human agency, not least through a focus on temporal sequencing, contingent causation and comparative analysis. This enables us at least to begin to understand what works where and when, and the factors that underlie positive outcomes. In this spirit, in evaluating specific pieces of research, it is important to remember that, for all the advanced analytical and technical tools now at our disposal, we live in a challenging and imperfect world. There are no sacred cows and we should be responsive to reasoned criticisms of our work in the evaluation process. This transparency in health research should enable individuals, organizations and governments to work towards improved health outcomes, using the evaluative opportunities explored in this chapter.

As with dissemination, putting in place packages of relevant training for evaluation – particularly for staff leading such initiatives – may assist with rolling out the tasks concerned. In the case of evaluation, these might usefully cover the general principles involved, as well as specific underpinning techniques operationalized in the health field, such as meta-analysis and cost–benefit analysis, discussed in Chapter 4 and Chapter 16 of this book. Along with mentorship and coaching from experienced personnel, a firm platform of development would then be provided for those taking forward the next critical steps in researching health.

Conclusion

To conclude, in conducting research into health and health care, dissemination and evaluation are very important if the field is to develop further. Given the many players in the health arena, both inside and outside the university context, knowledge of what others are working on and collaboration between researchers is essential. A shared knowledge of the vocabulary of health research and an understanding of what particular research methods can and cannot do will assist productive collaboration. We trust that this chapter has improved your insights into the many different dimensions of dissemination and evaluation and that these – together with other related chapters in this volume – will make you more aware of their significance and become more effective health researchers. An exercise follows that is designed to hone further your skills in these two vital areas of research.

Exercise 27.1   Disseminating and evaluating health research

Disseminating health research

In a research project of your choice, consider how you might best disseminate the findings, paying particular attention to factors such as:

- Any funders of the study and their requirements
- The audience you wish your research to reach
- The media of communication that you would use
- The resources that you possess.

Evaluating health research

Pick a research article on health from a journal that particularly interests you. Using the tools provided in this chapter, and elaborated in this book, undertake a detailed evaluation. This can very effectively be undertaken as a group exercise, in which each member evaluates the quality of the paper concerned and grades this on a scale from 0 (poor) to 10 (outstanding). A discussion of the comparative scores can then be undertaken, with a view to obtaining a consensual group ranking.

Recommended further reading

Drawing on high-level scholarship on dissemination and implementation, this book considers how science and health innovations can best be translated into everyday life:

Brownson, R. C., Colditz, G. A., Proctor, E. K. (eds) (2018) *Dissemination and Implementation Research in Health: Translating Science to Practice*, 2nd edition. Oxford: Oxford University Press.

This is a very useful article highlighting the complexities of evaluation in health and other areas:

Bryne, D. (2013) 'Evaluating complex interventions in a complex world', *Evaluation*, *19*(3): 217–28.

This recently reprinted book discusses the methodological issues, practical difficulties and associated problems in conducting evaluations of qualitative and quantitative social research, and specifically contains a helpful chapter on the evaluation of health care:

Clarke, A. (1999) *Evaluation Research: An Introduction to Principles, Methods and Practice*. London: Sage.

This book is a useful general guide to evaluating journal research papers:

Pyrczak, F. (2017) *Evaluating Research in Academic Journals: A Practical Guide to Realistic Evaluation*, 6th edition. London: Routledge.

References

Bastow, S., Tinkler, J. and Dunleavy, P. (2014) *The Impact of the Social Sciences: How Academics and Their Research Make a Difference*. London: Sage.

Bowling, A. (2014) *Research Methods in Health: Investigating Health and Health Services*, 4th edition. Maidenhead: Open University Press.

Brownson, R. C., Colditz, G. A. and Proctor, E. K. (eds) (2018) *Dissemination and Implementation Research in Health: Translating Science to Practice*, 2nd edition. Oxford: Oxford University Press.

Bryne, D. (2013) 'Evaluating complex interventions in a complex world', *Evaluation*, *19*(3): 217–28.

Chalmers, I. (1990) 'Under reporting research is scientific misconduct', *Journal of the American Medical Association*, *236*: 1405–8.

Chalmers, I. and Matthews, R. (2006) 'What are the implications of optimism bias in clinical research?', *The Lancet*, *367*: 449–50.

Chelimsky, E. and Shadish, W. R. (eds) (1997) *Evaluation in the 21st Century: A Handbook*. Thousand Oaks, CA: Sage.

Clarke, A. (1999) *Evaluation Research: An Introduction to Principles, Methods and Practice*. London: Sage.

Gingras, Y. (2016) *Bibliometrics and Research Evaluation: Uses and Abuses*. Cambridge, MA: The MIT Press.

Godlee, F. (2012) 'Research misconduct is widespread and harms patients', *British Medical Journal*, *344*: e14.

Goldacre, B. (2013) *Bad Pharma: How Medicine is Broken and How We Can Fix It*. London: Fourth Estate.

Greenhalgh, T. (2014) *How to Read a Paper: The Basics of Evidence-based Medicine*, 5th edition. Chichester: Wiley-Blackwell.

Hannaway, C. (2008) *Biomedicine in the Twentieth Century: Practices, Policies and Politics*. Fairfax: IOS Press.

Hargens, L. L. (1988) 'Scholarly consensus and rejection rates', *American Sociological Review*, *53*: 139–51.

Kara, H. (2012) *Research and Evaluation for Busy Practitioners: A Time Saving Guide*. Bristol: Policy Press.

Owen, A. (ed.) (2018) *Writers' and Artists' Yearbook*. London: Bloomsbury.

Parsons, D. (2017) *Demystifying Evaluation: Practical Approaches for Researchers and Users*. Bristol: Policy Press.

Poth, C., Lamarche, M. K., Yapp, A., Sulla, E. and Chisamore, C. (2012) 'Towards a definition of evaluation within the Canadian context: Who knew it would be so difficult?', *Canadian Journal of Program Evaluation, 29*(3): 1–18.

Pyrczak, F. (2017) *Evaluating Research in Academic Journals: A Practical Guide to Realistic Evaluation*, 6th edition. London: Routledge.

Rawat, S. and Meena, S. (2014) 'Publish or perish: Where are we heading?', *Journal of Research in Medical Sciences, 9*(2): 87–9.

Research Excellence Framework (2012) *Panel Criteria and Working Methods*. Bristol: HEFCE.

Rivas, C. and Pandya-Wood, R. (2014) 'Dissemination', in D. Walker (ed.), *An Introduction to Health Services Research*. London: Sage.

Saks, M. (2012) 'The challenge of implementing social science research', *Portuguese Journal of Social Science, 11*(1). Available at: http://pjss.iscte-iul.pt/index.php/pjss/article/view/113

Saks, M. (2015) 'Engaging the university administration', in R. Dingwall and M. B. McDonnell (eds), *The Sage Handbook of Research Management*. London: Sage.

Saks, M. (ed.) (2020, forthcoming) *Support Workers in the Healthcare Workforce: International Perspectives on the Invisible Providers of Health Care*. Bristol: Policy Press.

Saks, M. and Allsop, J. (2007) 'Social policy, professional regulation and health support work in the United Kingdom', *Social Policy and Society, 6*(2): 165–77.

Saks, M., Allsop, J., Chevannes, M., Clark, M., Fagan, R., Genders, N., Johnson, M., Kent, J., Payne, M., Szczepura, A. and Unell, J. (2000) *Review of Health Support Workers: Report to the UK Departments of Health*. Leicester: De Montfort University.

Tazzyman, A., Ferguson, J., Hillier, C., Boyd, A., Tredinnick-Rowe, J., Archer, J., de Bere, S. R. and Walshe, K. (2017) 'The implementation of medical revalidation: An assessment using normalisation process theory', *BMC Health Services Research, 17*: 749.

Key Concepts in Health Research

Action research A form of collective self-reflective inquiry undertaken by participants in social situations in order to improve the rationality and justice of their own situation, policy and practice.

Analysis Derived from the Greek word meaning 'to unravel tangles'.

Analytical induction A method for systematic qualitative data analysis where the researcher identifies themes that provide an explanation for a phenomenon with the progressive refinement of theory until no disconfirming evidence can be found.

Bias The danger that research data may be skewed for known or unknown reasons leading to false estimates of the effect of an intervention. Common sources of bias are in recruitment, selection, performance, detection, attrition or by researchers or participants.

Bioethics Usually refers to the more philosophical abstract version of health ethics.

Biomedical model of disease Where the patient may be seen as a physical/mechanistic entity that can be measured, controlled and ultimately manipulated. In research, the body and body parts are taken as objects for research.

Bivariate analysis Questions that address the possible relationship between two variables in statistical analysis.

Black box An area of life that cannot be accessed by researchers.

Blind trial Used to detect the specific effects of an intervention by removing any prior 'expectation' that the researcher or participant may have of the trial results from the active or placebo treatment. It maintains equipoise.

Boolean operators Terms such as 'and', 'or' and 'not' are used to refine or combine search terms to retrieve the most relevant articles for a literature review.

Bubbling A search engine that is set to guess what a user may want based on their search history and according to other factors such as their geographical location.

Case Refers to a particular empirical entity that is at the same time both a part and a product of a research project.

Case study design The case is the unit of analysis (an organization, place or person) and the focus is on the circumstances, dynamics and complexity of a single or a small number of cases.

Case-control study Compares the characteristics of a particular phenomenon in the group of interest to a control or reference group.

Cochrane Collaboration An international collaboration established to organize medical research findings to facilitate evidence-based decision-making by health professionals, patients and policy makers.

Coding frame Pre-constructed in quantitative research to pre-code closed questions. Researchers construct the coding for open questions or qualitative data.

Cohort studies A selected population is studied over time to investigate the effect of a particular factor on health outcomes.

Comparative design A design where the same phenomenon, institution, custom, tradition or culture is compared within two or more contrasting socio-cultural settings.

Comparative health research A method that may be exploratory, explanatory or evaluate differences and similarities against criteria of relative success or failure.

Complementary and alternative medicine (CAM) A diverse range of therapies outside the political mainstream which tends to ideologically take a holistic approach where the subjective views of clients and mind–body links are seen as central to treatment.

Concept A summary of an abstract idea or generalization based on phenomenon observed in the real world.

Confounding Occurs when a third variable – an unknown factor – intervenes between two variables that then appear to be associated, but the relationship between them is false.

Constant comparison Associated with grounded theory where the researcher compares new data with existing data to develop their coding categories.

Construct validity The robustness of an indicator when tested against the outcome measure used in previous studies.

Constructivism A theory that knowledge about social phenomena is constructed by research subjects and is embedded in society and culture.

Content validity The extent to which an indicator measures what participants think it should measure.

Convenience sample A technique for obtaining a sample by contacting known, rather than randomly selected, informants.

Conversational analysis A detailed analysis of recorded talk collected in a naturalistic setting.

Co-production A set of principles for all stages of the research that include researchers and a range of participants.

Covert research When research data are collected without the subject/participant's knowledge and consent.

Cross-over study A type of trial design that involves one treatment in a first phase, a washout period with no treatment and then a second randomized treatment with a control group.

Cross-sectional design A study that requires the collection of data from a number of subjects/objects over a specified time with the aim of establishing an association between variables.

Culture A multi-layered concept that includes many aspects of belief and behaviour, some learned and some linked to cherished aspects of identity.

Data analysis A crucial stage in the research process when the information collected is reduced to produce research findings.

Data extraction form A form created by researchers undertaking a literature review to systematically record key information from articles and books.

Deductive reasoning An approach where the researcher draws on a body of theory and knowledge to develop a hypothesis or proposition that can be tested through empirical research.

Delphi method A technique that collects opinions through questionnaires or other methods to find out views on problems or issues. It can include more than one round.

Deontology The discussion of moral principles and rules related to duties and obligations.

Descriptive statistics The numerical, graphical and tabular techniques for organizing, analysing and presenting data.

Deviant/divergent cases Those that differ from most other cases.

Discourse analysis An approach that analyses talk in natural settings to identify the rules of talk in context to show how social phenomena are constructed through language exchange.

Disease An abnormal condition affecting the body or body parts. Within bio-medicine disease refers to named clusters of signs and symptoms of pathology and anatomy.

Dissemination A process of sharing information and knowledge in research to improve access.

Documentary research Research that draws on human artefacts of one or more pages (or computer files) that contain information in the form of words, numbers, diagrams, drawings and/or illustrations.

Double-blind trial A type of randomized controlled trial where neither the investigators nor the trial participants (volunteers/patients) are aware of who is receiving the active or placebo treatment.

E-health The cost-effective and secure use of information communication technologies in support of health and health-related fields, including health care services, health surveillance, health literature, and health education, knowledge and research.

Economic evaluation A measure of the utility or value of particular combinations of inputs to achieve health outcomes. It includes cost–benefit analysis, costing studies, cost minimization analysis, cost-effective analysis, and cost and utility analysis.

Empirical research Research based on data collection of observations of phenomena.

Empowerment Aims to enable participants to take part in all aspects of the research process.

Epidemiology The study of variations in the pattern of disease and wellbeing in populations and their causes.

Epistemology The philosophical study of the nature of knowledge, the origins and legitimate routes to acquiring knowledge.

Equipoise A term used in clinical trials to indicate where researchers/clinicians have an equal belief in the treatments being compared and no grounds for recommending one form of treatment over another.

Ethics Defined as the formal moral standards set by professional associations and other institutions to help to maintain and evaluate high standards. 'Ethics' is also used interchangeably with the broader term 'morals', which are concerned with the principles of right and wrong behaviour.

Ethnicity A concept that refers to a socially defined group of people who may be characterized by such factors as culture and language or myth of origin.

Ethnography A method for collecting data from communities and groups through observation, interview and the analysis of cultural artefacts to develop theories and explanations.

Ethnomethodology An approach based on taking informants' stories and interactions as accounts of how social order is accomplished.

Evaluation The systematic assessment of the design, implementation or results of an initiative to assist learning or decision-making.

Experiment A research design based on the scientific method to test changes by having a treatment and control group which aims to establish a relationship between cause and effect. In the health field they are more common in the clinical sciences, psychological studies and, more recently, in policy intervention.

Experimental (or scientific) method An umbrella term that includes a variety of techniques that aim to maintain scientific rigour by testing a hypothesis, reducing bias and ruling out alternative explanations.

Face validity Refers to the relevance of the outcome measure or finding to the study questions.

Focus group A specific research technique derived from market research where a number of people are brought together to discuss a topic in a 'focused' way. In social research it is synonymous with a group interview.

Frequency table A table recording the number of times each value of the variable appears in a distribution.

Gender A concept that is part of situated experience and a fundamental organizing principle in society and science.

Gender-sensitive health research A term used to draw attention to gender bias in health care and the unfair and unequal treatment of men and boys, women and girls.

Generalizability A concern for the external validity of research findings and the possibility of applying the findings to other groups.

Gillick judgement A judgement made in 1985 that children's informed and 'wise' decisions must be respected in decisions about their care and treatment.

Governance A term referring to the arrangements to set, assess and monitor standards to safeguard the quality of research and promote good practice.

Grey literature A literature published independently by, for example, specialist research units rather than mainstream publishers.

Grounded theory A set of analytical strategies that can be applied to a variety of data collection techniques. Research begins in a general area of interest rather than with a hypothesis and moves on to identify concepts and theoretical connections emerging from the data.

Hawthorne effect A term derived from a classic research study, this refers to the possibility that the researcher's presence influences the behaviour observed.

Health An absence of illness or an ideal state of physical and mental wellbeing. In social science, it is seen variously as a socially constructed moral norm of social functioning or a subjective definition by individuals.

Health care user A person who uses health care services, either as a patient or carer.

Health needs assessment An assessment of one or more of the following: expressed needs, normative needs (defined by experts), comparative needs (in relation to other groups) or felt needs.

Health outcome assessment Measures of health status, such as the Short Form 36 (SF-36) and Measure Yourself Medical Outcome Profile (MYMOP).

Health technology assessment (HTA) A tool to evaluate evidence from different countries in order to identify what medical technologies or care pathways work best through systematic evaluation.

Heteroskedasticity A statistical term indicating that sub-populations have a varying scatter of variables.

Hippocratic Oath The oath relating to ethical standards for those engaged in medical work devised by the Greek philosopher Hippocrates.

Holistic medicine An approach adopted by practitioners to include the views of clients and mind–body links.

Hypothesis A proposition that underpins a research question to be tested by further research.

Identity Based on the idea that the notion of the 'self' is linked to identification with certain social groups. It may be associated with social class, ethnicity, age, gender or other communities.

Illness In social science, the obverse of health or as a subjectively defined condition by individuals and significant others.

Indicator Refers to a concept if there is no direct measure available. It is a method for operationalizing theory in surveys.

Inductive reasoning A process that begins with observation and/or data collection, finds patterns or associations and builds a theory, or explanation, on the basis of the evidence available.

Informed consent A participant freely agrees to participate in research and fully understands the consequences of this agreement.

Interdisciplinary research A collaborative form of research where a range of professions, occupations and users work together to address a research question.

Interpretivism An epistemological position that assumes that knowledge about the world derives from human perception and understanding.

Interval/ratio scale Sometimes called a metric scale, this is a scale which ranks results from highest to lowest but also measures the differences, or intervals, between them.

Kantian ethics A form of ethics based on principles that determine duties and obligations.

Literature review A stage in the research process where the aim is to identify, analyse, assess and interpret a body of knowledge related to a particular topic.

Longitudinal design The study of phenomena over time.

Measures of central tendency Indicates the typical or average value for a distribution. Three common measures are the mode, median and mean.

Measures of dispersion Descriptive statistics that indicate the spread or variety of scores in a distribution.

Meta-coding Where concepts and categories are linked conceptually.

Meta-ethnography The method for cross-checking qualitative studies on a matrix and to identify new interpretations of existing data.

Methodology A strategy with guidelines and principles used to address a research question by gathering information and assessing evidence.

Methods Tools or techniques used to collect data. Examples include experiments, surveys, observations and interviews.

Mixed methods research Research where both quantitative and qualitative methods are used to study a phenomenon and not simply a range of methods within the same paradigm.

Morbidity Any departure, subjective or objective, from a state of physiological or psychological wellbeing.

Mortality rate The incidence of death in a population.

Multidisciplinary research Teams of researchers that work alongside each other, such as health economists, epidemiologists and clinicians and social scientists. Collaborative working between the social and medical sciences is currently favoured in health research.

Narrative analysis A method that explores the structure of texts and the ways in which the narrator uses the narrative.

Narrative review A literature review that identifies key concepts, specific terms and the theoretical approaches adopted by different authors to understand a phenomenon.

Naturalism In the social sciences, a research technique that collects data in everyday settings with a minimum use of intrusive methods. In the sciences, it can mean the use of the scientific method.

Netnography Online research which is based on the principles of ethnography.

Nominal group technique A method that draws on a group to identify research questions, choose methods and make decisions on design.

Nominal scale Classifies cases into categories that have no quantitative ordering.

Non-probabilistic sampling The probability that each individual in a population will constitute a part of the sample and will not be known.

Normal distribution This is the most common form of distribution of a variable. It is sometimes called a bell curve as it is shaped like a bell. The peak of the curve reflects the mean of the median. It is symmetrical and tails off on either side.

Normalization Process Theory A middle-range theory that provides a framework to analyse the factors that have been shown to support the implementation of new policy interventions.

Ontology A philosophical term that refers to the study of reality and nature of being.

Opportunity cost An economic concept: every choice represents a value forgone.

Ordinal scale A ranking of cases according to the quantity or intensity of the variable expressed by each case.

Ordinary least squares (OLS) A method for estimating unknown parameters used in linear regression analysis.

Orthodox medicine Sometimes referred to as mainstream medicine, it draws on a body of knowledge learned during professional training and constitutes legitimated practice.

Paradigm A cluster of beliefs or set of assumptions about the nature of knowledge that influences what should be studied and how research should be done.

Paradigm wars The conflict between researchers taking different positions about concepts, methods and methodology. It has been used to describe the different positions on the nature of knowledge taken by positivist and interpretivist researchers.

Participant A person involved in research, and used in preference to research subjects, patients or volunteers. It implies active involvement and a shared control of the research process.

Participant observation A research method used where the researcher spends an extended period of time in a natural setting participating in, and observing, particular classes of activity.

Pathology The study of the causes and effects of diseases and a specialist area in medicine.

Patient narratives Accounts of the patient pathway through the illness and treatment process.

Patient pathway The treatment process through which the patient passes through the health system.

Phenomenology An interpretivist methodology that aims to study how individuals themselves make sense of their world.

Placebo A non-active treatment used in a trial.

Positivism An epistemological position that favours the use of scientific methods in conducting research. Positivism aims to identify general laws and objective facts in the natural and social world by using methods that are quantitative.

Pragmatic trial or study A trial or study undertaken to assess whether a therapy will work in everyday practice.

Probability sampling A sample where each member (a unit or element) has a specifiable chance of being selected.

Protocol A written plan of a clinical research project to cover aims and process to justify a proposal for peer review.

Public and patient involvement The involvement of members of the public in research where this is being carried out 'with' or 'by' members of the public rather than 'to', 'about' or 'for' them.

Purposive sampling A method where informants are selected because they have specific knowledge about the research question.

Quality Adjusted Life Year (QALY) A measure of a benefit in terms of one added year of perfect health. This measure must be set against the costs of treatment to assess clinical cost-effectiveness.

Quasi-experimental design A research design that includes a non-randomized control group, a before-and-after study and an interrupted time series design.

Quota sampling A non-probability technique for sampling commonly used in market research. It involves selecting sample elements according to a predetermined distribution across certain defined categories.

Randomized controlled trial (RCT) The RCT sets out to evaluate the effects of a particular treatment or management strategy in a population by comparing the outcome with a control group where no intervention has been made. The population must be well defined and carefully selected.

Reflexivity The 'tacit' or assumed knowledge of researchers when undertaking a project. Researchers should be aware of their role in the construction of knowledge at all stages for the research process and not make unwarranted assumptions about their informants' views.

Regression analysis Depicts the relationship between an independent variable and one or more dependent variables in the form of a regression equation.

Reliability The extent to which research instruments and concepts are stable and able to yield an unvarying measurement.

Replicability The degree to which the results of a study can be reproduced by a trained researcher.

Research ethics A means of setting standards in areas such as the relation to sponsorship, the relationships between researchers and participants, and the dissemination of research findings.

Sampling The science and practice of selecting information from a population. In quantitative research, this allows defensible inferences to be drawn from those data that apply to whole populations. In qualitative research, purposive and non-purposive sampling methods are used.

Sampling frame A list of units or elements, such as people, households or hospitals, in the population from which the sample will be selected that are assumed to best define the target or survey population.

Saturation In qualitative research, the point at which no, or very little, new information would be obtained from collecting additional data.

Secular trend Factors can include an unpredicted external influence or the effect of changes that occur naturally over time in the process of health care.

Semi-structured interview A flexible method used in qualitative research to collect data with an interview schedule of questions rather than a structured questionnaire.

Sensitive issues Topics likely to raise strong emotions for research participants.

Sex A biological characteristic, unlike gender, to which cross-reference may be made.

Snowball sampling A sample drawn by asking one informant to suggest another.

Social network analysis Investigates social structures through the use of networks and graph theory.

Statistical Package for the Social Sciences (SPSS) A widely used computer program for managing and analysing quantitative data.

Stratification An explicit method to ensure the desired distribution of a sample across certain groups in the population.

Structural analysis When considering documents, the term refers to the examination of the ways in which documents are created and how they achieve their effect.

Survey A quantitative method to collect data from a population sample at one point in time. The cases or units of analysis provide a structured data set. Surveys can be *ad hoc*, cross-sectional, national or longitudinal.

Survey analysis This can be descriptive or, when a questionnaire is used, may aim to establish associations or relationships between variables by establishing correlations between independent and dependent variables. Associations can infer cause but do not establish a causal link.

Symbolic interactionism A theoretical perspective that sees social interaction as based on the meanings that actors attach to action or events.

Synchronic reliability When observations are consistent conceptually within the same time period.

Systematic review A review that is based on a hierarchy of evidence and may include the findings from studies using quantitative, qualitative or both methods based on a synthesis of what is known and not known. In clinical research, they typically focus on the efficacy of a particular intervention based on the most robust evidence available.

Target population The population 'of interest' for a proposed investigation.

Theoretical model An abstract depiction of the possible relationship between variables.

Theoretical or theoretic sampling In qualitative methods it involves the collection, coding and analysis of data to develop theory.

Theories Ideas that have been developed to explain a specific phenomenon.

Translational research The use of research findings to develop new devices or technologies in health care.

Triangulation A navigational term based on using two bearings to locate an object. In social research it refers to claims that the aggregation of data from different sources can validate a particular truth, account or finding. It is also used to suggest that a greater understanding of a phenomenon can be achieved using both quantitative and qualitative methods.

Type 1 error An error due to chance findings.

Type 2 error An error due to a poorly designed trial.

Typology An abstraction drawn from an observation in the real world that simplifies, but helps to clarify, complexity.

Univariate analysis An interest in the distribution of a single variable for statistical analysis.

Unstructured interview An in-depth, open-ended narrative or long interview generally used to explore sensitive issues or vulnerable informants.

Utilitarian approach A justification that a course of action benefits a majority in society.

Validity The 'truthfulness' or accuracy of research findings. It is used in quantitative methods to test whether an indicator is measuring the concept it is intended to measure. *See also* face validity, content validity, construct validity and criterion validity.

Index